Introduction to Massage Therapy

Introduction to Massage Therapy

THIRD EDITION

Mary Beth Braun, BA, CMT, NCTMB

Stephanie J. Simonson, BS

Wolters Kluwer | Lippincott Williams & Wilkins
Health

Acquisitions Editor: Jonathan Joyce
Product Manager: Paula C. Williams
Marketing Manager: Leah Thomson
Production Project Manager: Marian Bellus
Designer: Stephen Druding
Manufacturing Coordinator: Margie Orzech
Compositor: Absolute Service, Inc.

Third Edition

Library of Congress Cataloging-in-Publication Data

Braun, Mary Beth, author.
   Introduction to massage therapy / Mary Beth Braun, Stephanie J. Simonson. -- Third edition.
       p. ; cm.
   Includes bibliographical references and index.
   ISBN 978-1-4511-7319-2
   I. Simonson, Stephanie J., author. II. Title.
   [DNLM: 1. Massage. WB 537]
   RM721
   615.8'22--dc23
                               2013022149

DISCLAIMER
Care has been taken to confirm the accuracy of the information present and to describe generally accepted practices. However, the authors, editors, and publisher are not responsible for errors or omissions or for any consequences from application of the information in this book and make no warranty, expressed or implied, with respect to the currency, completeness, or accuracy of the contents of the publication. Application of this information in a particular situation remains the professional responsibility of the practitioner; the clinical treatments described and recommended may not be considered absolute and universal recommendations.

The authors, editors, and publisher have exerted every effort to ensure that drug selection and dosage set forth in this text are in accordance with the current recommendations and practice at the time of publication. However, in view of ongoing research, changes in government regulations, and the constant flow of information relating to drug therapy and drug reactions, the reader is urged to check the package insert for each drug for any change in indications and dosage and for added warnings and precautions. This is particularly important when the recommended agent is a new or infrequently employed drug.

Some drugs and medical devices presented in this publication have U.S. Food and Drug Administration (FDA) clearance for limited use in restricted research settings. It is the responsibility of the health care provider to ascertain the FDA status of each drug or device planned for use in their clinical practice.

To purchase additional copies of this book, call our customer service department at **(800) 638-3030** or fax orders to **(301) 223-2320**. International customers should call **(301) 223-2300**.

***Visit Lippincott Williams & Wilkins on the Internet*: http://www.lww.com.** Lippincott Williams & Wilkins customer service representatives are available from 8:30 am to 6:00 pm, EST.

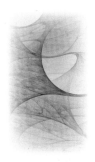

For Horace Davis
and all those instructors
who have taught me
how to be a better massage therapist
and instructor.

—MARY BETH BRAUN

In memory of Horace Davis,
who taught me that
there are many ways to learn,
and even more to teach.

—STEPHANIE J. SIMONSON

Preface

I ntroduction to Massage Therapy, Third Edition, is primarily a textbook for entry-level massage therapy students who are seeking fundamental and practical knowledge for becoming professional massage therapists. It integrates functional anatomy and physiology information with massage therapy techniques and introduces students to the foundations of history, medical terminology, documentation and communication skills, and business and self-care practices for massage therapists.

This book also serves as a functional approach reference for practicing massage therapists. Practicing therapists need a functional understanding of the anatomy and physiology as it pertains to the soft tissues, and they need to understand the various components of a massage therapy practice. This text is designed to provide practical information regarding the assessment and treatment of clients. In doing so, the special muscle section serves as an excellent guide to treating clients for their particular areas of concern.

This book was born from our desire for a more functional and practical curriculum for beginning massage therapy students as well as our need for a text that provides guidance and support for massage therapy instructors. With extraordinary care and teamwork, we have created a massage therapy textbook that enables the reader to translate the fundamental knowledge base for massage into practical applications both inside and outside the classroom.

Unique Organization and Features

This book helps the reader learn how to build a massage therapy business while maintaining health and energy through self-care.

The third edition has been refined to better prepare students for the National Certification Exam for Therapeutic Massage and Bodywork. Using the NCE's content outline as a reference, various topics from the second edition were updated or rearranged. There is a new chapter covering kinesiology and biomechanics to highlight that aspect of therapeutic massage.

The approach of this book is extraordinarily visual, with a wealth of illustrations and photos to facilitate comprehension of basic information and hands-on practice. Additionally, the book contains many outstanding features, including the following:

- Step-by-step procedure boxes enable the reader to practice techniques both in and outside the classroom.

- Progressive case studies walk the reader through the documentation process as sample clients are presented at different stages of a massage session.

- Critical Thinking Scenarios help the reader develop decision-making skills for applying different techniques in specific conditions.

- Special muscle section (at the end of Chapter 4) presents an easy-to-reference format to help the reader assess specific body movements and identify muscles that may be involved in a client's soft tissue area of concern. This section is also linked to a group of extraordinary art plates from *Basic Clinical Massage Therapy: Integrating Anatomy and Treatment* by James H. Clay and David M. Pounds (Lippincott Williams & Wilkins).

- Key points emphasize information that is particularly important for practical application and client education.

- Research boxes present evidence-based references that apply the latest research to practice.
- Pathology in-brief boxes provide a "nutshell" description of conditions relevent to massage therapists.
- **Alert** boxes point out precautions to take in situations that may arise in a massage therapist's practice.
- Contraindication boxes, also new to the second edition, highlight specific conditions and situations in which massage should not be used or when a specific stroke may be harmful.
- Key terms are defined at the beginning of each chapter as well as in the glossary to emphasize basic terminology associated with massage therapy.
- Chapter exercises help students review and retain the information they have encountered in each chapter.
- Video icons have been added to the third edition that lead the student to view the video on ThePoint companion web site. The videos aid the student in visuallly bringing the concept alive to foster deeper learning of the concepts and flows in the book.

For Schools and Instructors

The book contains a solid core of basic information that is flexible enough to use in any massage therapy program. For example, a program with a clinical focus can use advanced clinical massage and anatomy and physiology books to support its curriculum whereas a program that focuses more on spa massage can supplement this text with hydrotherapy, aromatherapy, and esthetics textbooks. The material is presented in a format so instructors can develop a curriculum and teach with ease.

Additional Resources

Introduction to Massage Therapy, Third Edition, includes additional resources for both instructors and students that are available on the book's companion Web site at http://thePoint.lww.com.

Instructor Resources

Approved adopting instructors will be given access to the following additional resources:

- Answers to Chapter Exercises
- Critical Thinking Exercises
- Homework Activities
  - Terminology
  - Ethics Questions
  - Matching Exercises
- Test Generator Questions
- Lesson Plans
- PowerPoint Presentations
- Image Bank
- Learning Management System Cartridges

Student Resources

Students who have purchased *Introduction to Massage Therapy, Third Edition,* have access to the following additional resources:

- Videos of procedures and flow sequences including body mechanics, sheet draping, side-lying, seated massage, client supine art, client leg and foot, client prone back, lymph drainage, and reflexology.
- Animations
- Coloring Exercises
- Stedman's Vocabulary and Pronunciation Guide
- Case Studies
- Interactive Quiz Bank
- Study Guide

In addition, purchasers of the text can access the searchable full text online by going to the *Introduction to Massage Therapy, Third Edition,* Web site at http://thePoint.lww.com. See the inside front cover of this text for more details, including the passcode you will need to gain access to the Web site.

Final Note

The functional and practical approach of this text makes it appropriate for entry-level massage therapy students and practicing massage therapists alike. The step-by-step procedures will help students learn and practice basic massage techniques relatively easily. The special muscle section enables practicing massage therapists to use the book as a resource for client education and for treating specific client conditions. Supported by effective instruction, this text is an excellent way to prepare for the National Certification Exam for Therapeutic Massage and Bodywork.

We wish every reader success in learning about massage therapy, and we hope this book will serve as a valuable resource to practitioners in all settings.

Mary Beth Braun

Stephanie J. Simonson

How to Use This Book

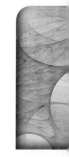

Introduction to Massage Therapy, Third Edition, provides the fundamentals you need to develop as a massage therapist. This exquisite text gives you a well-rounded and informed understanding that will help build your massage therapy skills—including anatomy and physiology, pathology, pharmacology, biomechanics and kinesiology, basic techniques, fundamentals of history, assessment, documentation, ethics, self-care, and more. This User's Guide shows you how to put the book's features to work for you!

Objectives

Upon completion of this chapter, the student will be able to:

- Identify the four ancient river valley civilizations that used massage
- Describe the essence of the Hippocratic Oath and its relation to massage therapy
- Name at least three ancient Greek and Roman physicians who recommended massage
- Explain the difference between development of the arts, science, and massage in Europe and that in the Arab countries during the Middle Ages
- Describe how massage therapy was affected by the Renaissance period
- Identify the transition that occurred in American healthcare in the 19th century
- Describe the difference between massage and bodywork
- List the nine categories of bodywork modalities
- Name at least two indications that massage is evolving in the American healthcare system
- Identify at least two attributes of a massage therapist that are needed for successful employment in a spa
- Name at least three current trends in massage education

Key Terms

Anointing: Ritualistic or religious activity of rubbing oil into the skin.
Bodywork: Treatment that involves manipulation of the client's body as a way to maintain or improve health.
Gymnastics: Activity at ancient gymnasiums that included exercise, massage, and baths.
Massage: Manual therapy involving pressure applied with the hands (term started by the French explorers in the 1700s).
Mechanical effects: Therapist applies pressure or manipulation to physically change the shape or condition of the client's tissues.
Metabolic effects: Combined result of mechanical and reflex effects on the whole body.

Modality: A collection of manual therapies that tends to use similar applications of movement or massage strokes to reach a similar goal.
Movement Cure: American version of Ling's movement system.
Reflex effects: Therapist stimulates the client's sensory neurons, which triggers the client's nervous system to change the shape or condition of the tissues in areas that were addressed as well as other, related areas.
Swedish Gymnastics: A therapeutic movement system developed by Per Henrik Ling.
Swedish Movements: Europe's version of Ling's movement system.
Qi (CHEE): A dynamic, changing energy force that runs through the whole body, supplying and being supplied by body processes and activities.

LEARNING OBJECTIVES

Objectives listed at the start of each chapter clearly outline what you must accomplish upon completion of the chapter.

KEY TERMS

Terms with definitions at the beginning of each chapter (as well as in the glossary) introduce you to basic massage therapy terminology.

The skin is the main structure of the integumentary system, but there are also some specialized structures located in or near the skin, including hair, nails, and cutaneous glands. **The skin, sometimes called the integument, is the largest organ of the body.**

KEY POINTS

Key point sentences within the text are highlighted in red to emphasize information important for client education and practical application.

ALERT BOXES

Marked with a ⬧ Alert, these boxes warn you about special circumstances in which caution is necessary.

⬧ Alert

Massage techniques that are too aggressive may create fatigue-like symptoms or initiate a protective reflex contraction in the muscles.

CONTRAINDICATION BOXES

Marked with a , these boxes point out contraindications to specific conditions that your client may have.

> Deep pressure can damage lymphatic vessels, and damaged lymphatic vessels cannot drain lymph properly, which is why massage is contraindicated over areas of inflammation.

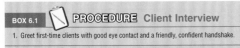

BOX 6.1 PROCEDURE Client Interview

1. Greet first-time clients with good eye contact and a friendly, confident handshake.

2. Explain your policies and intake form(s) and offer reasons for documentation.

3. Ask clients to fill out forms. Meanwhile, start filling out their SOAP note.

4. Interview clients:
   a. Clarify their purpose for coming to you for a massage.
      i. Is there any area in particular they want you to address or avoid?
      ii. Are there any techniques they prefer or dislike?
   b. Clarify their chief complaint, if there is one. This helps you better understand the client's current condition to know if any progress was made when you perform the posttreatment assessment.
      i. Is there anything that makes the pain worse or better?
      ii. Do they notice the discomfort all of the time, only during certain activities, or only after certain activities?
      iii. How long have they had this condition?
      iv. Ask them to try to rate the discomfort, using a scale of 1 to 10 or on a scale of mild to severe.
      v. Ask them to try to describe the discomfort (sharp, achy, numb, tingling, heavy, throbbing, etc.).

PROCEDURE BOXES

Offer step-by-step procedures for specific treatments or assessments for practice both in and outside the classroom.

RESEARCH BOXES

These boxes present evidence-based references that apply the latest research to practice.

BOX 9-6

RESEARCH Massage and Pain: The Gate Control Theory of Pain

In 1965, researchers Ronald Melzack and Patrick Wall published the now-famous Gate Control Theory that explained the pain mechanism. Afferent (sensory) nerve

Fibromyalgia in Brief

Pronunciation: fy-bro-my-AL-je-ah

What is it?
Fibromyalgia syndrome (FMS) is a chronic pain syndrome involving sleep disorders and the development of a predictable pattern of tender points in muscles and other soft tissues.

How is it recognized?
Fibromyalgia syndrome is diagnosed when other diseases have been ruled out and when 11 active tender points are found distributed among all quadrants of the body, along

IN-BRIEF BOXES

Provide a "nutshell" description of conditions relevent to massage therapists.

VIDEOS

Marked with a 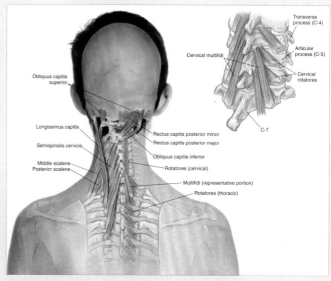, lead the student to view the video on thePoint companion Web site of the concepts and flows to foster deeper learning.

Components of Good Body Mechanics

Critical components of good body mechanics include efficient structural alignment of your body, proper stance, and ergonomics. The body should move fluidly, using gravity and the movement of the whole body to deliver the massage instead of using the muscles of the shoulders, arms, hands, fingers, and thumbs. Movement of the body as a whole improves the fluidity and rhythm of the massage.

Maximizing the amount of pressure and minimizing

Box 12-1 CRITICAL THINKING SCENARIOS ▪ CLIENT #1

Eastern physicians familiar with the practice of cupping have discovered a variety of additional benefits. Application of the cups usually creates short-term bruises, particularly if the patient is ill. To the practiced eye, this discoloration can be a valuable diagnostic clue. A skilled practitioner applying cups along the acupuncture meridians can recognize certain internal organ problems that may reside a considerable distance from the bruise.

Client Information

Eastern physicians familiar with the practice of cupping have discovered a variety of additional benefits. Application of the cups usually creates short-term bruises, particularly if the patient is ill. To the practiced eye, this discoloration can be a valuable diagnostic clue. A skilled practitioner applying cups along the acupuncture meridians can recognize certain internal organ problems that may reside a considerable distance from the bruise.

Recommendations

Eastern physicians familiar with the practice of cupping have discovered a variety of additional benefits. Application of the cups usually creates short-term bruises, particularly if the patient is ill. To the practiced eye, this

discoloration can be a valuable diagnostic clue. A skilled practitioner applying cups along the acupuncture meridians can recognize certain internal organ problems that may reside a considerable distance from the bruise.

Summary of Short Term Goals and Progress

Eastern physicians familiar with the practice of cupping have discovered a variety of additional benefits. Application of the cups usually creates short-term bruises, particularly if the patient is ill. To the practiced eye, this discoloration can be a valuable diagnostic clue. A skilled practitioner applying cups along the acupuncture meridians can recognize certain internal organ problems that may reside a considerable distance from the bruise.

Next Steps

Eastern physicians familiar with the practice of cupping have discovered a variety of additional benefits. Application of the cups usually creates short-term bruises, particularly if the patient is ill. To the practiced eye, this discoloration can be a valuable diagnostic clue. A skilled practitioner applying cups along the acupuncture meridians can recognize certain internal organ problems that may reside a considerable distance from the bruise. ▪

CRITICAL THINKING SCENARIOS

Provide a decision-making framework to help you develop a treatment plan to meet a particular client's unique needs.

CLEAR ILLUSTRATIONS AND PHOTOGRAPHS

Numerous high-quality illustrations and photographs throughout the book illustrate the most important information, make complex details easy to understand, and facilitate comprehension of basic information and hands-on practice.

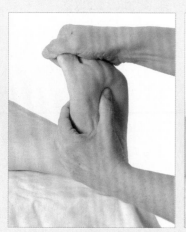
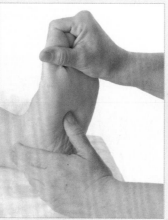

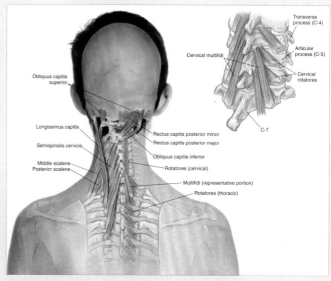

CASE STUDIES

Progressive case studies present sample clients and walk you through the documentation process for different stages of a massage session.

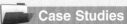

Case Studies

Introducing . . . The Case Studies

Three different case studies are presented throughout this text. The participants are introduced with brief biographies followed by the documentation forms used to record their information: health history and SOAP notes. The SOAP note will be highlighted differently in each chapter that includes the Case Studies, showcasing the information that is most appropriate for those chapters. Here, we introduce Rob Blackwell, Timothy Roberts, and Kirsten Van Marter.

Progressive Case Study 1:
Rob Blackwell

Rob Blackwell is a 42-year-old man who is trying massage for the first time and hopes to restore his sleep and reduce pain in his neck, shoulder, back, and knees so he can

with his activities the most. He complains that his sleep is affected by his pain, and his health history reveals osteoarthritis and tendinitis in his knees, multiple sprains in his ankles, sinus trouble, and multiple head injuries. Your interview determines that the osteoarthritis diagnosis was made more than 10 years ago. On a pain scale of 1 to 10, with 10 being the worst pain, Rob says all of his areas of concern are about 4. He soaks in the hot tub, which helps the pain, and he occasionally takes ibuprofen, which could affect his pain perception during massage. All of the information Rob tells you is subjective information, and you record anything that is pertinent to his chief complaints (Figs. 6-6 and 6-7).

The massage for Rob is designed to reduce pain and tension and find fascial adhesions, but you focus on the condition of the soft tissues in his shoulders. You use your standard massage flow, with the addition of some therapeutic techniques. After the massage, you perform the posttreatment assessment, prioritize Rob's functional limitations, and determine short- and

SPECIAL MUSCLE SECTION

Action Movement	Muscle	Origin	Insertion (bone that is moved is CAPITALIZED)	Nerve (spinal segment nerve numbers)	Plate(s)
SHOULDER					
Elevation	Levator scapula	Transverse processes of C1–C4	Medial border of SCAPULA	Cervical & dorsal scapular (C3,4,5)	Plate 4-1
	Rhomboid major	C7, T1–5	Medial border of SCAPULA	Dorsal scapular (C4,5)	Plate 4-1
	Trapezius (upper)	Occiput, ligamentum nuchae	Lateral end of clavicle, lateral spine of SCAPULA	Accessory (C2,3,4)	Plate 4-1
Depression	Serratus anterior	Outer surfaces of ribs 8–10	Anterior surface of medial border of SCAPULA	Long thoracic (C5,6,7)	Plate 4-2
	Subclavius	Junction of first rib and costal cartilage	Inferior surface of CLAVICLE	Branch of brachial plexus (C5,6)	Plate 4-3
	Trapezius (lower)	T4–12	Root of spine of SCAPULA	Accessory (C3,4)	Plate 4-1
Protraction	Serratus anterior	Outer surfaces of ribs 8–10	Anterior surface of medial border of SCAPULA	Long thoracic (C5,6,7)	Plate 4-2

MUSCLE TABLE

Special muscle section, at the end of Chapter 4: Kinesiology and Biomechanics, presents the specific movements and muscles involved in the soft tissue area of concern with reference to color plates to identify the muscle.

CHAPTER SUMMARIES

Review key topics and concepts of the chapter to understand and retain.

CHAPTER EXERCISES

At the end of each chapter, these exercises provide review questions to test your knowledge of the material.

CHAPTER SUMMARY

Massage therapists should always maintain a client-centered focus for care. The treatment plan for client care is part of that professional focus. With space and time constraints, you can write only brief notes in your massage treatment records, but you still need to document details accurately. Another therapist should be able to read your SOAP note and understand what the treatment plan includes, which self-care activities were recommended between sessions, and any referrals you may have made.

Self-care techniques give you a good topic of discussion for the next session, asking about which self-care techniques clients used or which ones were more effective. Soft tissue health and healing should always be the objective of self-care techniques recommended to clients. The effective and efficient documentation of treatment and self-care are vital aspects of a professional practice.

CHAPTER EXERCISES

1. Use abbreviations and symbols to rewrite the following treatment plans:
   a. 60-minute massages, twice a month, for 2 months. Try vibration over the left scapula, and stay away from the client's feet. Reevaluate AROM of left shoulder extension to see if the triceps stretches that were demonstrated and recommended once a day, every day, were helpful.
   b. 90-minute full body relaxation massages, once a month, for 3 months. Avoid proprioceptive neuromuscular facilitation and AROM evaluations, because the client does not like to actively participate during the session. Referred to Dr. Park for pain upon right elbow PROM.
   c. 30-minute massages, once a week, for 4 weeks. Only use supine, since client is claustrophobic and does not like to be prone. Discussed use of a bolster under the knees during sleep to relieve low back pain.

2. Develop and properly document treatment plans for the following sample clients:
   a. A 20-year-old man, at least 50 pounds overweight, quietly complains of bilateral knee pain. His physical activity is limited to his walk to and from work, 5 days a week. At work, he sits at a computer all day and drinks diet soft drinks all day long. He eats fast food every day and

does not like to drink water. Your general assessments discover bilateral symmetry with a forward posture, rolled shoulders, and knock-knees. He reports pain upon active and passive ROM of his knees, suggesting that some passive structures that are outside the massage scope of practice are involved.

   b. A 50-year-old man who appears in good physical condition explains that his friend got a massage from you and convinced him to try one even though he has no areas of concern. He swims for 30 minutes, at least five times a week, and drinks at least 60 ounces of water a day. He has a wife, three kids, and two dogs and is self-employed in an established and stable business. His posture is bilaterally symmetrical, but his head is forward, and he experiences occasional neck pain and tightness. You found fascial restrictions all around the cervical area, but did not have enough time to address it. He reports that he was able to relax but not until the massage was almost over and asks if massages can be longer than 60 minutes.

   c. A 70-year-old woman who has been coming to you regularly, once a month, for over a year. She is retired and enjoys her gardening club activities and worldwide travel. Every day, she drinks a glass of juice, a cup of tea, a glass of water, and a cup of coffee. Every day, she eats a lot of fruits and vegetables, very few carbohydrates, and a small amount of protein. In the past, she has always responded well to a full-body relaxation massage that includes some craniosacral work. She has not incorporated any self-care in the year you have been treating her, but she always asks about what she should do between sessions.

3. Explain the difference between an initial treatment plan and a treatment plan for the subsequent massage sessions.

4. List the six components included in the plan section of the SOAP note.

5. List at least five questions you can use to evaluate clients' internal healing environment to estimate their healing time and length of treatment.

6. Explain why it is not always better to recommend massage sessions that last longer and are more frequent.

7. Explain why it is not always better to recommend a lot of self-care activities.

Reviewers

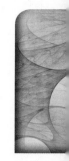

Kelley Aliffi, MA, CMT
Clinical Massage Therapist
Minneapolis, Minnesota

Erica Baern, BA, MA
Director of Education
East West College of the Healing Arts
Portland, Oregon

Carla Bashaw, BS, LMT, LA, LM
Licensed and Nationally Certified
    Massage Therapist
Ogunquit, Maine

Kathy Calise, BS
Program Coordinator
Continuing Education/
    Massage Therapy Program
Lane Community College
Eugene, Oregon

Julia Mims Edwards
Massage Therapist
Nashville, Tennessee

Beth B. Habig, AA
Licensed Massage Therapist
A Bodywork Center for Massage Therapy
Cary, North Carolina

Cher Hunter
Program Director
Massage Therapy
Community College of Baltimore County
Baltimore, Maryland

Carole Koenig, BA, MA
Massage Therapist
Los Angeles, California

Becky SanGregorio, Director
Laurel Highlands Therapeutic Academy
Edensburg, Pennsylvania

Matthew Sorlie, LMP
Director of Education
Cortiva Institute - Seattle
Seattle, Washington

Lori Vargas, Founder
Spa Vargas University
Bloomingdale, Illinois

Jean Wible, RN, BSN, NCTMB, CHTP
Assistant Professor of Massage Therapy
Community College of Baltimore County
Baltimore, Maryland

Acknowledgments

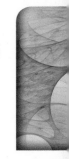

We extend our sincere appreciation to The Crew at Lippincott Williams & Wilkins for working tirelessly on this project since its inception. In particular, we want to thank:

- Paula Williams, LWW Product Manager
- Jonathan Joyce, LWW Senior Acquisitions Editor
- Stephen Druding, LWW Book Designer
- Freddie Patane, LWW Media Director
- Jennifer Clements, LWW Art Director
- Jessica Sillers, Project Manager

We also thank the follow people for their incredible work, who have played a significant part in making this such a visual and user-friendly textbook:

Artist: Rob Duckwall and Dragonfly Media Group

1st and 2nd edition photographer: Don Distel

3rd edition photographer: Mark Lozier

3rd edition video team: Directed by Freddie Patane, with support from Mike Licisyn, Ed Schultes, Jr.

3rd edition photography and video models: Kay Chen, Grace McKissick, Henry Lopez, and Lisa Kotokis

For the third edition, we thank Ruth Werner, friend and author of *A Massage Therapist's Guide to Pathology,* for her unwavering belief in our ability to complete this extraordinary text. We would also like to extend our gratitude to Diana Thompson, friend and notable author of *Hands Heal,* who helped us with the details of documentation.

This edition has been through an extensive review process by professionals in the massage therapy field (see the reviewer list), each of whom we thank for their time and input.

To best showcase some techniques and modalities, we invited several people to write about their particular field of expertise. Young Ki Park, DO, explained the philosophy and ancient practice of cupping. Debra Howard detailed the Asian bodywork therapies and described their overlap with massage therapy. Marybetts Sinclair provided an in-depth look at hydrotherapy and spa treatments. We sincerely appreciate these authors and value their input.

We thank everyone who served as models throughout the book and video: Rob Blackwell, Steve Benham, Jeff Braun, Leo Braun, Kylie Clevenger, Anne Jordan, Kathy Latimer, Stephen Lich, Kathleen Lich, Andy Simonson, Bob Simonson, Claire Simonson, Dr. Robert T. Simonson, Annie VanderLinden, and Kirsten VanMarter-Clevenger.

Mary Beth Braun would particularly like to thank her family, friends, and clients for their love, encouragement and support throughout this third edition of our beloved book project, including her husband, Tom Hanson, her parents, Leo and Mary Jane Braun; her brothers, Jim and Jeff Braun; Tracy Wilson, Kirsten VanMarter-Clevenger, Kathy Latimer, Steve Benham, Larry and Michelle Marietta, Christopher Sovereign, Eric Stephenson and Debra Koerner.

From Stephanie: Thank you to everyone who supported me throughout this endeavor. I could not have done it without your help.

Brief Contents

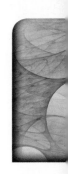

Preface vii

User's Guide xi

Reviewers xv

Acknowledgments xvii

CHAPTER 1: Welcome to the World of Massage Therapy! 1

CHAPTER 2: Ethics and Professionalism 30

CHAPTER 3: Body Systems 55

CHAPTER 4: Kinesiology and Biomechanics 146

CHAPTER 5: Pathology and Pharmacology 226

CHAPTER 6: Communication and Documentation 253

CHAPTER 7: Assessment 295

CHAPTER 8: Treatment Plan 326

CHAPTER 9: Massage Strokes and Flow 349

CHAPTER 10: Therapeutic Applications 419

CHAPTER 11: Complementary Modalities 466

CHAPTER 12: Special Populations 515

CHAPTER 13: Professional Massage Practice 535

Glossary 589

Index 595

Contents

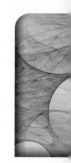

Preface vii
User's Guide xi
Reviewers xv
Acknowledgments xvii

CHAPTER 1: Welcome to the World of Massage Therapy! 1

History of Massage 2
    Ancient River Valley Civilizations
        (7000–1000 BCE) 3
    Ancient Greece
        (750 BCE–500 CE) 6
    Ancient Rome
        (750 BCE–500 CE) 7
    The Middle Ages
        (400–1400) 8
    The Renaissance (1450–1600) 9
    The 18th Century 11
    The 19th Century 11
    The 20th Century 14
    Contemporary Massage Therapy 14

Massage and Bodywork Modalities 14
    Swedish Modalities 16
    Deep Tissue Modalities 16
    Neuromuscular Modalities 17
    Circulatory Enhancement Modalities 17
    Energy Modalities 17
    Oriental/Eastern Modalities 18
    Structural and Postural Integration
        Modalities 18
    Movement Modalities 18
    Special Populations 18

Touch 19
    Touch Physiology 19
    Massage Research 19
    Interpretation of Touch 22

Massage as Part of the American Healthcare System 22
    Integrative Medicine Centers 22
    Oncology Massage 23

Massage in the Spa Industry 23
    History of the Spa Industry 24
    Medical Spas 24
    Spa Massage Education 24

Trends in Massage Education 26

Chapter Summary 26

Chapter Exercises 27

CHAPTER 2: Ethics and Professionalism 30

Characteristics of a Profession 31
    Education 31
    Body of Knowledge 32
    Scope of Practice 32
    Code of Ethics 33
    Standards of Practice 34

Scope of Practice 37
    Legal Regulations 37
    Education 38
    Competency 38
    Limits of Practice 40

Ethics 40
    Accountability 41
    Ethics for the Profession 41

Professionalism 43
    Conduct 43
    Business Practices 44
    Legal Requirements and Ethical
        Responsibilities 44
    Professional Associations 49

Relationships 50
   Physical Boundaries 50
   Conceptual Boundaries 50
   Client Relationships 52
   Professional Relationships 53

Chapter Summary 53

Chapter Exercises 54

CHAPTER 3: Body Systems 55

Terms for Structure and Function 56
   Anatomy 57
   Physiology 57

Cells and Tissues 58
   Cellular Functions 58
   Components of
     the Cell 59
   Tissues 63
   Tissue Membranes 74

The 12 Body Systems 76
   Integumentary System 76
   Skeletal System 82
   Muscular System 96
   Nervous System 104
   Cardiovascular System 119
   Lymphatic System 125
   Respiratory System 127
   Digestive System 130
   Urinary System 133
   Endocrine System 135
   Reproductive System 137
   Special Senses 142

Chapter Summary 143

Chapter Exercises 144

CHAPTER 4: Kinesiology and
Biomechanics 146
   Anatomical Terminology 147

Kinesiology 152
   Arthrology 152
   Range of Motion 156

Myology: The Study of Muscles 156
   Body Movements 162

Biomechanics 168
   Components of Good Body Mechanics 169
   Body Awareness 175
   Improper Body Mechanics 176

Chapter Summary 177

Chapter Exercises 225

CHAPTER 5: Pathology and Pharmacology 226
   Pathology 227
   Pharmacology 227

Pathology, Pharmacology, and Massage 230
   Abnormal Conditions of Cells and Tissues 230
   Integumentary (Skin) Conditions 231
   Skeletal System Conditions 233
   Muscular System Conditions 236
   Nervous System Conditions 240
   Cardiovascular System Conditions 243
   Lymphatic and Immune System Conditions 245
   Respiratory System Conditions 246
   Digestive System Conditions 248
   Endocrine System Conditions 248
   Reproductive System Conditions 250
   Conditions of the Special Senses 251

Chapter Summary 251

Chapter Exercises 251

CHAPTER 6: Communication and
Documentation 253

Medical Terminology 254
   Word Elements 255
   Translating Terms 261
   Spelling and Pronunciation 261

Communication 261
   Effective Communication and Interviewing
     Skills 263
   Documentation 268

SOAP 270
   Subjective Information 270
   Objective Information 274

Activity and Analysis Information 276

Plan Information 277

Putting the SOAP Together 278

Progressive Case Study 1: *Rob Blackwell* 283

Progressive Case Study 2: *Timothy Roberts* 284

Progressive Case Study 3: *Kirsten Van Marter* 284

Chapter Summary 284

Chapter Exercises 293

CHAPTER 7: Assessment 295

General Assessments 296

Wellness versus Therapeutic Massage Assessments 296

Fascia 297

Compensation Patterns 297

Assessment Documentation 301

Postural Assessment 302

Ideal Posture 304

Anterior Postural Assessment 305

Posterior Postural Assessment 305

Lateral Postural Assessment 305

Postural Deviations 306

Feet 308

Gait Assessment 308

Range of Motion Assessment 309

Active Range of Motion 310

Passive Range of Motion 311

Appearance of Tissues 313

Palpation Assessment 313

Assessment of Skin Temperature 314

Textures and Movement of Soft Tissues 314

Rhythms 314

Functional Assessments 315

Posttreatment Assessment 316

Progressive Case Study 1: *Rob Blackwell* 316

Progressive Case Study 2: *Timothy Roberts* 317

Progressive Case Study 3: *Kirsten Van Marter* 317

Chapter Summary 318

Chapter Exercises 324

CHAPTER 8: Treatment Plan 326

Planning Process 327

Initial Session 327

Subsequent Sessions 328

Future Treatment 329

Healing Time 329

Duration of Future Sessions 330

Frequency of Future Sessions 330

Length of Treatment 330

Techniques and Areas to Include or Avoid 331

Reevaluation 331

Self-Care Recommendations 331

Considerations for Self-Care 332

Hydrotherapy 332

Stretches 333

Rest 334

Nutrition 335

Body Awareness 335

Ergonomics 335

Referral to Other Healthcare Professionals 336

Follow-up Communication 336

Presenting the Treatment Plan 342

Treatment Recommendations 342

Progressive Case Study 1: *Rob Blackwell* 342

Progressive Case Study 2: *Timothy Roberts* 343

Progressive Case Study 3: *Kirsten Van Marter* 343

Chapter Summary 347

Chapter Exercises 347

CHAPTER 9: Massage Strokes and Flow 349

Client Positioning 350

Supine Position 351

Prone Position 352

Side-Lying (Laterally Recumbent) Position 353

Determining Client Positioning and Bolstering 354

Draping 354

Sheet Draping 355

Towel Draping 355

Communication for Client Positioning and Draping 359

Assisting Clients on and off the Table 360

General Effects of Massage 365

Components of a Massage Stroke 369

Stationary Massage Strokes 369
  Grounding 369
  Centering 370
  Resting Stroke 371

Basic Massage Strokes 371
  Compression 372
  Effleurage 373
  Petrissage 376
  Tapotement 378
  Friction 380
  Vibration 381

Joint Movement 382

Endangerment Sites 383

Flow 385
  Flow Sequences for Different Client
    Positions 385

Sample Flow Sequences for Specific Areas 397
  Supine: Chest, Neck, and Head 397
  Supine: Arm 400
  Supine: Abdomen 400
  Supine: Leg and Foot 403
  Prone: Back 404
  Prone: Leg and Foot 404
  Closing Sequence 404

Chair Massage 405
  Safety and Sanitation for Chair Massage 406
  Corporate Chair Accounts 413
  Indications and Contraindications for Chair
    Massage 413

Chapter Summary 413

Chapter Exercises 416

CHAPTER 10: Therapeutic Applications 419

Mechanisms of Injury and Tissue Repair 420
  Healing: Phase I 421
  Healing: Phase II 422
  Healing: Phase III 422

Pain 423
  Pain–Spasm Cycle 423

Principles of Therapeutic Techniques 424
  Fascia 425
  Direction of Ease 425
  Lengthening and Stretching 426

Circulatory Enhancement 426
  Arterial Enhancement 427
  Venous Enhancement 427
  Lymph Drainage 428

Neuromuscular Techniques 439
  Proprioceptive Neuromuscular Facilitation
    Techniques 439
  Myofascial Techniques 449
  Trigger Point Techniques 455

Chapter Summary 457

Chapter Exercises 460

CHAPTER 11: Complementary Modalities 466

Hydrotherapy 467
  Effects of Hydrotherapy 468
  Applications of Hydrotherapy 471
  Medication and Hydrotherapy 481

Asian Bodywork Therapy 481
  The Asian Bodywork Therapy Profession 481
  Chinese Medicine 482
  Principles of Treatment 489
  Self-Care 494

Ayurvedic Healthcare 496
  Five Elements 497
  Doshas 497
  Energy and Chakras 498

Reflexology 500
  Incorporating Reflexology into a Massage
    Session 501
  Indications and Contraindications for
    Reflexology 501

Polarity Therapy 511

Chapter Summary 513

Chapter Exercises 513

CHAPTER 12: Special Populations 515

Athletes 516
    Event Sports Massage 517
    Restorative Massage 521
    Maintenance Massage 523
    Treatment Massage 524
    Common Athletic Injuries 525
    Self-Care for the Athlete 525

Pregnant Women 525
    First Trimester 526
    Second Trimester 526
    Third Trimester 527
    Considerations for Pregnancy (Prenatal) Massage 527
    Postpartum Massage 528

Infants 528
    Infant Massage 529

Geriatric Clients 529
    Geriatric Massage 529

Chronically Ill Patients 531

Hospice Massage 531

Disabled Clients 531
    Visually or Hearing Impaired 531
    Physical Disabilities 532
    Paralysis 532
    Amputation 532
    Psychological Issues 533

Chapter Summary 533

Chapter Exercises 533

CHAPTER 13: Professional Massage Practice 535

Equipment 536
    Equipment Specifications 536
    Tables 537
    Massage Chairs 543
    Massage Mats 544
    Bolsters 544
    Massage Tools 544

Lubricants 545
    Oils 546
    Lotions, Creams, Gels 546
    Powders 546
    Lubricant Storage 546
    Application of Lubricants 547

Hygiene and Sanitation 547
    Disease 548
    Preventing Transmission of Pathogens 550
    Cleaning and Sanitizing Procedures 553

Safety 555
    Fire Safety 555
    Primary Assessment in an Emergency Situation 555
    Artificial Respiration 556
    Cardiopulmonary Resuscitation 556
    Choking 556
    Weather-Related Conditions 557

Becoming a Professional Massage Therapist 558
    Professional Concepts 558
    Employment and Business Options 560
    Business Start-up 563
    Choosing a Place of Business 568
    Advisors and Mentors 572
    Finances 572
    Marketing and Promotion 575
    Networking—The Importance of Building Relationships 577
    Long-term Business Development 578
    Self-Care 580

Chapter Summary 585

Chapter Exercises 585

Glossary 589
Index 595

Pathology in Brief

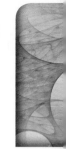

Plantar Fasciitis in Brief   231
Acne Vulgaris in Brief   232
Scar Tissue in Brief   232
Fungal Infections in Brief   233
Postural Deviations in Brief   233
Sprains in Brief   235
Osteoarthritis in Brief   235
Spasms, Cramps in Brief   237
Myofascial Pain Syndrome in Brief   237
Fibromyalgia in Brief   238
Strains in Brief   239
Tendinopathies in Brief   240
Headaches in Brief   242
Thoracic Outlet Syndrome in Brief   243
Varicose Veins in Brief   244
Hypertension in Brief   245
Edema in Brief   245
Fever in Brief   246
Common Cold in Brief   246
Sinusitis in Brief   247
Asthma in Brief   247
Irritable Bowel Syndrome in Brief   248
Peptic Ulcers in Brief   248
Diabetes Mellitus in Brief   249
Breast Cancer in Brief   249
Prostate Cancer in Brief   250

Welcome to the World of Massage Therapy!

Key Terms

Anointing: Ritualistic or religious activity of rubbing oil into the skin.

Bodywork: Treatment that involves manipulation of the client's body as a way to maintain or improve health.

Gymnastics: Activity at ancient gymnasiums that included exercise, massage, and baths.

Massage: Manual therapy involving pressure applied with the hands (term started by the French explorers in the 1700s).

Mechanical effects: Therapist applies pressure or manipulation to physically change the shape or condition of the client's tissues.

Metabolic effects: Combined result of mechanical and reflex effects on the whole body.

Modality: A collection of manual therapies that tends to use similar applications of movement or massage strokes to reach a similar goal.

Movement Cure: American version of Ling's movement system.

Reflex effects: Therapist stimulates the client's sensory neurons, which triggers the client's nervous system to change the shape or condition of the tissues in areas that were addressed as well as other, related areas.

Swedish Gymnastics: A therapeutic movement system developed by Per Henrik Ling.

Swedish Movements: Europe's version of Ling's movement system.

Qi (CHEE): A dynamic, changing energy force that runs through the whole body, supplying and being supplied by body processes and activities.

Welcome to the world of massage therapy! You are about to embark on a most rewarding journey, discovering what is involved in becoming a professional massage therapist. This chapter covers the history of massage and events that led to the current practice of massage. We define massage and distinguish it from bodywork because so many different bodywork techniques have been developed, and there is a lack of clarity regarding the difference. Whereas bodywork is a manipulative treatment of a client's body that is intended to maintain or improve health, massage requires manual pressure on the client's tissues, applied with the therapist's touch, to maintain or improve health. We identify nine categories and briefly summarize some of the massage modalities that have developed over time. The active development of so many kinds of specialized bodywork is partly due to the latest touch research. We introduce the concept of touch and illustrate the increased interest in scientific research on the topic. As the academic and scientific world proves the value of touch, massage becomes more a part of the American healthcare system. Continued involvement in the medical and healthcare communities is accompanied by some changes in massage education, also discussed in this chapter. A general understanding of these concepts can provide a solid foundation for you as you build your professional massage practice.

History of Massage

Throughout thousands of years and a myriad of cultures, people have used massage for communicating, relieving pain or discomfort, healing, protecting, or improving one's overall health. Most people have experienced the instinctive or intuitive use of massage when stopping to rub or hold an injury, bruise, or area of discomfort on the body.

Historical references to massage have been found in cultures around the world. To better comprehend that massage is found in many cultures, you can examine the different terms used to describe the same or similar activity (see Table 1-1). Even cultures without written language have passed down the tradition of massage and techniques,

Table 1-1 "Massage" Roots and Terms from Around the World

Root/Term	Meaning	Culture/Person
Amma	to calm by rubbing, or press-rub	Chinese
Anatripsis	to rub up	Greek/Hippocrates
Anma	to calm by rubbing, or press-rub	Chinese
Anmo	to calm by rubbing, or press-rub	Chinese
Kampo	"the Chinese way"	Japanese
Makeh	to press softly	Sanskrit
Mass	to press softly	Arabic
Mass'h	to press softly	Arabic
Massa	to touch, handle, squeeze, knead	Latin
Massein	to touch, handle, squeeze, knead	Greek
Masser	to knead by hand	French
Masso	to touch, handle, squeeze, knead	Greek
Mordan	to rub	Indian
Samvahana	hand rubbing	Indian

shown by the notes of early explorers who "discovered" these native people.

In the most primitive civilizations, medicine was ritualistic and oftentimes combined with magical or mystical activities, as people believed that illness came from demons, spirits, or sins. Shamans and priests used massage, among other practices, to help rid people of these evil entities. The spiritual and medical traditions were passed on from generation to generation, perpetuating the practice of massage. Evidence of this is found everywhere from Australia to Africa, including ancient Egypt, to the Pacific Islands, Russia and the Ukraine, and North and South America.

Ancient civilizations used massage in conjunction with many variations of water therapy to cleanse and purify the body of disease-causing spirits: bathing, steam rooms, hot springs, and sweat lodges. These rituals that combined massage with water therapies persisted throughout history and still exist today.

Ancient River Valley Civilizations (7000–1000 BCE)

The oldest civilizations were created by groups of people who were able to feed and house large populations efficiently. Large-scale agricultural practices were developed; complex architectural structures were designed and built; political and religious organizations were established; the arts, sciences, and medicine were explored; and written records were kept. One of the most important requirements for civilization was a dependable source of water. Large rivers were able to sustain large populations and, as a result, there are four areas in the world where ancient river valley cultures were established: the Yellow River, the Indus River, the Tigris and Euphrates Rivers, and the Nile River (see Fig. 1-1).

The exact dates that these river valley civilizations were established are controversial because it is unclear from the remaining ancient records when they were actually written. Additionally, records have been translated and rewritten a number of times, occasionally making the original intent and message questionable. For the purpose of this book, civilizations in these four areas developed during the same time period, many thousands of years ago.

Tracing massage history accurately is complicated because ancient references to massage do not use contemporary terminology or techniques. Early records of massage being used in healthcare can be found in documents from all of the ancient cultures. Some of the earliest records of massage refer to "anointing" (ah-NOYN-ting), which is a process of rubbing oil into the skin, often used to banish evil influences that caused disease, again demonstrating the spiritual and religious basis for healthcare. This section of the chapter introduces massage as it evolved in different areas of the globe over time, eventually developing into the current massage therapy profession.

Ancient China

The Yellow River valley culture is also referred to as Shang China, or Ancient China. There is widespread and extensive massage information found in ancient Chinese records. One of the ancient Chinese documents of disputable age is the *Cong Fou*, which includes information on the use of medicinal plants, controlled breathing, and a system of exercises and positions for healthcare. It is questionable whether massage treatment was actually included, but many assume it was. Possibly started around 2700 BCE, the *Cong Fou* may have been completed over several generations.

The *Nei Ching* is the Yellow Emperor's classic of internal medicine and is one of the oldest medical references that still exist. Some claim that it was written around 2600 BCE because of its association with the Yellow Emperor of China, who died at about the same time. Others suggest that it was written from 475 BCE to 220 CE as a series of entries by many different persons but linked to the famous and honorable emperor to establish its authority and bring it fame. The *Nei Ching* is more of a medical dialogue or discussion than a medical reference

Figure 1-1. The four ancient river valley civilizations.

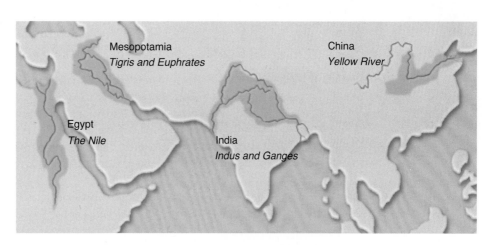

book and serves as the foundation for traditional Chinese medicine. Its main topics include the theory of five phases and the balance of yin and yang. These concepts are introduced in Chapter 11, entitled "Complementary Modalities," which compares Eastern and Western approaches to healthcare.

In the Chinese language, words are represented by contextual pictograms. Translating, reading, and writing the words in English letters can be subjective and vague. A Chinese word written in English is an attempt to spell the pronunciation of the word. One of the oldest Chinese terms for a therapy involving massage-like activity is commonly written as moshuo (moh-SZH-woh). This term can be found in the *Nei Ching* in the context of massage and finger pressure used to energize someone or treat paralysis, chills, fever, and poor circulation of blood. As the Chinese language developed through time, massage techniques were called anmo (AHN-moh), to press and rub, and Tui-na (TOOY-nah), to push and hold.

From China, bodywork made its way into Japan and provided a source of employment for blind people. Since the Japanese culture tends to shun the disabled, few professions were available to the blind outside of acupuncture and massage therapy. With refined perceptions of touch, blind acupuncturists and massage therapists were very successful and able to gain respect. While the Japanese developed many different forms of bodywork, Shiatsu is the best known. Figure 1-2 is a photo taken prior to 1895 of a blind massage therapist performing Shiatsu on a client.

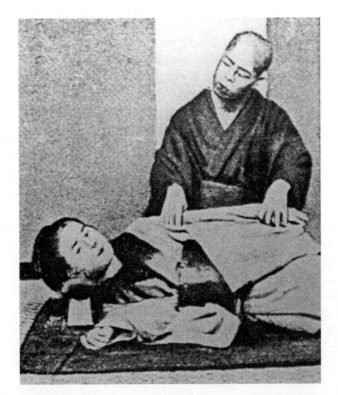

Figure 1-2. Blind Japanese masseur treating a patient. (Reprinted from Kellogg JH, Harvey JK. The Art of Massage. Battle Creek, MI: Modern Medicine, 1929.)

Ancient India

The Indus River is the site of the largest ancient river valley civilization discovered in the 20th century. This area of ancient India is near current day Pakistan. Unlike the others, the Indus Valley civilization did not leave a lot of written records to provide clues to their culture. There are four original scriptural texts, the Vedas, which may have been written over 5,000 years ago. It is believed that these lengthy, complex verbal messages from the gods were spoken directly to sages and only shared by word of mouth for generations. Eventually, these messages were written down in poetic, lyrical form as the Rik Veda, Sama Veda, Yajur Veda, and Atharva Veda. Because the words were passed down only verbally for so many generations, the rhyming patterns may have been instrumental in the accuracy of the translation.

The Ayur Veda, a supplement to the Atharva Veda, discusses pharmacology and health. Its age is questionable, some claiming it was written around 3000 BCE, and others, 1000 BCE or later. The teachings of the Ayur Veda provided the basis for Ayurvedic healthcare, which is gaining popularity in the Western world. The holistic approach attempts to balance the body, mind, and spirit to maintain health and prevent illness. Some of the many therapies employed in this natural system of healing include herbs, diet, fasting, aromatherapy, massage, meditation, yoga, color, and metal therapy.

Ayurvedic references made to massage include samvahana (hand rubbing), mordan (to rub), and most importantly, shampooing. Shampooing was a medical treatment done with a brush and the hands for treating health problems. Massage was and continues to be used regularly in the Indian culture.

Ancient Mesopotamia

The area of ancient Mesopotamia lies between the Tigris and Euphrates Rivers, in the area that is now called the Middle East, near Iraq. The earliest people may have arrived in Mesopotamia somewhere around 7000 BCE, but civilization began around 3000 BCE.

Ancient Mesopotamians developed a written language called cuneiform. A series of wedge-shaped dents were made in wet clay, and when the clay dried, the clay tablets were portable, storable, and long lasting. Clay tablets and paintings on the walls of tombs have shown evidence of massage being used for healthcare. See Figure 1-3 for a photo of an ancient Babylonian clay tablet, circa 300 BCE, which includes a reference to massage.

Physicians and priests both practiced medicine in Mesopotamia, another example of the relationship between illness and evil spirits. Even so, Mesopotamians had some understanding of anatomy and were able to diagnose and prescribe treatment for many specific medical conditions as well as perform surgeries. Babylonian King Hammurabi established a set of laws called the Code of Hammurabi,

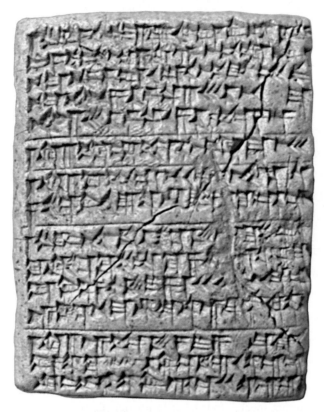

Figure 1-3. Clay tablet of medical text from Babylonia, 300 BCE. (Reprinted with Martin Schøyen's permission from the Schøyen Collection MS4575, Oslo and London.)

which includes the oldest code of medical ethics. It recommends an "eye for an eye" philosophy that is certainly questionable by today's standards.

Ancient Egypt

Located on the Nile River, the fourth of the ancient river valley civilizations is now called Northern Africa. The history of ancient Egypt follows a timeline similar to that of China and Mesopotamia. Instead of using pictograms on walls and cuneiform on clay tablets to convey messages, the Egyptians developed a more complex writing system of hieroglyphics and invented papyrus (puh-PAHY-rus) paper.

The papyrus plant was a reedlike plant found along the banks of the Nile that was used to fabricate, among other things, a useful and durable paper with a secret recipe that no other culture could replicate. Produced in lengths of 35 feet or longer, the papyrus paper could be rolled up for storage and transport, unlike the Mesopotamian clay tablets. Unfortunately, the Egyptians used up the local supply of papyrus, their secret recipe was lost, and papyrus paper was not made again for thousands of years.

Many of the ancient papyrus records have been discovered, named, and translated. Topics covered all aspects of the culture, including literature, governmental tax records, religion, magic, and medicine. As in other early ancient civilizations,

medicine was handled by priest-physicians who typically attributed health conditions to the work of gods and goddesses. Prayers, spells, amulets, herbal salves, and poultices were treatments often used in hopes of a cure. Additionally, records of intricate surgeries and more advanced medical knowledge were also found. The Kahun Papyrus, written around 1800 BCE and found in fragments in 1889 CE, focuses on gynecological matters. One of the passages specifically indicates the use of massage for a woman whose legs ache (see Fig. 1-4).

Medical conditions, prescriptions, diagnoses, and surgical treatments were documented in various papyri, as were details about the mummification process leading the deceased safely to the afterlife. The child king Tutankhamun's famous tomb and mummy demonstrate the extensive mummification process of the ancient Egyptians. The process required the removal of internal organs, leading the Egyptians to a thorough understanding of anatomy.

There is evidence of massage being used in ancient Egyptian healthcare from as early as 4000 BCE, when the mortal goddess Queen Isis included massage as treatment for health and healing. There is no evidence from the other ancient river valley cultures of any female healers, so it is probable that she was the first. She also trained her priestesses to perform the duties of a physician, massage being one of them.

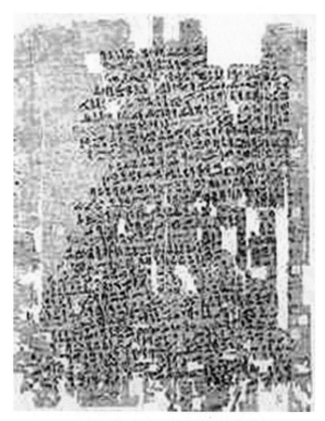

Figure 1-4. Kahun medical papyrus from 1825 BCE. (Reprinted from Griffith FL. The Petrie Papyri: Hieratic Papyri from Kahun and Gurob. London: Bernard Quaritch, 1898. © Petrie Museum of Egyptian Archaeology, University College London UC 32057.)

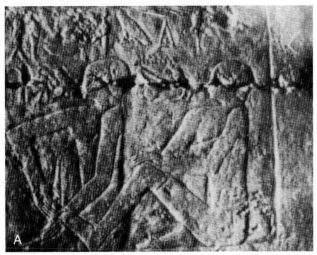

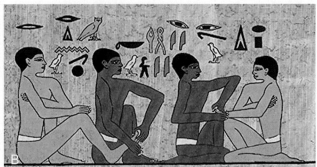

Figure 1-5. Ankhmahor's tomb illustrating bodywork. **(A)** Photo of the tomb wall (by Trudy Baker, taken from www.foot-reflexologist.com/ EGYPT). **(B)** An artistic rendition of inscription, sometimes claimed to be a painting from the tomb.

The tomb of Ankhmahor, dated somewhere around 2350 BCE, has been called the Tomb of the Physician. His title as a physician has been disputed; one theory suggests that he was only a ka-priest who had farming duties and served the king. Regardless, Ankhmahor's tomb has images of foot manipulation and surgical operations such as circumcision. There are many who believe that the images depict foot reflexology, but it is also possible that foot surgery is being shown. The hieroglyphs accompanying the pictograph have been translated with the patient saying "Do not cause pain," and the therapist responding "I will act so you shall praise me" (Fig. 1-5).

Ancient Greece (750 BCE–500 CE)

Although not one of the original river valley civilizations, there is evidence of human activity in Greece thousands of years ago. Written records can be found from about 2000 BCE, but what little has been deciphered does not reveal any advanced works of literature like those of the other civilizations of the time. Early evidence of the Greek alphabet dates from around 750 BCE.

Massage in Ancient Greece

The Greek health regimen included exercise, massage, fresh air, rest, diet, and cleanliness. Exercise and competitive athletics were so much a part of the culture that the Olympic Games were held every 4 years as part of a religious festival. These games were very important to the Greeks, who even stopped wars to compete in them. Physical training was critical to good performance, giving rise to gymnasiums all over the country. Athletes and military of the day received their

academic, art, and physical training at the gymnasiums. Baths, also an important aspect of the health regimen, were attached to or located near the gymnasiums. In time, the baths and gymnasiums served the general public as social, spiritual, mental, and physical gathering places.

Massage was one of the primary treatments provided at the Greek gymnasiums and baths throughout their existence. Athletes received special massage treatments to minimize exhaustion and tone the muscles. The aliptae were servants who provided this ritual before and after competition and became very knowledgeable about the muscles, the condition of muscles, and muscular activity during exercise. In a way, the aliptae were the predecessors to physical or athletic trainers. Massage was used so commonly in the gymnasiums that the term "gymnastics" referred to the combination of exercise, massage, and baths. Although ancient Greek records do not contain an abundance of specific information about massage, some detailed references to massage were made by the famous Hippocrates, who was also responsible for important scientific and medical advancements around 400 BCE.

Hippocrates of Cos

Hippocrates (hih-PAH-kruh-teez) was an ancient Greek physician who lived between 460 and 370 BCE. He is considered the "Father of Medicine" for a couple of reasons. He was the first influential physician to observe health and disease as a result of natural causes and establish medicine as a science, rejecting the theory of health and medicine as the work of magic and gods. Also, he was the first to introduce a medical code of ethics different from the eye for an eye philosophy outlined in the Laws of Hammurabi.

The Hippocratic Corpus is a series of 60 treatises discussing medicine and medical principles. Its several different styles of writing and many contradictory statements led to the belief that Hippocrates started the project but its completion occurred long after he was gone. Within the Corpus, the Hippocratic Oath is a statement in which physicians swear to respect, honor, and share knowledge with their teachers; promise to treat their patients to the best of their ability and only with good intentions; swear that they will not prescribe a deadly drug or treatment under any circumstance; and vow patient confidentiality in hopes of enjoying life and gaining respect from others. This is the philosophy with which Hippocrates practiced medicine, and it continues to be the foundation of the ethical codes for many health-care professions including massage therapy. **The Hippocratic Oath to "do no harm" provides the basis for professionalism, which is discussed in the next chapter.**

See Box 1-1 for a translation of the Hippocratic Oath.

BOX 1-1

A Translation of the Hippocratic Oath by Francis Adams

I swear by Apollo the physician, by Aesculapius, Hygeia and Panacea, and I take to witness all the gods, all the goddesses, to keep according to my ability and my judgment the following oath:

To consider dear to me as my parents him who taught me this art; to live in common with him and if necessary to share my goods with him; to look upon his children as my own brothers, to teach them this art if they so desire without fee or written promise; to impart to my sons and the sons of the master who taught me and the disciples who have enrolled themselves and who have agreed to the rules of the profession, but to these alone, the precepts and the instruction.

I will prescribe regimen for the good of my patients according to my ability and judgment and never do harm to anyone. To please no one will I prescribe a deadly drug, nor give advice which may cause his death. Nor will I give a woman a pessary to procure abortion.

But I will preserve the purity of my life and my art. I will not cut for stone, even for patients in whom the disease is manifest; I will leave this operation to be performed by practitioners (specialists in this art). In every house where I come I will enter only for the good of my patients, keeping myself far from all intentional ill-doing and all seduction, and especially from the pleasures of love with women or with men, be they free or slaves. All that may come to my knowledge in the exercise of my profession or outside of my profession or in daily commerce with men, which ought not to be spread abroad, I will keep secret and never reveal.

If I keep this oath faithfully, may I enjoy my life and practice my art, respected by all men and in all times; but if I swerve from it or violate it, may the reverse be my lot.

BOX 1-2

Evidence of Massage in the Hippocratic Corpus, volume III, "On the Articulations" and "On the Surgery," translated by Francis Adams

"On the Articulations" is a discussion of a dislocated shoulder suggesting in Part 9:

. . . the shoulder should be rubbed gently and softly. The physician ought to be acquainted with many things, and among others with friction; for from the same name the same results are not always obtained; for friction could brace a joint when unseasonably relaxed, and relax it when unseasonably hard; but we will define what we know respecting friction in another place. The shoulder, then, in such a state, should be rubbed with soft hands; and, moreover, in a gentle manner, and the joint should be moved about, but not roughly, so as to excite pain. Things get restored sometimes in a greater space of time, and sometimes in a smaller.

"On the Surgery" states in Part 17:

Friction can relax, brace, incarnate or attenuate: hard braces, soft relaxes, much attenuates, and moderate thickens.

Hippocrates' original holistic methods included exercise, massage, fresh air, rest, diet, and cleanliness. **Hippocrates promoted the concept that the body is capable of curing itself.** As you move through your massage education, you will discover that massage techniques help the body to cure itself or to encourage self-healing. Human touch is an incredibly powerful part of this process.

Although there is only brief mention of massage in the Hippocratic Corpus, the information is detailed and specific. Anatripsis (to rub up) was developed by Hippocrates as a method of rubbing toward the heart, from the extremity to the core, to increase circulation. His technique for increasing circulation is still taught today and is one of the major benefits of massage. He recommended that all physicians be trained in anatripsis because it could promote healing; adjust the tension at a joint; and tighten, relax, or build muscle. See Box 1-2 for translation of the part of the Hippocratic Corpus that refers to massage.

Ancient Rome (750 BCE–500 CE)

Legends tell of illegitimate twin brothers, Remus and Romulus, who were left to die in the Tiber River but were rescued and raised by a wolf. One of the stories ends with Romulus murdering Remus and founding Rome in 753 BCE. Another story describes the two brothers founding the city of Rome together. With the beginning of Rome being based on myth, it is difficult to know what the ancient Roman lifestyle was truly like. Records dating to 500 BCE provide dependable history, but before that time, Roman lifestyle is somewhat of a mystery.

It is clear that the Greek culture influenced Roman religion, entertainment, sports, and medicine. The Greek physicians, considered superior to the Roman physicians, gained status and recognition within the Roman culture by serving Roman royalty. With Greek medicine came the Greek health regimen and its terminology. Exercise, massage, and baths were collectively called "gymnastics" back in 400 BCE, and that term has maintained its association with massage throughout history.

Greek Physicians in Ancient Rome

Asclepiades of Bithynia (124–40 BCE) was a Greek physician who settled in Rome and promoted diet, exercise, bathing, and massage. His approach to medicine differed from Hippocrates' because his theory for health was based on a balance between tension; relaxation; and movement of very small, individual particles within the body called atoms. He believed that free, fluid movement of the atoms promoted health, and irregular, inharmonious movement caused disease. To restore atomic harmony, he used movement therapies such as massage, swinging, and vibration. His methods were so popular that many other physicians adopted and practiced his theory.

Aulus Cornelius Celsus (25 BCE–57 CE) was another prominent figure in ancient Roman medicine and massage. A follower of Hippocrates, he wrote a series of eight texts called *De Medicina*, which covered many different facets of health and medicine. Its preamble reviews the philosophies of Celsus' contemporaries and follows with a summary of his own approach to the art of medicine. First, he describes how health providers should act, then he shares his observations of diseases, and finally he discusses treatments. There are numerous references to massage throughout the work, indicating its use in the treatment of the following[1]:

- A weak body or tense body, headaches, paralysis (Book II: Chapter 14)

- Fevers (Book III: Chapters 9, 11, 12, 14)

- Paralysis, headaches, head cold (IV:5); neck spasm (IV:6); asthma (IV:8); cough (IV:10); flatulence, ulcers (IV:12); stomach pain (IV:13); lung disorders (IV:14); liver disorders (IV:15); spleen disorders (IV:16); intestinal distress (IV:20–23); diarrhea (IV:26); menstrual cramps, urinary disorders (IV:27); joints (IV:29, 30); healing (IV:32)

- Eye disorders (VI:6); ear disorders (VI:7); nose disorders (VI:8); fractures (VI:10); gum disorders (VI:13)

- Dislocations (VIII:11)

At the time it was written, somewhere around 30 CE, *De Medicina* was just another piece of medical literature. However, in the late 1400s, the work was rediscovered in Italy, printed, published, and circulated and now is celebrated as one of the earliest remnants of Western medicine.

Claudius Galenus (130–201 CE), also known as Galen, is possibly the most famous of the Greek physicians in Rome. Another follower of Hippocrates, Galen revolutionized medicine not only by his many works on anatomy and medicine but also by developing the experimental method of scientific investigation. He encouraged physicians to practice dissection to discover anatomy and improve their surgical skills. One of his books, *Hygiene*, includes a discussion on morning and evening massage, a description of massage strokes and muscle fibers being rubbed in every direction, as well as an explanation of anointing with oil for health and well-being.

The Fall of Rome

The culture of the Greeks continued to influence Rome until around 150 CE, when the fall of Rome began. In a series of events, including loss of territory and control to other cultures and religions, the power and glory of the Roman Empire finally faded out around 500 CE.

The Middle Ages (400–1400)

Once the last of the Roman emperors was ousted, Europe expanded northward with wars and battles for power and control, and world history was changing. This period, which lasted from the year 400 until 1400, is called the Middle Ages. Understandably, European history took a unique path, different from that of the rest of the world. Europe was significantly affected by the expansion and resultant wars, and the Church took control of society and education. The Arab world, however, was not involved in the European conflicts and was not under the influence of the Church.

Middle Ages in Europe

The Middle Ages in Europe are sometimes referred to as the Dark Ages. There was an absence of art, literature, science, medicine, and cultural development, and many written records were lost or destroyed amid the chaos of war. Gone was the luxurious lifestyle of the Romans. Despite the territorial battles, the Church maintained a strong presence throughout Europe. By salvaging and preserving some of the historical material, the Church became one of the primary sources of learning during the Middle Ages and became a powerful influence over society.

The Christian influence affected European culture for a thousand years. Teachings of the Church were strongly enforced; heretics were severely punished; independent, creative, progressive thought was discouraged; and development of the arts and sciences came to a screeching halt. Public baths and gymnasiums were abolished by the Church because of the increase of sexual improprieties. Women who provided healthcare were often accused of being witches with supernatural or magical activities and burned at the stake, some theorize because they posed a threat to the male doctors. With the advent of the Christian era, massage became synonymous with witchcraft, and the practice declined in Rome and most of Europe.

Fortunately, there were women who managed to keep touch alive during the Dark Ages. The Church operated hospitals in which nuns were granted permission to provide basic care to victims of war. Women from all walks of life eventually joined the nuns at the hospitals to care for patients, and massage and baths remained inexpensive treatments that women could provide. Incidentally, these oppressed women made great advances in women's rights toward the end of the Middle Ages, getting involved in politics, land ownership, science, literature, medicine, and education.

The Middle Ages in the Arab World

Women in the Arab world were also participating in healthcare during the Middle Ages, even if only serving as slaves who provided massage in the Turkish baths. While Europe suffered a thousand years with little progress, the Arab world continued to build upon the Greco-Roman knowledge base. The Arab countries were not constrained by the rules of the Church, which allowed them to use creativity, invention, and progressive thinking. They performed dissection on human cadavers, which was unacceptable in the Christian realm, and were able to advance anatomical knowledge. Al-Razi and Ibn Sina are Arabs who used massage and are famous for their contributions to medicine.

Al-Razi (854–935 CE), known in Latin as Rhazes, was an Islamic philosopher and physician. He wrote a medical encyclopedia that included knowledge from Arabic, Roman, and Greek physicians. He was especially interested in the interaction between psychology and physiology, gathering very detailed medical histories from his patients prior to diagnosing or prescribing. Because Al-Razi understood that health was affected by the state of mind, he considered preventive health maintenance very important. He perpetuated the use of massage as part of the health regimen as well as a treatment for disease.

Ibn Sina (980–1037 CE) is also known by his Latin name, Avicenna. He was a scholar, physician, and follower of the philosopher Aristotle. He wrote hundreds of books on a variety of subjects, but his greatest accomplishments were medical treatises. His *Canon of Medicine* is a systematic, useful, encyclopedic medical text that builds upon Galen's theories and observations. When revived after his death, it was quickly recognized as an excellent teaching text that was translated and used in medical schools across Europe for over 500 years.

Ibn Sina recommended health maintenance that included the original Greek regimen of exercise, baths, and massage. He also included massage as a treatment for relieving pain, for increasing blood flow, and for facilitating the healing process.

The Renaissance (1450–1600)

As Europeans tired of the cultural stagnation imposed by the Church, their curiosity and interest in the arts and sciences was revitalized. The Renaissance (French for rebirth) period started with this renewed burst of progressive thinking. During the Renaissance, medicine and art developed simultaneously, as renowned artists of the day studied and illustrated human anatomy and physiology.

Leonardo da Vinci's (1452–1519) illustrations of the human body and anatomy drawn during this period still exist today as some of the most admired medical illustrations. His studies of the human anatomy were often done in secret, since human dissection was not yet widely accepted in Europe. Figure 1-6 shows an example of Leonardo da Vinci's anatomical art.

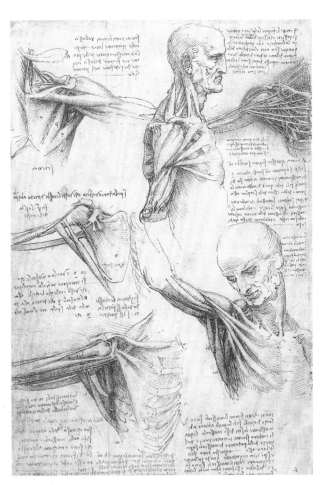

Figure 1-6. Leonardo da Vinci's anatomical illustrations. (Reprinted from Clayton M. Leonardo da Vinci: A Singular Vision. New York: Abbeville Press, 1996.)

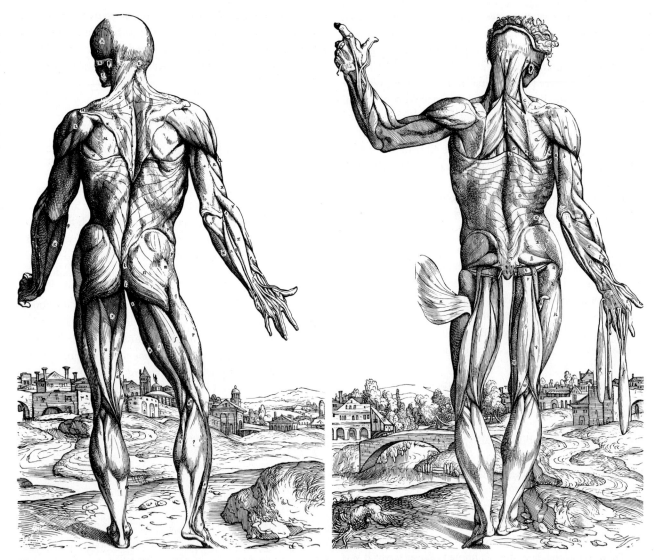

Figure 1-7. Anatomical illustrations by Andreas Vesalius showing muscular detail. (Reprinted from Saunders JB de CM, O'Malley CD. The Illustrations From the Works of Andreas Vesalius of Brussels. New York: Dover Publications, 1973.)

Another anatomical artist from the Renaissance is Andreas Vesalius (1514–1564) of Belgium. As a child, he felt compelled to learn anatomy, dissecting any unfortunate animals he could find. He found himself dissatisfied with his education at a medical school in Paris, partly because the teachers were fixed on Galen's philosophies and were still dissecting animals to understand human anatomy. He returned to Belgium so passionate about learning human anatomy that he stole a cadaver to dissect the body. Vesalius paid special attention to the muscles and their attachments and actions, making his contribution to massage history especially notable. Figure 1-7 shows an example of the anatomical art of Andreas Vesalius.

In his distinguished book *De Humani Corporis Fabrica*, published in 1543, Vesalius states, "It was when the more fashionable doctors in Italy, in imitation of the old Romans, despising the work of the hand, began to delegate to slaves the manual attentions they deemed necessary for their patients . . . that the art of medicine went to ruin."[2] This significant statement resonates with society today. Many people feel frustrated and disappointed with the medical community's personal disconnection and professional distancing, which fails to create a trusting relationship. Massage is a complementary therapy that can bridge the healthcare gap between clinical doctors who barely know their patients and the very personal and reassuring attention that human touch can provide.

The dualism theory of Rene Descartes (1596–1650), "I think, therefore I am," began the exploration into mind–body connection. In his book *Meditations VI*, he claims that the human body is like a machine: "so likewise if the body of man be considered as a kind of machine, so made up and composed of bones, nerves, muscles, veins, blood, and skin, that although there were in it no mind, it would still exhibit the same motions which it at present manifests involuntarily."[3] He drew a distinction between the mechanical body and the emotional mind but also claimed that they were interconnected. He was the first to differentiate between the human body and a human being, which continues to be a philosophical argument of medical ethics even today.

The 18th Century

The rediscovery of ancient cultures lasted until the next era, called the Age of Enlightenment or the Age of Reason, which occurred during the 1700s. The dogma and tradition of the Church were challenged, the sense of reason was explored and applied to different philosophies, humanitarianism blossomed, and education for everyone became a cultural norm. In America, reason, rationale, and education remained strong themes, but politics were the bigger part of history. The Declaration of Independence was signed, America became a free country, and the political system was established. The political and philosophical changes of the century bred inventions such as the bicycle, cotton gin, lightning rod, microscope, steam engine, telegraph, telescope, and thermometer.

Medical history was marked by the discovery of vaccination and inoculation. The ancient Chinese medical reference the *Cong Fou* was translated into French by Jesuit P. M. Cibot in 1779. The text, which recommended controlled breathing and a system of exercises and positions for healthcare, was accompanied by illustrations in the French version. It is very likely that this text served as the inspiration for Per Henrik Ling's Swedish Gymnastics.

Per Henrik Ling

Per Henrik Ling of Sweden (1776–1839) started a bodywork revolution during the transition from the 18th to 19th century. Throughout his travels across Europe teaching, translating, and writing poetry and plays, Ling learned to fence. He noticed the repetitive motions and one-sided physical activity of fencing and their effects on his body. To balance the physical activity, he incorporated gymnastics into his health regimen and consequently relieved his chronic elbow pain. He never became a doctor, but he studied anatomy and physiology extensively and developed Swedish Gymnastics, a movement system with four categories:

- Aesthetic—giving expression to feelings, emotions, and thoughts
- Educational—developing the innate potential of the body with good posture and control
- Medical—correcting bodily defects with active, passive, and duplicated movements
- Military—strengthening and toughening the body

The system included classifications of active, passive, or duplicated movements. Active movements were defined as activities in which patients exercised or moved their own bodies. Passive movements required the patients to be relaxed and have their bodies moved by the attendant or to be relaxed and receive manipulation by the attendant. The terms "active" and "passive" are still used with the same definitions to describe movement today. Duplicated movements required physical work from both the patient and the attendant, in which the attendant physically resisted the patient's efforts to move his or her own body. Dr. Mathias Roth, an English physician, wrote one of the first books published in English about Swedish Gymnastics, *The Prevention and Cure of Many Chronic Diseases by Movements*, in 1851. His book included drawings of treatments and showed the use of the low table, which was originally introduced by Ling. As the popularity and effectiveness of Ling's techniques spread across Europe and Russia, they were called the Swedish Movements, or the Swedish Movement Cure.

The use of the term "Swedish massage" likely stemmed from the Swedish Movements, even though the inclusion of actual massage techniques as we know them today is questionable. Because of the popularity of the Swedish massage technique, Ling has been credited with leading the revival of the massage profession and is considered by some the "Father of Swedish Massage." The contribution of Ling's work is certainly better known than that of other historical figures, but there are some people who are equally, if not more, important in massage history.

The 19th Century

Bodywork made a significant step forward into the 19th century with the help of Ling. His ability to demonstrate the validity of Swedish Gymnastics as an independent therapy quickly spurred other forms of manual therapy. Specific massage and bodywork techniques were created, promoted, and published in Europe and America.

Massage in 19th Century Europe

Following the development of the Swedish Movements, there were people who specifically promoted the field of massage therapy. Dr. Johan Georg Mezger (1838–1909) of the Netherlands coined some terms for massage techniques that are still used today: effleurage (EF-luhr-ahzh), petrissage (PEH-trih-sahzh), and tapotement (tuh-POHT-ment). It may seem odd that a Dutchman would choose French words for terminology, but the French words "massage," "masseuse," and "masseur" were already gaining popularity. Table 1-2 lists massage terms with French roots.

Until Dr. Mezger's influence, gymnastics were primarily Ling's exercises and movements that sometimes included massage techniques. Dr. Mezger was the first to identify classic massage strokes and differentiate them from gymnastics and Swedish Movements. He reinforced and popularized his terminology, which is still used as the standard worldwide.

Table 1-2 Massage Terms with French Roots

French Word	French Pronunciation	English Translation	English Pronunciation (If Applicable)
Masser	MAH-say	to rub or knead with hands	
Masseur	mah-SUHR	male person who kneads with hands	muh-SOOR
Masseuse	mah-SUHZ	female person who kneads with hands	muh-SOOS
Massage	MAH-sahzh	a method of kneading with the hands	Muh-SAHZH
Effleurer	EF-luhr-ray	to touch lightly	
Effleurage	EF-luhr-rahzh	a method of light touching or stroking	EF-luhr-ahzh
Pétrir	pay-TREER	to knead	
Pétrissage	PAY-trih-sahzh	a method of kneading	PEH- trih-sahzh
Tapoter	TAH-poh-tay	to tap	
Tapotement	TAH-poht-mahn	a method of tapping or patting	tuh-POHT-ment

The word "massage" was first found formally in a French-German dictionary in 1812, but French colonists in India may have started using the term in the mid-1700s. When they found natives rubbing each other for therapy, they described the activity in their journals, using their own French language. The terms "massage," "masseuse," and "masseur" are still used in many cultures, but in the United States, as the profession has evolved, the term "massage therapist" or "massage practitioner" has become the norm.

In 1888, Swedish physician Dr. Emil Kleen studied the effects of effleurage, friction, pétrissage, and vibration on circulation and lymph flow. He documented his results in *Handbook of Massage*, in which he also emphasized the inclusion of massage and manual therapy in medical treatment. At the same time, he discouraged laypersons from practicing massage because of its medical applications. He identified medical gymnastics as a form of exercise or movement of the muscles and differentiated it from massage, which he defined as a manual therapy that is not exercise and is applied by another individual. He stressed the importance of anatomical and physiological education, palpation skills, hands-on techniques, and the use of mechanical instruments for assistance in some situations. He also included some guidelines for therapist self-care and acceptable lubricants and provided a general outline for a massage session.

In the late 1800s, some British doctors made some unfortunate discoveries in the field of massage. They were noticing false claims of education and abnormally high fees for massage treatment. As a result, the British Medical Association ordered an inquiry and revealed patterns of inconsistency in the massage profession. Schools with unqualified teachers and nonstandardized courses were recruiting girls from poor neighborhoods and preparing students inadequately. They were giving students false impressions regarding employment opportunities, and many

graduates were finding themselves unemployed. Some schools opened massage school clinics and would forgive school debts to students who would work in their clinics. At best, these girls gave poor-quality massages. At worst, these clinics were considered houses of prostitution that deteriorated the reputation of massage practitioners. The rapid growth of the practice resulted in an excess of therapists who were unqualified and damaged the profession as a whole.

Legitimization of Massage

The negative repercussions of unregulated practice were accompanied by some clear advantages. Massage in hospitals and doctor's offices became more prevalent because the only massage therapists who were considered safe were directly associated with a doctor or hospital. Additionally, qualified massage therapists started organizing professional associations to protect the practice. The historical importance of this period relates to the steps that were taken to provide more legitimacy to the practice and to develop massage as a profession instead of an amateur trade.

Eight women founded the Society of Trained Masseuses in Britain in 1894 in an attempt to set a standard of high-quality massage therapists. They modeled their organization after the medical profession, where members had to meet specific academic requirements, pass an examination by a board of professionals including at least one physician, and receive training from a recognized school that received regular inspection and only hired qualified instructors. In 1900, it became the Incorporated Society of Trained Masseuses. When it expanded its membership to 12,000, it became the Chartered Society of Massage and Remedial Gymnastics. Massage practice was back on its way to being recognized as a legitimate profession.

Massage in 19th Century America

Healthcare made a transition in America during the 19th century from heroic, folk medicine and treatment to professional medical care. Massage first gained notice in the United States in the 1850s with Dr. George H. Taylor and his natural approach to medicine. He brought the Swedish Movements to the American medical community, integrated them into his practice, and eventually founded the Remedial Hygienic Institute in New York. Patients were taught a holistic approach to their health and disease, including an education regarding the nature of their illness, good nutritional habits, and an explanation of the treatment regimen, including water and massage therapies. Dr. Taylor's Movement Cure was later combined with Dr. Mezger's massage terms and techniques, one of which had the client lie on a table for the entire session, creating a scene similar to the present-day massage session.

Dr. John Harvey Kellogg (1842–1953) was an American physician who pioneered the health food movement, encouraging people to eat dry cereals for breakfast as part of a healthy vegetarian diet. He became the superintendent of the Battle Creek Sanitarium, a medical and surgical center where patients were taught that a proper diet, exercise and massage, fresh air, good posture, and sufficient rest result in good health. The sanitarium specialized in water therapies and massage and became famous for being "the place where people learn to stay well."[4]

Dr. Kellogg made some very important contributions to the history of massage. He conducted extensive massage research at the sanitarium, defining and examining the mechanical, reflex, and metabolic effects of massage on the different systems of the body. Table 1-3 explains the physiological effects of massage determined by Dr. Kellogg.

Table 1-3 Dr. John Harvey Kellogg and His Determination of the Physiological Effects of Massage

	Effect	Description	Example
	Mechanical	Client's tissues remain passive while the therapist applies pressure or manipulation to physically change the shape or condition of the client's tissues	Strokes directed toward the heart encourage venous blood flow
	Reflex	The therapist stimulates the client's sensory neurons, which triggers the client's nervous system to change the shape or condition of the tissues in both areas that were addressed and other, related areas	Light touch on the sole of the foot causes a reflex contraction of the rectus femoris, flexing the hip and pulling the foot away
	Metabolic	A combination of mechanical effects and reflex responses in which the whole body is affected	Sustained touch of massage activates the parasympathetic nervous response that lowers heart rate and encourages digestion

Photo courtesy of Robert Calvert, World of Massage Museum.

He found significant effects on the nervous, muscular, skeletal, circulatory, respiratory, integumentary, and digestive systems as well as thermal regulation, cellular metabolism, and kidney and liver activity. In 1895, Kellogg wrote about these effects in his book *The Art of Massage*. The book is an excellent reference with detailed and accurate information regarding anatomical structures, physiological effects, massage techniques, therapeutic applications, joint movement, massage for specific body regions and diseases, rules for practice, and correct terminology. This text was published again in 1909, 1919, and 1923 because of its superior presentation of information.

The 20th Century

Early in the 20th century, massage continued to establish a strong foundation for growth. Associations of massage professionals evolved to provide more legitimacy to the profession. The medical community respected the practice enough to allow it to continue in British hospitals and to be used as a form of rehabilitation for soldiers in World Wars I and II. In London, hospitals combined massage, physical exercise, physiotherapy, and orthopedic medicine departments. Massage services were particularly desired by private patients, so there was an increase in the number of nurses who took massage courses, studied for a Massage Certificate, and became nurse masseurs. Other students studied for the examination of the Chartered Society of Massage and Remedial Gymnastics, which later became the Chartered Society of Physiotherapy.

Social conservatism, the advancement of physiotherapy, physical therapy, and the use of electronic devices restrained the use of massage to some degree. Despite the negative connotations and technological progress, massage remained a part of healthcare. The later part of the 20th century brought much change to the massage profession, especially as bodywork techniques were developed all over the world. There are so many forms of bodywork generated in the later part of the 20th century that we consider it a separate period in massage history (Fig. 1-8).

Contemporary Massage Therapy

Bodywork has a long and rich history as a mode of physical, mental, and spiritual healing in various cultures and arenas that provides a solid foundation for the current massage therapy profession. For as much as bodywork has evolved over the previous thousands of years, massage has grown exponentially in the last 50 years. The rapid growth shows the popularity and validity of the practice, but it could also lead to the downfall of the massage profession. Although there is disagreement among current practitioners about standardization and governmental regulation, it encourages the safest and most dependable environment for massage clients.

Contemporary massage therapy in America began in the 1960s, when the younger generation rejected conservative habits and conformity in search of self-discovery. The Esalen Institute in Big Sur, California, became one of the major places to explore the "human potential," or the world of unrealized human capacities. Founded in 1962, Esalen became famous for its beautiful landscape; its blend of Eastern and Western philosophies; its experiential workshops; and the steady influx of philosophers, psychologists, artists, and religious thinkers. Esalen is one of the first modern places where massage was taught; there, bodywork is considered a pathway to well-being and transpersonal growth. The Esalen massage is a fluid and flowing combination of the structured Swedish Movements with massage strokes delivered in a sensitive, personal way.

The very popular human potential movement resulted in numerous books written to accompany the explosion of new bodywork techniques. Since then, many people have contributed to the advancement of the massage profession by conducting research studies to prove its therapeutic legitimacy and writing books that include scientific proof. As a result, massage is regaining acceptance with the public and the medical community as a valid therapy. Contemporary massage is recapturing the historic roots of massage as a preventive and rehabilitative medical approach and is reviving the rich tradition of bathing and anointing in the progressive spa industry.

Massage and Bodywork Modalities

Historically, massage techniques were based on the practices of anointing and bathing as well as variations of gymnastics and the Swedish Movements. Since then, numerous massage and bodywork modalities have emerged (Fig. 1-8). Keeping with the distinction that was made by Dr. Mezger and Dr. Kleen in the 1800s, massage is an activity that requires the therapist to apply manual pressure to the client's tissues. Bodywork can be characterized as treatment that involves manipulation of the client's body as a way to maintain or improve health. In other words, all forms of massage may be considered bodywork, but not all forms of bodywork may be called massage.

3000 BCE	Ancient Chinese medical texts, the *Cong Fou* and the *Nei Ching* are written Ancient forms of bodywork: anmo, anointing, mordan, samvahana, Tui-na
2500 BCE	Ancient Indian scriptures, the Vedas, are written
2350 BCE	Ankhmahor's tomb is inscribed with Egyptian drawings of bodywork
1825 BCE	Egypt's Kahun Medical Papyrus is written
1700 BCE	Babylonian laws called the Code of Hammurabi include "eye for an eye" medical ethics
1000 BCE	Ancient Greek health regimen included massage and baths
400 BCE	Hippocrates writes Hippocratic Corpus
30 CE	Aulus Cornelius Celsus writes *De Medicina*
175	Greek physician Claudius Galenus (Galen) of Rome develops early scientific research method
400–1400	The Middle Ages in Europe, influenced by the Church, is marked by cultural emptiness that results in a decline of massage in Europe The Middle Ages in the Arab world, less affected by the Church, generates the belief that health is affected by state of mind
1450–1600	The Renaissance brings anatomical art from Leonardo da Vinci and Andreas Vesalius René Descartes develops theory of mind–body connection, "I think, therefore I am"
1700s	Humanitarianism, reason, and education flood society, and many scientific inventions are created
1779	Jesuit P.M. Cibot translates the *Cong Fou* into French
1800s	Sweden's Per Henrik Ling creates Swedish Gymnastics The Netherlands' Dr. Johan Mezger standardizes massage terminology and differentiates massage strokes from movement therapies Dr. George Taylor popularizes the Movement Cure in America Dr. John Kellogg pioneers the health food movement in America, researches the physiological effects of massage, and writes *The Art of Massage*, which is still an excellent reference British inquiry reveals unethical activity in the field of massage, which provides the stimulus for legitimization
1894	The first professional massage organization, the Society of Trained Masseuses, is founded in Britain
1913	Dr. William Fitzgerald develops Zone Therapy, a precursor to reflexology, based on reflex zones
1914-1918	Swedish massage rehabilitates injured soldiers in WWI
1920	The Society of Trained Masseuses grows, incorporates, and becomes the Chartered Society of Massage and Remedial Gymnastics Dr. Mikao Usui of Japan originates Reiki
1927	The first American massage association, New York State Society of Medical Massage Therapists, is founded
1939	The Florida State Massage Therapy Association, Inc. (FSMTA) organizes 85 charter members
1940	British osteopath James Cyriax creates deep transverse friction
1940s	Therese Pfrimmer creates cross-fiber muscle therapy, later called Pfrimmer Deep Muscle Therapy
1943	American Association of Masseurs and Masseuses (AAMM) formed in Chicago with dues of 50 cents The first Massage Act is passed by the Florida Legislature
1949	Massage Registration Act formulated by AAMM
1950s	Francis Tappan and Gertrude Beard write significant books and articles on massage techniques Dr. Randolph Stone develops Polarity Therapy
1952	Janet Travell researches trigger points
1958	AAMM becomes the American Massage and Therapy Association (AM&TA)
1960s	Esalen Institute establishes itself as a center to explore human potential
1960	Jin Shin Jyutsu, the Japanese art of circulation awakening, was brought to America by Mary Iino Burmeister
1964	Applied Kinesiology was founded by chiropractor George Goodheart
1970s	John F. Barnes, physical therapist, introduces his therapy called Myofascial Release to the public
1972	Moshe Feldenkrais develops his own method of movement therapy
1977	Paul St. John, LMT, develops the St. John Method of Neuromuscular Therapy
1978	Joseph Heller develops Hellerwork, a structural bodywork
1980	Dr. Milton Trager opens the Trager Institute and teaches the Trager Approach to movement therapy
1981	Dr. Lawrence H. Jones develops Strain Counterstrain neuromuscular techniques for relieving trigger points
1983	AM&TA becomes the current American Massage Therapy Association (AMTA)
1987	Associated Bodywork and Massage Professionals (ABMP)
1992	Dr. Tiffany Field opens the Touch Research Institute AMTA creates the National Certification Board for Therapeutic Massage and Bodywork (NCBTMB) National Institutes of Health establish the Office of Alternative Medicine

Figure 1-8. Timeline of bodywork and massage.

Table 1-4 Bodywork Modalities and Some Examples of Each

Modality	Examples	Modality	Examples
Swedish	Swedish massage Relaxation massage Health maintenance massage Esalen massage	Energy	Polarity therapy Reiki Therapeutic Touch Touch for Health Magnet therapy Zero Balancing
Deep tissue	Connective tissue work Myofascial work Pfrimmer Deep Muscle Therapy Cross-fiber friction techniques Craniosacral work SOMA Neuromuscular Integration	Oriental/ Eastern approaches	Acupressure Shiatsu Jin Shin techniques Tui-na Thai massage Watsu Qigong Lomi Lomi
Neuromuscular	St. John Method of Neuromuscular Therapy (NMT) Trigger point therapy Muscle energy techniques Proprioceptive neuromuscular facilitation Reflexology Ortho-Bionomy	Structural integration	Rolfing Hellerwork Aston-Patterning
		Movement	Feldenkrais Alexander Technique Trager work
Circulation enhancement	Manual lymph drainage (MLD) Vodder techniques Arterial enhancement Venous enhancement	Special populations	Athletes Corporate massage Prenatal massage Infant massage Elderly massage Physically disabled Stone therapy

A **modality** is a collection of manual therapies that tends to use similar applications of movement or massage strokes to reach a similar goal. There has been inconsistency in the categorization of the various bodywork modalities, partly because so many of the modalities fit more than one category. This text separates and identifies the following nine categories of bodywork: Swedish, deep tissue, neuromuscular, circulation enhancement, energy, Oriental/Eastern approaches, structural/postural integration, movement bodywork, and special populations (see Table 1-4). These categories are briefly introduced in this chapter, and many are covered in detail later in the text. The techniques not covered in detail likely require extensive study, training, and special certification.

Swedish Modalities

Swedish massage is the most widely recognized and commonly used category of massage. While the public commonly identifies it as a gentle and superficial massage, the techniques vary from light to vigorous. Generally, Swedish includes a combination of long gliding (effleurage), kneading (petrissage), tapotement (percussion), and friction strokes applied to the superficial tissues of the body. They can be applied separately or mixed and matched to adapt to the needs of the client during the massage session. Oftentimes, these strokes are combined with active and passive movements to create a fluid, relaxing, circulatory-enhancing massage session.

Relaxation massage and health maintenance massage are considered Swedish modalities. Their mechanical and reflexive benefits are primarily intended to increase circulation of the blood and lymphatic fluid throughout the body as well as increase joint range of motion. These techniques and their effects are covered extensively in Chapter 9.

Deep Tissue Modalities

The deep tissue modalities are intended to affect the tissues that are deep within the body and are often difficult to palpate. They are usually applied slowly and specifically and typically use long, sustained gliding strokes, prolonged direct pressure, and strokes that travel across the muscles, perpendicular to the muscle fibers. This category of massage modalities includes, but is not limited to, connective tissue, myofascial, Pfrimmer, cross-fiber friction, and craniosacral techniques.

Connective tissue, myofascial, and Pfrimmer work are frequently used when there is some kind of restriction in the fascia or muscle. These restrictions, sometimes called adhesions, can form as a result of injury or chronic muscular tension patterns, may limit movement, create pain, and result in postural compensation patterns. These techniques may be uncomfortable for some clients, but by breaking up the restrictions and restoring space to the tissues, circulation and lymphatic flow are increased and health can be restored.

Dr. James Cyriax was an English physician who is considered the "Father of Orthopaedic Medicine." He developed the connective tissue technique of cross-fiber (deep transverse) friction that can be used to help heal muscular, tendinous, and ligamentous dysfunctions resulting from injury and overuse.

Deep tissue modalities often consist of applications of intense, localized pressure to access the deep tissue layers, but there are also some very subtle techniques that can accomplish the same thing. It may seem counterintuitive that a subtle technique could be a deep tissue modality, but there is a common misconception that "deep" means "hard." Consider the effect of vibrations. When you feel the rumbling of loud thunder or the booming bass of a car stereo or you strike a tuning fork and hold it against your skin, you may feel the vibrations resonate deep in your chest or throughout your whole body. Likewise, the deeper tissue layers can be affected with minimal energy and very little pressure by applying vibration or other subtle techniques such as craniosacral therapies or many of the energy modalities described later in this section.

Craniosacral therapy is a subtle technique that can affect deep tissues and have very profound effects. Practitioners palpate and manipulate the rhythmic flow of cerebrospinal fluid that bathes the brain and spinal cord. Altering the rhythm of the flow can rearrange the fascia, restore space to the tissues, and increase lymph and blood flow to the area. The technique is applied very lightly, which is why it is sometimes considered an energy modality, but this text classifies it as a deep tissue modality due to the cerebrospinal fluid being deep within the body, as well as its effects on the deep fascia.

Neuromuscular Modalities

Neuromuscular modalities engage the relationship between the nervous and muscular systems to create reflex responses. The organ systems of the body are separate but very interdependent processes. All of the activity of the muscular system depends on the nervous system, which is the main control system of the body. By using the physiological relationship between nerves and muscles, we can change muscle length and kinesthetic perception. Some of the neuromuscular modalities use massage, but this may be considered more of a bodywork modality. St. John Method of Neuromuscular Therapy (NMT), trigger point therapy, muscle energy techniques, proprioceptive neuromuscular facilitation, and reflexology can be categorized as neuromuscular modalities.

Circulatory Enhancement Modalities

Circulatory enhancement modalities are massage techniques that use purely mechanical effects to manipulate the movement of blood, lymphatic fluid, and waste within the body. The flow of blood through the cardiovascular system can be enhanced through the arteries as well as the veins. Basic massage strokes are used in specific patterns to accomplish both arterial and venous enhancement.

Lymphatic fluid from the body tissues is collected and transported through the lymph vessels and is eventually emptied into the heart. The flow of lymph can also be encouraged with specific manual techniques such as manual lymph drainage (MLD) or the Vodder method.

Energy Modalities

Energy modalities are often associated with a sense of mystery and doubt, mostly because their validity may be unproven by scientific methods. There are several types of energy bodywork, most of which use very light touch or off-the-body application to manipulate the human body's energy fields. Polarity therapy and Reiki are two of the more common energy techniques.

The famous physicists Albert Einstein, Prince Louis de Broglie, and Max Planck suggested that matter is composed of an essence of energy, having electromagnetic fields and positive and negative poles. Polarity therapy, based on the concept that the human body creates an energy field, suggests that the human energy field is affected by internal and external inputs, including emotions, touch, sounds, and movement. While the central nervous system is the main component of our electrical or energetic existence, a whole host of biochemical reactions play a part as well. Basically, if biochemical reactions are hindered, the efficiency of nerve transmission and other body systems is diminished. Theoretically, if the blockages are removed, function can be restored. Polarity therapy addresses the electrical field of the body, attempting to balance it out in an attempt to allow normal electrical activity to occur.

Reiki is an energy modality that restores flow to the life force energy with spiritual guidance. The life force energy, or **Qi** (CHEE), is a dynamic, changing energy force that runs through the whole body, supplying and being supplied by body processes and activities. It can be vaguely compared to the flow of energy that you feel when you are enlightened, optimistic, or motivated. Unlike most bodywork modalities, Reiki is a technique that is transferred as a gift from one practitioner to another, requiring no intellectual or spiritual education. A very simplified explanation of Reiki portrays it as a spiritually guided manipulation of the life force energy.

Oriental/Eastern Modalities

In traditional Eastern philosophies, the Qi travels through a series of pathways called meridians. The philosophies teach that a balanced, unrestricted flow of Qi is required for the body to maintain good health, and disruptions or blockages to Qi cause disharmony in the body. Theoretically, removal of the disruptions and restoration of a balanced energy flow can restore health. The Oriental bodywork modalities manipulate the Qi mechanically to restore normal function and health to the body. These techniques use external, visible applications of pressure and manipulation, which classifies them as massage techniques. In addition to mechanical pressure, these techniques also use internal, energetic manipulations that are not visible. The internal work is the more profound of the two, which leads to the consideration of the Oriental techniques as forms of art as opposed to science. Acupressure, Shiatsu, Jin Shin techniques, and Tui-na are just some of the many Oriental modalities that use mechanical pressure from fingers, hands, thumbs, elbows, knees, and feet.

Structural and Postural Integration Modalities

Structural and postural integration modalities, such as Rolfing and Hellerwork, may be considered massage techniques. They generally focus on realigning the skeletal system to relieve pain from postural compensations. Posture can significantly affect health, and although it often takes a lot of bodywork that may be accompanied by discomfort, structural realignment can be very beneficial. The Assessment chapter of this text, Chapter 7, discusses the relationship between posture and health in further detail.

Movement Modalities

These bodywork modalities use movement to reorient the body for more optimal function. Feldenkrais (FEHL-den-krahys), Alexander Technique, and Trager (TRAY-ger) are examples of movement modalities.

Dr. Moshe Feldenkrais was a physicist, engineer, martial arts master, and teacher who developed his own bodywork method in the mid-1900s. Feldenkrais is a movement therapy that teaches body awareness, coordination, and flexibility through movement techniques. Habitual activities that may create dysfunctional movement patterns are studied and then neuromuscularly reprogrammed by practicing precise movement patterns that are balanced. The neuromuscular component of this modality leads some to categorize it as a neuromuscular therapy, but its focus is on movement.

The Alexander Technique was developed by Frederick Matthias Alexander, a Shakespearean actor from the early 1900s. His technique studies the client's balance, coordination, flexibility, and support structure and encourages the client to be aware of reactive, habitual movements. The practitioner uses palpation skills and gentle movements to relieve muscular tension while the client demonstrates simple activities. By reprogramming the body to make conscious movement choices instead of reactive, reflexive motions, the technique creates ease of movement and improves overall health.

Milton Trager, MD, developed a bodywork approach in the mid-1900s that uses active and passive components similar to ancient gymnastics. The client lies on a table for the passive component while the practitioner moves him in gentle, natural rocking and shaking patterns that are intended to feel unrestricted and effortless. The intent is to relieve chronic patterns of muscular tension. The active portion of the approach requires clients to shake and loosen their bodies to reinforce the practitioner's table work. Giving the clients exercises to use on their own allows them to take an active part in their healthcare and can have longer lasting or permanent results.

Special Populations

There are groups of clients who have special conditions or require special considerations to receive massage and bodywork comfortably or safely. This text refers to these groups as special populations, and the therapist must understand their specific needs to determine which techniques are appropriate and which should be avoided. Some special populations a therapist may encounter include athletes, corporate, geriatric, prenatal, infant, and physically disabled clients. Essentially, the same massage strokes are used, but special considerations are given to session duration, pressure, areas to avoid, positions to avoid, precautions to take, and equipment to use. These special populations are covered in more detail later in the text.

Touch

Touch is one of the most basic of human needs and occurs in every culture. Touch can be used as a method of communication and learning, for comfort, and to provide self-esteem. Scientific research has indicated that it is required for healthy growth, development, and immune function. It has also been scientifically proven that deprivation of touch can cause significant developmental barriers in humans and animals. In essence, the sense of touch is required for our very survival.

From the time you are in the womb, you depend on touch to learn about the world. Infants commonly explore objects by putting them in their mouths, discovering the shapes, textures, and temperatures of objects in their world. When babies cry, they are comforted when they are picked up and held, stroked, or kissed. This comforting aspect of touch continues into adulthood. When you are upset, you often seek touch for comfort and validation. Handshakes, pats on the back, hand holding, hugs, and kisses are different forms of touch that provide comfort and validation, and they are also used as modes of communication. Adults use touch to communicate, evaluate, and navigate through the world. Again, touch is very powerful and, when used appropriately, can have incredibly positive outcomes on the human experience.

Touch Physiology

The average person is covered with 18 square feet of skin, making the skin the largest sensory organ of the body. Unlike the other sensory organs, the skin remains in a constant state of readiness, sending pressure, temperature, and pain sensations to the central nervous system for the appropriate response. This function is especially critical when a person is blind or deaf or when other physiological changes affect sensory input. The skin is the major structure of the integumentary system and is covered in more detail in the chapter on body systems.

Massage Research

Various forms of touch have long been a part of many cultures throughout history, but the formal, scientific study of touch is relatively new. As the massage profession continues to evolve, research is vital for validating the effects of massage. The hard scientific proof is helping the medical profession understand and accept the value of touch. Several medical schools, including Duke, Harvard, and Johns Hopkins, offer integrated medicine electives and research opportunities to study the effects of touch and other bodywork modalities.

One very early example of touch research is the classic study conducted in 1958 by University of Wisconsin psychologist Harry Harlow. Infant rhesus macaque monkeys were taken from their real mothers, isolated in metal cages, and offered different objects for sources of comfort and security. Harlow showed that the infants preferred cuddling with a soft cloth, artificial mother to a wire model with a head and face that held food (Fig. 1-9). In fact, when the cloth model had the food as well, the infant monkeys did not go to the wire model at all, suggesting that infants may instinctively prefer cuddling and tactile stimulation to food nourishment. There are so many people who believe in the power of touch that the government and private interest groups have funded research to prove its efficacy.

Government-Sponsored Research

The National Institutes of Health established the Office of Alternative Medicine in 1992 to study and recommend

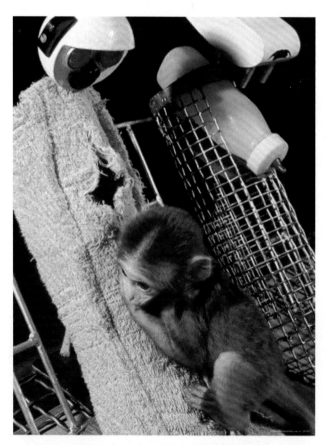

Figure 1-9. Harlow's rhesus monkey clinging to the soft cloth figure instead of the wire figure that holds nourishment.

further research on unconventional medical treatments. In 1998, it expanded to become the National Center for Complementary and Alternative Medicine (NCCAM). "It is dedicated to exploring complementary and alternative healing practices in the context of rigorous science, training complementary and alternative medicine (CAM) researchers, and disseminating authoritative information to the public. To fulfill its mission, NCCAM supports a broad-based portfolio of research, research training, and educational grants and contracts, as well as various outreach mechanisms to disseminate information to the public."[5]

A growing number of Americans are using complementary approaches to healthcare and medical treatment and are seeking healthcare providers who treat the whole person instead of just an illness. As a result, then President Bill Clinton established the White House Commission on Complementary and Alternative Medicine Policy (WHCCAMP) by issuing Executive Order 13147 on March 7, 2000. The commission is composed of no more than 15 individuals who are knowledgeable in conventional, complementary, and alternative medicine. These representatives were appointed by the president and were asked to address the following issues:

- Research on CAM practices and products
- Delivery of and public access to CAM services
- Dissemination of reliable information on CAM to healthcare providers and the general public
- Appropriate licensing, education, and training of CAM healthcare practitioners

In March 2002, the WHCCAMP issued a final report covering all their charged issues. The following is the overview of the report, as written:

"Although heterogeneous, the major CAM systems have many common characteristics, including a focus on individualizing treatments, treating the whole person, promoting self-care and self-healing, and recognizing the spiritual nature of each individual. In addition, many CAM systems have characteristics commonly found in mainstream health care, such as a focus on good nutrition and preventive practices. Unlike mainstream medicine, CAM often lacks or has only limited experimental and clinical study; however, scientific investigation of CAM is beginning to address this knowledge gap. Thus, boundaries between CAM and mainstream medicine, as well as among different CAM systems, are often blurred and are constantly changing."[6]

Dr. Tiffany Field and the Touch Research Institute

Tiffany Field, PhD, is the pioneer of modern massage research and remains one of the foremost authorities on

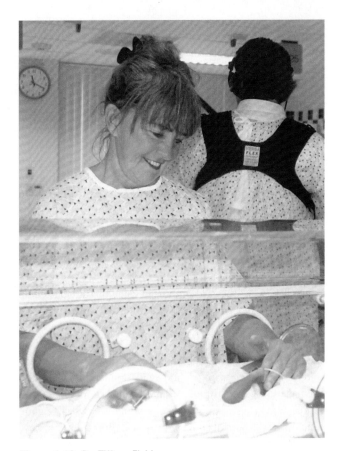

Figure 1-10. Dr. Tiffany Field.

scientific proof of the benefits of massage (Fig. 1-10). Her interest in touch therapy began when her daughter was born prematurely. She conducted her first study as a psychology graduate student in 1982, determining that "infants given pacifiers during their tube feedings gained more weight, went off tube feedings earlier, did better on newborn behavior and neurological examinations, and were discharged earlier, at a much lower hospital cost, than infants not given pacifiers."[7]

Her remarkable work won her a start-up grant from Johnson & Johnson in 1992 to create the Touch Research Institute (TRI) at the University of Miami's School of Medicine. It was the first center in the world devoted to studying the scientific aspects and medical applications of touch, designing research studies that can prove how touch promotes health and can be used to treat disease. The outcomes of these critical research studies will help validate the beneficial effects of massage. In fact, the TRI has already shown that massage is medically beneficial for premature infants and fibromyalgia, asthma, and diabetes patients. TRI research has shown that massage enhances the immune system by increasing production of natural killer cells and increases alertness and computational accuracy. See Research Box 1-1 for specific research studies performed by the TRI.

RESEARCH BOX 1-1

General Information about TRI Research

(Taken directly from the TRI web site: http://www.miami.edu/touch-research/index.html)

The Touch Research Institutes have conducted over 90 studies on the positive effects of massage therapy on many functions and medical conditions in varied age groups. Among the significant research findings are enhanced growth (e.g., in preterm infants), diminished pain (e.g., fibromyalgia), decreased autoimmune problems (e.g., increased pulmonary function in asthma and decreased glucose levels in diabetes), enhanced immune function (e.g., increased natural killer cells in HIV and cancer), and enhanced alertness and performance (e.g., EEG pattern of alertness and better performance on math computations). Many of these effects appear to be mediated by stress hormones. Several of these findings have been reviewed in the TRI newsletter ("Touchpoints") and in the volumes *Touch Therapy* (Harcourt Brace) and *Touch* (MIT Press).

References are cited below the subject/topic. Articles can be obtained by taking the reference to your local university library (not a public library) and asking the librarian to help you find a journal article. References listed as "in press," "in review," or "ongoing" are not yet available. To order a packet of articles from the Touch Research Institute, please go to the order form under "Touchpoints." You can select studies to receive for $20 per 4 articles.

Back Pain Massage lessened lower back pain, depression, and anxiety and improved sleep. The massage therapy group also showed improved range of motion, and their serotonin and dopamine levels were higher.

Hernandez-Reif M, Field T, Krasnegor J, Theakston T. Low back pain is reduced and range of motion increased after massage therapy. Int J Neurosci 2001;106:131–145.

Breast Cancer Massage therapy reduced anxiety and depression and improved immune function including increased natural killer cell number.

Hernandez-Reif M, Ironson G, Field T, et al. Breast cancer patients have improved immune functions following massage therapy. J Psychosom Res, in review.

Diabetes Following 1 month of parents massaging their children with diabetes, the children's glucose levels decreased to the normal range and their dietary compliance increased. Also the parents' and children's anxiety and depression levels decreased.

Field T, Hernandez-Reif M, LaGreca A, et al. Massage therapy lowers blood glucose levels in children with diabetes mellitus. Diabetes Spectrum 1997;10:237–239.

Early Stimulation Research is reviewed on the critical nature of rubbing the rat pup and the preterm newborn for their growth and development.

Schanberg S, Field T. Sensory deprivation stress and supplemental stimulation in the rat pup and preterm human neonate. Child Dev 1987;58:1431–1447.

Father–Infant Massage Fathers gave their infants daily massages 15 minutes prior to bedtime for one month. The fathers in the massage group showed more optimal interaction behavior with their infants.

Cullen C, Field T, Escalona A, Hartshorn K. Father–infants interactions are enhanced by massage therapy. Early Child Dev Care 2000;164:41–47.

Fibromyalgia Fibromyalgia patients slept better (showed lower activity levels, suggesting more deep sleep), and had lower substance P levels and less pain following a month of biweekly massages.

Field T, Diego M, Cullen C, et al. Fibromyalgia pain and substance P decrease and sleep improves after massage therapy. J Clin Rheumatol 2002;8:72–76.

Leukemia Twenty children with leukemia were provided with daily massages by their parents and were compared with a standard treatment control group. Following a month of massage therapy, depressed mood decreased in the children's parents, and the children's white blood cell and neutrophil counts increased.

Field T, Cullen C, Diego M, et al. J Bodywork Movement Ther 2001;5:271–274.

Migraine Headaches Massage therapy decreased the occurrence of headaches, sleep disturbances, and distress symptoms and increased serotonin levels.

Hernandez-Reif M, Field T, Dieter J, et al. Migraine headaches were reduced by massage therapy. Int J Neurosci 1998;96:1–11.

Massage Therapy Foundation

The American Massage Therapy Association (AMTA), covered in more detail in Chapter 2, created the AMTA Foundation in 1990. Its original goal was to generate and apply knowledge regarding the benefits of massage therapy and to disseminate the information to all aspects of society. The current mission also includes support of scientific research, community education, and community service. The organization, which has since been renamed the Massage Therapy Foundation, relies on donations from individuals, schools, massage therapy product vendors, and the AMTA to grant funds for research, community service, educational scholarship, and conferences. It also educates massage therapists about current research and provides direct consultation to the medical and research communities.

In 1998, the Foundation established the Massage Therapy Research Database with hopes that it would become the primary source for massage-related articles with a focus on information from peer-reviewed research journals. It currently contains thousands of records and journal citations dated through 2006 as well as up-to-date, current citations from the non-Medline resources *Journal of Bodywork and Movement Therapies, Journal of Soft Tissue Manipulation, Massage and Bodywork, Massage Magazine* and *Massage Therapy Journal.* Some of these sources of data are not included in standard medical indexes but are important for the field of massage. The Massage Therapy Research Database page offers a link to live PubMed, which allows the user to look for current medical research citations.

Interpretation of Touch

While the physiological mechanisms for the touch response are basically the same in every human being, individual interpretation of touch can be vastly different. Influenced by emotion, gender, age, culture, spirituality, and religious customs, each person's unique intention and perception of touch make it one of the most powerful forms of communication.

There is a fine and often fuzzy line between all aspects of giving and receiving. In the world of massage therapy, the therapist gives his or her own form of touch to the client, and at the same time receives tactile input from the client that relays information pertaining to muscular tension or reduced range of motion. These inputs are a form of communication between therapist and client. Any time a client is receiving massage or bodywork, the therapist must be aware of the many ways a client's body can convey its reaction to the work. Clients may express discomfort by wincing, pulling away, getting quiet or talking excessively, holding the breath, or tensing the body. On the other hand, clients who are enjoying the bodywork might sigh or let out a big breath, their whole body might relax and go limp, breathing could slow down, or they could become quiet or go to sleep. All of these responses, which can be noticed by the therapist, are body language messages that might be telling the therapist to adjust the bodywork. Therapists must not let their own emotions, belief systems, or reactive responses influence sensory input from the client's body. This separation of the therapist's life experiences from the client's body is sometimes referred to as grounding, which is discussed later in the text.

Massage as Part of the American Healthcare System

Contemporary massage therapy is evolving within and outside the American healthcare system. The practice of massage and bodywork is now considered a major component of complementary and integrated healthcare, as is evidenced by government-sponsored research and development. Medical schools are incorporating complementary health education into their programs, and doctors are graduating with a general understanding of complementary healthcare. Hospitals are incorporating massage therapy into their services for both staff and patients, and massage is becoming more prevalent in medical clinics, pain clinics, and doctors' offices.

Even more exciting is the fact that insurance companies are beginning to recognize massage as a legitimate treatment instead of a luxury that has no medical benefit. Currently, American insurance companies are often looking to spend as little money as possible, they are notorious for delaying payment or denying claims, and they tend to raise premiums while reducing benefits. With the abundance of research to prove the benefits of massage, insurance companies are beginning to see that the low cost of massage may significantly reduce their overall costs. Massage may minimize or eliminate the need for pharmaceuticals, reduce the length of hospital stays, and reduce the number of physical therapy sessions a patient may need. Better yet, the side effects of massage do not require additional medical treatment, which often happens with prescription medications. Continued scientific research to validate the benefits of massage will help the public, healthcare community, and insurance companies validate the efficacy of touch.

Integrative Medicine Centers

The current American healthcare system includes integrative medicine centers, some of which provide training for medical professionals in the complementary therapies in addition to patient services. These centers also conduct massage research in a scientific method that is accepted in the professional healthcare environment, which is one of the reasons they are so important to the massage profession as it grows.

- The Arizona Center for Integrative Medicine concentrates on clinical care, education, and research. Clinical integrative medical care offered at the University of Arizona ranges from preventive healthcare options to treatments for cancer and chronic conditions such as heart disease or diabetes. The educational opportunities in integrative medicine are available to all levels of students, both online and onsite. They developed the first integrative medicine residency program, and they now offer a variety of opportunities in integrative medical education for doctors. Though their educational opportunities are outstanding, one of the primary goals of the Center is to contribute rigorous scientific research on the integration of complementary and alternative therapies with traditional Western medicine. They support a CAM research fellowship that is offered through the University of Arizona's Family and Community Medicine department, and currently have several research projects under way.

- The Duke Integrative Medicine program aims to heal patients physically, emotionally, and spiritually by incorporating medical treatment, acupuncture, exercise, meditation, mind–body techniques, nutrition, supplements, and therapeutic massage. It offers fourth-year medical students an integrative medicine elective rotation that includes botanicals, homeopathy, mind–body connection, naturopathy, nutrition, traditional Chinese medicine, osteopathy, and energy medicine, as well as integrative medicine research. Their staff conducts research as part of their dedication to understand the efficacy of integrative healthcare, and the clinical outcomes help guide their development of innovative systems of care. They even cite several research studies when promoting massage as an effective treatment to relieve pain, reduce swelling, and reduce anxiety.

- Mayo Clinic's Complementary and Integrative Medicine program helps patients integrate CAM such as acupuncture, Ayurvedic treatments, herbal medicine, hypnosis, massage, meditation, resilience training, stress management, and traditional Chinese medicine into their conventional Western medical

care. Most importantly, their staff conducts dozens of clinical research studies each year to determine which treatments work best. This kind of ongoing research helps identify effective therapies and bring them into clinical practice. In fact, one of the four areas of research that the program focuses on is massage and manual therapies, and positive results have been found in both pre- and postcardiovascular surgery patients as well as breast disease patients.

- The Integrative Medicine Service at Memorial Sloan-Kettering Cancer Center offers their services and therapies, including acupuncture, creative therapies, mind–body therapies, nutrition, and touch therapies to anyone receiving cancer care, anywhere. They also offer workshops and programs to educate patients, caregivers, and healthcare professionals about alternative and complementary treatments, including massage therapy. The integrative medicine research program has a branch of research devoted to quality of life studies and, in one collaborative effort with the Memorial Sloan-Kettering's Pain and Palliative Care Service, is constructing a controlled trial to evaluate the benefits of massage therapy for terminally ill patients.

Oncology Massage

Oncology massage, or massage for cancer patients, is a rapidly growing specialty. There are several options for training, some with independent instructors and others with clinics associated with hospitals and universities. If a therapist wants to focus on or specialize in oncology massage, it may be beneficial to pursue oncology massage certification. These certification programs help train the therapists to work within a hospital environment and as part of a healthcare team; understand hospital charts to determine an appropriate, safe plan of massage treatment; follow doctor's orders; and thoroughly understand the physiology and progression of cancer, the medical treatments, and their possible side effects. The more qualified massage therapists there are practicing in hospital environments and delivering safe, appropriate, and effective massage treatment, the more the profession is advanced within the American healthcare system.

Massage in the Spa Industry

In addition to the increased use in the healthcare system, the spa industry has greatly increased its interest in massage and bodywork over the last few years. The spa industry has a

long history that includes massage and bodywork, and massage is offered in almost every spa in America now. In fact, it seems massage and water treatments have come full circle and are currently gaining extraordinary popularity as therapeutic treatments.

History of the Spa Industry

The ancient Romans discovered the therapeutic properties of hot mineral springs in the village of Spa, Belgium, and used them to heal wounded soldiers. The soldiers took their knowledge back to Rome, and the Roman baths were born. As the natural hot springs quickly became a standard part of health maintenance and improvement, the spa business was refined. Physicians recognized the therapeutic effects of spas and commonly set up practice in or near the spas to treat their patients. By 14 CE, there were over 150 spas in Rome being used by the general public for rest, relaxation, and stress reduction. Massage was one of the many rituals of the spa experience.

Native Americans were using hot springs for healthcare long before America was discovered by the Europeans. In 1790, Saratoga Hot Springs in Saratoga, Wyoming, was the first commercial spa to be established in America. Spas have since become a standard community business. As stated above, massage and water treatments have come full circle and are currently gaining extraordinary popularity as therapeutic treatments.

The International Spa Association (ISPA) was founded in 1991 to provide a network for professional spa associates. ISPA's goals are to educate, set standards, provide resources, influence policy, and build coalitions for the spa industry worldwide. It has identified 10 elements of the spa experience, including a touch component for massage and bodywork (Fig. 1-11).

Medical Spas

For years, American spas focused on providing beauty and relaxation for their patrons, with little or no involvement of medical personnel. The 10 elements of a spa experience were incorporated into the services offered. The current industry trend, however, is showing a slow but steady increase in medical spas. With the philosophy that health and healing can be improved with a positive state of mind, medical spas offer a special approach toward healthcare by integrating client comfort and relaxation with conventional medical treatments.

Dentists, dermatologists, obstetricians, oncologists, and plastic surgeons are some of the medical professionals who can be found working at spas. The presence of these doctors and their services raises the profile of a beauty-related spa to

a professional, health and medical treatment spa. The doctors offer medical and spa services to segments of the population who might not normally be able to take advantage of a spa. For example, an oncologist could determine which massage lubricants would not damage the skin or complicate the condition of a client undergoing chemotherapy. Likewise, an obstetrician would be able to recommend aromatherapy products that are safe during pregnancy, allowing the mother to enjoy a massage with therapeutic essential oils. The medical doctors on staff can ensure that all other spa services are safe for their patients and can monitor healing progress in addition to their patients' health.

Spa Massage Education

Currently, spas are the largest employer of massage therapists. As American spas become more professional and medically oriented, massage training must be geared to support this direction. Self-employment tends to be the focus for most massage education, but many massage therapists work as employees for hospitals, clinics, fitness centers, and spas. Many of these jobs require group interaction, teamwork, and a willingness to take on other responsibilities.

Spas are now finding that they must spend time and resources training massage therapists to work as part of the team. Spa owners are looking for therapists who are team players. To fill this demand, esthetician schools, beauty schools, and cosmetology schools are starting to offer massage therapy training. These schools are graduating therapists who may be more adept at working in a spa, but who have insufficient knowledge of anatomy, physiology, pathology, and pharmacology. The market will be better served by massage schools adding spa therapy training to their programs, preparing students for the hospitality environment and group interaction.

Group environments require cooperation, good communication skills, and an appreciation for the success of the business being a result of good teamwork. In addition to doing their own job very well, each person in the group must be aware of the other business activities and be willing to support and help the others accomplish those tasks. There are many occasions when therapists are asked to handle retail sales, housekeeping, front desk reception, body wraps, showers, and other spa services. When massage therapy is only one part of an assortment of business activities, it is important to work efficiently, keep appointments on schedule, cooperate, and support everyone else on the team.

Some massage therapists are so passionate about the benefits of massage that they sound like they are bragging, making it seem like massage is better than any other spa treatment, and may unintentionally offend others in a group. Touch is so

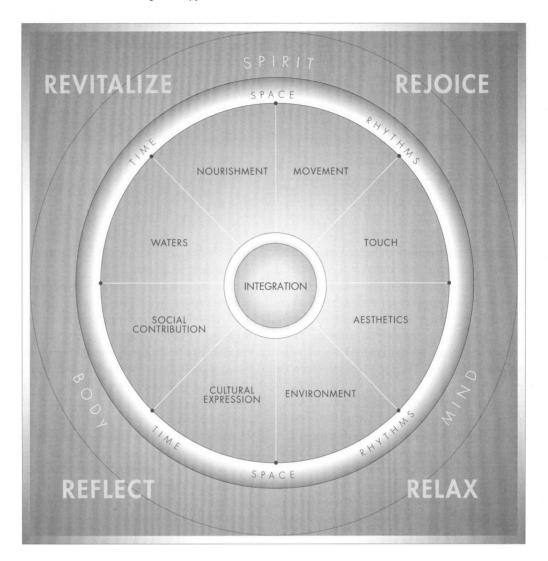

Waters: The internal and external use of water in its many forms.

Nourishment: What we feed ourselves: food, herbals, supplements, and medicines.

Movement: Vitality and energy through movement, exercise, stretching, and fitness.

Touch: Connectivity and communication embraced through touch, massage, and bodywork.

Integration: The personal and social relationship between mind, body, spirit, and environment.

Aesthetics: Our concept of beauty and how botanical agents relate to the biochemical components of the body.

Environment: Location, placement, weather patterns, water constitution, natural agents, and social responsibility.

Cultural Expression: The spiritual belief systems, the value of art and the scientific and political view of the time.

Social Contribution: Commerce, volunteer efforts, and intention as they relate to well-being.

Time, Space Rhythms: The perception of space and time and its relationship to natural cycles and rhythms.

Circle concept created by R. Zill for ISPA 2001

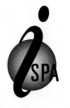

ISPA would like to thank the ISPA education committees past and present.

Figure 1-11. ISPA's 10 elements. (Reprinted with permission from the International SPA Association. Circle concept created by R. Zill for ISPA 2001.)

personal and individual that someone who receives the same simple stroke from two different therapists may find that the strokes feel completely different. Keep this in mind as you give and receive massage in class, comparing the feel of one person's touch to that of another and considering how different you feel after each massage. Outside school, you may find that your massage may not suit a particular client. To maintain a client-focused business, you can refer that client to a different therapist or to a different kind of treatment. Ego and a sense of superiority can be detrimental, so it is important to separate your ego from your massage treatments for the benefits of you, your clients, and your coworkers.

Trends in Massage Education

When the "hippie" movement popularized massage in the 1960s, American massage education took an informal and nonscientific approach. People who felt gifted with touch often learned techniques from early texts, such as Dr. Kellogg's *The Art of Massage*. For the next 20 years, there was a rebirth of the massage industry in America. Many people were learning techniques from individuals who specialized in massage, and the number of schools was steadily increasing.

Today, massage schools can be found across the country, with various levels of academic, technique, and business education. The more formal, extended study program is becoming increasingly more popular as the country embraces regulation and standardization of the practice.

There is not necessarily a trend in the method of teaching human anatomy to massage students, but there is definitely a wide range of teaching techniques. Some schools go to the extreme, using human cadavers to teach anatomy. This is without question a beneficial and unique educational experience, but cadaver laboratories are very expensive. Most schools teach anatomy from textbooks, hands-on models, and video presentations, and generally speaking, these teaching techniques are sufficient. This variation in teaching technique presents a challenge to the standardization of massage education, especially considering the rising cost of education in today's economy.

Insurance companies and their excessive trails of paperwork introduce an aspect to the practice that needs to be addressed. Medical coding, documentation, and billing procedures must be done correctly for insurance companies to even consider disbursing payment. Medical offices have higher incomes to offset the slow payment from insurance companies, but massage therapists often depend on fast payment to pay monthly bills. It may expedite payment from an insurance company if you are familiar with medical codes, paperwork, and billing procedures. It is not clear whether massage schools should be responsible for teaching students how to manage insurance billing or not, but it is certainly worth considering as massage education moves forward. Most massage schools have not incorporated medical billing into their standard curriculum, but numerous courses are available through massage and bodywork associations and independent educators.

As the integrative medicine approach to healthcare becomes more mainstream, so does the need for massage therapists to understand the research findings that pertain to massage. "Massage research literacy" is a term that describes the ability to find and understand the research studies that focus on massage, to evaluate the information, and to apply it in a massage setting. There may be some difficulty incorporating research literacy into existing massage programs, partly because most massage instructors have little training in research literacy, and partly because the scientific-based approach to massage only appeals to a portion of most massage students. In an attempt to reduce the education gap, the Massage Therapy Foundation offers a Teaching Research Literacy course to massage school faculty. This program helps schools incorporate research literacy into a curriculum by teaching how to help students understand the language and terminology that is commonly used in research, how to write case reports that are ready for publication, and how to develop scientific evidence–informed practices. It is important that massage students be able to sort through many research studies to find ones that are scientifically sound, especially if they plan on incorporating the results into their practice. Whether or not the inconsistency in teaching research literacy is ever addressed with regulations, it remains an important trend in massage education.

Remember that academic education is only one part of the therapist's skills. Solid, substantial knowledge of science is necessary, but palpation and communication skills are just as important. Massage therapy is a hands-on activity that must be taught and learned with hands-on practice. One hopes that the future will bring regulations and standardization to all aspects of massage therapy, including education.

CHAPTER SUMMARY

To better understand massage, it helps to understand the profession as it evolved through history. Basically, bodywork has existed as long as humans have walked the earth, used in both the spiritual and medical realms. The practice of massage has consistently been delivered by religious figures, laypersons, and folk healers, but the medical community exhibits a fluctuating pattern of acceptance and resistance of massage. Currently, the field of massage therapy is gaining acceptance in the medical community, and many people are suggesting that medical massage is a new modality. There is a push to separate medical massage treatment from spa massage, but this is really a moot point as the physiological effects of massage are the same for the client regardless of the setting. In fact, some massage therapists work at both medical clinics and day spas, providing individualized treatment to all of their clients. Therapists who have sufficient academic education accompanied by adequate hands-on training can deliver the appropriate massage in any environment.

Throughout history, the associated use of massage and water therapies has also fluctuated in popularity. At this point, there is a renewed use of water and massage therapy as evidenced by hydrotherapy and spa treatments. These patterns of coexistence can be used as a guide to understand trends in the use of massage as a healthcare treatment.

Scientific research continues to prove the efficacy of massage as a medical treatment for a number of conditions and to contribute to its growth in popularity. Science is showing the world the importance of touch in its many forms. Regardless of the science, there is a powerful human requirement for touch, and massage will continue to be used both intuitively as well as professionally.

History can guide us into a successful future for the world of massage therapy. Excessive growth in the field of massage in the 1800s flooded society with inadequately trained therapists. Lack of regulation and standards of practice damaged the reputation of massage, but the decline was stopped because steps were taken to legitimize the practice. Understanding historical lessons, you can better appreciate the importance of standardization and regulation to legitimization of massage therapy (Box 1-3).

CHAPTER EXERCISES

1. List at least three ancient Greek and Roman medical texts and their references to the use of massage treatment.

2. Identify at least three examples throughout history where massage was associated with the spiritual realm. Are there any scenarios in today's culture that illustrate a connection between massage and the spiritual realm?

3. Name at least four factors that influence a person's interpretation of touch. Write a paragraph describing a tactile experience with another person in which your interpretation of the event differed from theirs.

4. Match the following individuals listed in the left column with their historical contributions listed in the right column:

a. Kellogg	__wrote *De Medicina*
b. Vesalius	__developed terminology for massage: "effleurage" "petrissage" "tapotement"
c. Hippocrates	__popularized Movement Cure in America
d. Cibot	__originated theory of mind–body connection "I think, therefore I am"
e. Ling	__created Swedish Gymnastics
f. Mezger	__identified physiological effects of massage in his book *The Art of Massage*
g. G. Celsus	__promoted medical ethical code to "do no harm"
h. H. Taylor	__translated the *Cong Fou* from Chinese to French
i. I. Field	__promoted medical ethical code to treat "an eye for an eye"
j. J. Hammurabi	__created anatomical illustrations focusing on musculature
k. K. Descartes	__established the Touch Research Institute

BOX 1-3
Suggested Web Sites for Further Information

- The Massage Therapy Foundation: www.massagetherapy foundation.org
- National Library of Medicine's PubMed: http://www.ncbi .nlm.nih.gov/pubmed/
- NCCAM: www.nccam.nih.gov
- WHCCAMP final report: www.whccamp.hhs.gov/
- *De Humani Corporis Fabrica* by Andreas Vesalius: http://www.stanford.edu/class/history13/Readings /vesalius.htm
- *De Medicina* by Aulus Cornelius Celsus: http://historical .hsl.virginia.edu/treasures/celsus.html

Figure 1-12. Global map for Exercise 7.

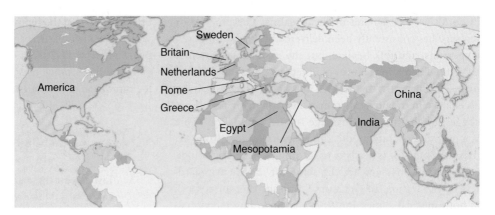

5. Choose one of the following events from the history of massage. Write a paragraph about its effect on history and how history might have been different without it.

   Hippocrates writes the Hippocratic Corpus

   Dr. Mezger popularizes French massage terms

   Dr. Kellogg studies the physiological effects of massage

   The British Medical Association finds inconsistency and inadequacy in the field of massage therapy

   Dr. Tiffany Field opens the Touch Research Institute

6. Organize the following historical events in chronological order and number the list:

   Kahun Medical Papyrus is written in Egypt

   Doctors find inconsistent and inadequate massage practices in Britain

   Code of Hammurabi's medical ethics are written in Mesopotamia

   Greek ritualistic health regimen included massage

   Dr. Mezger initiates massage terminology in the Netherlands

   Per Henrik Ling develops Swedish Gymnastics in Sweden

   Ancient texts, the *Cong Fou* and the *Nei Ching*, written in China

   The New York State Society of Medical Massage Therapists is the first professional American massage association

   Ancient Indian scriptures, the Vedas, are written

   Galen of Rome develops scientific method for research

7. Trace the history of massage across the world by using the map and events from Exercise 6. Identify the location of each event by writing its number on the map in Figure 1-12.

8. There is currently a lot of touch research being conducted in the public and private sectors. List at least three examples of massage research that you would want someone to do and explain why. (For example: I am interested in seeing how massage influences a person's physical coordination because of the neuromuscular effects on proprioceptors.)

9. Identify at least five doctors who were notable in the history of massage therapy and describe their contributions.

10. List the nine categories of bodywork, identify each one's classification as a bodywork or massage modality, and explain why it has been classified as such.

REFERENCES

1. Celsus AC. *De Medicina.* http://www.intratext.com/X/LAT0382.HTM, accessed 03.23.13
2. Vesalius A. *De Humani Corporis Fabrica.* http://www.stanford.edu/class/history13/Readings/vesalius.htm, accessed 03.23.13
3. Descartes R. *Meditations.* Veitch J (transl), 1901. http://www.wright.edu/cola/descartes/mede.html, accessed 03.23.13
4. Kellogg JH. *The Art of Massage.* http://www.heritagebattlecreek.org/index.php?option=com_content&view=article&id=95&Itemid=73, accessed 03.23.13
5. http://www.nccam.nih.gov, accessed 03.23.13
6. http://www.whccamp.hhs.gov/finalreport.html, accessed 03.23.13
7. Field T. *Touch.* Cambridge, MA: MIT Press, 2001.

SUGGESTED READINGS

Aten J. *A Part of Something Great.* Carthage, IL: Good Apple, 1980.
Crabtree C, Nash GB, Gagnon P, et al. *Lessons from History, Essential Understandings and Historical Perspectives Students Should Acquire, A Project of the National Center for History in the Schools.* A Cooperative UCLA/NEH Research Program. Los Angeles: National Center for History in the Schools, 1992.
DeBaz P. *The Story of Medicine.* New York: Philosophical Library, 1975.

Field T. *Touch*. Cambridge, MA: MIT Press, 2001.

Field TM, Ingatoff E, Stringer S, et al. Nonnutritive sucking during tube feedings: Effect on preterm neonates in an intensive care unit. *Pediatrics* 1982;70(3):381–384.

Finney S, Kindle P. *China Then and Now, Dynasties to Dragon Boats, Pagodas to Pavilions*. Carthage, IL: Good Apple, 1988.

Garrison FH. *An Introduction to the History of Medicine, with Medical Chronology, Suggestions for Study and Bibliographic Data*. 4th ed. Philadelphia: WB Saunders, 1929.

Harlow H, Zimmerman RR. The development of affectional responses in infant monkeys. *Proc Am Philos Soc* 1958;102:501–509.

Jackson R. *Holistic Massage, the Holistic Way to Physical and Mental Health*. New York: Sterling Publishing, 1987.

Kellogg JH. *The Art of Massage*. Battle Creek, MI: Modern Medicine Publishing, 1975.

Knasta M. *Energy, Eastern style*. Massage Ther J 1998; Fall.

Libby W. *The History of Medicine in its Salient Features*. Boston: Houghton Mifflin, 1922.

Partin RL. *The Social Studies Teacher's Book of Lists*. Englewood Cliffs, NJ: Prentice Hall, 1992.

Saunders JB de CM, O'Malley CD. *The Illustrations from the Works of Andreas Vesalius of Brussels*. New York: Dover Publications, 1973.

Tappan FM, Benjamin PJ. *Tappan's Handbook of Healing Massage Techniques, Classic, Holistic, and Emerging Methods*. Old Tappan, NJ: Appleton & Lange, 1998.

Taylor GH. *A Sketch of the Movement Cure, with Illustrative Cases*. New York: New York Institute for Movement Cure, 1860.

Van-Why RP. *The Bodywork Knowledgebase: Lecture on the History of Massage in Four Parts*. Richard P. Van-Why, 1991.

Waltz SK. *Handbook of Instructional Devices for Intermediate Social Studies*. Darien, CT: Teachers Publishing Corporation, 1968.

http://books.mirror.org/gb.hippocrates.html, accessed 3.5.06.

http://digilander.libero.it/debibliotheca/Arte/Leonardoana_file/page_01.htm, accessed 3.5.06.

http://emuseum.mnsu.edu/prehistory/egypt/dailylife/papyrus.html, accessed 3.5.06.

http://integrativemedicine.arizona.edu/, accessed 7.8.11.

http://orientalmedicine.com/acupuncture_faq.htm, accessed 3.5.06.

http://ragz-international.com/sumeria.htm, accessed 3.5.06.

http://scriptorium.lib.duke.edu/papyrus/texts/world.html, accessed 3.5.06.

http://spas.about.com/cs/massagetherapy/l/aa030199.htm, accessed 3.5.06.

http://spas.about.com/library/weekly/aa063002ga.htm, accessed 3.5.06.

http://www.amednews.com/2002/prca0128, accessed 3.5.06.

http://www.aota.org, accessed 3.5.06.

http://www.apta.org/AM/Template.cfm?Section=Physical_Therapy&Template=/TaggedPage/TaggedPageDisplay.cfm&TPLID=217&ContentID=24249, accessed 3.5.06.

http://www.ayurvedicscience.com/clinic_intropage.htm#what, accessed 3.5.06.

http://www.bbc.co.uk/history/historic_figures/galen_claudius.shtml, accessed 3.5.06.

http://www.body-balancing.com/Massage_and_Spa_History.htm, accessed 3.5.06.

http://www.cmtbc.bc.ca/index.shtml, accessed 3.5.06.

http://www.cmto.com/index.html, accessed 3.5.06.

http://www.compwellness.com/eGuide/deept.htm, accessed 3.5.06.

http://www.csp.org.uk/director/about.cfm, accessed 3.5.06.

http://www.dukeintegrativemedicine.org/index.php/200407076/about-us/news1.html, accessed 7.8.11.

http://www.experienceispa.com, accessed 3.5.06.

http://www.famousamericans.net/georgehtaylor/, accessed 3.5.06.

http://www.fonetiks.org, accessed 3.5.06.

http://www.foot-reflexologist.com/EGYPT_1.HTM, accessed 3.5.06.

http://www.geocities.com/Athens/Oracle/9840/kellogg.html, accessed 3.5.06.

http://www.geocities.com/unclesamsfarm/drtaylor.htm, accessed 3.5.06.

http://www.ijtmb.org/index.php/ijtmb/article/viewArticle/138/169, accessed 7.12.11.

http://www.intratext.com/X/LAT0382.HTM, accessed 3.5.06.

http://www.iskcon.com/about/philosophy.html, accessed 3.5.06.

http://www.itmonline.org/arts/japacu.htm, accessed 3.5.06.

http://www.massagetherapyfoundation.org/literacy.html, accessed 7.12.11.

http://www.mayoclinic.org/general-internal-medicine-rst/cimc.html, accessed 7.8.11.

http://www.mendiseasestcm.com/translatione.htm, accessed 3.5.06.

http://www.meridianinstitute.com/eamt/files/articles/artfasse.htm, accessed 3.5.06.

http://www.miami.edu/touch-research, accessed 3.5.06.

http://www.mskcc.org/mskcc/html/1990.cfm, accessed 7.11.11.

http://www.mskcc.org/mskcc/html/97317.cfm, accessed 7.8.11.

http://www.naprapathicmedicine.edu/, accessed 3.5.06.

http://www.naturalchoice.net/glossary.htm, accessed 3.5.06.

http://www.nb.no/baser/schoyen/5/5.5/#4575, accessed 3.5.06.

http://www.ncbtmb.com/applicants_corner.htm#application, accessed 3.5.06.

http://www.nccam.nih.gov, accessed 3.5.06.

http://www.nefertiti.iwebland.com/timelines/topics/medicine.htm, accessed 3.5.06.

http://www.pbs.org/wgbh/aso/databank/entries/bhharl.html, accessed 3.5.06.

http://www.petrie.ucl.ac.uk/digital_egypt/lahun/ucarchivelahun/uc32057page1-2small.gif, accessed 3.5.06.

http://www.petrie.ucl.ac.uk/digital_egypt/med/birthpapyrus.html, accessed 3.5.06.

http://www.qigonghealing.com/html/qigong.html, accessed 3.5.06.

http://www.stanford.edu/class/history13/Readings/vesalius.htm, accessed 3.5.06.

http://www.state.mn.us/portal/mn/jsp/content.do?subchannel=536882721&id=-536882720&agency=BMP, accessed 3.5.06.

http://www.thebodyworker.com/history.htm, accessed 3.5.06.

http://www.unani.com/avicenna%20story%202.htm, accessed 3.5.06.

http://www.wga.hu/frames-e.html?/html/l/leonardo/10anatom/index.html, accessed 3.5.06.

http://www.whccamp.hhs.gov/finalreport.html, accessed 3.5.06.

http://www.wischik.com/marcus/essay/med2.html, accessed 3.5.06.

http://www.wright.edu/cola/descartes/mede.html, accessed 3.5.06.

2

Ethics and Professionalism

Key Terms

Accountability: The quality of accepting the consequences of your actions and claiming responsibility for your decisions.

Body of knowledge: The essential knowledge, concepts, skills, and attitudes of a profession, as defined by the relevant professional association, which must be mastered to achieve success.

Certification: The act of issuing someone a certificate of completion or validation of authenticity.

Client-centered: When attitudes, decisions, and activities of a practice are in the best interest of the client's health and well-being.

Code of ethics: Commonly accepted guidelines or principles of conduct that govern professional conduct.

Confidentiality: The principle that client information revealed to a health professional during an appointment is to be kept private and has limits on how and when it can be disclosed to a third party.

Ethics: Conduct rules based on integrity and differentiating right from wrong.

Informed consent: A client's agreement to participate in an activity after the purpose, methods, benefits, risks, and rights to withdraw at any time have been explained.

Licensure: Legal authority or permission to practice massage when the state laws or regulations require it.

Professionalism: Ethical conduct, goals, and qualities characterized by a profession.

Registration: The act of enrolling in a system or database that keeps track of recorded information.

Scope of practice: A practitioner's service limits and boundaries as determined by legal, educational, competency, and accountability factors.

Standards of practice: Specific rules and procedures for professional conduct and quality of care that are to be followed by all members of a profession.

Ethics and professionalism are the cornerstones of a successful massage practice. The massage therapy profession follows a set of guiding principles based on right and wrong, commonly referred to as ethics. They provide guidelines for appropriate and safe decisions and behaviors. The fundamental ethical principle for massage therapy is client-centered care, which focuses all of the attitudes, decisions, and activities on whatever is best for the client's health and well-being. Client-centered care is a key component of a therapist's professionalism, which is the combined qualities of integrity, competency, effective communication and interpersonal skills, respectful behavior, and good business practices. Ethics and professionalism are closely intertwined and sometimes inseparable as they reinforce and support each other. The relationships you develop as a professional can be complicated and rewarding, but ethics and professionalism provide guidance. The specific concepts outlined in this chapter can help you establish and maintain appropriate, professional relationships. Combining ethics and integrity with professionalism establishes a foundation for developing yourself as an effective, successful, professional massage therapist.

Characteristics of a Profession

A profession is an occupation that requires a specialized academic education and is characterized by a body of knowledge, a scope of practice, a code of ethics, and standards of practice. The massage therapy profession requires a lot of academic knowledge and hands-on training, and each of these components is of equal importance. You can learn massage from a book without practicing on a person; however, without adequate anatomy, physiology, kinesiology, and pathology knowledge, your massage may be harmful to your clients. A body of knowledge is the essential knowledge, concepts, skills, and attitudes of a profession, as defined by the relevant professional association, which must be mastered for successful practice. A scope of practice outlines the limits of a massage therapist's service determined by legal, educational, and competency factors. The scope of practice for massage therapy has yet to be standardized, but the determining factors could lead to the development of two separate scopes within the profession: a wellness massage scope of practice and a therapeutic massage scope of practice. There is a code of ethics, or commonly accepted guidelines or principles of conduct, that governs professional conduct. Standards of practice are specific rules and procedures for professional conduct and quality of care that all members of a profession should follow. These standards involve the public image of a practitioner as well as the legal and ethical obligations that protect both clients and therapists. Unfortunately, the current massage therapy profession has not been standardized, and as a result, there is some confusion within and from outside the profession regarding education, scope of practice, code of ethics, and standards of practice. The professional characteristics outlined by some of the current professional massage associations are fairly similar and are used as a basis for the information in this chapter.

Education

Massage is a hands-on activity that requires hands-on training. Massage also requires scientific education because therapists need to understand what tissues are being touched and how the body responds to the touch. Both of these aspects of a high-quality massage education are equally important, but you may find one easier than the other. Some students find that when they have their hands on a person to practice techniques, everything makes sense and comes easily, but when they read the textbooks and do the homework, it is a struggle. Others sail through the academic work without trouble, but find that when they put their hands on a practice client, nothing makes sense. In both of these situations, there may be frustration and disappointment. Remember that this is a learning process that will take time and effort. Although it may not be easy, your massage education will help you understand more about yourself and will provide a solid foundation for building a successful practice.

Historical Perspective of Massage Education

Recognizing the historical events in massage therapy education can be used to guide future education in a better direction by preventing similar unfortunate outcomes. Very early on, many ancient medical practices were passed down from generation to generation or from masters to apprentices. Massage and other forms of natural treatment were taught as part of the medical treatments. Later, as massage became more popular with patients, the hospitals developed specific educational programs for massage, and British nurses started studying massage therapy. The reputation of massage was so quickly rising that it became a very popular occupation. Unfortunately, along with the many massage therapists with a good education, there were also a number of poorly trained therapists flooding the market. At the time, lack of regulation resulted in unqualified teachers, inferior schools, incompetent therapists, and unscrupulous practices. There was a downfall in the reputation of massage therapy that led to a split between professional massage therapists and those with little or no formal training. The division allowed massage to continue its acceptance within the medical community, and the lack of regulation started a movement toward legitimizing the practice.

As described in Chapter 1, massage therapy prevailed, and several techniques of massage and bodywork were created during the 19th century (see Fig. 1-8, Timeline of bodywork and massage). In the 1960s, massage experienced a revival in America. Although the long-time tradition of passing massage techniques from person to person was becoming more prevalent, standardized massage education resurfaced at the Esalen Institute in Big Sur, California. History was repeated as massage education became a widely variable experience.

Current Perspective of Massage Education

As the popularity of massage continues, there are a myriad of avenues for massage education today. You can find courses that only take a couple of days to programs that last 2 years. You will see programs that offer absolutely no anatomy or physiology, and you will find programs that study human cadavers to learn human anatomy. Some therapists receive a certificate of completion and consider themselves "certified," and others are required to pass a national written exam to be considered certified. Regulation of the profession exists in some states, but not all, and you will find that the level of education and professional requirements varies from state to state. Standardizing massage education will benefit therapists, clients, and the profession.

In states without massage regulation, massage continues to be taught through apprenticeship or by schools and instructors that may have different levels of experience and/or varied qualifications. That is not to say that unregulated states have unqualified or incompetent educators, but you cannot assume that the educators are qualified. In fact, there are some excellent massage training programs in unregulated states.

Currently, it is difficult to determine the information that is fundamental to the entry-level massage therapist, but learning anatomy, physiology, kinesiology, and pathology will provide a good foundation. With enough motivation and support, massage education will continue to evolve toward a more specific knowledge base requirement for entry into the profession.

Education should not end once you have entered the profession. You can continue to develop professionally by taking continuing education classes. There are hundreds, possibly thousands, of courses offered around the world that teach various specialties of massage and bodywork. By continuing the educational process, you show your dedication to the wealth of knowledge that exists in the field of massage. In turn, you may share that knowledge and expertise with your clients. **Knowledge is power!**

Body of Knowledge

Most acknowledged professions have a well-articulated foundational understanding of who they are and what they do, also called a body of knowledge. The massage therapy profession has yet to establish this in a cohesive manner. In January 2007, the American Massage Therapy Association (AMTA) initiated a collaborative effort to reach a consensus on definitional and scope of practice issues for massage therapy. Several entities from the accreditation, certification, education, regulatory, advocacy, and research arenas made up the initial group. In July 2008, Associated Bodywork & Massage Professionals (ABMP) joined the group along with several organizations representing accreditation and other bodywork, movement, and somatic disciplines. Over time, participating organizations transitioned into an autonomous Massage Therapy Body of Knowledge Stewardship group comprising representatives from AMTA, ABMP, Federation of State Massage Therapy Boards (FSMTB), Massage Therapy Foundation, and National Certification Board for Therapeutic Massage and Bodywork (NCBTMB).

Establishing a body of knowledge collaboratively is important because several different perspectives will all be focused into a single, unified vision that is stronger and more influential that any one organization can construct. The profession is at a key stage in its development and this Stewardship group will drive the recognition and growth of massage therapy with the long-term goal of advancing the profession. To develop and adopt a well-articulated body of knowledge for the massage therapy profession will provide a living resource of competencies, standards, and values that inform and guide the domains of practice, licensure, certification, education, accreditation, and research.

Scope of Practice

Boundaries exist in all aspects of life, and although they are seen by some as constraints, they give everyone the same ground rules and provide everyone with an aspect of safety by giving us a better idea of what to expect. Massage therapists provide a service that is limited by legal, educational, and competency factors. Collectively, these boundaries are called the scope of practice, and they paint a clear picture of which services are and are not acceptable for massage therapists to provide.

Most states have created legislation to regulate the massage therapy profession. In those states, the scope of practice outlines specific activities that determine what is and what is not considered a part of that practice. The scopes of practice vary from state to state, and Box 2-1 identifies web sites that list nationwide massage therapy laws. Box 2-2 shows Pennsylvania's legal description of scope of practice for massage.

Currently, the scope of practice for massage therapy is not standardized, but the factors that determine it may lead to the development of two separate scopes within the profession. Wellness massage is provided for general relaxation and health maintenance. Its primary intent is to increase circulation for general physiological benefit. The therapist typically uses only basic massage strokes and does not address specific muscular conditions or client complaints. Therapeutic massage, sometimes referred to as medical massage, requires a higher level of education and uses advanced massage techniques. These techniques are covered in the Hands On and Therapeutic Applications chapters, 9 and 10 respectively. With a thorough understanding of anatomy, physiology, and kinesiology, and with practical knowledge of specific techniques, the scope of practice for therapeutic massage is wider. It allows therapists to treat clients with specific muscular or soft tissue conditions and complaints of pain or dysfunction.

BOX 2-1
Web Sites for Further Information

Professionalism:
- AMTA: www.amtamassage.org
- ABMP: www.abmp.com
- NCBTMB: www.ncbtmb.org

Nationwide massage therapy laws:
- http://www.massagetherapy.com/careers/stateboards.php
- http://www.amtamassage.org/about/lawstate.html

State and federal listings for laws regarding abuse and neglect:
- http://www.prevent-abuse-now.com/govhome.htm

BOX 2-2
Pennsylvania's State Board of Massage Therapy Scope of Practice for Massage

SCOPE OF PRACTICE

(a) Massage therapists apply a system of structured touch, pressure, movement, holding and treatment of the soft tissue manifestations of the human body in which the primary intent is to enhance the health and well-being of the client. Massage therapy includes:

(1) The external application of water, heat, cold, lubricants, and other topical preparations.

(2) Lymphatic techniques.

(3) Myofascial release techniques.

(4) The use of electro-mechanical devices which mimic or enhance the action of the massage techniques.

(b) Massage therapy practice does not include:

(1) The diagnosis or treatment of impairment, illness, disease, or disability.

(2) Medical procedures.

(3) Chiropractic manipulation—adjustment.

(4) Physical therapy mobilization—manual therapy.

(5) Therapeutic exercise.

(6) Ordering or prescribing drugs or treatments for which a license to practice medicine, osteopathic medicine, nursing, podiatry, optometry, chiropractic, physical therapy, occupational therapy, or other healing art is required.

(7) The application of high velocity/low amplitude force further defined as thrust techniques directed toward joint surfaces.

(8) The use of equipment or devices that require a prescription (e.g., ultrasound, diathermy or electrical neuromuscular stimulation).

(c) Licensure under the act may not be construed as requiring new or additional third-party reimbursement or otherwise mandating coverage under 75 Pa.C.S. Chapter 17 (relating to financial responsibility) or the Workers' Compensation Act (77 P. S. § § 1—1041.4 and 2501—2506).

Code of Ethics

In the same way that a scope of practice limits the services a massage therapist can perform, a code of ethics is a set of principles or guidelines for decisions and professional conduct that all massage therapists should follow. It serves as a

BOX 2-3
American Massage Therapy Association Code of Ethics

PRINCIPLES OF ETHICS

The Principles of Ethics form the first part of the Code of Ethics. They are aspirational and inspirational model standards of exemplary professional conduct for all members of the association. These Principles should not be regarded as limitations or restrictions, but as goals for which members should constantly strive.

Massage therapists/practitioners shall:

1. Demonstrate commitment to provide the highest quality massage therapy/bodywork to those who seek their professional service.
2. Acknowledge the inherent worth and individuality of each person by not discriminating or behaving in any prejudicial manner with clients and/or colleagues.
3. Demonstrate professional excellence through regular self-assessment of strengths, limitations, and effectiveness by continued education and training.
4. Acknowledge the confidential nature of the professional relationship with clients and respect each client's right to privacy within the constraints of the law.
5. Project a professional image and uphold the highest standards of professionalism.
6. Accept responsibility to do no harm to the physical, mental and emotional well-being of self, clients, and associates.

RULES OF ETHICS

The Rules of Ethics are mandatory and direct specific standards of minimally-acceptable professional conduct for all members of the association. The Rules of Ethics are enforceable for all association members, and any members who violate this Code shall be subject to disciplinary action.

Massage therapists/practitioners shall:

1. Conduct all business and professional activities within their scope of practice and all applicable legal and regulatory requirements.
2. Refrain from engaging in any sexual conduct or sexual activities involving their clients in the course of a massage therapy session.
3. Be truthful in advertising and marketing, and refrain from misrepresenting his or her services, charges for services, credentials, training, experience, ability or results.
4. Refrain from using AMTA membership, including the AMTA name, logo or other intellectual property, or the member's position, in any way that is unauthorized, improper or misleading.
5. Refrain from engaging in any activity which would violate confidentiality commitments and/or proprietary rights of AMTA or any other person or organization.

Effective Date May 1, 2010

---

basis for establishing and maintaining the reputation of massage therapists as honest, respectable professionals. Codes of ethics are often established by professional organizations as guidelines for their members to use in their practices. At the same time, a code of ethics helps the public understand the expected behavior of professional massage therapists. The AMTA is the largest nonprofit professional massage organization for massage therapists, massage students, and massage schools. Its code of ethics is a two-part summary of the principles and rules of ethics that all members must follow (Box 2-3).

The ABMP is a membership organization for bodywork, massage, and somatic therapists. Its professional code of ethics covers client-centered care, quality service, confidentiality, self-assessment, and exclusion of sexual activity; specifies professional behaviors that are acceptable and not acceptable; specifies scope of practice limitations; specifies a physiological understanding to determine when to use and when not to use techniques; and stresses professional public image, public education, and honest advertising: client relationships, professionalism, scope of practice/appropriate techniques, and image/advertising claims. Box 2-4 shows the ABMP code of ethics.

As you can see by the examples, these codes look different on a quick glance, but their content is similar. It may seem like common sense to follow these codes, but ethical conduct is not always clear cut. There are many situations in which the ethical decision between one choice and another is unclear and difficult. Codes of ethics are not just the rules and regulations set forth by a profession to dictate what is right or wrong, they are living documents that continually evolve and serve to guide you in your words and actions.

Standards of Practice

Standards of practice give the members of a profession a specific set of rules and procedures that help provide clients with a law-abiding, safe environment in a professional atmosphere. Basically, they include everything that contributes to high-quality care and client safety: professionalism, legal responsibilities, relationships, business practices, sanitation, hygiene, and safety. Professionalism, legal and ethical issues, and relationships are covered in this chapter, whereas

BOX 2-4
ABMP Code of Ethics

As a member of Associated Bodywork & Massage Professionals, I hereby pledge to abide by the ABMP Code of Ethics as outlined below.

Client Relationships

- I shall endeavor to serve the best interests of my clients at all times and to provide the highest quality service possible.

- I shall maintain clear and honest communications with my clients and shall keep client communications confidential.

- I shall acknowledge the limitations of my skills and, when necessary, refer clients to the appropriate qualified health care professional.

- I shall in no way instigate or tolerate any kind of sexual advance while acting in the capacity of a massage, bodywork, somatic therapy or esthetic practitioner.

Professionalism

- I shall maintain the highest standards of professional conduct, providing services in an ethical and professional manner in relation to my clientele, business associates, health care professionals, and the general public.

- I shall respect the rights of all ethical practitioners and will cooperate with all health care professionals in a friendly and professional manner.

- I shall refrain from the use of any mind-altering drugs, alcohol, or intoxicants prior to or during professional sessions.

- I shall always dress in a professional manner, proper dress being defined as attire suitable and consistent with accepted business and professional practice.

- I shall not be affiliated with or employed by any business that utilizes any form of sexual suggestiveness or explicit sexuality in its advertising or promotion of services, or in the actual practice of its services.

Scope of Practice / Appropriate Techniques

- I shall provide services within the scope of the ABMP definition of massage, bodywork, somatic therapies and

skin care, and the limits of my training. I will not employ those massage, bodywork or skin care techniques for which I have not had adequate training and shall represent my education, training, qualifications and abilities honestly.

- I shall be conscious of the intent of the services that I am providing and shall be aware of and practice good judgment regarding the application of massage, bodywork or somatic techniques utilized.

- I shall not perform manipulations or adjustments of the human skeletal structure, diagnose, prescribe or provide any other service, procedure or therapy which requires a license to practice chiropractic, osteopathy, physical therapy, podiatry, orthopedics, psychotherapy, acupuncture, dermatology, cosmetology, or any other profession or branch of medicine unless specifically licensed to do so.

- I shall be thoroughly educated and understand the physiological effects of the specific massage, bodywork, somatic or skin care techniques utilized in order to determine whether such application is contraindicated and/ or to determine the most beneficial techniques to apply to a given individual. I shall not apply massage, bodywork, somatic or skin care techniques in those cases where they may be contraindicated without a written referral from the client's primary care provider.

Image / Advertising Claims

- I shall strive to project a professional image for myself, my business or place of employment, and the profession in general.

- I shall actively participate in educating the public regarding the actual benefits of massage, bodywork, somatic therapies and skin care.

- I shall practice honesty in advertising, promote my services ethically and in good taste, and practice and/ or advertise only those techniques for which I have received adequate training and/or certification. I shall not make false claims regarding the potential benefits of the techniques rendered.

business practice, hygiene, sanitation, and safety are detailed in Chapter 13

The ABMP does not have a separate document for its standards of practice because it has addressed the topics of professionalism and relationships within its code of ethics.

The AMTA has established its standards of practice to help its members provide safe and consistent care,

determine quality of care, develop a practice, and protect and preserve client and therapist rights. It also gives the public a general understanding and expectation of professional massage therapy. Included are the topics of professional conduct, sanitation and safety, relationships with clients and other professionals, record keeping, marketing, legalities, and research. Box 2-5 includes the AMTA standards of practice.

BOX 2-5

AMTA Standards of Practice Document

Purpose Statement: These American Massage Therapy Association (AMTA) Standards of Practice were developed to assist the professional massage therapist to:

- provide safe, consistent care
- determine the quality of care provided
- provide a common base to develop a practice
- support/preserve the basic rights of the client and professional massage therapist
- assist the public to understand what to expect from a professional massage therapist

This document allows the professional massage therapist to evaluate and adapt performance in his/her massage/bodywork practice. The professional massage therapist can evaluate the quality of his/her practice by utilizing the Standards of Practice in conjunction with the Code of Ethics, the Bylaws and Policies of AMTA, and precedents set by the AMTA Grievance, Standards, and Bylaws Committees.

1. **Conduct of the Professional Massage Therapist or Practitioner, hereinafter referred to as "Practitioner"**

   1.1 AMTA members must meet and maintain appropriate membership requirements.

   1.2 Individual AMTA members who engage in the practice of professional massage/bodywork, shall adhere to standards of professional conduct, including the AMTA Code of Ethics.

   1.3 The Practitioner follows consistent standards in all settings.

   1.4 The Practitioner seeks professional supervision/consultation consistent with promoting and maintaining appropriate application of skills and knowledge.

2. **Sanitation, Hygiene and Safety**

   2.1 Practitioner provides an environment consistent with accepted standards of sanitation, hygiene, safety and universal precautions.

   2.2 Pathophysiology (Contraindications)

   2.2.1 The Practitioner maintains current knowledge and skills of pathophysiology and the appropriate application of massage/bodywork.

   2.2.2 The Practitioner monitors feedback from the client throughout a session.

   2.2.3 The Practitioner makes appropriate referrals to other reputable healthcare providers.

3. **Professional Relationships with Clients**

   3.1 The Practitioner relates to the client in a manner consistent with accepted standards and ethics.

   3.2 The Practitioner maintains appropriate professional standards of confidentiality.

   3.3 The Practitioner relates to the client in a manner which respects the integrity of the client and practitioner.

   3.4 The Practitioner ensures that representations of his/her professional services, policies, and procedures are accurately communicated to the client prior to the initial application of massage/bodywork.

   3.5 The Practitioner elicits participation and feedback from the client.

4. **Professional Relationships with Other Professionals**

   4.1 The Practitioner relates to other reputable professionals with appropriate respect and within the parameters of accepted ethical standards.

   4.2 The Practitioner's referrals to other professionals are only made in the interest of the client.

   4.3 The Practitioner's communication with other professionals regarding clients is in compliance with accepted standards and ethics.

   4.4 A Practitioner possessing knowledge that another practitioner:

   (1) committed a criminal act that reflects adversely on the Practitioner's competence in massage therapy, trustworthiness or fitness to practice massage therapy in other respects;

   (2) engaged in an act or practice that significantly undermines the massage therapy profession; or

   (3) engaged in conduct that creates a risk of serious harm for the physical or emotional well being of a recipient of massage therapy; shall report such knowledge to the appropriate AMTA committee if such information is not protected or restricted by a confidentiality law.

5. **Records**

   5.1 Client Records

   5.1.1 The Practitioner establishes and maintains appropriate client records.

   5.2 Financial Records

   5.2.1 The Practitioner establishes and maintains client financial accounts that follow accepted accounting practices.

6. **Marketing**

   6.1 Marketing consists of, but is not limited to, advertising, public relations, promotion and publicity.

   6.2 The Practitioner markets his/her practice in an accurate, truthful and ethical manner.

7. **Legal Practice**

   7.1 American Massage Therapy Association members practice or collaborate with all others practicing professional massage/bodywork in a manner that is in compliance with national, state or local municipal law(s) pertaining to the practice of professional massage/bodywork.

8. **Research**

   8.1 The Practitioner engaged in study and/or research is guided by the conventions and ethics of scholarly inquiry.

   8.2 The Practitioner doing research avoids financial or political relationships that may limit objectivity or create conflict of interest.

Scope of Practice

The scope of practice for massage therapists is important to understand, especially as massage therapy evolves as a profession. The scope of practice identifies the limits and boundaries for a practitioner and is determined by several factors, including the law, education, and competency. The massage therapy scope of practice outlines:

- Which activities are allowed
- When specific methods are used
- Where specific methods are applied
- How specific methods are applied
- Why specific methods are used

Generally, massage therapists are allowed to perform manipulation on the soft tissues or energetic fields of the body; however, they are prohibited from diagnosing medical conditions or prescribing specific treatments, and they are prohibited from intentional joint manipulation and skeletal realignment.

Legal Regulations

Government agencies and professional associations establish regulations for the practice of massage therapy. Since the United States has not standardized the scope of practice for massage, scopes vary from state to state. For example, some states include Reiki in the massage therapy scope of practice and require Reiki practitioners to conform to the same regulations as massage therapists. Other states exclude Reiki from the massage therapy scope, which gives the practitioners more freedom. Regulation is not intended to remove freedoms from practitioners, but many people equate regulation with restraint. Actually, the intention is to separate professional massage therapists from those who have unscrupulous or unsafe practices. Some regulations even specify appropriate and inappropriate locations for practicing massage. Regulation aims to provide the public with a more dependable and qualified pool of massage therapists and motivate the profession to maintain high educational and ethical standards.

State, county, and local governments regulate the scope of massage therapy practice through the processes of licensure, certification, and registration. These terms are used interchangeably with vague and sometimes combined definitions, so it is especially important to learn about your own local laws and regulations before starting a practice. There are generally accepted definitions for licensure, certification, and registration that we have outlined below, but again, check your local regulations before assuming these definitions.

Licensure is the process of obtaining a license from the state government. Some states require that you have a license to practice massage therapy, making it illegal to practice massage without a license in those states. Licensure is intended to identify a level of proficiency that the state considers acceptable and safe. Typically, licensure requires a certain level of educational training or experience and the successful completion of some form of evaluation or testing. Licensure may also include title protection, which gives people who hold a license the exclusive use of particular titles such as "massage therapist," "massage practitioner," and "licensed massage therapist."

Certification is also a process of validation and authentication that may be voluntary or required. Certification programs are offered either via the government or nongovernmental agencies or organizations as a way to identify practitioners who have advanced knowledge or skills. As with licensure, certification requires evaluation by the organizational body as well as sufficient education or experience. Certification is a form of title protection in which only persons who hold a certificate can identify themselves as "certified," but this can lead to some confusion. Unfortunately, there are persons who receive a certificate of completion for a 2-day course and consider themselves certified. True certification is typically granted by an organization that did not provide the education and can make an objective evaluation of the practitioner.

Registration is a process that allows an organization to keep track of therapists in a database. Some state government agencies, such as the Texas Department of Health, require massage therapists to hold a certificate of registration to practice massage therapy. To be eligible for registration, there are educational requirements, fees, and examinations, making the process very similar to licensure in other states. In essence, the registration policy in Texas is more of a licensure policy, differing mostly in terminology. Texas outlines the scope of practice for massage therapy that determines who is required to register as a massage therapist. Texas also includes an ineligibility statement that precludes a therapist from being registered if there is any kind of sexual misconduct conviction on public record. In addition to the other requirements, massage therapists in Texas have continuing education criteria. By keeping track of its registered massage therapists, the state has more control over who is practicing massage. Again, some may consider governmental regulation to be overbearing and controlling, but it is implemented with a client-centered philosophy.

Certification and licensure are the primary forms of regulation that promise consumer protection by requiring therapists to renew their credentials periodically with specific requirements for renewal and by creating an agency that can verify credentials, investigate and process grievances, and enforce discipline when necessary. Table 2-1 highlights licensure versus certification.

Table 2-1 Licensure versus Certification

Licensure	Certification
Authentication by governmental agency	Authentication by nongovernmental agency
Sets a scope of practice whose application legally requires practitioner to hold a license	Sets a scope of practice for illustrative purposes only
Some practitioner titles legally require a license	Some practitioner titles legally require certification
Restrictive levels of practice are established, such as wellness and therapeutic massage applications	Certification at higher levels of education could be built over a licensure program
It is mandatory, which implies that local laws are automatically preempted by state regulation	
It is mandatory, so practitioners who engage in related professions may need to be identified for exemption from licensure	It is voluntary, so it does not create exemption for other practices
It is mandatory, so any new licensing laws usually allow preexisting practitioners to be grandfathered into the new laws	It is voluntary, so there are no grandfathering provisions necessary for any new laws

Education

There is a basic level of knowledge required to practice massage that determines the scope of practice. With the varied lengths and types of massage education and training programs, it has been difficult to establish consistent massage therapy regulations for scope of practice. Generally, massage programs teach some anatomy and physiology, pathology, massage techniques, hygiene and sanitation, ethics, and business practices, but the depth to which these topics are studied and the emphasis put on different topics is unique to each school. Regulation may define the number of hours required for training, but it does not guarantee the same knowledge base from graduates of different schools. In states without regulation, the common knowledge base may be even more difficult to determine.

Some states have specific requirements for establishing educational institutions, making it necessary for the massage schools or massage training programs in those states to be accredited by a state education agency. Basically, the state tries to determine a school's legitimacy by investigating funding, intended location, property procurement, short- and long-term business plans, as well as the qualifications of the person interested in starting the school. Today, accredited massage training programs are offered by proprietary vocational schools, community colleges, cosmetology schools, and massage therapists turned educators.

Additionally, there are a myriad of continuing education options available following graduation. While regulations serve as a guide for initial training, adopting specialties through continuing education creates a unique scope of practice for each therapist. For example, a massage therapist who takes continuing education classes in neuromuscular therapy and craniosacral therapy may have a clientele and an approach to bodywork that differs from someone who takes classes in polarity and Reiki. These two therapists have different scopes of practice because of their education and competency.

Competency

In addition to education, scope of practice is influenced by the issue of competency. Competency raises two particularly poignant questions: What skills should an entry-level therapist have? What determines competency? At the time of publication, formal education hours and written and practical examinations are used to determine the laws and regulations for competency. The educational requirement for entry-level therapists in most regulated states generally begins at 500 hours and goes up from there. States that require licensure, certification, or registration may require continuing education courses and renewal examinations, both of which promote competency.

Academic knowledge is simple enough to test and evaluate, but as discussed in Chapter 1, touch is influenced by age, gender, experience, and emotions. Massage is especially difficult to measure objectively because of the perception of touch and the unique experience that each person experiences with touch. Practical examinations may determine general competence because the person who receives the massage can judge the therapist's knowledge, technique, and concern for safety. Some aspects of a practical examination are subjective, but it is difficult to fake competence when giving a massage.

While the determination of competency for entry into the massage profession is more established at this time, determining competency within specialized studies remains an issue. There are continuing education courses and workshops ranging in duration from a few hours to several years. The massage therapy profession is currently faced with the question of how to determine when a therapist is considered competent in a particular or specialty method. Polarity therapy, Reiki, craniosacral therapy, and Shiatsu are some examples of bodywork modalities that are often introduced in massage school, but specialized, intense certification programs with hundreds of hours of education are available in each of these modalities. Some therapists consider the introductory education sufficient, but others argue that advanced certification is required to ensure competency.

National Certification Board for Therapeutic Massage and Bodywork

In 1992, the AMTA created the NCBTMB, which has since become its own, independent organization. The mission of the NCBTMB is to "define and advance the highest standards in the massage therapy and bodywork profession by establishing and improving the basic competency parameters, providing a standard of proficiency, and promoting professionalism for massage therapists in the United States."[1] The NCBTMB offers two examinations for national certification: the National Certification Examination for Therapeutic Massage (NCETM) and the National Certification Examination for Therapeutic Massage and Bodywork (NCETMB). These have become the standard tests for licensure in most of the states that regulate massage.

Currently, therapists must meet the eligibility requirements in one of three ways in order to take the national exam: educational/training process, portfolio review process, or the national exam for state licensing option. The educational eligibility criteria, which are the same for NCETM and NCETMB, are as follows[2]:

1. A minimum of 500 hours of instruction as follows:
    a. 125 hours of body systems (anatomy, physiology, and kinesiology)
    b. 200 hours of massage and bodywork assessment, theory and application, in-class and supervised
    c. 40 hours of pathology
    d. 10 hours of business and ethics (minimum of 6 hours in ethics)
    e. 125 hours of additional instruction in an area or related field that theoretically completes the massage program of study
2. Graduate of an NCBTMB Assigned School Code with a current valid transcript submitted to NCBTMB.

In 2011, nearly 90,000 massage therapists had their NCBTMB certification, and it is the closest thing there is to a national standard for massage therapy. Massage therapists who want to portray a professional image should consider becoming nationally certified.

The NCBTMB started developing a National Certification for Advanced Practice in 2011. This voluntary accreditation will build on the educational, experiential, and ethical requirements of the current national certification by testing a practitioner's ability to utilize outcome-based approaches that require more education and hands-on experience. The advanced certification will nationally recognize therapists who have critical thinking skills necessary for treating complex conditions, which translates into greater credibility, marketability, and job mobility.

Federation of State Massage Therapy Boards

In 2005, ABMP convened a meeting of massage educators from around the country as well as representatives from seven regulated states to address the need for an organization to formally bring the regulatory community together. By September 2005, the FSMTB was formally established with a mission to provide safe and effective massage to the public. As part of this mission, the FSMTB developed a licensing examination called the Massage & Bodywork Licensing Examination (MBLEx) to determine entry-level competence. Anyone can apply to take the exam, but licensure is still dependent on state requirements, so applicants must check with their state licensing board or agency to learn their particular requirements. There are no educational requirements to take the MBLEx because the FSMTB did not want to pick an arbitrary number of hours of education as a minimum eligibility requirement. Therefore, each state board is still responsible for determining its own educational standards. The content of the MBLEx reflects the broad spectrum of knowledge and core competencies identified by the profession for safe and effective entry-level practice[3]:

*   Anatomy and physiology
*   Kinesiology
*   Pathology, contraindications, areas of caution, and special populations
*   Benefits and physiological effects of techniques that manipulate soft tissue
*   Client assessment, reassessment, and treatment planning

- Overview of massage and bodywork history, culture, and modalities
- Ethics, boundaries, laws, and regulations
- Guidelines for professional practice

Limits of Practice

Although the specifics of massage therapy's scope of practice vary from state to state, there is enough consistency to understand the general limits of practice. Still, without specific limits, you have to make judgment calls regarding acceptable activity, which can lead to confusion. Limiting the practice can benefit clients by giving them an opportunity to seek treatment from several different people, all with different specialties and different scopes of practice. Often, it may be in the client's best interest to rely on a team of healthcare professionals instead of one person. There is no cure-all, and likewise, there is no individual who provides all facets of healthcare.

Given the factors that determine scope of practice, including legal, educational, and competency, the limits of practice can be applied within the field of massage therapy.

Wellness Massage Scope of Practice

Wellness massage uses basic massage strokes to promote circulation, encourage relaxation, and reduce stress. The therapist's basic education will include general anatomy, physiology, kinesiology, and pathology as well as basic techniques for normalizing and treating soft tissue to promote homeostasis in the body.

Therapeutic Massage Scope of Practice

Therapeutic massage intertwines the normalization of soft tissues with rehabilitative treatment. In addition to the basic knowledge for wellness massage, therapists will understand physical assessment, injury and tissue repair mechanisms, structural compensation patterns, and treatment techniques for soft tissue rehabilitation. This type of training allows therapists a wider scope of practice that includes treatment of specific soft tissue conditions and pain patterns.

Clients seeking therapeutic massage treatment may be under the care of another healthcare professional. If so, the therapist has an ethical responsibility to work cooperatively with the other caregivers to make sure that everyone is aware of all concurrent treatments, as they may compromise or enhance each other. **Overtreating is worse than not treating at all and may make the condition worse.**

This concept is important for you to know when there are numerous treatments being used at the same time. The interactions can affect the client's well-being, and sometimes not for the better. This goes for pharmaceutical medications as well as complementary therapies, which is evidenced by the computer cross-checking procedures that pharmacies install to avoid dangerous drug interactions that could go unnoticed.

In both wellness and therapeutic massage, one must be able to evaluate a client's condition to determine whether a more thorough examination or medical diagnosis may be necessary and whether the client can safely receive massage. If a condition exists that is contraindicated for massage, a client may need to be referred to another healthcare professional or refused massage treatment at the time. A massage therapist who is only qualified for wellness massage has an ethical responsibility to stay away from the therapeutic massage scope of practice by recognizing and respecting the limits of wellness massage. The scope of practice for therapeutic massage has more educational requirements and a higher competency level, allowing the therapist to provide more services to more clients. Additionally, it is important to remember that if you are trained in therapeutic massage there are still limits, and as an ethical and professional therapist, you will not go beyond your scope of practice either.

Ethics

Everyone has a conscience. It is an internal feeling or regard for fairness or a sense of obligation to do the right thing. In essence, your conscience makes ethical decisions by helping you determine whether your behavior is acceptable or not. The decisions and behaviors regulated by your conscience are called ethics. You make ethical choices in your decisions and daily activities in your personal life, but you also use ethics in your professional life.

Ethics are one of the cornerstones of a successful massage practice, as they help you distinguish right from wrong and are established to keep you within your scope of practice and maintain client-centered care. An ethical practice is one that demonstrates the code of ethics in its attitudes, policies, procedures, and relationships. It not only serves the client and therapist's best interest, it supports and maintains the reputation of the profession as a whole. Remember, a code of ethics is only a guideline for behavior. The extent to which you follow the code depends on your conscience and your willingness to be responsible for your behavior.

Accountability

Accountability is the quality of accepting the consequences of your actions and claiming responsibility for your decisions. Accountability requires that you look beyond the immediate moment or situation and consider all the consequences that may be your responsibility. Ethical behavior is influenced by our accountability when we choose to behave a certain way and are willing to accept the results of that behavior. Professional massage therapists understand the generally accepted scope of practice, they understand the repercussions of unacceptable behavior, and they make their own choices about what happens in the treatment room. In addition to holding yourself accountable for your behavior, you can also be held accountable by your clients, by a professional organization, by the profession as a whole, by your community, or by the law.

You have to be honest with yourself and others regarding the techniques and services you provide. Going outside your scope of practice is unethical behavior and, depending upon the situation, may be illegal. For example, telling a client to take ibuprofen for inflammation from an injury may be considered diagnosing, prescribing, or even practicing medicine without a license. These activities are out of the massage therapist's scope of practice, and it is against the law to perform them. On the other hand, recommending that the client apply ice to an area that has received specific massage treatment is most likely within the scope of practice for massage therapy.

Rules exist in all aspects of life, but it is an individual's choice to follow them. It is your responsibility to keep yourself within the limits set by regulation, certification, scope of practice, or membership in a professional organization. Your words and actions will affect the world around you and the massage therapy profession as a whole. Make thoughtful decisions based on accountability to maintain your integrity and stay within your scope of practice.

Ethics for the Profession

Professional ethics are rules for acceptable behavior that are set forth for all members of a profession to follow to ensure a client-centered philosophy and maintain the integrity of the profession. You not only have a responsibility to use professional ethics in your own practice but also have a responsibility to make sure your peers are practicing professional

ethics. The reputation of the entire profession is at stake, and unethical behavior on the part of one massage therapist can quickly spread through a community and damage the reputation of massage for years.

At some point during your career, you may suspect a colleague of unethical or illegal behavior. This can be an awkward and difficult position. Sometimes we have been taught to mind our own business and that nobody likes a tattletale, and sometimes we feel compelled to rectify an inappropriate, unfair, or improper situation. If you suspect that a colleague has behaved unethically or illegally in some way, you have to decide whether you will attempt to investigate the situation further. It may be possible to resolve the situation without help, but it is probably better to let an outside source, such as a professional organization or the government, resolve the issue.

Reporting Unethical Activity

Professional organizations want to uphold their codes of ethics and are willing to spend time and resources to make sure that their members maintain a good reputation. The AMTA and the ABMP both have formal grievance procedures. The first step usually requires you to submit a description of the facts and nature of the suspected violation in writing. Once the grievance has been filed, the therapist in question will be informed of the suspected incident. From there, the rest of the resolution process is kept confidential, usually handled by the board of directors unless objective mediation or legal action is deemed necessary.

Resolving an ethical dilemma can be complicated if the therapist in question is not a member of a professional organization. You may need to look into the local or state laws that apply to massage therapy. In the states that do not regulate massage therapy with licensure, local regulations govern the practice of massage therapy. State licensure laws usually supersede the local regulation, meaning that the state laws carry more weight and are more consequential than the local laws. Each locale or state has its own process for filing and handling complaints and suspected illegal activity.

An example is Washington State's Department of Health Complaint and Disciplinary Process, which designates more than a dozen people to be the decision makers.[4] They review incoming complaints and determine whether public safety or a person's health may be affected by the situation in question. If health or safety is in danger, an investigation will be made. Disciplinary action can be applied in the form of a lawsuit, fines, limitations imposed on the practice, or suspension from practice. The Washington State Department of Health claims responsibility to public protection by imposing the disciplinary action and also attempts to rehabilitate the healthcare professional with counseling and retraining.

To locate other information regarding the governmental regulation of massage therapy, you can search the internet with state name + regulation + massage. If you prefer to have a hard copy version of this information, you can contact your local department of health to see if they can direct you to the appropriate regulatory body. Additionally, your massage school or training program will most likely be aware of the appropriate regulatory agencies you will need to contact upon graduation.

Resolving Ethical Dilemmas

There will most likely come a time when you, as a professional massage therapist, will be faced with making an ethical decision regarding your practice. Codes of ethics serve as guidelines for these decisions, but they do not guarantee that the decisions will be easy to make. When faced with an ethical dilemma, it is helpful to make a decision that is based on the highest good for all. The decision-making process outlined below, which is only one of many equally helpful methods, involves a series of steps for resolving ethical dilemmas:

1. Identify the problem or situation and gather any relevant information.

2. Identify the nature of the conflict: legal, moral, ethical, or a combination.

3. Identify the person, condition, or results that will be affected by the decision.

4. Brainstorm different decisions and the potential outcomes of each.

5. Consider different perspectives: your intuition, community, peers, legal.

6. Determine whether rules, codes of ethics, or laws invalidate any of the decisions.

7. Determine the best course of action. Will the client or you be harmed? Is it the most helpful thing to do?

Box 2-6 shows an example of using the 7-step guideline to ethical resolution.

BOX 2-6

An Example of Ethical Resolution Using the 7-Step Guideline

DILEMMA

A client insists that you use a skeletal adjustment technique that you have not learned. How should you handle this situation?

1. Identify the problem or situation and gather any relevant information
   You have to decide whether to try an unfamiliar technique or disappoint your client.
2. Identify the nature of the conflict: legal, moral, ethical, or a combination
   The technique is outside your scope of practice, which makes it a possible legal conflict, and you are unfamiliar with a technique, making it ethically wrong to try it because it may harm the client.
   However, your client is insisting that you use the technique, and your client-centered philosophy encourages you to serve the client's needs.
3. Identify the person, condition, or results that will be affected by the decision
   Your client could get hurt, your professional membership could be revoked, or your practice could be suspended by law if you attempt the technique.
   However, the client might not return because you will not address his or her needs, thus affecting your practice.
4. Brainstorm different decisions and potential outcomes of each
   a. You could explain your professional and ethical commitments to scope of practice and hope the client understands.

   b. You could attempt the technique and hope that it works and that the client does not get hurt.
   c. You could pretend to perform the technique and hope the client does not continue to push you.
   d. You could adamantly state that you will not attempt the technique because it is not a massage technique and tell the client that if he or she is not happy with your massage services, he or she can go elsewhere.
5. Consider different perspectives: your intuition, community, peers, legal
   Intuition tells you to explain things to the client and hope for understanding, which is probably the same thing your peers and community will suggest.
   The law does not have a preference how you handle it, as long as you do not attempt the technique.
6. Determine whether rules, codes of ethics, or laws invalidate any of the decisions
   By law, skeletal adjustments are outside the scope of practice for massage therapy, so you may not attempt the technique.
   Pretending to perform the technique and lying to the client about the technique not working is unethical.
7. Determine the best course of action: Will the client or you be harmed? Is it the most helpful thing to do?
   The best course of action is probably to gently explain scope of practice and hope for understanding. It protects the client from being hurt, it protects your practice from being sued or suspended, and it allows you to practice your ethics.

Professionalism

Professionalism is defined as the conduct, goals, and qualities that generally characterize a profession. There is often a sense of maturity, patience, and awareness that accompanies professionalism. Typically, professionalism refers to conduct, business practices, legal and ethical responsibilities, and membership in professional associations that create your public image. You never get a second chance to make a first impression, so the image you portray when people first come in contact with you on a professional level should be a good one.

Conduct

A respectable and reputable professional image is influenced by appropriate conduct. There are codes of ethics to provide guidelines for professionalism, which are discussed above, but there are other factors that contribute to your public image. Any input people receive with their eyes, ears, and nose will be used to develop an image of you as a professional, so your conduct includes the visual, auditory, and olfactory cues you project.

Visual Cues

Clients will see facial expressions, eye contact, posture, cleanliness, what you wear, and how you dress. Your facial expressions can convey emotion, exhaustion, stress, distraction, interest, or disinterest. Eye contact can express interest or disinterest, confidence, patience, and self-esteem. Posture can indicate your level of exhaustion, self-esteem, depression, shyness, or self-consciousness. Cleanliness of the practice, treatment room, equipment, your body, and your clothing may illustrate the level of pride in your practice or how careful you are.

Clothing is always used to evaluate people, both what they wear and how they wear it, so keep that in mind as you consider your professional image. The following are some guidelines for appropriate clothing and appearance for a professional massage therapist:

- Short sleeves
- Breathable fabrics
- Loose, comfortable clothes
- Long hair tied back
- Minimal or no jewelry
- Clean, intact clothes and shoes

Why short sleeves? Long sleeves interfere with massage strokes and pushing sleeves up throughout the massage is disruptive. Why breathable fabric? Massage is physical work that creates body heat, and cotton, linen, or cotton blends are cooler and more comfortable. Why loose clothing? Tight, form-fitting clothes restrict movement and can distract the client from the professional atmosphere. Why tie back long hair? Pushing hair out of your face throughout a massage is distracting, and you do not want your hair to accidentally touch the client during the treatment, for sanitation and hygiene reasons. Why limit jewelry? Excessive jewelry is a visual distraction that can also interfere with massage strokes and scratch skin. Why clean and intact clothes? Holes, tears, and stains are visually distracting. Visual input is the primary ingredient for a professional image. Figure 2-1 shows examples of professional attire.

There are some visual aspects of the practice that will also contribute to your professional image. Business cards and brochures are intended for public use, and they significantly influence your image. The quality of these marketing tools is measured by the paper, the colors, the layout, and the included information. Business marketing tools are covered in more detail in the professional massage practice chapter.

Auditory Cues

The words you speak; the tone you use; the volume, pace, and clarity of your speech; and the emotions you convey with your speech all contribute to a client's perception of your professional image. From the moment you exchange the first spoken words, whether over the phone or in a face-to-face meeting, you are creating a professional image that your client will associate with you. The fact that communication skills are critical may seem like common sense, so we address this topic very broadly. Discuss your policies and procedures with your clients and make sure there is no

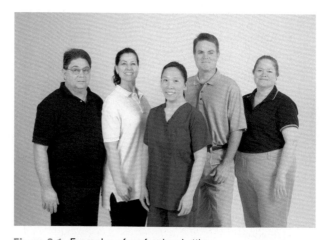

Figure 2-1. Examples of professional attire.

confusion. Use your answering machine, voice mail box, or email as a communication tool. Let your clients know that you will return their messages within 24 to 48 hours, or let them know if you are unavailable for an extended period of time. Tone and attitude can be interpreted through your voice, so be careful to speak clearly and audibly, with a friendly and professional tone.

The sounds of your practice's environment add to your professional image. Traffic noise, nearby conversation, clocks, alarms, televisions, radios, bathroom noises, and pets may be distracting and detract from a professional image. Gentle music with a slow tempo and the natural sounds of water, birds, and wind can provide a more tranquil atmosphere that will encourage clients to relax and let go of their stress.

Olfactory Cues

Odors can evoke strong, emotional responses. Try to stay aware of any odors that might be present in your practice. Body odor, breath odor, and foot odor are especially offensive to a lot of persons, so check throughout the day and take preventive measures to avoid these problems. Many persons are sensitive to scented products, so perfumes and colognes should be used sparingly, if at all. Environmental smells will also affect your professional image. Garbage, food, pets, air fresheners, and chemical cleansers have odors that will be noticed, and not necessarily in a good way. You may want to ask a friend with an objective nose to check the surroundings of your practice and identify any odors that should be eliminated.

Business Practices

Standards of practice for massage therapy include everyday business practices such as record keeping, sanitation, hygiene, safety, and marketing. These topics are detailed in Chapter 13, but they are outlined below.

The following are some aspects of your practice that require record keeping:

- Appointments
- Client information
- Client health history
- Massage session notes
- Meetings
- Work-related travel
- Business-related purchases (e.g., equipment, lubricants, business cards)
- Business-related expenses (e.g., laundry, professional memberships, utilities)
- Income

Sanitation, hygiene, and safety are concepts that support massage therapy's client-centered philosophy. Sanitation is the act of keeping your practice clean enough to prevent disease transmission. Professional standards of practice dictate a sanitary environment for the benefit of you, your clients, and the general public. A similar concept is hygiene, which is the act of keeping things clean to promote health. Safety is the condition that prevents physical harm to a person and applies to everything your clients will use: parking area, walkway, steps, bathroom, treatment room, equipment, floors, and furniture. Fire safety is specifically addressed by law, covering fire extinguisher placement, fire escape route, maximum capacity of people in a building, the use of open flames, and smoke detectors. You can learn about sanitation and safety regulations from your local regulatory agency and fire department.

Marketing your business can be as low or high budget as you want. Word-of-mouth advertising is possibly the least expensive, and although it can be very effective, it is limited by the people who recommend your services. Business cards are an inexpensive but almost necessary marketing tool. Self-promotion involves you, sharing and educating people about the benefits of your services through demonstrations and public speaking. Promotional brochures and pamphlets are useful and attractive, but they can be expensive. Local media can provide some other avenues for marketing your services, including newspaper articles, television interviews or demonstrations, and radio shows or commercials. Whatever method(s) of marketing you choose should be professional and ethical.

Legal Requirements and Ethical Responsibilities

There are legal requirements and ethical responsibilities associated with standards of practice that influence the foundation of the therapeutic relationship. We have covered legalities in terms of local or state regulations, including licensure, certification, and registration, scope of practice, and fire safety. Additionally, there are the two important principles of informed consent and confidentiality.

Informed Consent

Informed consent, sometimes called patient rights, is a client's agreement to participate in an activity after the benefits and risks of the activity have been explained and the client understands that he or she has the right to withdraw at any time. Basically, clients who are informed about a treatment give their consent to try it. The concept of informed consent was started in the medical profession as a way to empower patients by attempting to prepare all parties involved and avoid any unpleasant surprises. Educating persons about their healthcare and allowing them to make an educated decision about whether they want to participate or not gives them a sense of comfort and control instead of feelings of vulnerability and powerlessness. Utilizing informed consent in a massage practice gives clients an opportunity to be engaged in the massage treatment and can facilitate a teamwork approach to healthcare in a client-centered practice. Informed consent benefits and protects clients because it:

- Provides the client the opportunity to ask questions
- Allows the client to completely understand the rules and policies of the massage therapy session
- Clarifies what the massage session will and will not include
- Identifies the benefits and possible contraindications of massage or a particular technique
- Provides the opportunity to participate willingly in their healthcare by choosing to receive massage or specific techniques
- Allows the client to refuse treatment or stop treatment at any time
- Provides the opportunity to validate and verify the therapist's credentials

For the therapist, informed consent provides a signed statement that represents the therapist's good intentions and the client's education and awareness about massage. See Figure 2-2 for different examples of informed consent.

Clients are given the right of refusal and the control for session termination. While the therapist is ultimately responsible for maintaining boundaries and respecting limits, the client also has the capability and responsibility to do the same. Clients and therapists must adhere to the policies and procedures of the office, and both maintain the right to terminate or refuse treatment if there is reasonable cause. Specific conditions that would prompt session termination are often stipulated in the therapist's policies and procedures, which the client should have read and accepted during the initial intake. Generally, these situations include anything that violates or could interfere with safe and ethical treatment. Any activity that sexualizes the massage treatment is grounds for termination: sexual or lewd comments, gestures with a sexual connotation, intentional genital exposure, or intentional sexual contact of any kind. Clients who are repeatedly late or who repeatedly cancel appointments demonstrate a lack of respect for the therapist's practice and can be refused treatment if the therapist feels it is justified. The client must feel comfortable and agree to participate with a particular therapist, but it is equally important for the therapist to feel comfortable and agree to work with a particular client.

Confidentiality

Confidentiality is the principle that information revealed to a massage therapist during an appointment is to be kept private except under limited circumstances when that information is to be disclosed to a third party. Keeping client information confidential, or private, helps establish trust and respect between the client and the therapist. If clients want to tell people what is said or experienced in the therapeutic setting, it is up to them to do so. It is ethically, and maybe legally, wrong for you to share that information without the client's permission because you have promised to keep the information private. It is professionally wrong because you have agreed to uphold the professional standards of practice, which include confidentiality. Generally, as long as there is no direct or implied association to any specific person's identity, the shared information is probably allowed. There are many situations in which confidentiality may need to be broken, and each such circumstance will require that you make an ethical decision.

For example, you may want to discuss a client's condition or treatment plan with another healthcare professional and would need to share specific and thorough details about the client's condition. The best course of action would be to have a conversation with your client, explain your intention, and obtain the client's permission to disclose the information. The client should identify the details that can be shared, including names, dates, locations, conditions, treatments, or outcomes, as well as any limitations on where, when, or how you plan to use the information. To allow professionals to exchange information, you can ask the client to sign a standard release form. See Figure 2-3 for examples of release forms.

You must break confidentiality in any situations that indicate a clear and imminent danger to someone's life, such as intended suicide, murder, personal endangerment, or abuse or neglect of a child, elderly person, or mentally challenged individual. It is your ethical responsibility to report these situations, but many states have established laws that require certain professionals to report suspected abuse.

Courts of law can subpoena any of your client files. Names, contact numbers, health histories, treatment notes, and account balances are all subject to being surrendered by subpoena. This situation does not occur frequently, but it does happen. Records should always be accurate, organized, and thorough, and extraneous and irrelevant notes, such as client's emotional state or comments on behavior, should never be kept in client files.

There are confidentiality issues to manage outside the treatment room as well. Unless clients approach you in public first, try to refrain from greeting them. They may not want people to know that they are receiving massage treatment, or they may not want their relationship with you to be public. Take your cues from the clients. If they openly acknowledge their professional relationship with you,

I understand that the massage therapy given here is for the purpose of stress reduction, relief from muscular tension, spasm or soft tissue injury, or for increasing circulation and energy flow. I understand that massage therapists **do not** diagnose illness or disease, nor do they prescribe any medical treatments or perform spinal manipulations. I acknowledge that massage **is not** a substitute for medical examination or diagnosis, and it is recommended I see a healthcare professional for that service. I have stated all medical conditions and will update the massage therapist with any changes in my health status. I understand that sexual advances and/or comments will result in immediate termination of the massage session with full payment due. I understand that massage sessions are available by appointment only, and if I am unable to keep my appointment, I will inform the massage therapist within 3 hours of the appointment or I will be charged a cancellation fee.

Signature: _____ Date: _____

I understand that massage therapy is intended to maintain and improve my general health by increasing circulation, reducing stress, and promoting relaxation. In order to minimize any health risks, I have provided all my known medical information and will inform the therapist of any new medical information I acquire as long as I am under the therapist's massage treatment. I acknowledge that manual therapy is not a substitute for medical treatment and that the massage therapist cannot diagnose or prescribe any medical conditions.

Signature:_____ Date: _____

I promise to participate fully in my healthcare as part of a team of professionals. I will make choices about my treatment based on the information provided regarding the benefits, risks, and procedures involved. I agree to help choose and participate in any self-care activities that may be recommended in order to promote health and healing. I promise to inform my therapist(s) if I feel uncomfortable or that my health is being compromised during any treatment. In turn, I expect my therapist(s) to provide safe and effective, knowledgeable care that is in the best interest of my health and well being. I promise to keep my therapist(s) informed of any health or medical concerns, conditions, or treatments while I am receiving massage therapy in order to minimize any risks.

Signature: _____ Date: _____

Figure 2-2. Examples of informed consent.

PATIENT'S RELEASE OF HEALTH CARE INFORMATION

Patient's Name _Darnel G. Washington_

Social Security Number _123-45-6789_ Date of Birth _4-22-37_

Health Care Provider/Facility _John Olson, LMP, GCFP_

is hereby authorized to release health care information, including intake forms, chart notes, reports, correspondence, billing statements, and other written information to my attorneys, employees, and designated agents of my attorneys, to wit:

Attorney's Name _B. Charma Storro, JD_ Phone _(612) 555-2337_

Address _5 Hive Lane_

City _Minnehaha_ State _MN_ Zip _55987_

This request and authorization applies to:

_✓_ Health care information relating to the following treatment, condition, or dates of treatment: _MVA 1-6-01_

____ All health care information:

____ Other: _____

Revocation of Prior Authorization: All medical authorizations by the patient or patient's authorized representatives given before the date of this release for any reason whatsoever are hereby revoked.

Information is not to be disclosed to any other person, including insurance agents or adjusters or other attorneys or their employees or agents, without my attorney's prior permission.

Effect of photocopy of this release shall have the same force and effect as a signed original.

Authorization expires 90 days from date of signature. Thereafter, no authorization exists unless an updated release is provided by: _B. Charma-Storro, JD_

Darnel G. Washington _2-15-01_

Signature of Patient or Patient's Authorized Representative Date

Figure 2-3. Examples of release forms. (Reprinted with permission from Thompson D. Hands Heal: Communication, Documentation, and Insurance Billing for Manual Therapists. 2nd ed. Baltimore: Lippincott Williams & Wilkins, 2002.)

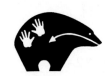

Helena LaLuna, CR
123 Sun Moon and Stars Drive
Capital Hill, WA   98119
Tel   206 555 4446

HEALTH INFORMATION

Patient Name _Zamora Hostetter_   Date _4-4-01_

Date of Injury _3-31-01_   Insurance ID# _C98-7654321_

A. Patient Information

Address _63 18th Ave. W_

City _Capitol Hill_   State _WA_ Zip _98119_

Phone: Home _(206) 555-1221_

   Work _555-2112_ Cell/Pgr _555-1122_

Date of Birth _5-22-80_

Employer _Howling Moon Cafe_

Occupation _Chef_

Emergency Contact _Mary Lou Hostetter_

Phone: Home _(206) 555-0909_

   Work _555-9090_ Cell/Pgr _555-9900_

Primary Health Care Provider

Name _Manda Rae Yuricich, DC_

Address _4041 Bell Town Wy, Ste. 200_

City/State/Zip _Capitol Hill WA 98119_

Phone: _555-3535_   Fax _555-4646_

I give my manual therapist permission to
consult with my referring health care provider
regarding my health and treatment. _& P.T._

Comments _re: work injury only_

Initials _ZH_   Date _4-4-01_

B. Current Health Information

List Health/Concerns Check all that apply

Primary _shoulder pain_

☐ mild ☐ moderate ☒ disabling

☒ constant ☐ intermittant

☒ symptoms ↑ w/activity   ☐ ↓ w/activity

☐ getting worse ☐ getting better ☒ no change

treatment received _ER-x-rays, sling_

Secondary _back pain_

☐ mild ☒ moderate ☐ disabling

☒ constant ☐ intermittant

☒ symptoms ↑ w/activity   ☐ ↓ w/activity

☐ getting worse ☒ getting better ☐ no change

treatment received _ER, DC-adjust._

Additional _neck pain & headaches_

☒ mild ☐ moderate ☐ disabling

☐ constant ☒ intermittant

☒ symptoms ↑ w/activity   ☐ ↓ w/activity

☐ getting worse ☒ getting better ☐ no change

treatment received _ER, DC_

Have you ever received Manual Therapy
before? ☐ Y ☒ N Frequency? _____

List all conditions currently monitored by a
Health Care Provider _none_

List the medications you took today
(include pain relievers and herbal remedies)
arnica, calcium, vitamins

List all other medications taken in the last 3
months _none_

List Daily Activities

Work   _standing, lifting, cooking, chopping_

Home/Family _cooking, cleaning, yardwork_

Social/Recreational _biking, roller hockey, dancing_

Circle the activities affected by your condition,
☒ all of the above

Check other activities affected: ☒ sleep
☐ washing ☐ dressing ☒ fitness

How do you reduce stress? _sports, being outdoors_

Pain? _arnica, ice packs, visualization_

What are your goals for receiving Manual
Therapy? _get back to work & sports_

C. Health History

List and Explain. Include dates and treatment
received.

Surgeries _none_

Accidents _Broken arm ®, fell out of tree
house in 1987, cast for 8 wks_

Major Illnesses _none_

Figure 2-3. *(continued)*

respond with a professional demeanor. If you make eye contact with clients who do not openly recognize or acknowledge a relationship with you, let them go. It is possible that they do not remember you, but it is also possible that they are not interested in a public relationship.

Confidentiality is a standard of care that is imperative to the professional therapeutic relationship by guaranteeing the clients that whatever happens in the therapeutic setting is private and protected. There are ethical and legal responsibilities that massage therapists should be aware of and understand.

Professional Associations

A professional image is often supported by membership in professional organizations. The original massage associations were established to protect the massage profession, and they have since evolved to provide a number of benefits to their members. Different levels of insurance coverage, marketing and promotional media, networking groups, and continuing education are just some of the options available to members of professional massage associations.

Professional Associations in Britain

Chapter 1 described the British Medical Association's discovery of unethical massage practices and how the massage profession prevailed, despite its tarnished reputation. At that time, if a massage therapist was associated with a physician or hospital, the massage was still considered legitimate. A group of four women in Britain decided to protect the massage profession by forming the Society of Trained Masseuses in 1894. Lucy Marianne Robinson, Rosalind Paget, Elizabeth Anne Manley, and Margaret Dora Palmer founded the society using the standards for the medical profession as their model. They established academic prerequisites for training, outlined criteria for qualified instructors, and inspected schools on a regular basis. Massage instructors and graduates were required to take written and practical examinations before a board, which included a physician. They maintained high standards and set membership regulations, requiring the massage professionals to only accept physicians' referrals and to avoid advertising through the media.

Many members abided by the many rules and regulations of the society, but there were still a number of massage therapists who continued to practice unethically. By 1900, the group became the Incorporated Society of Trained Masseuses. In 1920, a Royal Charter was granted, the group joined forces with the Institute of Massage and Remedial Gymnastics, and the Chartered Society of Massage and Remedial Gymnastics was established. With several branches throughout Britain, the widely respected society reached a membership of 12,000. In 1944, the society changed its name to the Chartered Society of Physiotherapy, which remains its name today.

Professional Associations in America

Soon after the British started the movement toward professional massage therapy, a flurry of professional activity began in the United States as well:

- 1927—The New York State Society of Medical Massage Therapists was America's first professional massage association to be established
- 1939—The Florida State Massage Therapy Association was organized with 85 charter members
- 1943—The first Massage Act was passed by the Florida legislature
- 1943—The American Association of Masseurs and Masseuses (AAMM) was formed in Chicago
- 1949—AAMM established the Massage Registration Act, a state law requiring massage therapists to register with the state
- 1958—AAMM became the American Massage and Therapy Association (AM&TA)
- 1983—AM&TA became the current AMTA
- 1987—ABMP was founded in Colorado

The AMTA still exists today, providing massage therapists with professional liability and other insurance, membership standards for education and continuing education, a code of ethics, and standards of practice. The AMTA promotes research studies, supports involvement in regulatory efforts, and prints promotional information, among other benefits. The AMTA's state chapters offer opportunities for community education, continuing education, and volunteer involvement in the organization. Therapists can volunteer in any capacity, from handling registration at a chapter meeting to being a national committee chairperson or director on the board.

In 1987, two massage therapists formed the ABMP organization in Evergreen, Colorado. The ABMP philosophy centers on the credo of "expect more" and helps massage, bodywork, somatic, and esthetic (skin care) practitioners build and sustain successful practices. The primary selling point for the ABMP is its claim to support the needs of its members by providing the necessary products or services. Currently, there is a companion magazine publication, an insurance program, and a business handbook for members in addition to its massage school relations program and support for regulation.

Relationships

Relationships can be complicated in any situation, but massage therapy can make them even more complex. Every relationship, whether personal or professional, is characterized by physical and conceptual boundaries. Physical boundaries describe the physical area that defines a person's comfort zone, and conceptual boundaries are the attitudes and behaviors that affect a person's level of comfort. The comfort provided by physical and conceptual boundaries can create a safe space for clients that allows a healthy professional relationship to grow.

Professional relationships are made with clients, with other healthcare professionals, and in any situation in which you are representing yourself as a massage therapist. The physical and conceptual boundaries will play a part in each one of these relationships, so you must be aware of boundaries and respect them to maintain professionalism.

Physical Boundaries

There is physical space around a person that is a boundary for outsiders. Anthropologist Edward T. Hall pioneered the field of proxemics, or the human behavioral use of space, in the 1960s. He defined the immediate space around a person as having four different zones:

- Intimate—for whispering and embracing, within 18 inches of your body
- Personal—for conversing with close friends, 18 inches to 4 feet away from your body
- Social—for conversing with acquaintances, 4 to 10 feet away from your body
- Public—for interacting with strangers, 10 to 25 feet away from your body

Personal space is like a protective bubble that insulates us from persons and things around us. You should respect others' personal space and stay out of it unless invited. When a person comes within a zone that is inappropriate for the relationship, Hall suggests that it makes the person being invaded feel uncomfortable and vulnerable and triggers an avoidance response. Americans typically require a space about 6 feet in diameter, or a little further than an arm's distance away, for social or comfortable public situations. This space is commonly called personal space, and the size of it varies with cultural, emotional, physical, and sexual experiences.

As mentioned above, personal space may vary individually depending on perceived comfort and safety. During a massage session, you will be moving into different zones of your clients' space and need to be aware of their comfort level to make sure that you do not trigger avoidance or resistance. Understanding and maintaining physical boundaries is essential for preserving the therapeutic process before, during, and after the massage. Accountability is a quality that can help you maintain a safe personal space for your clients. It can be challenging to know for sure whether you are too far into a client's personal space, so do not hesitate to ask periodically during the massage and suggest that the client respond. You can adjust the pressure and techniques according to the client's responses. In fact, you can inform clients prior to the treatment that during the massage you may ask about their comfort and can make the appropriate adjustments to the massage. In addition to the physical space that we use for protection and comfort, there are conceptual boundaries that do the same.

Conceptual Boundaries

Conceptual boundaries, sometimes called comfort zones, provide us with a sense of safety or comfort. The intimate nature of massage can easily create a feeling of vulnerability, discomfort, nervousness, or hesitancy. Clients who feel safe, comfortable, and trusting will ultimately receive more benefit from a massage than clients who feel unsure and uncomfortable. Comfort levels with the issues of emotions, intellect, energy, and sexuality are all forms of conceptual boundaries.

Emotions

Emotional boundaries determine the extent to which we expose emotions and feelings based on perceived levels of trust, safety, and comfort. The term "openness" expresses a person's willingness to share his or her emotions openly. Massage therapists must respect emotional boundaries as much as physical space boundaries. If you push clients to expose more emotion than they want to share or if you share too many of your own emotions with your clients, you may be met with resistance and avoidance. Clients' emotions and the issues that surround them may be interesting and can certainly affect the healing process, but managing them is not within the scope of massage therapy.

Intellect

Intellectual boundaries protect a person's thoughts, opinions, and belief systems. Culture, religion, spirituality, politics, nutritional habits, age, and gender can influence belief systems, so all of those topics should be respected and handled carefully without judgment. In a basic example, it may be challenging for a massage therapist who is a strict vegetarian to refrain from judging a junk food eater's nutritional habits. Even if the vegetarian therapist strongly believes that it is wrong to eat animal products, it is inappropriate for that therapist to think less of a client who disagrees. Another example of an intellectual boundary is a person sharing religious beliefs with his or her therapist. Therapists must respect the client's ideas even if they seem absurd to them. Consider how a client in that situation would feel if the therapist responded with disbelief and surprise, saying "You actually believe that God does not exist!?"

Energy

Within human beings are endless chemical reactions and energetic transfers that create various energy fields in and around the body. Massage therapy affects physiological activities and consequently changes the energetic fields. Emotions can also affect physiological activity and energetic fields. Energy flows and patterns can influence each other, which is easily demonstrated by a magnet's ability to attract or repel, depending on the energy patterns of different objects. With increased awareness, you can prevent energetic influence from occurring between you and your clients.

In the beginning of your career as a massage therapist, you may become aware of increased physical stress on your body as a result of working with a client. For example, a client may come in with neck pain, and after the session, you feel discomfort in your neck. While this may seem strange, many therapists experience this phenomenon. It can also occur in reverse, with a transfer from the therapist to the client. Either way, it can affect the therapist's and the client's health and well-being. Some grounding and centering techniques that can minimize the effect of these seemingly energetic influences are covered later in the text. Everyone who works with human bodies and receives work on his or her body is affected by the energy of another, so do what you can to protect yourself and your clients from negative effects.

Sexuality

Massage is an intimate and personal activity, and it is ultimately the therapist's responsibility to maintain a professional boundary. This is both a physical and conceptual boundary, but the conceptual limits are more sensitive and subtle than the physical limits. The therapist should be very clear in the informed consent process that sexualizing the treatment session is unacceptable and will result in immediate termination of the session. The treatment can be sexualized with a simple inappropriate comment, and there are also cases in which clients have asked for genital massage and for a sexual encounter. It should be very clear that there are absolutely NO exceptions to this boundary.

The intention of touch can significantly influence how a person perceives the touch, which is why you must make your professional policies absolutely clear prior to the session. In the somewhat puritanical American culture, any form of touch can be perceived as sexual. A client who is trying to sexualize the session can change a safe, ethical, and therapeutic touch into something that could be interpreted as sexual touch. Sexualizing a treatment session is the ultimate violation of professional boundaries, and it is undeniably unethical and probably illegal. If reported, you will most likely lose your right to practice and may face legal recourse.

With that in mind, you should know that sexual arousal may occur during a treatment session. Massage provides a lot of sensory stimulation in many different ways. Sometimes the slow massage strokes paired with a safe and caring touch can create feelings of intimacy and sexuality. Even if the feelings are unintentional, they can result from this excessive tactile experience and sometimes cause sexual arousal. The process of sexual arousal is a complex physiological and emotional response to many stimuli. We will cover this response very basically so you can be aware of what may occur during a treatment session and have an idea how to handle it if it does occur.

Sexual arousal may result from one or a combination of increased sensory stimulation, increased activity of the parasympathetic nervous system, and stimulation of the limbic system, which is the part of the brain that controls emotions. The primary intention of massage is to promote relaxation, which can be caused by the parasympathetic nervous system's response to some basic massage strokes. Many physiological changes occur during the parasympathetic response that allow the body to fall into a "rest and digest" mode, such as reduced heart rate, reduced blood pressure, dilation of the pupils, and increased blood flow to the digestive system and reproductive organs. The female's clitoris and the male's penis both become erect as a result of the parasympathetic response, but we all know that male erections are more apparent. The point here is that an erection does not necessarily mean that your client has sexual intent.

There are several thoughts and methods on how to handle this situation if it occurs, but in the end, you want to act with a client-centered frame of mind.

1. The first way to handle this situation takes place BEFORE any sexual arousal occurs. Your informed consent process can be used to educate clients about the parasympathetic system and its potential effect of sexual arousal.

2. You can speed up the tempo of the massage and switch to brisk, percussive strokes to induce the opposite physiological response, which will make the erection subside.

3. You can ignore an erection if you believe your client is either unaware of it or if you believe your client has no sexual intent.

4. If the client mentions or asks about his erection and you believe that he has no sexual intent, you can explain the physiology briefly and assure him that it is a natural response and that his body is relaxing.

5. If a male client's erection is accompanied by inappropriate sexual gestures or comments, you must address the situation directly. You could temporarily stop the session, remind your client about your professional policies and intolerance of sexual behavior, and continue with the massage. You could also terminate the session, explain your professional intolerance for sexual behavior, excuse yourself from the room, ask the client to get dressed, and escort him to the door.

You may be embarrassed, upset, and afraid or confused when a client has an erection during a massage session. The way you handle the situation is a personal, professional, and ethical decision depending on the subtleties of the situation. Trust your intuition, respect the sexual boundaries of your clients and yourself, and keep professionalism in mind.

Safe Space

Safe space refers to the physical and emotional atmosphere of your practice. It provides an environment that is welcoming, comforting, noninvasive, safe, and secure, so clients can relax and get the most beneficial massage session. Security and safety in your practice can be conveyed by:

- A safe location in the city
- A clean and well-maintained building
- An easily accessible treatment room
- Privacy in the treatment room
- Freedom from disruptive noises or odors
- Adequate lighting
- Appropriate music
- Proper draping techniques
- Professional image
- Professional knowledge, competence, compassion, and communication

Client Relationships

The therapeutic relationship between the massage therapist and client is an important standard of practice to examine closely. The therapeutic relationship begins with your initial contact with the client and continues for as long as you and the client agree to work together. When the therapeutic relationship begins, there is usually an immediate power differential when the client assumes that the healthcare professional is an expert. Clients who seek massage treatment assume you have the training and knowledge to handle their condition appropriately. To emphasize the differential, massage clients take off some or all of their clothes and, while they are covered with appropriate draping, are in a more vulnerable position than the therapist. It may be easy to forget this power differential exists, so keep in mind that you are a person who represents authority and may seem more powerful in the client's eyes.

Dual Relationships

Dual relationships, which occur when personal and professional roles overlap, can enhance or detract from the therapeutic relationship depending on how they are handled. **It is always the responsibility of the therapist to determine and communicate the risks, boundaries, and impact of dual or multiple relationships.**

When two people who are personal friends have a professional relationship of some kind, they have what is called a dual relationship. The overlap between professional and social interaction can jeopardize the personal and the professional relationships. Another issue that can complicate client relationships is transference. Basically, it is the experience in which expectations and behaviors from one relationship are placed on another relationship, and it has a significant impact on your professional relationships.

This may be especially important when working with family and friends who become your massage clients. Family and friends do not intentionally take advantage of you as a professional, but they are more comfortable about canceling appointments at the last minute, not paying promptly, asking for massage outside the office and in social situations, and assuming that you will treat them anytime, anywhere. Some therapists describe these kinds of situations and let their friends and family know that if any of those situations occur, the professional relationship will be terminated. You may have to set definitive professional boundaries with them, and although it is not easy to do, it will make the professional relationship easier in the long run.

When assessing the risks of dual relationships, examine the impact it would have on the professional relationship. Since you are ultimately accountable for the therapeutic relationship, you must assess whether there is mutual benefit for establishing the secondary relationship and whether there could be any negative impact on your business and professional image. If you and the client decide that the risks are minimal, it is important to establish clear boundaries regarding the additional roles.

Transference

The concept of transference is found mostly in therapeutic relationships involving psychotherapy and healthcare relationships, and it is frequently present in massage therapy. You should be aware of the concept and understand the mechanism enough to recognize when it surfaces.

Transference is the process in which clients transfer expectations and behaviors of another relationship onto their therapeutic relationship with you. They may transfer or project unresolved feelings, needs, and issues onto you without good reason. Some examples of transference in the massage setting:

- The client brings you gifts in addition to your normal fees at every appointment.
- The client repeatedly asks for personal psychological advice.
- The client seems to linger in your office, unwilling to leave.
- The client frequently tells you how much you look like another person.
- The client repeatedly calls you at home despite your request that you only be called on your business phone.
- The client always pushes for a longer session for the same price, despite your insistence that the session is finished.

Professional Relationships

Similarly, there are social and professional relationships that may develop from the therapeutic relationship. You might cross paths with clients in social circles, business settings, or even in the dating scene. Dating and sexual activity with clients is unacceptable and unethical, but establishing a friendship is less definitive. It is especially important to stay within your scope of practice as a massage therapist, even if your clients ask you for help in the areas of psychological evaluation or nutritional advice. If you suspect the client needs additional expertise in an area in which you are not qualified, it is your ethical and professional responsibility to refer your client to the appropriate professional.

Countertransference

Countertransference is similar to transference, except it occurs when you, as the massage therapist, transfer or project feelings or needs from another relationship onto your client. Some signs that you may be displaying countertransference include:

- Disappointment when your client does not praise you
- Thinking that you are the best therapist for a particular client and that all other therapists only do more damage than good
- Feeling frustrated with a particular client for a vague reason
- Feeling strong emotions toward a particular client
- Thinking that a client is ungrateful because he or she mentioned that there was little improvement after the last session
- Frequently reaching out to clients for social interaction outside the practice

In a massage practice, the therapist is ultimately responsible for maintaining the therapeutic relationship. If you recognize transference or countertransference in your practice, it is your responsibility to examine the situation and decide what to do. You may need to terminate the professional relationship or discontinue the social relationship. You could discuss your awareness of the situation with your client and explain that the therapeutic relationship is being compromised. If you are uncomfortable with handling the situation directly, you may want assistance from a professionally trained counselor, a social worker, or a psychotherapist who has expertise in this arena.

CHAPTER SUMMARY

The principles of ethics and professionalism are used as a guide in the massage therapy profession and promote and maintain the reputation of massage therapy. Understanding the professional standards of practice for a client-centered practice and having the accountability to follow the currently accepted codes of ethics will influence your thoughts and actions in creating and sustaining a successful massage therapy practice.

Legal regulations and scope of practice determine practice and technique parameters as well as the amount of education required to be considered a competent and professional massage therapist. Currently, the use of terminology is inconsistent and confusing, which makes it especially important to understand the specific requirement of your local and state laws.

The relationships you establish will present physical and conceptual boundaries that are different for every person, but if you are sensitive to and respect the limits, you can develop ethical and professional relationships. Massage therapy presents some complications to dual relationships and having a basic understanding about transference and countertransference can help you sort through those difficulties. Ultimately, being accountable for your behavior and actions and consistently behaving with a client-centered philosophy serve the best interest of everyone.

CHAPTER EXERCISES

1. Define the following terms and explain their importance in massage therapy:

    a. Ethics
    b. Code of ethics
    c. Standards of practice
    d. Body of knowledge
    e. Informed consent
    f. Scope of practice

2. Explain what a client-centered philosophy is and why it is important to the massage profession.

3. Describe the following terms as they apply to the relationships of a massage therapist: dual relationships, transference, and countertransference.

4. What is scope of practice for

    a. Wellness massage
    b. Therapeutic massage

5. Explain what the NCBTMB aims to establish.

6. Define accountability and describe an experience from your own life in which your accountability influenced a decision you had to make.

7. Give at least five examples of boundaries that influence relationships.

8. What is the ultimate boundary violation and why?

9. How can you portray yourself as a professional massage therapist?

10. Use the 7-step process learned in this chapter to resolve the ethical dilemmas in each of the following scenarios:

    a. You accept free concert tickets from a client, but at the next appointment, your client expects a free session. What do you do?
    b. A new client makes sexual jokes during the massage session. What do you do?
    c. A long-time client who has recently been separated from his spouse begins scheduling more frequent appointments and repeatedly refers to his search for companionship throughout his massage sessions. What do you do?

REFERENCES

1. NCBTMB mission statement. http://www.ncbtmb.org/about_mission.php, accessed 8.2.11.
2. NCBTMB educational eligibility. http://www.ncbtmb.org/applicants_what_you_need_to_know.php, accessed 8.2.11.
3. MBLEx content outline. http://fsmtb.org/downloads/examContentOutline.pdf, accessed 8.12.11.
4. Washington State's Health Department Complaint and Disciplinary Process. http://www.doh.wa.gov/hsqa/complaint.htm, accessed 8.2.11.

SUGGESTED READINGS

Alpert A. Defining boundaries. *Assoc Bodywork Massage Professionals Massage Bodywork Magazine* (Evergreen, CO: Associated Bodywork and Massage Professionals) 1999;June/July:76–78.

Benjamin B, Jordan D, Polseno D. Issues on sexuality. *Am Massage Ther Massage Ther J* (Evanston, IL: AMTA) 2000:Summer: 52–93.

McIntosh N. *The Educated Heart*. Memphis, TN: Decatur Bainbridge Press, 1999.

Polseno D. Informed consent. *Am Massage Ther Massage Ther J* (Evanston, IL: AMTA) 2001:Spring:136–141.

Rattray F, Ludwig L. *Clinical Massage Therapy: Understanding, Assessing and Treating over 70 Conditions*. Toronto, Ontario: Talus Incorporated, 2000.

Sohnen-Moe C, Benjamin B. *The Ethics of Touch*. Tucson, AZ: Sohnen-Moe Associates, 2003.

Torrenzano S. Ethics: The heart of the matter: Part 2. *Assoc Bodywork Massage Professionals Massage Bodywork Magazine* (Evergreen, CO: Associated Bodywork and Massage Professionals) 1999;June/July:62–70.

Torrenzano S. The heart of ethics. Lecture presented at: The American Massage Therapy Association National Convention; 2001; Quebec, Canada.

http://www.abmp.com, accessed 8.12.11.

http://www.amtamassage.org, accessed 8.12.11.

http://www.asinc.ca/en/services/licensure.html, accessed 3.5.06.

http://www.careeratyourfingertips.com/laws.htm, accessed 3.5.06.

http://www.fsmtb.org, accessed 8.12.11.

http://www.law.cornell.edu/statutes.html, accessed 3.5.06.

http://www.mdmassage.org/Stat%20and%20Regs.htm, accessed 3.5.06.

http://www.mtbok.org, accessed 8.12.11.

http://www.m-w.com, accessed 3.5.06.

http://www.ncbtmb.org, accessed 8.12.11.

http://www.pacode.com/secure/data/049/chapter20/chap20toc.html#%C2%A7%C2%A0%C2%A020.41., accessed 8.1.11.

http://www.prevent-abuse-now.com/govhome.htm, accessed 3.5.06.

http://www.stedmans.com, accessed 3.5.06.

Body Systems

Objectives

Upon completion of this chapter, the student will be able to:

- Describe the relationship between anatomy and physiology
- Define homeostasis
- Name the 12 body systems
- Name the major structures of each body system
- Name the major functions of each body system
- Identify at least five effects of the sympathetic and parasympathetic nervous systems

Key Terms

Anatomy: The study of the structures of plants and animals.

Artery: A tube that carries blood away from the heart.

Bony landmark: Site for muscle attachment or safe passageway for nerves and blood vessels; bony landmarks can usually be externally palpated.

Fascia (FASH-uh): A fibrous band or sheetlike tissue membrane that provides support and protection for the body organs.

Homeostasis (HOH-mee-oh-STAY-sis): The process by which the body continually adjusts to changes in order to maintain chemical, physiological, and structural balance.

Joint: The mechanical structure where neighboring bones are attached, often with connective tissue and cartilage.

Lymphatic fluid (lymph): The interstitial fluid that is taken from the all over the body into the lymphatic system.

Metabolism: The overall cellular activity that breaks down nutrients to generate energy to build essential molecules.

Motor neuron (efferent neuron): Neuron that carries messages away from the central nervous system to the muscle or organs that must react.

Motor unit: One motor neuron and all of the muscle cells it stimulates.

Muscle: A specially organized and packaged group of muscle cells, connective tissue wrappings, and blood vessels.

Nerve: A specially organized and packaged bundle of neurons, connective tissue wrappings, and blood vessels.

Nerve plexus: Large network of intertwined nerves.

Neuron (nerve cell): The basic unit of the nervous system.

Parasympathetic response: Autonomic nervous system response that stimulates organs to work in a relaxing "rest and digest" mode.

Physiology: The study of the functions of a living organism or any of its parts.

Proprioceptor (PROH-pree-oh-SEP-tor): Sensory nerve cell sensitive to body position, muscle tone, or equilibrium.

Sensory neuron (afferent neuron): Neuron that receives sensory input and transmits that information to the central nervous system.

Stretch reflex: A protective muscle contraction that occurs when the tissues are stretched too far and/or too fast.

Sympathetic response: Autonomic nervous system response that prepares the body for a stressful situation, sometimes called the "fight or flight" response.

Tendon reflex: A reflex that relaxes a muscle when a muscle and its tendon are subjected to slow and gentle tension.

Tissue: An organized group or layer of cells with similar structure and function.

Vein: A tube that transports blood from the capillaries of the body back to the heart.

The human body is complex, to say the least. This chapter starts out with the foundation of all living matter, cells and tissues. The basic building blocks of living organisms are cells. Combined in specific ways, these cells create specific kinds of tissues that are then organized into various structures in the body. Understanding the structure of the cell and the different mechanisms that occur in the cell provides a foundation for learning about tissues, which then lends itself to a more thorough understanding of the structures and functions of the larger body systems.

The basic structures and functions of the human body are then presented as 12 separate body systems: Integumentary System, Skeletal System, Muscular System, Nervous System, Cardiovascular System, Lymphatic System, Respiratory System, Digestive System, Urinary System, Endocrine System, Reproductive System, and Special Senses.

The 12 body systems must function with each other in order to sustain life and maintain health. The body continually adjusts to changes in its environment to maintain chemical, physiological, and structural balance—a critical life process called homeostasis (HOH-mee-oh-STAY-sis). When an imbalance occurs, the overall health of the tissues or body may be compromised. Massage can contribute to the homeostatic balance by enhancing the flow of body fluids (via mechanical effects) and affecting chemical activity in the body (via reflexive effects).

The benefits of massage are strongly supported by empirical evidence, which is evidence based on observation or experience, but there is limited scientific research proving the changes that occur in the body during massage therapy or how those changes directly influence health. Since the empirical evidence is so compelling, many research studies are being conducted to determine the science behind the benefits of massage (See Box 3.1). While additional evidence is being gathered, it is still important for you to understand the effects of massage on each body system, so these effects are identified for each body system.

This chapter serves only as an introduction to the body systems and is intended to give you a basic idea about the human body, what it is made of, and how it works. The aim is to provide a functional understanding of how the structures and body systems relate to massage.

BOX 3-1

NCCAM-Funded Research on Massage Therapy

Recent studies sponsored by the National Center for Complementary and Alternative Medicine (NCCAM) have been investigating:

- The effects of massage on chronic neck and low back pain

- Massage to treat anxiety disorder, alleviate depression in patients with advanced AIDS, and promote recovery in women who were victims of sexual abuse as children

- Massage to relieve fatigue in cancer patients undergoing chemotherapy, reduce treatment-related swelling of the arms in breast cancer patients, and alleviate pain and distress in cancer patients at the end of life

- Whether massage improves weight gain and immune system function in preterm infants

- Whether massage given at home by a trained family member helps reduce pain from sickle cell anemia

---

Terms for Structure and Function

Anatomy is the study of the structures of plants and animals. Massage therapists need to know the correct terms for different structures of the body for the work they do, for record keeping, and for communication. In addition to learning the name of a structure, such as a specific organ, muscle, or bone, you need to learn its function or functions. Physiology is the study of the functions of an organism or any specific part of an organism.

Anatomy

The word anatomy is derived from the Greek roots "ana," meaning up or again, and "tomy," meaning cutting or dissection. The term refers to the first anatomists, who had to cut open cadavers to discover anatomical structures. Science and technology have brought us a long way since then, and we now have amazing capabilities when it comes to looking at the human body. MRI and computed tomography scans let us look at the hard and soft tissues inside the body with excellent clarity. In addition to the visible anatomical structures, there are invisible components that we cannot see with any current technology.

The structures of all living organisms are made up of individual components that can be organized from the simple to complex. The smallest element of structure is the invisible atom. Bonded together in specific arrangements, these atoms make up molecules. Various molecules combine to create cells. The cell is the basic building block for all living things. Groups of specialized cells are organized into tissues, each with a specific function. Different tissues coordinate their individual functions and form organs. Organs that all have a similar purpose are grouped together as organ systems, also called body systems. Finally, the most complex level of organization is the organism, which depends on all the organ systems working together (Fig. 3-1).

Physiology

Learning the individual structures of the body naturally leads to the discovery of the processes or responsibilities of those parts, called physiology. Massage therapists have to know at least the major anatomical structures and their physiological functions to provide safe and beneficial treatment. Likewise, they need to know the physiological effects of massage to administer the appropriate treatments. You will need to know the normal structures and functions to recognize abnormal ones that may need to be avoided. Most importantly, massage therapists specialize in the muscular system, so they need to know a lot about skeletal muscles:

- Structural components of muscle
- Names of the major skeletal muscles
- Attachment points of different muscles
- Actions of different muscles
- Cooperative movement of muscle groups
- Neuromuscular control of muscle contraction
- Fascial involvement
- Interaction between the muscular system and other body systems

These components are explained in greater detail in Chapter 4, Kinesiology and Biomechanics.

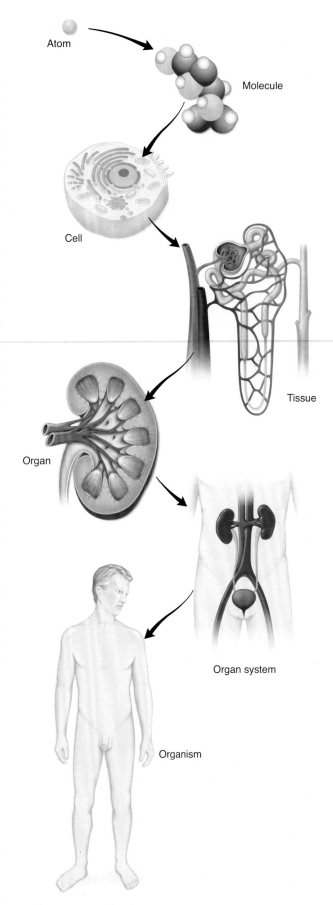

Atom

Molecule

Cell

Tissue

Organ

Organ system

Organism

Figure 3-1. Levels of organization.

Cells and Tissues

All living matter is made up of a variety of parts that range in size and complexity. The cell, which comes in many specialized forms, is the basic building block for structures of living things. A **tissue** is an organized group or layer of cells that have similar structure and function. Organs are groups of tissue that perform specialized body functions. Tissues and organs that work closely together, cooperating to perform a particular function, are collectively called a body system, or organ system. Each body system works specifically to sustain a certain function in the body. Together, they work to sustain the life of the organism.

A basic cell has several different structural components, each with its own specific function. However, all of the components work together toward a common goal of maintaining the life of the cell. This section introduces the functions of the cells and the functions of the individual components of cells, and it identifies the different kinds of tissues that are created by cells.

Cellular Functions

A living cell is a powerhouse of chemical and molecular activity. There are three general functions of the cell: growth, maintenance, and reproduction. The physical and chemical processes of metabolism (meh-TAB-oh-liz-m) allow cells to grow. Maintenance and control of the metabolic processes is accomplished with homeostasis. Cells reproduce by a series of steps called cell division, which consists of two major activities called "mitosis (mahy-TOH-sis) and cytokinesis (SAHY-toh-kih-NEE-sis). The general functions of a cell are made possible by cooperative work of the cell's independent components.

Metabolism

Metabolism is the overall cellular activity that both breaks down large molecules into smaller molecules to generate energy and also builds large, essential molecules from smaller ones, consuming energy. Catabolism (kah-TAB-oh-liz-m) is the destructive metabolic process that breaks down complex substances and releases energy for cellular activity, often in the form of adenosine triphosphate (ATP). Anabolism (an-AB-oh-liz-m) is the constructive metabolic process that requires energy to build larger, more complex molecules from simpler ones. When all of the metabolic processes are working properly and efficiently, the cell functions normally.

Homeostasis

The body is constantly monitoring and adjusting metabolic processes in an effort to maintain an internally balanced state of equilibrium. This process is called homeostasis: through the dynamic process of responding to changes in the external environment, the body keeps fluid and chemical levels within very narrow limits, body temperature within a narrow range of safety, and oxygen demands of the tissues satisfied. Homeostasis is primarily controlled by negative feedback mechanisms that trigger the body to increase or reduce certain metabolic activities when abnormal levels of chemicals, body temperatures, or pressures are detected in the body. Blood pressure, body temperature, oxygen level in the blood, carbon dioxide content, and heart rate are all controlled by negative feedback mechanisms. For example, the body is constantly monitoring its internal core temperature, which it typically maintains between 96.8° and 98.6°F. When the core temperature is too low, the body constricts the blood vessels in the skin to conserve heat and initiates shivering to generate heat when the environment is especially cold. As soon as the core temperature is detected within the normal range, the body stops shivering and the blood vessels in the skin dilate. Another example of homeostasis is the body's ability to maintain sufficient levels of oxygen in the blood. Every one of our cells requires a certain amount of oxygen in order to function properly, but when the levels are insufficient, such as when muscular contraction uses up extra amounts of oxygen, the body makes adjustments to deliver more oxygen to the blood.

Cell Division

Cells can replicate themselves through the process of cell division, which occurs in a series of steps that replicate the genetic material of the cell and divide the components of the cell. Mitosis is the part of cellular division that divides the nucleus. The nucleus, which is an organelle inside the cell that holds the genetic material, is discussed below in this section. Cytokinesis divides the original cell and its contents into two separate cells. Cell division is preceded by interphase, which is the part of the cell cycle in which there is no division taking place. Interphase prepares the cell for mitosis by replicating the genetic material called deoxyribonucleic acid (DNA). Following interphase, cell division occurs in the following four stages (Fig. 3-2):

1. Prophase—The chromosomes, which carry the now-duplicated DNA, thicken and resemble limp Xs that

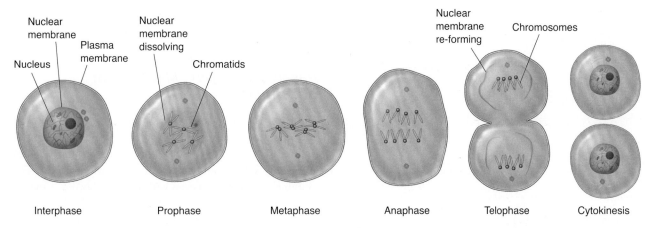

Figure 3-2. Stages of cell division.

are identical pairs of chromatids. A chromatid is one of two daughter strands of a duplicated chromosome, joined together at a single centromere. The nuclear membrane, which encloses the DNA inside the nucleus, breaks down and disappears.

2. Metaphase—The paired chromatids group together and arrange themselves along the midline of the cell.

3. Anaphase—The chromatids separate, sending each of the identical parts to opposite sides of the cell. Once the chromatids reach the opposite ends of the cell, they are again called chromosomes.

4. Telophase—The chromosomes lengthen and become thinner. Nuclear membranes form around each set of chromosomes to create two separate nuclei. At the same time, cytokinesis divides the rest of the cell into two separate cells, each with its own nucleus.

The entire process of cell division can last anywhere from several minutes to several hours, depending on the type of tissue. At the end of telophase, the original cell has become two cells that are slightly smaller than the original, but are genetically identical to it. The metabolic processes help the cell grow, and homeostatic processes maintain cell growth and life by adjusting metabolic activity. Interestingly enough, and contrary to popular belief, many scientists currently believe that not all cells divide.

The cellular function of homeostasis keeps cells safe, healthy, and alive, which keeps the tissues, organs, organ systems, and the whole body safe, healthy, and alive. A cellular imbalance will affect cell growth, maintenance, and cell division and can even result in cell death. This concept can be applied to massage when dealing with a hypertonic (excessively tight) muscle. Hypertonic muscles constrict blood flow, limiting the cell's ability to receive nutrition and eliminate waste. Insufficient oxygen or energy creates an imbalance in the cell and decreases the efficiency of cellular activity. Excessive buildup of

waste does the same. Massage techniques can improve the circulation of the blood, which can restore cellular activity to a normal level and, consequently, restore the health of the organism.

Components of the Cell

The metabolic and homeostatic functions of cells are carried out by a number of different structures. A cell is a powerhouse of activity that serves as the basis for all anatomy and physiology. The basic components of a cell are the cell membrane, the cytosol, and the organelles. The cell membrane, or plasma membrane, is the outer barrier of the cell and holds the contents of the cell. The cytoplasm is a fluid that suspends the many organelles, which are like separate little machines, each with specific functions to help keep the cell alive and functioning.

Cell Membrane

The cell membrane, sometimes called the plasma membrane, is the outer layer of the cell that protects the contents and activities of the cell. The membrane is primarily composed of phospholipids, which are phosphate molecules attached to fatty acid chains. The structure is also referred to as a lipid bilayer. Scattered throughout the membrane are proteins and their receptor sites (Fig. 3-3). The membrane provides a selective transport barrier that helps maintain a stable internal environment within the cell. The plasma membrane allows nutrients to enter the cell, allows waste material to exit, and maintains appropriate chemical and fluid levels. When those levels are out of balance, cellular activity is affected and extra energy is required to maintain homeostasis.

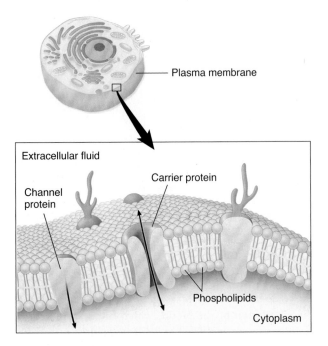

Figure 3-3. Structure of the plasma membrane.

   The most important function of the semipermeable plasma membrane is to be the "gatekeeper" of nutrient and waste exchange between the cell and the world outside it. If cells do not adequately receive nutrition or eliminate waste, cell growth is hindered and cell death is possible. The semipermeable quality allows some, but not all, things to pass through the membrane, depending on shape, size, and chemical properties. The exchange can occur passively, without energy, or actively, requiring energy. Diffusion (dif-YOO-zhun), osmosis (oz-MOH-sis), and filtration are passive transport processes that occur without energy expenditure.

Processes that require energy to take place, such as exocytosis (EK-soh-sahy-toh-sis) and endocytosis (EN-doh-sahy-toh-sis), are called active transport processes.

Passive Transport Mechanism of Diffusion

Diffusion is a process in which chemical ions and some chemical molecules move from an area of higher concentration to an area of lower concentration until the molecules are evenly spread out throughout a solution or area. For example, over time and even without being stirred, a spoonful of sugar will dissolve and become evenly distributed throughout a glass of water through the process of diffusion. The lipid bilayer structure of the membrane gives it some of its abilities to repel molecules that are fat insoluble (cannot dissolve in fat). It also allows fat-soluble molecules and gases to diffuse through. Water-soluble chemicals, even ones as small as sodium and hydrogen ions, must be assisted through the membrane by specialized proteins. This differentiation of fat-soluble and water-soluble transport allows the cell to control its permeability by opening or closing specific kinds of channels. Fats and fat-soluble vitamins can be absorbed into cells via diffusion through the plasma membrane, oxygen and carbon dioxide molecules can diffuse across the respiratory membranes, and sodium ions cross via action potentials in which the membrane opens its channels for a millisecond to allow sodium ions to pass through (Fig. 3-4A).

Passive Transport Mechanism of Osmosis

There are occasions when chemicals that cannot pass through the semipermeable membrane are concentrated differently on either side of the membrane. To maintain homeostasis and keep everything balanced, the body moves

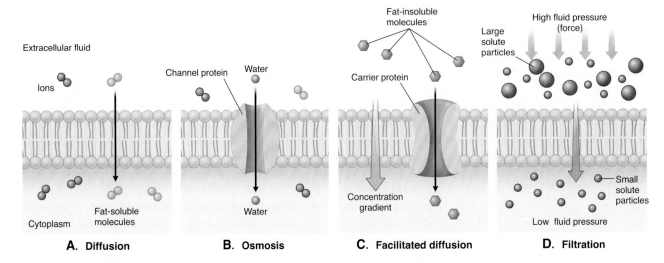

A. Diffusion   **B. Osmosis**   **C. Facilitated diffusion**   **D. Filtration**

Figure 3-4. Mechanisms of passive transport. **(A)** Diffusion. **(B)** Osmosis. **(C)** Facilitated diffusion. **(D)** Filtration.

water from the side that has a lower concentration of these molecules to the side with the higher concentration. The addition of water effectively lowers the concentration of these chemicals. Most people recognize that oil and water do not mix. Because of its molecular structure, water is not soluble in oil or fat. Although water is not a fat-soluble molecule and it would typically be repelled by the lipid bilayer, water moves through the semipermeable cell membrane. Osmosis is the specific passive transport mechanism by which water crosses the membrane through channel proteins to balance concentrations on either side of the membrane. The best way to remember which direction water moves through the membrane is the phrase "Water follows concentration" (Fig. 3-4B). If there is a higher concentration of solutes outside the cell, water will move out of the cell in an attempt to balance the solutions on either side of the membrane. Conversely, if there is a higher concentration of solutes inside the cell, water will flow into the cell to achieve a balance.

Solutions possess tonicity, the amount of dissolved particles in the solution. A solution whose tonicity is the same as that within our cells is called an isotonic (AHY-soh-TAHN-ik) solution. When an isotonic solution surrounds our cells, water levels within the cells do not change. Intravenous fluids such as Ringer's lactate and 0.9% saline solution are isotonic solutions that have the same concentrations as our cells, so when they are injected into the bloodstream, the cells do not absorb or eliminate water.

When solutions that do not have the same concentration as dissolved substances in our cells are introduced into our bodies, the water content within the cell is adjusted to maintain a balance on either side of the cell membrane. This homeostatic mechanism is used therapeutically when medical professionals give patients intravenous fluids. Hypotonic (HAHY-poh-TAHN-ik) solutions have a lower osmotic pressure (are less concentrated) than the fluid inside our cells and result in water moving into the cell by osmosis. Conditions of dehydration are sometimes treated with hypotonic solutions, which force water to move into and rehydrate the cells. Hypertonic (HAHY-per-TAHN-ik) solutions are used to treat edema, which is swelling due to an excess of fluid between the cells. The hypertonic solution, often 3% to 5% sodium chloride solution, causes water to move toward the higher concentration, outside the cells, and into the bloodstream (Fig. 3-5). The excess fluid is then processed by the kidneys and excreted as urine.

Passive Transport Mechanism of Facilitated Diffusion

Facilitated diffusion is a special form of passive membrane transport. Molecules that are too large or that would be repelled by the lipid bilayer use carrier proteins scattered along the membrane as trap doors that allow them to pass through easily. A carrier protein molecule will attach to the oversized molecule, possibly altering its shape or enveloping it, and will pull it through the membrane (see Fig. 3-4C). A good example of facilitated diffusion is the passage of glucose through a cell membrane. Glucose is a large molecule used for cellular metabolism that is not fat soluble but can use a carrier protein to get through the membrane.

Passive Transport Mechanism of Filtration

Filtration is another mode of passive transport whereby water and dissolved substances (solutes) are pushed through a membrane by fluid pressure. This process moves the solution from an area of higher pressure to an area of lower pressure, again part of the homeostatic process of keeping a balance on either side of the membrane (see Fig. 3-4D). An example of filtration is urine formation in the kidneys, where the fluid pressure in the blood capillaries is higher than that in the kidney tubules. The difference in pressures forces the solution out of the blood capillaries and into the kidney tubules for elimination.

Figure 3-5. Effects of osmosis on red blood cells in different concentrations: isotonic, hypotonic, and hypertonic solutions.

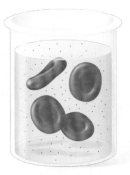
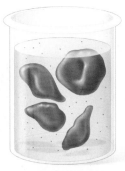
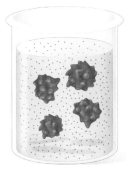

Normal
(isotonic)
solution

Hypotonic
solution

Hypertonic
solution

Active Transport Mechanisms

Active transport processes require ATP as a source of energy to move chemicals through a membrane. There are several different situations in which molecules cannot be transported passively and energy must be used to move them:

- Molecules that are too large to pass through the membrane and cannot take advantage of carrier proteins

- Molecules that have to move against the concentration gradient, or from an area where they are lower in concentration to an area of higher concentration

- Molecules that are not fat soluble and cannot take advantage of carrier proteins

Solute pumping is the active transport process that uses energy from the breakdown of ATP to help protein carriers pull amino acids, some sugars, and many ions through the membrane.

Bulk transport is an active transport process that uses energy to package molecules and carry them across the membrane. Exocytosis is the bulk transport mechanism that takes cellular products from the inside of the cell to the outside of the cell. The products in the cytoplasm are packaged in a sac, the sac is incorporated into the membrane, and the contents of the sac are released into the extracellular fluid (the fluid that surrounds the cell). Mucus is released outside the cell via exocytosis (Fig. 3-6B).

Endocytosis is another bulk transport mechanism that works in the opposite direction of exocytosis. Substances outside the cell are engulfed, transported inside the cell, and usually digested by enzymes (Fig. 3-6A). Bacteria and dead body cells are managed by the specific form of endocytosis called phagocytosis (FAY-goh-sahy-TOH-sis). When liquids that contain dissolved proteins or fats cannot diffuse through a cell membrane, pinocytosis (PEE-noh-sahy-toh-sis) is the special form of endocytosis that moves them into the cell. The prefix "exo-" means to "move out" and "endo-" means to "move in."

The cell membrane is a very active component of the cell that is involved in homeostasis, but there are a number of other structures that are equally important.

Cytoplasm

The cytoplasm is the liquid substance inside the plasma membrane that houses most of the cellular activity, composed of a gel-like substance called cytosol that contains nutrients, minerals, enzymes, and cytoplasmic organelles suspended in it. The cytoplasm makes up 50% of the cell's volume and contains everything necessary for protein synthesis as well as the enzymes for building and breaking down molecules (Fig. 3-7).

Cytoplasmic Organelles

The cytoplasmic organelles are the metabolic machinery of the cell that keeps the cell alive and dynamic. Organelles, including the nucleus, nucleolus, ribosomes, endoplasmic reticulum, mitochondria, Golgi apparatus, lysosomes, and

Figure 3-6. Bulk transport mechanisms. **(A)** Endocytosis. **(B)** Exocytosis. (Reprinted from Premkumar K. The Massage Connection: Anatomy & Physiology. 2nd ed. Baltimore: Lippincott Williams & Wilkins, 2004.)

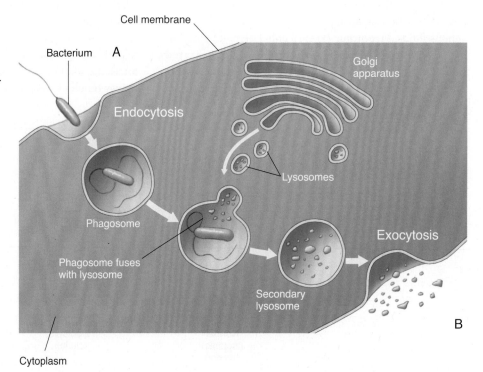

Human cell

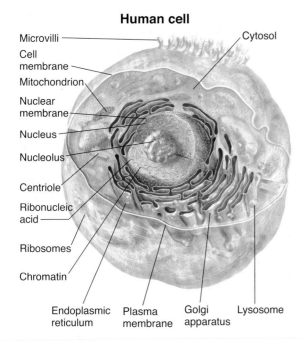

Microvilli

Cell membrane

Mitochondrion

Nuclear membrane

Nucleus

Nucleolus

Centriole

Ribonucleic acid

Ribosomes

Chromatin

Endoplasmic reticulum

Plasma membrane

Golgi apparatus

Lysosome

Cytosol

Figure 3-7. Components of a cell. (Asset provided by Anatomical Chart Co.)

centrioles, are all suspended in the cytosol. They have different shapes and functions, and any disruption of their activity will affect the homeostasis of the cell.

The largest organelle is the nucleus (NOOK-lee-us), located somewhere near the center of the cell. The nucleus is the control center for the cell. It is enveloped in a double-layered membrane that is perforated with pores that allow some molecules to pass between the nucleus and the cell. Within the nucleus is a small, spherical structure called a nucleolus (nook-lee-OH-lus) that builds the molecules required for protein synthesis. Occasionally, cells have two nucleoli, if there is a heavy demand for proteins. Among other molecules, the nucleus contains DNA, which is necessary for building all proteins. Proteins are necessary components for building cell structures and carrying out cell functions including cell reproduction.

Outside the nucleus are many organelles suspended in the cytosol that carry out other cellular operations. There are many ribosomes (RAHY-boh-zohmz) that serve as the factory where proteins are put together with the help of enzymes. Some ribosomes are suspended in the cytosol, and some are attached to the rough endoplasmic reticulum. Within the cytosol, there are one or more endoplasmic reticula, which are networks of tubes that modify and direct newly made proteins to other cell organelles. The endoplasmic reticula also manufacture membrane lipids, synthesize and break down cholesterol, and metabolize fat.

Also within the cytosol are several elongated oval organelles called mitochondria (MAHY-toh-KON-dree-uh). As the powerhouses of cellular function, mitochondria break down nutrients and release energy. Some of the energy is released as heat, but most of the energy is converted to ATP molecules through the process of cellular respiration, which is the primary source of energy for cellular metabolism. Because oxygen is required for cellular respiration, the process is sometimes referred to as aerobic respiration. Without oxygen, cells will suffer and eventually die. Generally, the more active the cell, the more oxygen and energy it requires and the more mitochondria it will have. Muscle cells that get regular exercise increase their numbers of mitochondria to generate more energy for the muscle cell.

The Golgi apparatus is an organelle that resembles a stack of flattened sacs that are suspended in the cytosol. Serving as a sort of packaging plant, the sacs receive proteins by way of the endoplasmic reticulum. The proteins are modified, sorted, and gathered in sacs until the sacs swell to the point that they pinch themselves off and become secretory vesicles. The final destination of the vesicles depends on their contents. Vesicles that contain substances destined for the blood or a body tube fuse with the plasma membrane and expel their contents outside the cell, illustrated above as the active transport mechanism of exocytosis (see Fig. 3-6). Some vesicles contain proteins and phospholipids that are taken to the plasma membrane and become part of its structure.

Some of the smaller cytoplasmic organelles include lysosomes (LAHY-soh-zohmz) and centrioles (SEN-tree-ohlz). Varied in size, lysosomes are essentially vesicles containing digestive enzymes. Inside the cell, lysosomes engulf and digest cellular waste, bacteria, and unwanted foreign substances. Centrioles are rod-shaped organelles located close to the nucleus that aid in chromosome separation during cell division. Some cells have cilia, which are small, hairlike extensions of the plasma membrane on the outside of the membrane that help sweep objects past the cell. They are located in respiratory and reproductive tracts to push mucus or an egg in a specific direction. An extra-long form of cilium called a flagellum (fluh-JEL-uhm) is a whiplike extension that propels the cell itself. The human sperm cell has a single flagellum that moves the sperm from one place to another.

The many structures of a cell, with their many activities, work cooperatively to maintain the life cycle of the entire cell. As part of the whole picture, cells are the tiny building blocks that make up tissues, organs, organ systems, and the organism.

Tissues

A tissue is a group of cells that have a similar structure and work together to accomplish a similar function. There are four basic tissue types, each with a unique structure, a specific function, and its own rate of healing. Structure and function are closely related, following the rule of "form follows function." Much of healing depends on nutrient delivery and waste removal, so the healing rate tends to be related to the tissue's blood supply. Epithelial (EH-pih-THEE-lee-uhl) tissue, connective tissue, muscle tissue, and nervous tissue are woven together within the body to provide coverings, support, movement, and control, respectively (Table 3-1). All tissues produce hormones. For example, skin makes vitamin D, fat makes leptin (to regulate appetite), bone makes osteocalcin (to stimulate insulin and testosterone production) and growth factors, and kidneys make erythropoietin.

Epithelial Tissue

Epithelial tissue, or epithelium (EH-pih-THEE-lee-uhm), covers the outside of our bodies, lines cavities and tubes inside our bodies, and forms the glands in the body. Protection, absorption, filtration, excretion, and secretion are functions specific to individual types of epithelia. All epithelial tissues share some common characteristics:

- Epithelial cells fit closely together without many gaps, forming epithelial tissue that is a continuous sheet of tightly joined cells.
- The top surface of epithelium is unattached and exposed to an open space (or was at some point during its development), either the environment or an internal body cavity.

- The bottom surface of epithelium lies on a basement membrane, which is a material secreted by the epithelial cells and has no structure.
- There are no blood vessels in epithelia (they are avascular), so they rely on diffusion of nutrients through the basement membrane.

Epithelia are classified according to the arrangement and shape of the cells within the tissue. By arrangement, epithelia are classified by the number of layers of cells. Simple epithelium is formed with only a single layer of cells. Stratified epithelium has more than one layer of cells in its structure, making it more durable. By cell shape, the classifications include squamous (flat), cuboidal (cube-like), and columnar (column-like). The different types of epithelia are generally identified by their structural layers and cell shape (Fig. 3-8):

- Simple squamous—found in air sacs of the lungs, walls of capillaries, and serous membranes
- Simple cuboidal—in glands and their ducts
- Simple columnar—in mucous membranes and the lining of the digestive tract
- Pseudostratified columnar—in parts of the respiratory tract
- Stratified squamous—in the mouth, outer portion of skin, and esophagus
- Stratified cuboidal—not very common, but found in the ducts of large glands
- Stratified columnar—not very common, but found in the ducts of large glands
- Transitional—highly modified epithelium found in the lining of the urinary bladder, ureters, and part of the urethra

There is a special type of epithelium that does not have lining or covering functions. Glandular epithelium develops into glands, which produce and secrete fluids that contain special proteins. Exocrine (EK-soh-krihn) glands use ducts to deliver their secretions to the top surface of the epithelium. Sweat and oil glands are examples of exocrine glands that release their secretions outside our bodies. The liver and the pancreas are exocrine glands that release their secretions inside our bodies. Endocrine (EN-doh-krihn) glands, which also develop from glandular epithelium, are ductless, so their secretions diffuse directly into the bloodstream. The thyroid, adrenal, and pituitary glands are examples of endocrine glands.

Connective Tissue

Connective tissue serves many different functions and is located throughout the body. It connects one part of the body to another, it provides a gentle support structure to various parts of the body, it protects internal organs, and it

Table 3-1 Types of Tissue

Tissue Type	Function	Location
Epithelium	Lines Covers Produces secretions	Skin, organs, glands
Connective tissue	Connects Protects Supports	Blood, bone, cartilage, fascia, fat, ligament, lymph, tendon
Muscle tissue		
Cardiac	Contracts the heart	Heart
Skeletal	Moves and stabilizes	Attached to skeleton
Smooth	Produces peristalsis	Organs
Nervous tissue	Communication and control	Brain, spinal cord, nerves

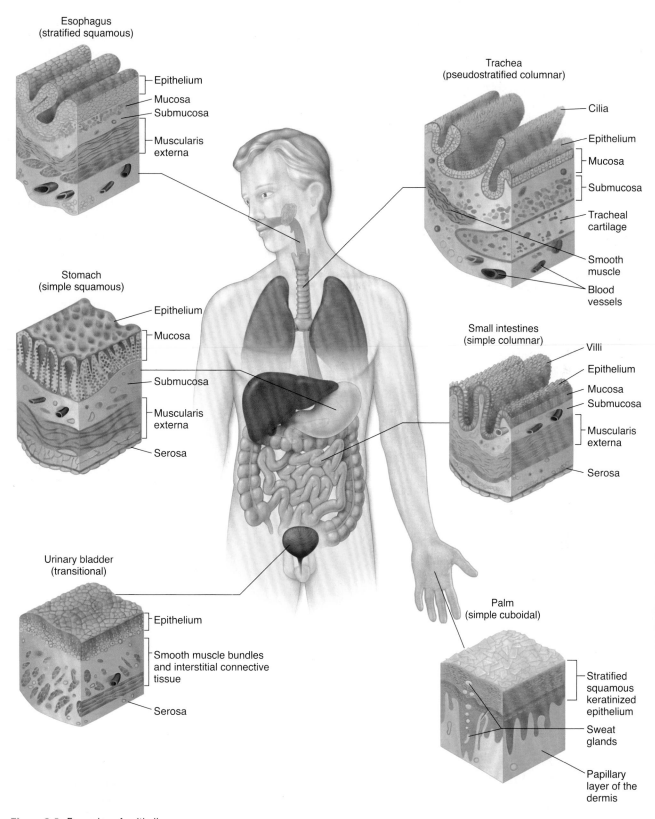

Figure 3-8. Examples of epithelia.

serves as a defensive barrier against disease. It is composed of living cells suspended in their own secretion of a non-living structural material called the ground substance. The ground substance is made up of water, protein fibers, and sometimes hard minerals, collectively called the extracellular matrix. The consistency of the matrix can range from fluid to solid, depending on the density of living cells in the matrix, the kinds and quantities of protein fibers incorporated in the matrix, and the amount of minerals. The matrix can provide a pathway for blood vessels and nerves. Figure 3-9 illustrates connective tissues and their locations in the body.

The protein fibers secreted by the cells and incorporated into the extracellular matrix that provide strength, elasticity, and structural support to varying degrees include collagen (CAHL-uh-jen), elastin (ee-LASS-tin), and reticular (reh-TIK-yoo-lahr) fibers. Collagen fibers are white protein fibers that provide strength in structures such as the bones and tendons. Elastin is a yellow protein fiber with an elastic or stretchy quality that allows structures such as the vocal cords and walls of large blood vessels to return to their original length after being stretched. Reticular fibers are threads of a few collagen fibers that create a delicate, mesh-like web material often found in areolar tissue. The reticular fibers support large numbers of free blood cells in the spleen, lymph nodes, and liver. Figure 3-10 shows the difference between collagen and elastin protein fibers in the extracellular matrix of areolar connective tissue.

The density and arrangement of any one or a combination of these protein fibers contribute to the strength and elasticity of a particular tissue. Dense fibers tend to result in stronger, harder connective tissues. The more loosely these fibers are packed in the matrix, the more pliable the tissue. Fiber arrangements can be random or aligned. When the fibers are aligned

Figure 3-9. Examples of connective tissue in different locations in the body.

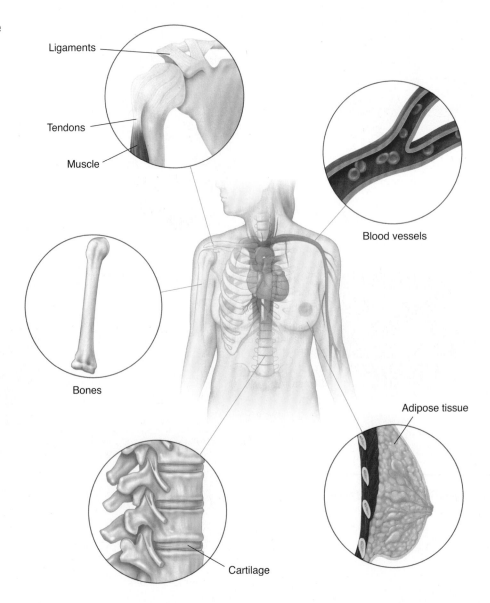

Ligaments

Tendons

Muscle

Blood vessels

Bones

Adipose tissue

Cartilage

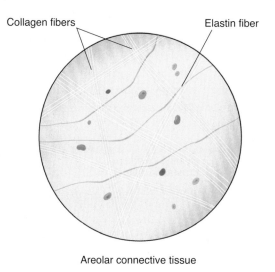

Areolar connective tissue

Figure 3-10. Collagen and elastin fibers in an extracellular matrix.

in the same direction, the tissue resembles ropelike cords, as in the tendons and ligaments. Scar tissue has a random arrangement and has a patchwork-like quality. Connective tissue can be categorized into four groups: hard, fibrous, soft, and liquid. Figure 3-11 illustrates the four types of connective tissues.

Hard Connective Tissue

The hard connective tissues are very firm and not very pliable, and some contain hardened minerals that further solidify their structure. The two forms of hard connective tissue in our bodies include cartilage and bones.

Cartilage

Cartilage is a form of hard connective tissue that is firm, smooth, and bendable. It is composed of living chondrocytes (KON-droh-sahytz), or cartilage cells, suspended in a non-living extracellular matrix that contains collagen and elastin protein fibers. It functions as a shock absorber that can bear mechanical stress without permanent distortion and reduce friction between moving parts, as in the knee joint. Cartilage can also be used as a material for structural support, as in the outer ear. Cartilage is avascular, which makes it slow to heal after injury. It can only receive nourishment via diffusion from capillaries in the adjacent tissues or from the synovial fluid that bathes and lubricates freely movable joints. While temporary cartilage forms the fetal skeleton and is later ossified and converted to bone, permanent cartilage remains throughout life. The three major types of cartilage are hyaline cartilage, fibrocartilage, and elastic cartilage (Table 3-2).

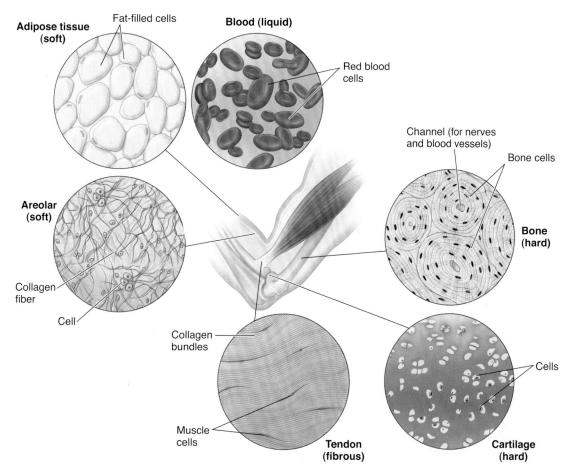

Figure 3-11. Examples of the four types of connective tissue: soft, liquid, hard, and fibrous.

Table 3-2 Types of Cartilage

Cartilage	Characteristics	Examples
Hyaline	Strong, not very flexible	Costal cartilage
Fibrocartilage	Strongest	Intervertebral discs
Elastic	Most flexible	Outer ear

Hyaline cartilage (costal cartilage)

Fibrocartilage (intervertebral discs)

Elastic cartilage (external ear)

Hyaline cartilage is the most common form of permanent cartilage and provides strength and shock absorption but not much flexibility. It appears white or whitish blue because of its avascularity and the predominance of white collagen protein fibers. It is found where two bones come together and need some padding, for example, where the ribs contact the sternum and at the growth zones at the ends of long bones. Hyaline cartilage also provides a structural framework in the walls of large respiratory passages that go from outside the body to the lungs, including the nose, trachea, and bronchi.

Elastic cartilage has an abundance of elastic fibers, which give it a yellowish color and make it the most flexible type of cartilage. It can be bent and return to its normal shape, providing a structural framework for parts of the body that are subjected to higher amounts of movement, such as the external part of the ear, the ear canal, the eustachian tube, and the epiglottis.

Fibrocartilage has dense collagen fibers surrounding rows or groups of chondrocytes, making it extremely resilient. Providing a cushion between bones that are only slightly movable, fibrocartilage is found between adjacent vertebrae (bones in the spine) and in the sutures between the cranial bones.

Bone

Bone is the other form of hard connective tissue. Calcium and phosphate salts that accompany the dense collagen fibers in the extracellular matrix create the hardness of bone. There are three different kinds of living cells suspended in the matrix of bone: osteoblasts (AHS-tee-oh-blastz), or bone-forming cells; osteocytes (AHS-tee-oh-sahytz), or mature bone cells; and osteoclasts (AHS-tee-oh-klastz), or bone-destroying cells. Figure 3-12 shows the difference between the matrix of bone and the matrix of hyaline cartilage.

Bones are much more than a compilation of proteins and minerals. Their structure is a highly organized series of bundles of osteocytes and blood vessels. Because of its high vascularity, bone heals quickly, relative to other tissues. Bone, which is the main component of the skeletal system, has many functions:

- Bones are the main storage place for calcium and other ions.
- Bones act as a lever system for converting muscle contraction into movement.
- Blood cells are formed inside many bones.
- Bones protect soft tissue structures in the body.

Fibrous Connective Tissue

Fibrous connective tissues, sometimes called dense connective tissues, are found as tendons, ligaments, and scar tissue. Most of the protein fibers in the extracellular matrix are collagen fibers that are all aligned in the same direction, giving the fibrous connective tissues a cord-like structure that is strong and flexible.

Tendons connect muscles to bones and, as part of the muscle–tendon (musculotendinous) unit, create skeletal movement. Almost every muscle has at least one tendon attached to it, and some muscles have more than one tendon. Because the tendons themselves do not actively contract or relax, they vary in tension, depending on the activity of the muscles to which they attach. For example, a tendon attached to a muscle that is working against a lot of resistance will feel tight and not very pliable, like an elastic band that has been stretched almost to its limit. A tendon attached to a muscle that is relaxed will feel looser, like a rubber band lying on a table. Specialized tendons that are broad and flat called are called aponeuroses (AP-poh-nur-OH-seez). They provide attachment for broad muscles to connect to bone or for one set of muscles to connect to another.

As a form of fibrous connective tissue, tendons have parallel collagen fibers that are dense and regular. The dense arrangement and poor blood supply make it difficult for the nutrient–waste exchange to occur. Because this exchange occurs mostly through diffusion from the surrounding tissues, injured tendons heal slowly.

Ligaments are fibrous connective tissue structures that connect bones to bones at a joint. They stabilize and strengthen the joints of the body that must withstand great mechanical force, such as the knee and the hip. As in tendons, most of the protein fibers are dense, regular, parallel strands of collagen. Ligaments are more flexible than tendons because there are more elastin fibers and the proportion of ground substance to protein is larger. Ligaments remain tight despite movement or various states of contraction and are more

Figure 3-12. Hard connective tissue matrix: hyaline cartilage and compact bone.

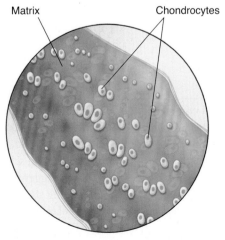

Matrix   Chondrocytes

Hyaline cartilage

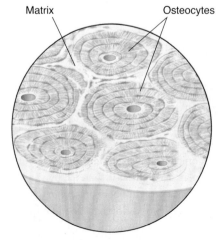

Matrix   Osteocytes

Compact bone

difficult to palpate because of their location within joints. Because of the minimal blood supply to the ligaments at their attachment sites, the healing process is very slow. ▶

Scar tissue is a special kind of fibrous connective tissue that forms when tissues are injured. It is unique because, unlike those in tendons and ligaments, the collagen fibers are not arranged in a parallel pattern. Because of the abundance of dense and irregular collagen fibers, scar tissue is strong but not as pliable as normal, healthy tissue. Serving as a replacement for other injured tissue, it cannot perform the functions of the tissue it replaces, and its blood supply is minimal. Extensive scarring can restrict normal movement, reduce or prevent normal circulation of blood and lymph, and impede or even prevent injured tissue from functioning properly. The structure of scar tissue depends on where the injury occurs, but it usually contains the same components as the original tissue, accompanied by an abundance of extra collagen fibers.

Soft Connective Tissue

Soft connective tissues are also called loose connective tissues. They have more living cells and fewer protein fibers in their matrix and are highly vascular, giving them a relatively fast healing rate.

Areolar (ah-REE-oh-lahr) tissue is a form of soft connective tissue that is highly vascular, delicate, and somewhat resistant to stress. Phagocytes, living cells that engulf bacteria or cellular debris, are present in the matrix, accompanied by few collagen and elastin fibers. Found just below the skin, in membranes around blood and lymph vessels, around organs, and between muscles, areolar tissue cushions and protects the structures it surrounds.

Adipose tissue, commonly called fat, is basically areolar tissue with adipose cells suspended in the matrix. Adipose cells can synthesize fat and store it as a large droplet of oil. When the body needs a source of energy, it can use fat released by adipose cells. Besides its function as a source of energy, adipose tissue acts as a thermal insulator. Heat is not conducted well through the fat, which means that if there are different temperatures on either side of the adipose tissue, those temperatures will be maintained. Adipose tissue also provides padding and protection for organs in its locations just beneath the skin in the superficial fascia, around organs, between muscles, in the marrow of the long bone shafts, and in the breasts and hips.

Liquid Connective Tissue

Blood and lymph are sometimes called liquid connective tissues because they have living cells suspended in a nonliving matrix and they "connect" different parts of the body. Technically, however, neither blood nor lymph has an extracellular matrix that is secreted by the living cells. Moreover, blood has protein fibers present in the matrix only during the process of blood clotting. Blood flows through the blood vessels of the cardiovascular system, and lymph flows through the lymphatic vessels in the lymphatic system. Blood and lymph are described in more detail in the sections on the cardiovascular system and the lymphatic system, respectively.

Muscle Tissue

Tissues are a group of cells with similar structure and function. Muscle tissue is a group of muscle cells that are grouped together with blood vessels and packaged with connective tissue in a specific organization, more commonly called a **muscle**. These cells have an elongated shape and are sometimes referred to as muscle fibers. Muscle cells have the special ability to contract and relax, resulting in their primary function of creating movement. Skeletal, cardiac, and smooth muscle tissues are the three types of muscle tissue that have slightly different characteristics and arrangements. Some have striations (strahy-AY-shunz), which are microscopic structural features that look like stripes. Some muscle cells contain more than one nucleus, and some muscle cells form branching networks of cells. The control mechanism for muscle cells can also differ. Some are involuntary, meaning that they contract without our conscious effort, and others are voluntary, which means that we have to consciously make an effort to contract the muscle to create movement. Table 3-3 characterizes the different types of muscle tissue. This section of the body systems chapter briefly introduces and compares the different kinds of muscle tissue. There is a comprehensive discussion of skeletal muscle tissue below in this chapter.

Skeletal Muscle

Skeletal muscle is tissue that attaches to the skeleton. The cells are long and cylindrical with multiple nuclei and heavy striations. Skeletal muscle tissue is under voluntary control, meaning that we consciously make skeletal muscles contract to move our bodies. When actively contracted, skeletal muscles are shortened and the muscles cells are closer together. As a result, blood vessels are constricted, and the delivery of nutrients and elimination of cellular metabolic waste is limited. Healthy muscles at their normal resting length have more space between the cells and the exchange of oxygen, nutrients, and waste is more efficient. Skeletal muscle tissue is responsible for producing body movement and holding our bodies up against the force of gravity. Simply, gravity is the force that pulls us to the earth, and except when we are lying down, we use skeletal muscles to hold ourselves upright.

Massage deals with movement, restriction of movement, and restoration of health to the skeletal muscle system. **Understanding skeletal muscle tissue and how it functions is fundamental to massage.** Massage can relax hypertonic (tense) skeletal muscles by using the help of the nervous system to stop triggering muscles to contract. Once the muscles stop receiving signals from the nervous system to contract, they can relax, and then other massage techniques can help return skeletal muscles to their normal resting lengths. Using massage to return skeletal muscles to their normal

Table 3-3 Different Types of Muscle Tissue, Characteristics, and Locations

Type of Muscle Cell	Cell Characteristics	Control	Function	Location
Smooth	Tapered at both ends Single nucleus Nonstriated	Involuntary	Slow, sustained contractions (peristalsis)	Blood vessels Intestines
	 Nucleus			
Cardiac	Branching networks Single nucleus Light striations	Involuntary	Pumps blood out of the heart	Wall of heart
	Intercalated discs Nucleus			
Skeletal	Long, cylindrical Multinucleated Heavy striations	Voluntary	Movement of skeleton	Attached to bones
	 Nucleus			

resting lengths allows sufficient space between muscle cells for adequate blood circulation and nutrient–waste exchange, thus enhancing the health of the tissues. Reflexive and mechanical techniques are covered in detail in the Massage Strokes and Flow and Therapeutic Applications chapters.

Cardiac Muscle

Cardiac muscle is another type of muscle tissue that is found only in the walls of the heart. It has light striations and only one nucleus per muscle cell, but the cells branch together at tight junctions and gap junctions called intercalated (in-TER-kuh-lay-ted) discs. The gap junctions allow the electrical impulses that signal muscle contraction to move quickly across the heart. Cardiac muscle contracts involuntarily, which is why our heart continues to beat while we are asleep and why we cannot consciously control the contractions.

Smooth Muscle

Smooth muscle, sometimes called visceral muscle, has cells that are nonstriated and tapered at both ends. Each smooth muscle cell has only one nucleus and is involuntarily controlled. Although it provides a weaker contraction than skeletal or cardiac muscle, it can sustain contractions for a longer time. Smooth muscle tends to be arranged in layers, and the fibers of each successive layer run in a different direction than those in the previous layer. Figure 3-13 illustrates smooth muscle layering in the stomach. These layers alternate contractions to produce peristalsis, which is the wavelike pulsating contraction that propels substances along a tube in the body. For example, the digestive tract has layers of smooth muscle that push its contents in one direction, from the mouth toward the anus, via peristalsis.

Nervous Tissue

Nervous tissue has a specialized structure that serves as the communication path for controlling activity within our bodies. The nervous tissues send electrochemical impulses to and from different parts of the body to receive stimuli and trigger bodily responses. The structural components that make up the brain, spinal cord, and nerves include two kinds of nervous tissue cells called neurons (NOO-rahnz) and neuroglia (noo-ROH-glee-uh).

Neurons

A **neuron**, or **nerve cell**, is a specialized cell that is the basic unit of nervous tissue. A neuron has a unique structure with three basic parts: a body, a single axon, and dendrites (Fig. 3-14). The body of the neuron is similar

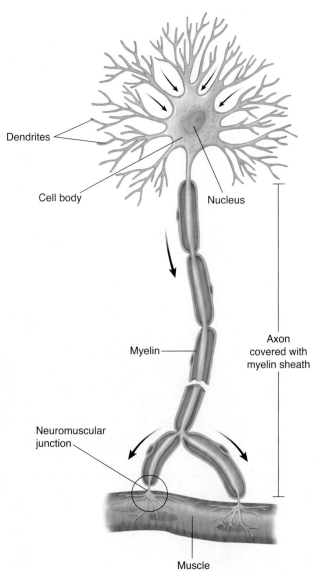

Figure 3-14. Basic nerve cell structure.

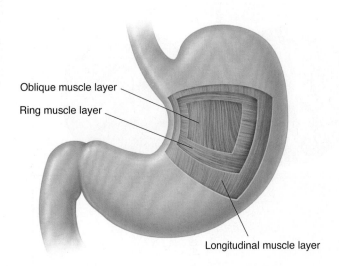

Figure 3-13. Layering of smooth muscle in the stomach.

to other cells because of its generally rounded shape that holds the nucleus and other cytoplasmic organelles. Unlike other cells, the cytoplasm and plasma membrane have long branches that protrude from the body of the cell that receive and send the electrochemical impulses of nerve signal transmission. Dendrites are the processes radiating out from the cell body that receive electrochemical nerve impulses from other neurons and carry them to the cell body. Neurons usually have a lot of dendrites and can receive input from many other neurons. The axon is a long, single process radiating out from the body of the neuron that conducts nerve impulses from the cell body to another cell. Axons can also branch to carry impulses to many cells at once. The process of nerve signal transmission is like a chain of communication in which the dendrites receive the signal and pass it along to the cell body, and then the axon carries the signal from the cell body to another neuron, where it is received by the dendrites of the second neuron, and so on. Massage activates this chain of communication in a number of ways. For example, when we first touch our clients, the tactile input stimulates

an electrochemical impulse to travel along the plasma membrane from the dendrites, toward the cell body, out the axon, and then to another neuron. The impulse continues to travel along the neurons until it reaches the central nervous system (CNS), at which point the client's body responds to the initial touch. The client's response will be influenced by your professionalism, standards of care, and respect for the client's physical and conceptual boundaries, discussed in the chapter covering Ethics and Professionalism.

Some neurons are covered with a white, fatty material called myelin. It functions as insulation, significantly increasing the speed of nerve impulses. When myelinated nerves lose their myelin or the myelin becomes hardened, nerve transmission may become problematic. Myelinated axons appear as white fibers that, when grouped together, are called white matter. Groups of unmyelinated nerve cells are called gray matter. Figure 3-15 is a cross section of the spinal cord, showing the gray matter of the nerve cell bodies and the white matter made of myelinated axons.

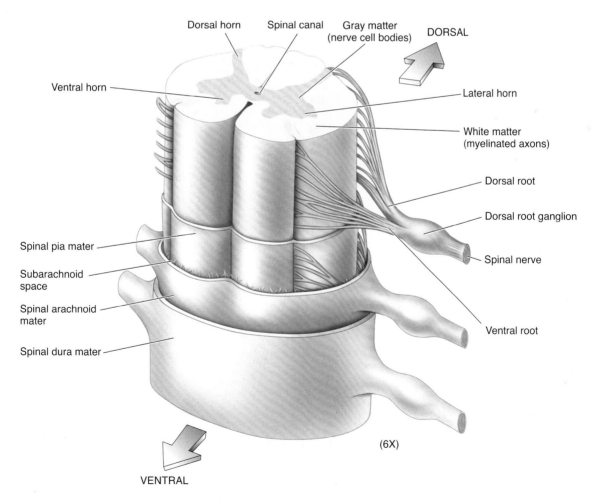

Figure 3-15. Cross section of the spinal cord, showing the gray and white matter. (Reprinted from Bear MF, Connors BW, Parasido MA. *Neuroscience: Exploring the Brain.* 2nd ed. Philadelphia: Lippincott Williams & Wilkins, 2001.)

Neuroglia

Neuroglia, also called glial (GLEE-uhl) cells, are connective tissue cells that support and protect neurons, connect them to blood vessels, produce myelin, destroy and remove pathogens and cellular debris, and help circulate the cerebrospinal fluid (CSF). They are structurally similar to neurons but cannot transmit impulses.

Tissue Membranes

Membranes are thin sheets of tissues with many different characteristics that give rise to different functions:

- Serve as a covering for the outside of the body
- Serve as a covering for organs
- Serve as an anchor for organs

- Act as a partition between structures
- Serve as a lining for tubes of cavities in the body
- Reduce friction between structures

Membranes can be fragile, tough, or transparent, and some contain cells that secrete lubricating fluids. There are two general classifications of membranes: epithelial and connective tissue membranes.

Epithelial Membranes

Epithelial membranes are constructed with an epithelium that is integrated onto an underlying layer of connective tissue. The connective tissue layer, in addition to the closely packed epithelial cells, creates strong and protective membranes. There are three types of epithelial membranes: serous (SEER-us), mucous (MYOO-kus), and cutaneous (kyoo-TAY-nee-us) (Fig. 3-16).

Figure 3-16. Locations of epithelial membranes. **(A)** Serous. **(B)** Mucous. **(C)** Cutaneous.

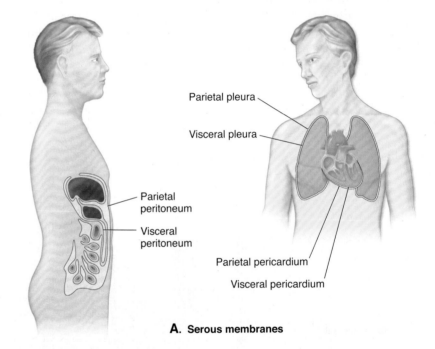

Parietal pleura

Visceral pleura

Parietal peritoneum

Visceral peritoneum

Parietal pericardium

Visceral pericardium

A. Serous membranes

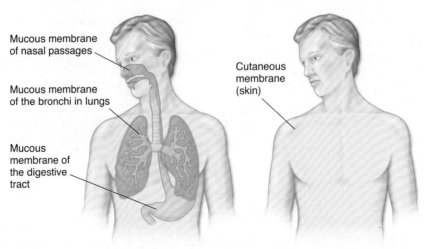

Mucous membrane of nasal passages

Mucous membrane of the bronchi in lungs

Mucous membrane of the digestive tract

Cutaneous membrane (skin)

B. Mucous membrane   **C. Cutaneous membrane**

Serous Membranes

Serous membranes are composed of a layer of simple squamous epithelial cells atop a thin layer of areolar connective tissue. The serous membranes line the ventral (anterior) body cavities and cover the organs within those cavities. Serous membranes contain cells that secrete serous fluid, a thin lubricant that allows organs to move and slip past each other with minimal friction during normal body movements. Serous membranes have a layered, folded construction that forms two different layers of each membrane. The parietal (puh-RAHY-eh-tuhl) layer of a serous membrane lines the wall of a body cavity, and the visceral layer of that same serous membrane covers the organs within that body cavity.

Three types of serous membranes, shown in Fig. 3-16A, are found in the human body: the pleura (PLUR-uh), the pericardium (PAIR-ih-KAR-dee-um), and the peritoneum (PAIR-ih-toh-NEE-um). The pleura, or pleural membranes, are located in the thoracic cavity. The parietal layer of the pleura lines the interior walls of the thoracic cavity, and the visceral layer covers the lungs. The pericardium is also located in the thoracic cavity, but its parietal layer forms the sac that encloses the heart, and its visceral layer covers the heart muscle itself. The peritoneum is located in the abdominal cavity. The parietal peritoneum lines the abdominal cavity walls and the visceral peritoneum covers, supports, and protects most of the organs and structures within the abdomen.

Mucous Membranes

Mucous membranes are epithelial membranes that line tubes and spaces that are exposed to the outside of the body. These membranes are made of simple and/or stratified epithelium resting on a layer of soft connective tissue and form continuous linings in the digestive, respiratory, reproductive, and urinary systems. The primary function of most of these wet membranes is to secrete mucus, a viscous and sticky substance that moistens and protects the membranes.

Examples of mucous membranes are shown in Fig. 3-16B. In the nasal passages and the bronchi in the lungs, mucus keeps the passages wet, despite exposure to external air. The mucus also traps pathogens that enter the respiratory pathway. Ciliated cells in the respiratory tract then sweep the mucus and foreign particles up and outward, away from the lungs, to protect us against infection and to get rid of pathogens that have already entered the respiratory tract. In the digestive tract, the mucus has several different functions. It acts as a protective barrier against the strong acids that break down food. When the mucus barrier breaks down, the acids can attack the organs, resulting in ulcers and irritation within the digestive tract. The mucous membranes located toward the end of the digestive tract secrete mucus that traps the nutrients made available as a result of our food being broken down.

Cutaneous Membrane

Cutaneous membrane, commonly called skin, has an outer layer of stratified squamous epithelial tissue over a layer of connective tissue (Fig. 3-16C). Functioning primarily to protect the body from the environment, the cutaneous membrane is the only kind that is dry. The skin is discussed in the section on the integumentary system.

Connective Tissue Membranes

Connective tissue membranes consist of sheets of connective tissue without an attached epithelium. The different forms of connective tissue membranes include synovial membranes, meninges, connective tissue sacs around organs, and fascia.

Synovial Membranes

Synovial (sin-OH-vee-uhl) membranes line the joint cavities, tendon sheaths, and bursae, which are the small cushioning sacs located in some of the larger joints. These membranes secrete synovial fluid, a thick, clear substance that has the consistency of egg white. This slippery secretion nourishes the articular cartilage and lubricates and reduces friction in the following locations:

- At the freely movable joints
- Between muscles
- Between a tendon and ligament
- Between a muscle and a ligament

Meninges

Meninges (men-IN-jeez) consist of multiple membrane layers that cover the brain and spinal cord. The dura mater, arachnoid mater, and pia mater are the three meningeal layers that function as protective coverings. These connective tissue membranes are discussed below, in the section on the nervous system.

Connective Tissue Coverings

Connective tissue surrounds many anatomical structures in the form of connective tissue sacs. The heart is encased in a fibrous membrane sac called the pericardium, the bones are covered with periosteum, and cartilage is covered with perichondrium.

Fascia

Fascia (FASH-uh), sometimes called the fascial sheath, is a fibrous band or sheetlike tissue membrane that provides support and protection for the body organs. **Fascia wraps around everything in the body, stabilizing, protecting, and supporting organs and muscles.** Fascia is very pervasive, forming a sort of three-dimensional meshwork throughout the body. A restriction or adhesion in the fascia is an area where the smooth membrane has been crumpled or kinked with some sort of trauma; additional collagen fibers are deposited in the area, and a scar is created that pulls the surrounding fascia toward it. This resultant tension and pulling action can even affect anatomical structures that are a significant distance away, causing a number of problems:

- Restricted movement
- Compensation patterns
- Reduced circulation
- Muscular tension
- Pain in areas that seem completely unrelated

This situation is common following surgery. For a couple of weeks after surgery, the area that was surgically repaired is usually subjected to minimal movement to give the incision a chance to heal. The fascia has already been disrupted, and without movement, the body's healing response deposits fascia on top of the disruption, essentially fixing the disruption into place with a fascial adhesion. The three-dimensional nature of fascia creates a situation where the rest of the fascia is pulled toward the adhesion. For example, clients who have ankle surgery may complain of tightness or restricted movement in the knee. Clients who have abdominal surgery could feel tightness in the neck or shoulder. Massage therapy can reduce fascial restrictions, helping to restore normal function to the body. Specific massage techniques have been especially designed to manipulate the fascia and are discussed in the Therapeutic Applications chapter.

Superficial fascia is a continuous sheetlike layer composed of mostly adipose connective tissue with some interspersed collagen and elastin fibers that provide:

- Energy from the fat stored in the adipose cells
- Protection for the skin

- A passageway for nerves
- A passageway for circulatory vessels
- Thermal insulation

Sometimes called the subcutaneous layer or the hypodermis, superficial fascia lies just beneath the surface of the skin. It is dense and anchors the skin firmly to underlying tissues.

Deep fascia is found in and around every skeletal muscle. It wraps almost every structure of a muscle, starting with the wrapping around a muscle cell, called the endomysium. Several wrapped fibers together form fascicles, which are wrapped in perimysium. The entire muscle, made up of several fascicles, is wrapped in the epimysium. Figure 3-17 shows the deep fascia surrounding structures of a muscle. Deep fascia contains no fat and is mostly composed of collagen fibers and some elastin, making it very strong and a little pliable. It functions to cover, separate, and protect the muscles. This tissue has a thixotropic quality, meaning that it is a gelatinous substance that without movement can thicken, contract, and become less pliable. When the deep fascia is stiff and contracted, it restricts muscle movement and circulation within the muscles. On the other hand, the thixotropic quality also means that deep fascia can be thinned to a more fluid or liquid state with mechanical manipulation. Massage therapy can provide the manipulation to thin the deep fascia and encourage movement and circulation. A special form of deep fascia, thicker than the muscular coverings and running transversely to the muscle fibers, is called a retinaculum. Found in small areas that contain numerous tendons, such as the wrist and ankle, retinacula hold the tendons down in a particular position or location.

The 12 Body Systems

Anatomy and physiology of the human body is a large and very complex topic that can easily overwhelm any student. For that reason, the information is often broken up into smaller pieces that are more approachable. As mentioned before, this text presents only an introduction to human anatomy and physiology, dividing the information into 12 separate body systems: integumentary, skeletal, muscular, nervous, cardiovascular, lymphatic, respiratory, digestive, urinary, endocrine, reproductive, and special senses.

Integumentary System

The integumentary (in-TEG-yoo-MENT-ah-ree) system includes the skin, hair, nails, and the glands that reside

in or near the skin. Massage therapists should know about the integumentary structures, particularly the skin, because the client's skin is the initial point of physical contact and is touched continually throughout the massage.

Functions of the Integumentary System

The main function of the integumentary system is to protect our bodies from the environment, but it also serves as a means of communication, helps regulate body temperature, provides a means of excretion, and participates in the formation of vitamin D.

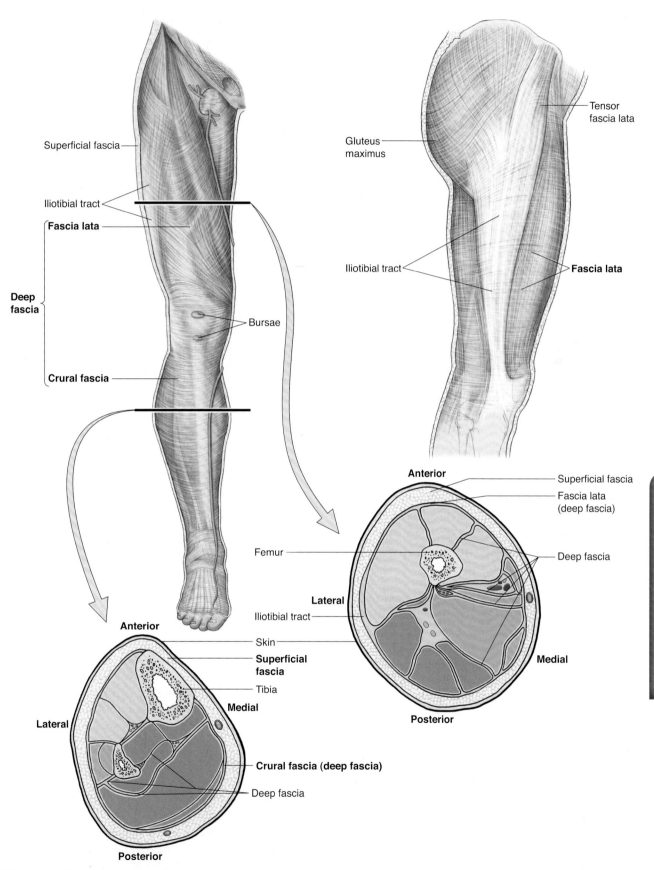

Figure 3-17. Deep fascia surrounding muscle.

Protection

The skin is waterproof and resistant to many chemicals and bacteria. Its strength and pliability make it tough to outside physical forces such as sharp edges. Essentially, it keeps the inside structures in and the outside substances out. Keratin is a protein in skin cells that makes our skin water repellant, so water cannot soak through it. Acidic skin secretions help resist chemical damage and help prevent bacterial growth. Additionally, the skin protects the body from ultraviolet radiation damage. Coloration cells in the skin are called melanocytes (meh-LAN-oh-sahytz). Exposure to sunlight increases the production of melanin, creating a suntan. The darkening of the skin helps shield the cell nucleus from ultraviolet damage, like sunglasses for the DNA.

Communication

Most essential for massage therapy is the skin's communication function. Cutaneous receptors in the skin detect touch, pressure, pain, and temperature and send their sensory signals to the brain and spinal cord for processing. These structures are made of nervous tissue. In addition to the skin's function of transmitting external stimuli to the inside of our bodies, the color and texture of the skin can reveal information about the processes going on inside the body. For instance, a liver dysfunction can lead to excessive amounts of liver chemicals that make the skin yellowish. Low levels of oxygen in the blood will cause the skin to look grayish.

Thermal Regulation

A very important function of the integumentary system is thermal regulation. The skin helps regulate body temperature via the capillaries, sweat glands, and fat. The body's thermostat recognizes a safe range for core body temperature. When the core temperature is too high, the body responds with vasodilation, or expanding blood vessels, in the skin. That allows heat to be dissipated by the large surface of the skin. When the core temperature drops too low, the body responds with vasoconstriction (blood vessel constriction) in the skin, which reduces blood flow to the skin in an effort to conserve heat in the body. Sweat glands diffuse water through the skin, and in a low-humidity environment, the water evaporates and helps cool the body. Evaporative cooling is less effective when humidity in the air is high, because the water from our bodies cannot diffuse into the air. Subcutaneous fat, or the fat in the superficial fascia, also acts as a thermal insulator, preventing heat from being transferred into or out of the body. In cold temperatures, fat keeps body heat in the body and does not allow the cold external temperatures to affect the internal organs,

which is usually a good thing. However, when it is hot, fat still keeps body heat in the body, which makes it harder for the body to dissipate heat and maintain the proper core temperature.

Excretion

Excretion (ehks-KREE-shun) is a minor role of the integumentary system. Metabolic processes create chemical wastes that the body cannot use. The body can eliminate unwanted salts and water from the skin via perspiration. Nitrogen wastes such as urea are also excreted in minimal amounts through the skin.

Vitamin D Formation

Vitamin D is critical in the process of absorption of calcium for proper bone growth and normal cell growth. The production of vitamin D is another important function of the skin. Although we can obtain vitamin D from food sources such as milk, this is one of two vitamins that can be produced by the body. A form of cholesterol located in the skin, when exposed to the sun's ultraviolet rays, is converted into vitamin D.

Structures of the Integumentary System

The skin is the main structure of the integumentary system, but there are also some specialized structures located in or near the skin, including hair, nails, and cutaneous glands. **The skin, sometimes called the integument, is the largest organ of the body.**

Skin

The skin has a two-layered structure consisting of the epidermis and dermis (Fig. 3-18). The skin, like all epithelial membranes, has a layer of epithelial tissue atop a layer of connective tissue. The epidermis is the epithelial layer, and the dermis is the connective tissue layer. The subcutaneous layer, also called superficial fascia or the hypodermis, is another connective tissue layer beneath the dermis and is sometimes considered part of the skin.

Epidermis

The outermost layer of our skin, the epithelial layer, is called the epidermis. It is nonvascular, like all epithelia, and is composed of up to five layers. From deepest to most superficial, they are the stratum germinativum, stratum spinosum, stratum granulosum, stratum lucidum, and stratum corneum. The epidermis is constantly being regenerated,

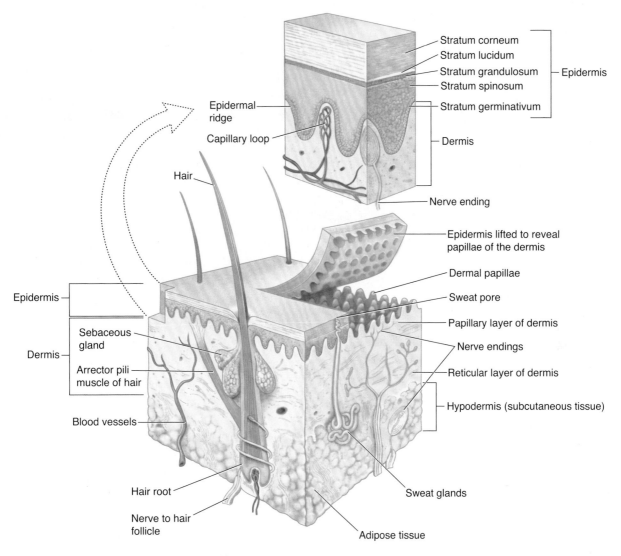

Figure 3-18. Cross-sectional illustration of skin.

which it does rapidly via cell division. Skin cells are formed in the stratum germinativum, the deepest layer that is closest to the blood vessels in the underlying dermis. The skin cells slowly progress upward and outward until they reach the external environment. As they migrate outward, they accumulate water-repelling keratin and get farther from the blood vessels that supply nutrients and oxygen. Fortunately for us, these deteriorated skin cells are sloughed off when they reach the external environment. It takes approximately 2 to 4 weeks for a cell to migrate through a layer of epidermis, meaning that in 2 to 4 weeks, a person has a completely new outer layer of skin. This process of renewal keeps our skin healthy and alive and gives us a water-repellant outer covering. This constant renewal also helps protect against cancer by ensuring that damaged cells die before cancer can develop.

Dermis

The dermis is the layer of connective tissue beneath the epithelium. It is constructed of two layers. The superficial papillary layer is named for its dermal papillae, which are like spiked mountains that stick up into the epidermis. The papillae are highly vascular structures that provide oxygen and nutrients to the epidermis that surrounds them. Pain receptors and tactile sensory receptors reside within the dermal papillae. Beneath the papillary layer is the reticular layer. It is a dense form of connective tissue that contains blood vessels, sweat glands, sebaceous glands, and the sensory receptors for cold, heat, and pressure. The specific sensory receptors are discussed in detail in the nervous system section, but Figure 3-19 illustrates the kinds of sensory reception in the skin. Collagen and elastin protein fibers give the dermis its toughness and elasticity. Collagen fibers are hydrophilic, meaning that they attract water molecules and hold onto them, keeping the skin

Figure 3-19. Five different kinds of sensory receptors in skin.

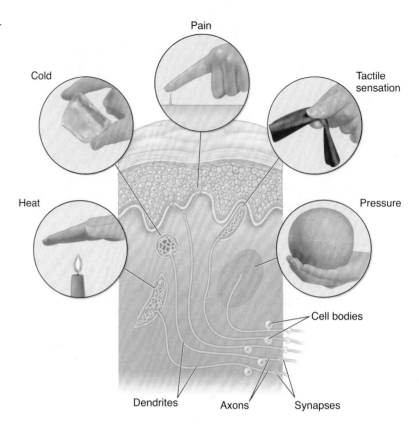

hydrated. Elastin fibers give skin elasticity, which is noticeable in young children. As we age, the collagen and elastin wear out and diminish, giving us wrinkled, dry skin.

Subcutaneous Layer

The subcutaneous (SUB-kyoo-TAY-nee-us) layer, also known as the hypodermis or superficial fascia, lies deep to the dermis. It is connected to the dermis with numerous bundles of elastin protein fibers, so it is difficult to tell where the dermis stops and the subcutaneous layer starts. This fascia binds the skin to the underlying organs and structures, provides shock absorption, serves as a thermal insulator, and provides energy storage. It is highly vascular, has many nerve endings, and contains adipose (fat) cells. The number of fat cells in a particular person's superficial fascia varies from one area of the body to another. For example, the superficial fascia in the breasts and hips tends to have more fat cells than the superficial fascia on the hands or elbows. With age or significant weight loss, subcutaneous fat in adipose cells tends to diminish, and the skin will start to sag.

Nails

Fingernails and toenails are special structures of the skin (Fig. 3-20A). The free edge of the nail and the body of the nail are made of hard keratin and are not alive. The nail body lies upon the nail bed, which is a very thin epidermal layer over the vascular dermis. This is the part that bleeds when someone tears a nail too far back. Nails grow from the root, and their growth rate can be affected by temperature. The general health of the body can be detected in the nails because they are the tangible, visible outcome of metabolic activity. A disease or dysfunction in the body affects homeostasis, and imbalances may show up as a difference in the quality of the nail. For example, nails that are thin and weak can be a result of poor nutrition. Nails that appear bluish can indicate poor circulation in the underlying dermis.

Hair

Hair is present almost everywhere on the body but is more visible in some areas than in others. It is a nonliving, keratinized protein structure that grows upward from follicles in the subcutaneous layer. The follicle receives its nutrients from the blood vessels surrounding it. When fully developed, hair extends from its root at the base of a long shaft up through the skin and out into the environment (Fig. 3-20B). Hair provides animals with an additional layer of protection, as a way of regulating body temperature and as a mechanism of safety when being faced by a predator. A tiny arrector pili muscle connects the follicle to the dermis, and when it contracts, it pushes the hair out farther to make the animal appear larger (see Fig. 3-18). The same mechanism can trap air and provide a layer of thermal insulation if the hair is thick enough. In humans, however, arrector pili muscle contraction usually produces the familiar "goose bumps" on the skin. What little purpose hair serves for humans includes light insulation and protection from sunburn. Incidentally,

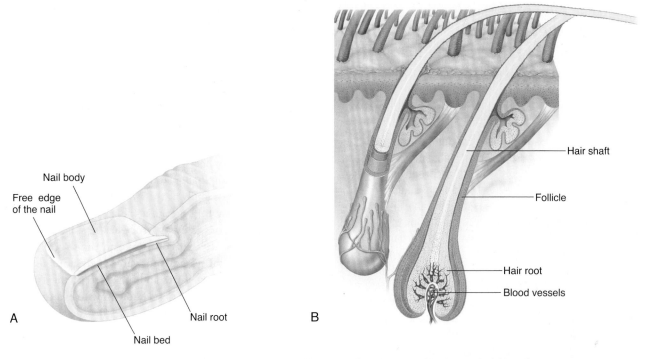

Figure 3-20. Structure of fingernail and hair root. **(A)** Nail. **(B)** Hair root. (Part B provided by Anatomical Chart Co.)

what people commonly call "pores" on the face are actually the openings of hair follicles.

Cutaneous Glands

The two types of glands in the integument are sudoriferous (SOO-doh-RIF-fer-us), which produce sweat, and sebaceous (seh-BAY-shus), which secrete oil. These exocrine glands release their secretions directly to the outer surface of the skin through ducts.

Sudoriferous glands, or sweat glands, can be classified even more specifically as eccrine or apocrine sweat glands. Eccrine sweat glands are simple coiled tubular glands that open to the surface of the skin with pores. They are found all over the body and are especially abundant in the soles of the feet, palms of the hands, and forehead, where there are not many hair follicles. These types of sweat glands secrete sweat, which is a thin fluid consisting mostly of water, some salts, and waste. When sweat reaches the surface of the skin, it evaporates and helps cool the body, which is a very important mechanism of thermal regulation.

The large, branched apocrine sweat glands are found mostly in the axilla (armpit) and genital area, but they are also located in the ear canal, eyelid, and mammary areola. They produce an odorless secretion triggered by puberty, stress, pain, and excitement, and their ducts open into the upper part of the hair follicles, but their function is not fully understood. If bacteria accumulate in the secretion, they break down the apocrine secretions and an unpleasant odor is released. Some apocrine glands are highly specialized to produce milk and are found in the mammary areola; ear canal glands are modified to produce earwax.

The sebaceous glands are exocrine glands, but their ducts do not reach the surface of the skin. Instead, sebaceous glands release their secretion into the hair follicle and it travels to the skin's surface through the follicle. They secrete sebum, which is a mixture of fats, waxes, oil, and cellular debris. It is transported to the surface of the skin via the hair follicles to soften the skin, hinder evaporation, and kill bacteria.

The skin does not "breathe" or serve as an exchange for gases. It is only an avenue for transportation of perspiration and oil from the sweat and sebaceous glands.

Effects of Massage on the Integumentary System

The skin is loaded with sensory receptors and is the point of contact between you and your clients. When you initially place your hands lightly on your client, the touch can trigger the sympathetic nervous system, or the stressful "fight or flight" response. However, if you sustain the light touch or moderately increase the pressure, a shift occurs and the parasympathetic nervous system is activated, which is the relaxation response (See Research Box 3.1). Sustained superficial techniques such as simply resting your hands on a client's skin, light strokes, and fine vibration can reduce anxiety, decrease pain, and decrease muscle tension.

RESEARCH BOX 3-1

Massage and the Parasympathetic Nervous System Response

Twenty healthy adults were randomly assigned to a moderate pressure or light pressure massage therapy group, and EKGs were recorded during a 3-min baseline, during the 15-min massage period, and during a 3-min postmassage period. EKG data were then used to derive the high frequency (HF), low frequency (LF) components of heart variability and the low to high frequency ratio (LF/HF) as noninvasive markers of autonomic nervous system activity. The participants who received the moderate pressure massage exhibited a parasympathetic nervous system response characterized by an increase in HF, suggesting increased vagal efferent activity and a decrease in the LF/HF ratio, suggesting a shift from sympathetic to parasympathetic activity that peaked during the first half of the massage period. On the other hand, those who received the light pressure massage exhibited a sympathetic nervous system response characterized by decreased HF and increased LF/HF.

Moderate pressure appears to be necessary for massage therapy effects. Studies comparing moderate and light pressure massage are reviewed and they suggest that growth and development are enhanced in infants and stress is reduced in adults, but only by moderate pressure massage. The stimulation of pressure receptors leads to increased vagal activity which, in turn, seems to mediate the diverse benefits noted for massage therapy.

Diego MA, Field T. Moderate pressure massage elicits a parasympathetic nervous system response. Int J Neurosci 2009;119:630–638.

Field T, Diego M, Hernandez-Reif M. Moderate pressure is essential for massage therapy effects. Int J Neurosci 2010;120:381–385.

Mechanically, massage warms the skin with friction and increases circulation of blood and lymph in the skin. The enhanced heat and circulation stimulate the sebaceous glands to produce more secretions that make the skin more supple and pliable, and increase sweat production, which has a cooling effect on the body when the sweat evaporates.

Adhesions in the subcutaneous layer, or superficial fascia, can constrict the circulatory vessels, reducing the local flow of blood and lymph and restricting movement of muscles and nearby tissues. Massage is an effective treatment for breaking down fascial adhesions to restore circulation and movement.

Skeletal System

The skeletal system, sometimes called the skeleton, is made up of the bones of the body, the joints between bones, and the connective tissue cartilage and ligaments. Bones come in all shapes and sizes. Because bones are sometimes viewed simply as the hard structural support of the body, it is easy to forget that they are alive. **Bones are living tissue.** There are living processes occurring within the individual bones that contribute to the overall functions of the skeletal system and whole-body homeostasis. Understanding the structures and functions of the skeletal system helps massage therapists know how to evaluate and assess their clients' bodies and provide the safest and most effective treatment.

Structures of the Bones

The bones have structural aspects at the cellular level that are only visible with a microscope. There is also an overall structural view of the bones that we can see with our eyes, including visible structures, shapes, and exterior projections or depressions. There are two types of bone tissue that are visibly distinguishable: spongy bone and compact bone.

Microscopic Structures of Bones

Different types of bone tissue have a different microscopic structure that contributes to their different overall appearance. Spongy bone, sometimes called cancellous bone, resembles a brittle sponge. Its airy, mesh-like structure looks similar under a microscope. Compact bone, however, looks dense and ivory-like until you see the microscopic structures. The basic unit of bone tissue is the osteocyte, literally translated as bone cell. The arrangement of the osteocytes in compact bone tissue is very different from that in spongy bone tissue. The osteocytes are microscopically arranged in visibly concentric rings called lamellae (lah-MEL-lee). The rings form around a central haversian canal, also called the central canal, which can contain blood vessels, nerves, and lymph vessels. The many central canals are interconnected with blood vessels that travel through Volkmann's canals, also called transverse canals. Radiating from the central canal, out through the lamellae, are canaliculi, which are minute canals containing osteocyte extensions that transport nutrients to every osteocyte. Figure 3-21 illustrates compact and spongy bone tissue.

Microscopic osteoblasts and osteoclasts participate in bone formation, growth, and remodeling. They are discussed below in this section on the skeletal system.

Figure 3-21. Structure of a long bone, including spongy bone and compact bone.

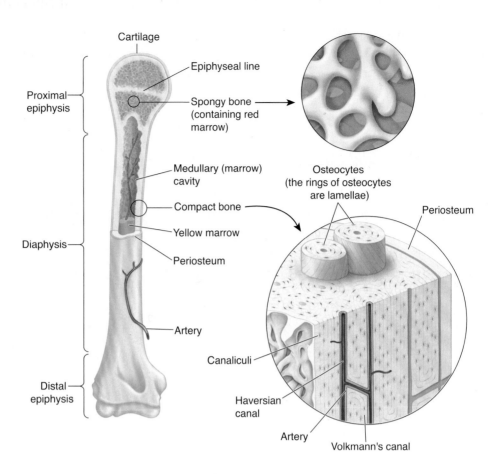

Visible Structures of Bones

The bones are covered outside with a periosteum (membrane), which is a tough fibrous sheath that covers all but the joint region of a bone. It is firmly connected to the bone with hundreds of connective tissue fibers and contains a network of nerves, blood vessels, and lymphatic vessels that supply the bone. Osteoblasts, involved in bone formation, are also present in the periosteum.

Bone Shapes

The human skeleton has bones of all shapes and sizes. They are classified as short, flat, irregular, and long bones. Figure 3-22 shows the four bone shapes.

Short bones are typically shaped like cubes or elongated cubes. The carpals of the wrist are short bones. Again, the periosteum covers all but their articular surfaces. A sesamoid bone, such as the kneecap, is a special kind of short bone embedded in tendons or ligaments.

Flat bones are platelike and often slightly curved. The ribs and cranial bones are flat bones. Red marrow fills cavities of spongy bone of the flat bones and makes red blood cells (RBCs).

The bones that do not fit into any of the other categories are called irregular bones. The vertebrae and facial bones are irregular bones.

Long bones are the ones most familiar to people. They are long and narrow with knobby ends and have a hollow inner cavity. The structure of a long bone is outlined below.

Structures of a Long Bone

Long bones are longer than they are wide, including bones such as the femur (FEE-mer) in the thigh and the humerus (HYOO-mer-us) in the upper arm. Their structure consists of a long, narrow shaft called the diaphysis (dahy-AFF-ih-sis) with two knobby ends called epiphyses (ee-PIH-fih-seez) (see Fig. 3-21 for the structure of a long bone). At the core of the compact bone diaphysis is the medullary cavity that contains bone marrow. The medullary cavity is filled with yellow marrow, which contains mostly fat. The epiphyses, the knobby ends of the long bones, are primarily made of spongy bone but are wrapped with a thin layer of compact bone. They are often part of a joint, articulating with other bones. Inside the epiphyses is red marrow that produces RBCs. Between the epiphysis and diaphysis is an epiphyseal line that looks like a thin strip of compact bone in the midst of spongy bone. The epiphyseal line is what remains of the hyaline cartilage epiphyseal plate in a child's growing long bone.

There is a periosteum on the outside and an endosteum on the inside of long bones. The endosteum is a membrane lining the interior of the compact bone that separates the medullary cavity from the compact bone and contains cells involved in growth and repair of the bone.

Bony Landmarks

The outer texture of bones can be smooth or rough and may contain projections, depressions, or hollows.

Figure 3-22. The four bone shapes.

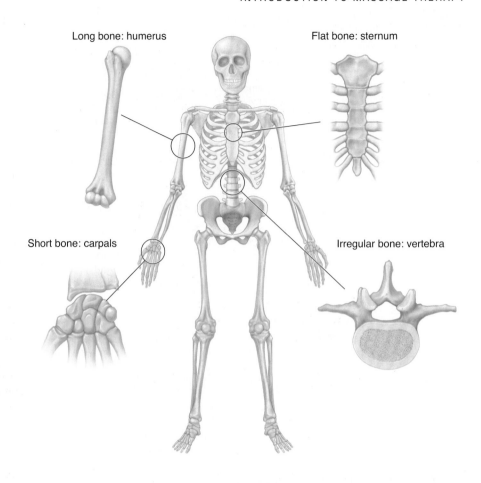

Long bone: humerus

Flat bone: sternum

Short bone: carpals

Irregular bone: vertebra

Bony landmarks, or bone markings, are the distinguishing features of bones that can usually be externally palpated and serve as sites for muscle attachment and safe passageways for nerves and blood vessels. Several specific bony landmarks are commonly used by healthcare professionals when referring to a client's anatomy. Generally, projections stick out from the bone to offer an attachment site for muscles, tendons, aponeuroses, and ligaments. Depressions, openings, and concave portions of the bone provide smooth articulating surfaces and holes or openings that are passageways for tendons, nerves, or blood vessels. Sometimes these formations also provide muscle attachment sites. Bony landmark projections and depressions are included in Table 3-4, with examples of each.

Skeleton

The skeleton normally contains 206 bones, cartilage, and joints. The bones of the skeleton can be defined as two separate groups called the axial and appendicular skeletons. Cartilage is discussed in the section covering cells and tissues, but we briefly review the skeleton-specific cartilage in this section. A **joint** is the mechanical structure where neighboring bones are attached, often with connective tissue and cartilage. There are a number of joints in the body that provide different amounts and different kinds of movement.

Axial Skeleton

The axial skeleton makes up the axis of the body, or the central support structure. It contains 80 bones, including those of the skull, the vertebral column, and the bony thorax.

Skull

The skull is made up of 8 cranial bones, 14 facial bones, 6 inner ear ossicles, and 1 hyoid bone. Its primary function is to protect the brain. It has cavities for the eyes, ears, nose, and mouth, and teeth and jaws for mastication (chewing). Some of the cranial bones are paired, such as the parietal and temporal bones, but the sphenoid, ethmoid, frontal, and occipital bones are not (Fig. 3-23). Most of the facial bones are paired, including the maxilla (upper jaw), zygomatic (cheekbones), nasal, lacrimal (tear ducts are here), palatine, and inferior nasal conchae. Unpaired facial bones include the mandible (the movable lower jaw) and the vomer bone of the nose. There are three tiny bones, called ossicles, in each middle ear.

One facial bone is unique. Although not considered a true skull bone, the hyoid (HAHY-oyd) bone is located just superior to the larynx and deep to the base of the tongue (See Plate 4-35 in the special muscle section at the end of Chapter 4 for an illustration of the hyoid bone). It is unique in that it does not articulate with any other bones. Instead, it acts as the attachment site for muscles involved in raising

Table 3-4 Bony Landmarks

Landmark	Description	Location	Example
Projections			
Condyle	Smooth, rounded	Articular ends of bones	Occipital condyles
Crest	Prominent ridge or border	Along an edge	Iliac crest
Epicondyle	Rough, rounded	Above or around a condyle	Lateral and medial epicondyles of humerus
Head	Rounded, knobby	End of long bone	Head of humerus, head of femur
Line	Long ridge	Shaft of bone	Linea aspera
Process	Fingerlike	Sticks out of a bone	Xiphoid process, olecranon process
Ramus	Slightly flattened, bar-like	Near joint	Pubic ramus
Spine	Sharp, bladelike	Muscle attachment site	Spine of scapula, ASIS
Trochanter	Blunt, rough, bump	Muscle attachment site	Greater and lesser trochanters of femur

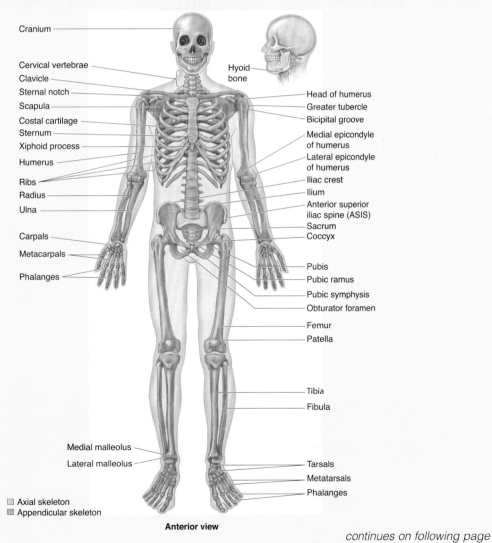

Cranium

Cervical vertebrae
Clavicle
Sternal notch
Scapula
Costal cartilage
Sternum
Xiphoid process
Humerus
Ribs
Radius
Ulna
Carpals
Metacarpals
Phalanges

Hyoid bone

Head of humerus
Greater tubercle
Bicipital groove
Medial epicondyle of humerus
Lateral epicondyle of humerus
Iliac crest
Ilium
Anterior superior iliac spine (ASIS)
Sacrum
Coccyx
Pubis
Pubic ramus
Pubic symphysis
Obturator foramen
Femur
Patella
Tibia
Fibula

Medial malleolus
Lateral malleolus

☐ Axial skeleton
☐ Appendicular skeleton

Tarsals
Metatarsals
Phalanges

Anterior view

continues on following page

3 Body Systems

Table 3-4 Bony Landmarks *continued*

Landmark	Description	Location	Example
Tubercle	Small, rough bump	Head of bone, for muscle attachment	Greater and lesser tubercles of humerus
Tuberosity	Rough bump	Neck portion of bone, for muscle attachment	Deltoid tuberosity
Depressions and openings			
Foramen	Hole	Through a bone	Obturator foramen, foramen magnum
Fossa	Concave	Articular bone surface	Supraspinous and infraspinous fossa of scapula
Groove	Small, concave, furrow-like	Muscle attachment site	Bicipital groove of humerus
Meatus	Short, tube-shaped passageway	Through a bone	Auditory meatus
Notch	Concave, half-moon	Cut-out in a bone	Sternal notch, sciatic notch of pelvis
Sinus	Air-filled cavity	Mucus-lined areas	Cranial bone (frontal sinus)

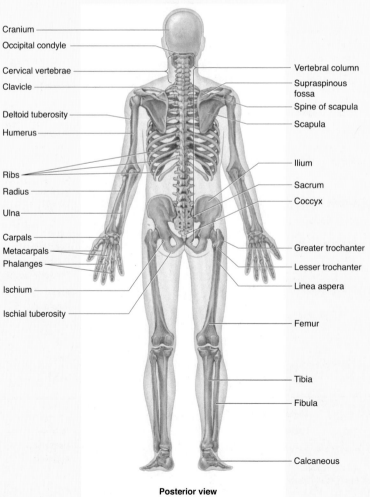

Posterior view

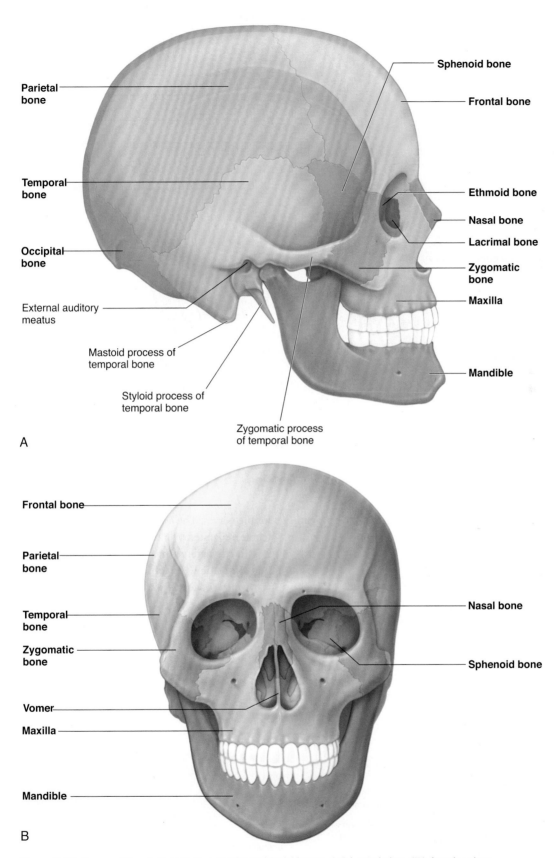

Figure 3-23. Bones of the skull, including cranial and facial bones. **(A)** Lateral view. **(B)** Anterior view.

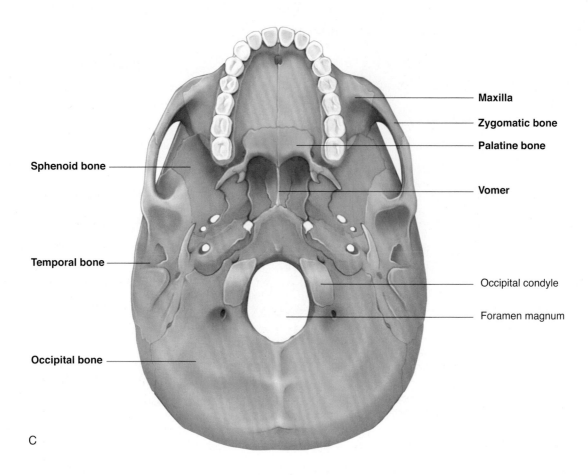

C

Figure 3-23. (*continued*) **(C)** Inferior view.

and lowering the larynx to provide speech and for moving the tongue in the process of swallowing.

Vertebral Column

The vertebral column, or spine, is made up of a series of irregularly shaped bones called vertebrae that act as a group to support the skull, protect the spinal cord, and provide passageways for the nerves. The average adult vertebral column has 26 vertebrae, separated by intervertebral discs of cartilage.

Each vertebra has specialized structures, including a body, foramen, vertebral arch, one spinous process, two transverse processes, and four articular processes (Fig. 3-24). The vertebral body resembles a hockey puck and bears weight. The foramen is a hole near the center of the vertebra

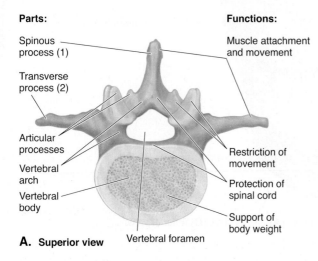

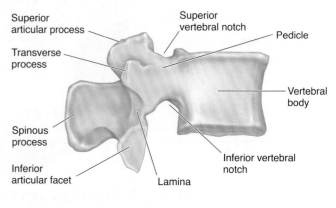

Figure 3-24. Structures and functions of a vertebra.

through which passes the spinal cord. The vertebral arch is the portion of the bone that arches around the posterior surface of the foramen, consisting of a pair of pedicles and a pair of laminae. The spinous process is the one that points out posteriorly and is most easily palpated. The transverse processes point out laterally. The four articular processes, sometimes called facets, are small bumps that allow the vertebrae to articulate with each other. Although each vertebra has the structures mentioned above, vertebrae in different regions of the spine also have specialized structures.

Unlike adults, newborn babies have as many as 34 vertebrae. The spine is the first bony structure to develop in the fetus and has concave thoracic and pelvic curves that protect the organs. Further along in postfetal development, the vertebral column acquires convex curves in the cervical and lumbar regions. The convex cervical curve matures as the infant begins to hold up its head, and the convex lumbar curve matures when the baby begins to stand and walk in an upright position (Fig. 3-25). These normal spinal curves, in addition to the cartilaginous intervertebral discs, give the spine the mechanical springlike properties of strength and flexibility.

Once completely formed, the spine has five distinct sections (Fig. 3-26):

- Cervical—7 vertebrae
- Thoracic—12 vertebrae

- Lumbar—5 vertebrae
- Sacral—5 vertebrae in childhood become a single fused bone in adults
- Coccygeal—3 to 5 vertebrae in childhood become a single fused bone in adults

The seven cervical (SER-vih-kul) vertebrae are relatively small and allow considerable neck movement. They are numbered C1 through C7, starting at the superior end. The first two vertebrae are often referred to as the atlas (C1), which allows us to nod the head "yes" and the axis (C2), which allows us to rotate the head side to side as in shaking the head "no." A common anatomical landmark is the spinous process of C7, which protrudes on the posterior side of the neck as the most prominent bump.

The 12 thoracic (thoh-RASS-ik) vertebrae are slightly larger than the cervical vertebrae and are similarly numbered T1 through T12. They have additional articulating surfaces that act as rib attachments for the posterior ends of the 12 pairs of ribs. The first intervertebral foramen occurs between C7 and superior to T1, allowing the spinal nerve C8 to exit the spinal cord.

The five lumbar vertebrae, numbered L1 through L5, are even heavier and larger to support the greater mechanical stress on the lumbar region. This section bears the weight of the rest of the spine and supports the trunk.

The sacral section of the spine, also called the sacrum (SAY-krum), is a single bone composed of five vertebrae that are normally fused together. The sacrum usually fuses anywhere from age 16 to 59, but occasionally fusion does not occur. This bone articulates superiorly with L5 and inferiorly with the coccyx (KAHK-sikz), but it also articulates laterally with the iliac bones of the pelvis to create the posterior wall of the pelvis.

The coccygeal section of the vertebral column is also called the coccyx. It is a single bone made of three to five vertebrae that are usually fused together. Located at the tail end of the spine, it is sometimes called the tailbone, and articulates with the sacrum at its superior surface. There are rare occasions when the sacrum has fused to the coccyx.

Bony Thorax

The bony thorax consists of the 12 pairs of ribs and the sternum. It functions as a protective cage for the lungs and the other organs of the thoracic cavity.

Like the thoracic vertebrae that they contact posteriorly, the ribs are numbered in pairs from 1 to 12 (Fig. 3-27). The first seven pairs are called true ribs because they also attach to the anterior portion of the sternum via the individual costal cartilages. The false ribs pairs 8 through 10, do not have their own individual anterior attachments. Instead, they all attach to the cartilage of the seventh true rib. The last two pairs are considered floating ribs because they have no anterior attachment. Between the ribs, in the intercostal spaces, there are muscles, blood vessels, and nerves.

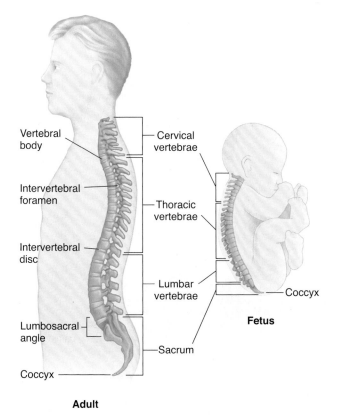

Vertebral body

Intervertebral foramen

Intervertebral disc

Lumbosacral angle

Coccyx

Cervical vertebrae

Thoracic vertebrae

Lumbar vertebrae

Sacrum

Coccyx

Fetus

Adult

Figure 3-25. Spinal curves of a fetus and an adult.

Figure 3-26. Anterior, lateral, and posterior views of the vertebral column.

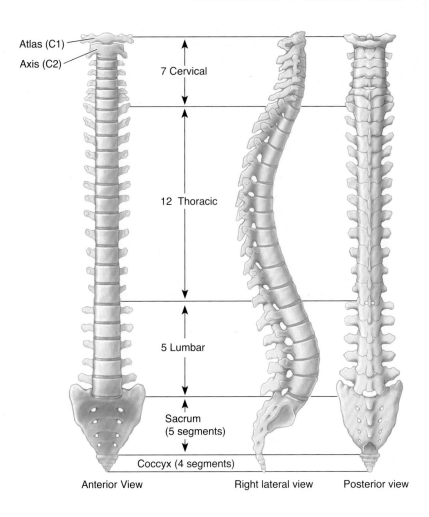

Figure 3-27. Bony thorax, anterior view.

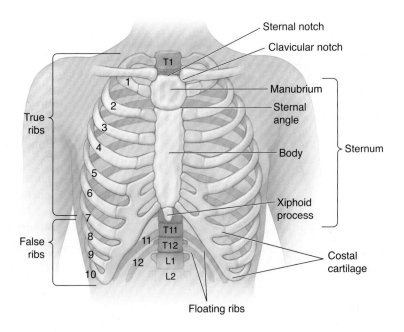

The sternum is the other integral portion of the bony thorax. The sternum lies in the middle of the anterior rib cage and is the attachment site for the true ribs via the costal cartilage. The sternum has three distinct portions: the manubrium (man-OO-bree-um), the body, and the xiphoid (ZAHY-foyd) process. The manubrium is the most superior portion of the sternum and has the bony landmark called the sternal (jugular) notch at its superior end. The body, sometimes referred to as the breastbone, joins the manubrium at the sternal angle. The sternal notch can be seen through the skin, but the sternal angle, which represents the location of the aortic arch, must be palpated.

The xiphoid process is a spear-like projection at the inferior edge of the body of the sternum. It is often used as a starting landmark when locating hand placement for chest compressions during CPR. The suggested placement is approximately three finger widths superior to the xiphoid process. Because it is sharp and can cause damage if fractured, compression or deep pressure at or near the xiphoid process should be avoided.

Appendicular Skeleton

The appendicular skeleton, which appropriately includes the bones of the appendages, or upper and lower extremities, contains 126 bones. This section contains all the bones peripheral to the axial skeleton: the shoulder girdle, the upper extremities, the pelvic girdle, and the lower extremities.

Shoulder Girdle

The shoulder girdle, sometimes called the pectoral girdle, consists of the clavicle and the scapula (Fig. 3-28). The clavicle, also known as the collarbone, is a long bone that is frequently broken. The scapula, often called the shoulder blade, is a flat bone with many bony landmarks that are commonly used in healthcare. The spine on the posterior surface of the scapula runs transversely and is easily palpated. Above the scapular spine is the supraspinous fossa, which is a long depression that runs the length of the spine. The large, flat area of the scapula below the spine is an infraspinous fossa, which is a slight depression. The acromion process at the lateral end of the spine protrudes like a knob. It, too, can be palpated easily as the bony point of the shoulder. Below the acromion process, on the lateral side of the scapula is the glenoid cavity, which cradles the head of the humerus in a ball-and-socket joint, a shallow marking that cannot be palpated. Medial to the glenoid cavity is the coracoid process that points anteriorly, like a fingertip. The coracoid process can be delicately palpated just inferior to the lateral clavicle.

Upper Extremities

The upper extremities include the bones of the arms, wrists, and hands. There are a total of 30 bones in each upper extremity: 3 arm bones, 8 wrist bones, and 19 hand bones (Fig. 3-29).

The humerus is the "upper arm" bone. Anatomically speaking, the upper arm is the arm, whereas the lower arm is called the forearm. Healthcare professionals reference several bony landmarks of the humerus. The head of the humerus is the ball at the proximal end that fits into the glenoid cavity of the scapula to form the shoulder joint. The greater and lesser tubercles, located more laterally on the proximal end of the humerus, provide muscle attachment sites. Between the tubercles is the bicipital (bahy-SIP-ih-tuhl) groove, sometimes called the intertubercular groove, which is a major site for muscle attachment. The deltoid tuberosity lies midway down the humerus, on the lateral surface, and serves as the attachment site for the deltoid muscle. On the distal end, the medial and lateral epicondyles of the humerus stick out as bumps, also for muscle attachment.

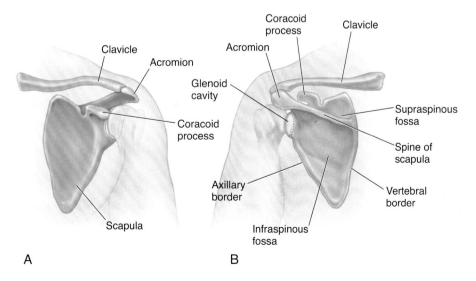

Figure 3-28. Shoulder girdle. **(A)** Anterior view. **(B)** Posterior view.

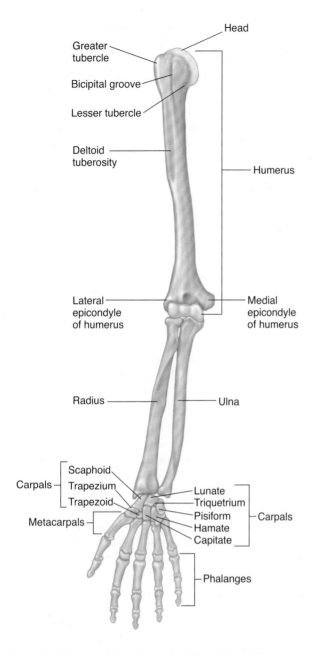

Figure 3-29. Bones of the wrist, arm, and shoulder girdle.

The radius and ulna are the two bones that make up the forearm. The radius is on the lateral side and the ulna is more medial. An easily palpable landmark of the forearm is the styloid process of the radius, located at the lateral, distal end. This landmark is often used when locating the radial pulse, which can be found just medial and slightly anterior to the styloid process of the radius. The ulna has some major landmarks of its own. The olecranon (oh-LEK-rah-nahn) process is a bony landmark of the ulna that is often mistaken for part of the humerus. It is very easily identified as the point of the elbow, sometimes feeling sharp, depending on the amount of subcutaneous fat in the area. The styloid process of the ulna is the bump located at the distal end, next to the wrist, on the posterior (dorsal) surface. It is most

easily seen and palpated with the forearm in a prone position, palm down.

The wrist comprises eight carpal bones: capitate, hamate, lunate, pisiform, scaphoid, trapezium, trapezoid, and triquetral. The carpals are short bones that fit together like puzzle pieces (see Fig. 3-29).

The hand is made up of five metacarpals and the phalanges (see Fig. 3-29). The metacarpals are numbered 1 through 5, with the thumb being the first and the "pinky" being the fifth. The phalanges consist of 14 bones, with 2 in the thumb and 3 in each of the others.

Pelvic Girdle

The pelvic girdle consists of three bones that are fused together: the ilium (ILL-ee-um), the ischium (ISH-ee-um), and the pubis (PYOO-bis) (Fig. 3-30). There are two major bony landmarks on the pelvic girdle that cannot be palpated. One is the acetabulum, literally translated to "vinegar bowl." Created at the intersection of the three fused bones, the acetabulum (ASS-sih-TAB-yoo-lum) is the cuplike socket that cradles the head of the femur. Another important bony landmark that cannot be palpated is the obturator foramen. This is a large hole encircled by the ischium and pubis that allows nerves and blood vessels to pass through.

The individual bones of the pelvis each have some identifiable, easily palpated landmarks. The posterior side of the ilium has a transverse ridge called the iliac crest, just inferior to the waist. The front of each hip has a prominent bump called the anterior superior iliac spine, commonly known as the "hip bone." The ischia have the ischial tuberosities that are sometimes called the "sit bones" because these protruding landmarks can be felt and may become uncomfortable when one sits on a hard surface. The pubic bones are joined anteriorly at the cartilaginous pubic symphysis. During the late stages of pregnancy, the cartilage softens to allow the pelvic girdle to expand for childbirth.

The male pelvis differs from the female pelvis in several ways. From the superior view, looking down through the pelvis, the opening within the female pelvis is circular, and the male's is shaped more like a heart. In the anterior view, the female pelvis has a less significant pubic arch than the male pelvis. The more pronounced arch in the male pelvis narrows the entire structure compared with the female pelvis, which is wider and gives women wider hips. The sacrum is fairly straight in the female and more curved in the male (compare Figs. 3-30 and 3-31).

Lower Extremities

The lower extremities of the appendicular skeleton consist of the thigh, knee, lower leg, ankle, and foot. There are a total of 30 bones in each lower extremity (Fig. 3-32).

The femur, or thighbone, is the largest bone in the body. Its major proximal landmarks include the head and neck, which fit into the acetabulum to create the hip joint,

Figure 3-30. Pelvic girdle, male.

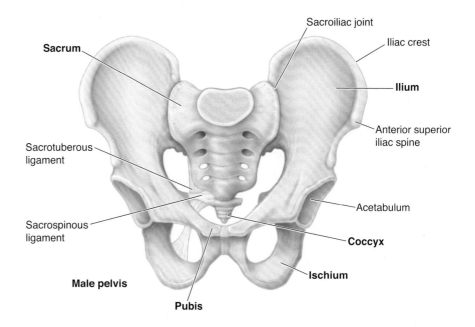

and the trochanters, which serve as sites for muscle attachment. The greater trochanter is the large, lateral protrusion that is easily palpated. The lesser trochanter is the smaller and more distal of the two, located medially, and is quite difficult to palpate. The lateral and medial epicondyles of the femur are located at the distal end, near the knee, just above the condyles that articulate with the tibia of the lower leg. The patella (puh-TEL-luh), also called the "kneecap," is a sesamoid bone embedded in the tendon of the quadriceps femoris muscle. The linea aspera (LIN-ee-uh ASS-per-uh) is a protruding line found on the posterior shaft of the femur that serves as a site for muscle attachment.

The tibia and fibula are the bones of the lower leg. The tibia is the larger and more medial of the two and is the weight-bearing bone. It has an anterior ridge that runs vertically, a tibial tuberosity on the anterior surface of the proximal end, and the medial malleolus (inner ankle bone) at the distal end. The tibia is part of the knee joint, along with the femur and the patella. The fibula is the smaller, more lateral bone of the lower leg that does not bear weight and is not part of the knee joint. Its landmarks are located on the lateral aspect of the lower leg. The head of the fibula is on the proximal end, and the lateral malleolus (outer ankle bone) is located at the distal end.

The seven tarsals that make up the ankle joint are the calcaneus (the largest of the seven, also known as the "heel"), talus, navicular, medial cuneiform, intermediate cuneiform, lateral cuneiform, and cuboid.

The structure of the foot is similar to that of the hand. The foot has five metatarsals that form the instep and the

Figure 3-31. Pelvic girdle, female.

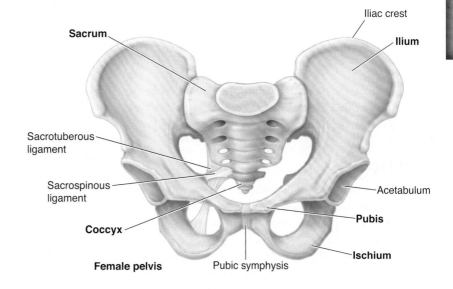

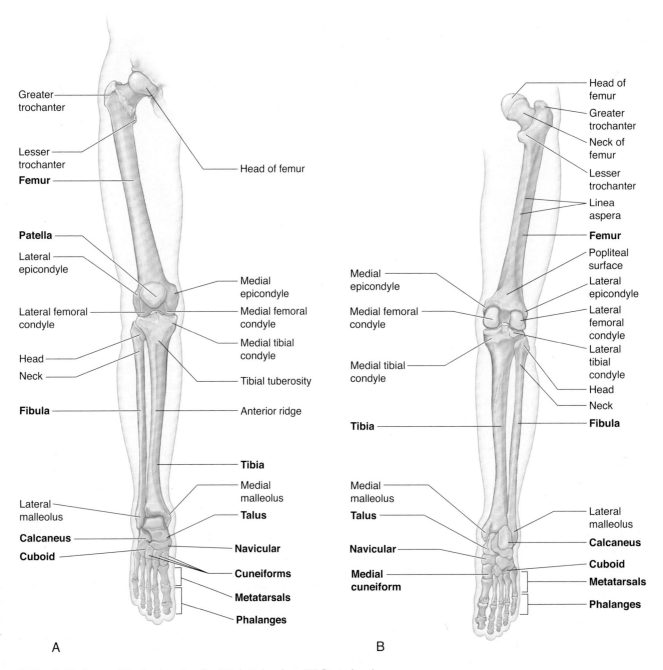

Figure 3-32. Bones of the lower extremity. **(A)** Anterior view. **(B)** Posterior view.

ball of the foot; the metatarsal behind the "big toe" is meta-tarsal 1, and behind the "baby toe" is metatarsal 5. The toes are made up of 14 phalangeal bones.

Cartilage

Cartilage is essential for bone formation early in life, and it provides cushion and support for various body structures. The three types of cartilage are elastic, hyaline, and fibrocartilage.

Hyaline cartilage is the most abundant in the body. It is translucent and pearly blue, and no nerves are found within

hyaline cartilage. It is firm but elastic, providing flexibility and support and allowing smooth, efficient movement at the joints. Examples of hyaline cartilage include the temporary cartilage in infants and children, the costal cartilages of the ribs, and articular cartilage. Figure 3-33 illustrates the location of articular cartilage.

Fibrocartilage, sometimes called white fibrocartilage, has much collagen that provides strength and structure but little flexibility. It is found in the intervertebral discs of the spinal column and in the temporomandibular joint (TMJ).

Elastic cartilage, also referred to as yellow cartilage, is more opaque and flexible than the other types. It consists of

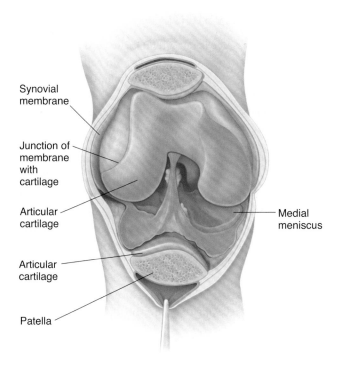

Synovial membrane

Junction of membrane with cartilage

Articular cartilage

Articular cartilage

Patella

Medial meniscus

Figure 3-33. Knee joint showing articular cartilage.

many elastin fibers within the collagen, giving strength to flexible structures. For example, the external ear is made up of elastic cartilage, as is the larynx.

Functions of the Skeletal System

The skeleton provides the basic support and general shape of the human body. Many of the bones serve as levers that are pulled by the muscles to create movement, and because muscles are the focus of the scope of practice for massage, the bones are a very important part of anatomy education. They also provide protection for organs, act as storage sites for calcium salts, and manufacture blood cells. Bone formation, growth, and repair are processes that are responsible for converting cartilage to bone, lengthening long bones, and remodeling bones in response to the levels of calcium in the blood and mechanical stresses on the bones.

Support

The calcium salts in the extracellular matrix of bones makes them especially hard. Their hardness provides a strong internal framework for our bodies that can hold us up and firmly anchor muscles and organs.

Protection

The hardness of bone also helps protect internal organs and structures. For example, the ribs protect the lungs and the heart in the thoracic cavity, and the vertebral column protects the spinal cord. The abdominal cavity has minimal protection from bones, and it is therefore the most vulnerable cavity of the body.

Movement

The skeleton provides the necessary leverage that the tendons and muscles use to create movement. Tendons attach bones to muscles, muscles contract to pull the bones, and the joints allow the neighboring bones to move in relation to each other.

Storage

Bones serve as storage sites for several different minerals as well as fat. Magnesium, phosphorus, sodium, and calcium are minerals stored in the bones. Much of the body's calcium is stored as calcium salts in the extracellular matrix of bones. Calcium is constantly being used as a necessary component for nerve conduction, muscle contraction, and blood clotting. The interior cavities of long bones store fat in the form of yellow marrow. The fat serves as a thermal insulator and a source of energy.

Hematopoiesis

Blood cell formation, or hematopoiesis (HEM-ah-toh-poh-EE-sis), is another function of the skeleton. The interior cavities of some flat bones contain red marrow, which is a site of RBC formation. RBCs are essential for life because they carry the oxygen required for everything from cellular respiration to healing. The blood cells and components of blood are discussed in the section covering the cardiovascular system.

Bone Formation, Growth, and Remodeling

Continuous regeneration and adjustments occur within the bones to ensure that the skeleton can support and protect our bodies adequately. This is an ongoing and dynamic process that begins prior to birth and continues throughout life as our bodies are subjected to gravity and other physical stressors. The process of bone formation converts cartilage to bone. Once all of the bones have ossified, they grow larger as we grow older. Bones undergo remodeling to maintain the proper levels of calcium in the blood and to change the shape of the bone in response to physical stressors. Hormones that regulate and encourage growth influence the continuous process of creating new bone. Without calcium and vitamin D, growth will not occur.

Bone Formation

Ossification, the process by which cartilage is turned into hardened bone, begins with osteoblast cells in the fetus. When the fetus is only 2 or 3 months old, the osteoblasts become active, manufacturing the matrix that surrounds them. The matrix is rich in collagen, a fibrous white protein that provides strength and resilience. After it is deposited, the matrix accumulates calcium and other minerals that contribute to the hardening of the bone tissue. Once hardened, osteoblast cells are called osteocytes, or mature bone cells. Most of the hyaline cartilage has been transformed into bone by the time babies are born.

Bone Growth

A small amount of hyaline cartilage remains in bones during childhood, in the epiphyseal (ee-PIH-fih-SEE-uhl) plates, or growth zones, of long bones. Located toward the knobby end of a long bone, the epiphyseal plates are where long bones grow longer. The hyaline cartilage acts as a model for bone growth. The epiphyseal plate first grows wider, and then bony matrix is deposited on the side closer to the center of the bone. By following the hyaline model, bones maintain their shape and proportion through the normal growth process. Lengthening continues through the late teenage years, and when it stops, the epiphyseal plates solidify and become inactive. They can then be identified on an x-ray film at the junction between the shaft (long part) of the bone and its knobby ends as thin lines called epiphyseal lines.

Bone Remodeling

Long bones increase in diameter as well but use the process of bone remodeling instead of the hyaline model. Bone remodeling is a process of moving bone material from one place to another for maintaining normal calcium levels in the blood, for bone growth, and for strengthening bone in response to physical stressors.

When there is not enough calcium in the blood, osteoclast cells in the bony matrix are activated by hormones to destroy bone tissue, a process called resorption. Bone breakdown releases calcium into the blood to maintain homeostasis. Conversely, if there is too much calcium in the blood, the body will deposit calcium salts into the bony matrix.

Bone remodeling maintains the general shape of the bones through their course of growth. To increase the width of long bones and to increase the overall size of bones other than long bones, growth follows the remodeling process. The process starts in the cavity at the center of the bone with resorption at the cavity wall. A rest period follows, and then bony matrix is deposited on the outside of the bone. The process creates a thicker, wider bone.

The rate of bone formation exceeds that of bone resorption during childhood and adolescence, allowing bones to become larger and denser. In young and middle adulthood, however, the rates tend to be fairly balanced. As a person enters old age, osteoclastic (breakdown) activity tends to exceed osteoblastic (creative) activity, resulting in weaker bones.

Effects of Massage on the Skeletal System

Even though massage is not intentionally used as treatment for the bones and joint structures, they do benefit. Massage enhances circulation of blood and lymph, thus increasing nutrient delivery to, and waste removal from, body tissues including the bones. The result is healthier bones and better healing of fractures and other bone injuries. Massage increases the number of red and white blood cells in the blood, which increases the body's ability to deliver oxygen to cells and fight germs. The bones house the red marrow, which is the site for RBC production, and higher numbers of blood cells benefit all of the tissues and organs of the body.

The joints of the body can also benefit from massage. Regular movement of some joints can increase the production of the fluid that lubricates the joints. Also, if joint pain is caused by excessive muscle tension or tissue adhesions near the joint, massage therapy may be able to relieve those conditions, thus relieving the joint pain.

Muscular System

Muscles make up almost half of an average person's body weight. Muscle tissue, like nervous tissue, does not reproduce as rapidly and regularly as other body tissues. Muscle cells can get larger or smaller, and can die, but muscle tissue is not constantly replenished. Because muscle cells have an elongated shape, they are often referred to as muscle fibers.

Types of Muscle Tissue

Classified by structure, function, and location, there are three types of muscle tissues: cardiac, smooth, and skeletal. These different types of muscle tissues all share the following features:

- Contractility—the elongated muscle fibers contract better than a square or round cell, thus creating tension
- Excitability—the fibers are capable of a forceful response to a nervous impulse
- Extensibility—muscles can be stretched beyond their normal resting length
- Elasticity—after being stretched or contracted, muscles can return to their original length

Cardiac Muscle

Cardiac muscles are only found in the walls of the heart and are responsible for pushing blood into the blood vessels. The muscle cells are striated, each cell has only one nucleus, they have

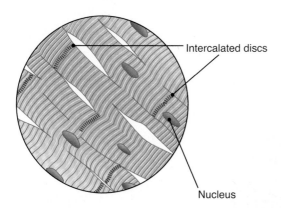

Figure 3-34. Cardiac muscle cells. (Reprinted with permission from Cohen BJ, Wood DL. Memmler's Structure and Function of the Human Body. 9th ed. Philadelphia: Lippincott Williams & Wilkins, 2009.)

a branching structure, and they contract involuntarily. Between cardiac muscle cells are intercalated discs. They are unique to cardiac muscle tissue and allow the electrical impulses that stimulate contraction to be conducted along the network of fibers, creating contractions that are strong and rhythmic (Fig. 3-34). These cardiac muscle contractions forcibly pump blood out of the heart with a rush that can be felt, referred to as the pulse.

Smooth Muscle

Smooth muscles are found in the walls of hollow organs, such as the stomach and intestines. They have no striations, each cell has only one nucleus, and they contract involuntarily (Fig. 3-35). Smooth muscle contracts as nerve impulses move from one fiber to the next, creating sequential, strong, slow contractions. Primarily arranged in sheetlike layers in which one runs along the length and the other encircles the tube like a belt, the layers take turns alternating contraction and relaxation. These coordinated contractions result in a wavelike movement called peristalsis that squeezes the organ to move substances through the system, such as food through the digestive tract. (Fig. 3-13 illustrates the layering of smooth muscle.)

Skeletal Muscle

Skeletal muscles attach to the skeleton in most cases. Made up of masses of muscle fibers wrapped in connective tissue organized in bundles, the muscle cells are long and thin (Fig. 3-36). Some are almost a foot long. They are striated and each muscle fiber has more than one nucleus. The more bundles of fibers there are, the thicker that particular muscle is. The contraction of an entire skeletal muscle can be fast and forceful. Contraction is controlled voluntarily, meaning that we can consciously make skeletal muscles contract. There are, however, nervous system reflexes that create involuntary skeletal muscle contractions, usually in response to a potentially dangerous situation. When you touch a burning hot surface, reflexes will contract a series of muscles to pull your arm away before you think about it.

In Western massage and bodywork, the best massage therapists are, in essence, muscle specialists. Just knowing the names of the muscles is not sufficient for a professional massage therapist. You should also know the attachment points of muscles, the actions of the muscles, how skeletal muscles work on a microscopic level, as well as how they work to create movement of the skeleton. Because skeletal muscles are the most relevant to massage therapy, they are the focus of this text (Fig. 3-37).

Structures of Skeletal Muscle

The structural aspect of skeletal muscle can be studied from a microscopic, cellular level as well as an overall view of a whole muscle. The basic muscle cell, or muscle fiber, is made up of several different components that influence the overall look of a whole muscle.

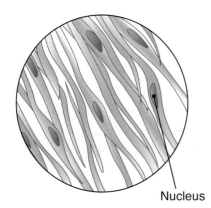

Figure 3-35. Smooth muscle cells. (Reprinted with permission from Cohen BJ, Wood DL. Memmler's Structure and Function of the Human Body. 9th ed. Philadelphia: Lippincott Williams & Wilkins, 2009.)

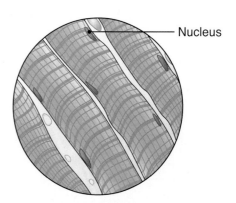

Figure 3-36. Skeletal muscle cells. (Reprinted with permission from Cohen BJ, Wood DL. Memmler's Structure and Function of the Human Body. 9th ed. Philadelphia: Lippincott Williams & Wilkins, 2000.)

3 Body Systems

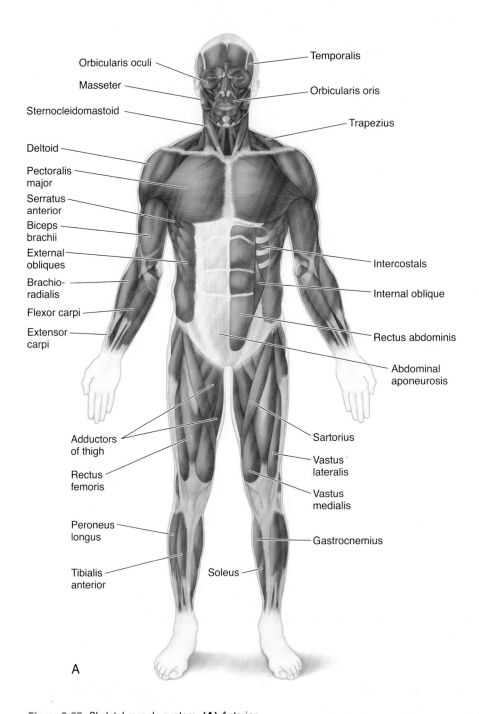

Figure 3-37. Skeletal muscle system. **(A)** Anterior.

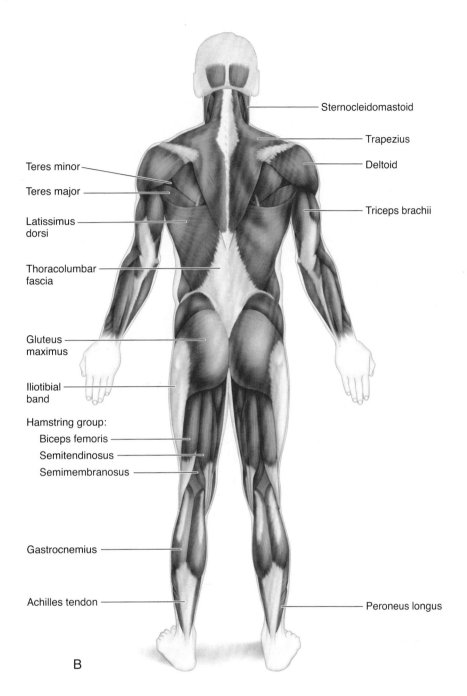

Sternocleidomastoid

Trapezius

Deltoid

Teres minor

Teres major

Triceps brachii

Latissimus dorsi

Thoracolumbar fascia

Gluteus maximus

Iliotibial band

Hamstring group:
   Biceps femoris
   Semitendinosus
   Semimembranosus

Gastrocnemius

Achilles tendon

Peroneus longus

B

Figure 3-37. (*continued*) **(B)** Posterior.

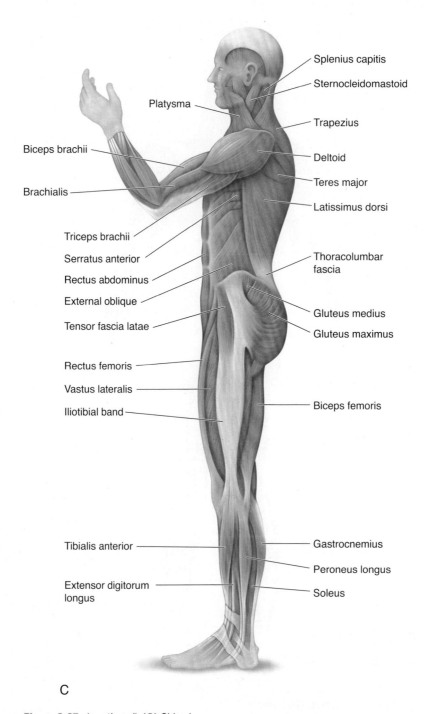

C

Figure 3-37. (*continued*) **(C)** Side view.

Microscopic Structures of a Skeletal Muscle Cell

The microscopic anatomy and physiology of skeletal muscle cells illustrates how they create movement. Muscle cells consist of a bundle of myofibrils, also called fibrils, encased in a plasma membrane called the sarcolemma (SAHR-koh-LEM-muh). The myofibrils are made of thick myofilaments called myosin (MAHY-oh-sin) and thin myofilaments called actin. Because bunches of dark myosin filaments alternate with

bunches of light actin filaments, the muscle fibers appear to have shaded bands, or stripes, which is why they are called striated muscle tissue. Multiple chains of these bands, called sarcomeres (SAHR-koh-meerz), are the contractile units of the muscle fiber.

Sliding Filament Theory

Although it has not been proven, the sliding filament mechanism is a widely accepted theory of how muscle contraction occurs. This theory suggests that the actin and myosin myofilaments remain the same length, but that the overall length of the sarcomere shortens because the myofilaments slide together. Calcium molecules first uncover sites on the actin where the myosin can attach. Once those sites are exposed, the myosin's cross bridges latch onto the actin filaments like Velcro. Temporarily connected, the actin filaments are pulled closer together, overlapping the myosin filaments. Figure 3-38 illustrates the sliding filament mechanism. The overlapped filaments create a shorter sarcomere,

resulting in a shorter fibril. When many fibrils shorten, the whole muscle cell shortens. Clearly, calcium is necessary for muscle contraction, which is one of the reasons calcium should be included in a balanced diet.

Muscular Control Mechanism

The sliding together of the myofilaments begins with a nerve impulse from the CNS via a somatic motor neuron. One somatic motor neuron can stimulate hundreds of

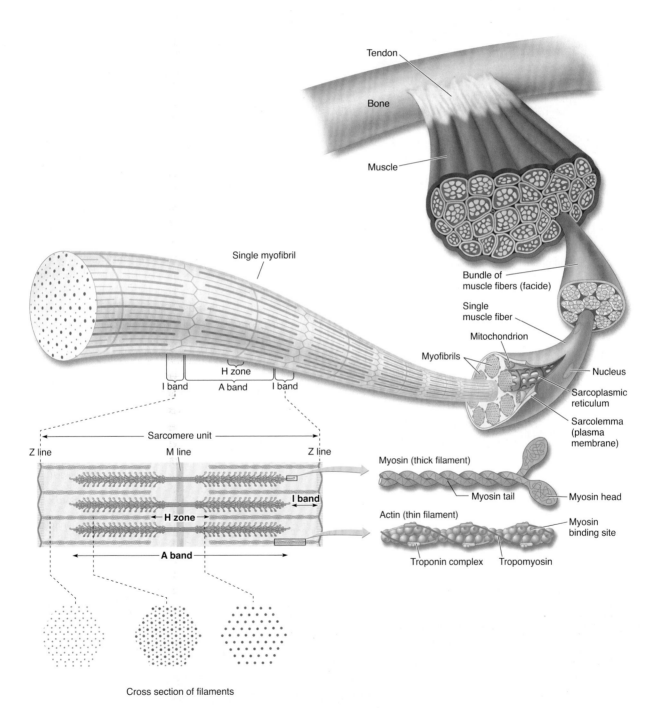

Figure 3-38. Sliding filament mechanism. (Reprinted with permission from McArdle WD, Katch FI, Katch VL. Exercise Physiology: Energy, Nutrition, and Human Performance. 5th ed. Baltimore: Lippincott Williams & Wilkins, 2001.)

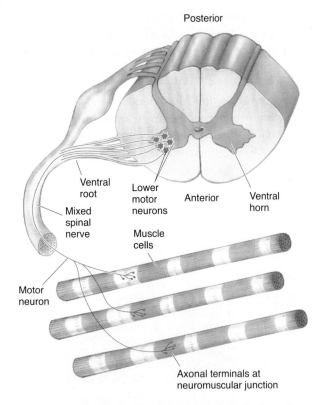

Figure 3-39. Motor unit. (Reprinted with permission from Bear MF, Connors BW, Paradiso MA. Neuroscience: Exploring the Brain. 2nd ed. Baltimore: Lippincott Williams & Wilkins, 2001.)

branches out with axonal terminals, like tree branches, as it nears the muscle cells. Each axonal terminal meets the motor end plate, the place on the muscle cell membrane that receives the nerve impulse, at a synaptic cleft, which is the space between the axon and muscle cell. This collection of structures, including the axonal terminal, the synaptic cleft, and the motor end plate, is called the neuromuscular junction. Figure 3-40 illustrates the neuromuscular junction.

The axonal terminal releases a chemical neurotransmitter called acetylcholine (ah-SEE-tuhl-KOH-leen) that is received by the motor end plate and triggers muscle contraction. (The series of events that occurs at the neuromuscular junction is described in detail below in the nervous system section.) As soon as the acetylcholine causes the muscle fiber to contract, it is broken down by a chemical in the synaptic cleft to prevent an unwanted sustained contraction. If more nerve impulses are conducted to the same muscle cell, it can sustain a prolonged contraction.

A minimal amount of current, called the threshold stimulus, is necessary to stimulate the contraction of a muscle cell. When the threshold is reached, the muscle cell reacts with complete contraction. All the muscle cells in a motor unit respond as one when stimulated. This response is commonly called the "all-or-none" principle, meaning the muscle cells contract completely or not at all. The all-or-none principle may seem counterintuitive, since we know muscle contractions can be precise or forceful. Remember, there are thousands of muscle cells in a whole muscle. The strength of the whole muscle contraction is determined by the number of muscle cells that have been stimulated to contract. In other words, a whole muscle contraction does not require every muscle cell to contract. The precision of a movement is determined by the number of muscle cells that are controlled by a single nerve cell. A motor unit that

muscle cells, but each muscle cell is controlled by only one somatic motor neuron. The more muscle fibers one nerve must supply, the less precise the movements. One motor neuron and all of the muscle cells it stimulates is called a motor unit (Fig. 3-39). The extension of this neuron that communicates to the fibril is called an axon (AK-sahn) and

Figure 3-40. Neuromuscular junction.

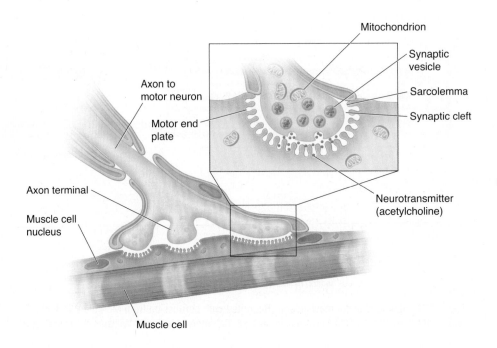

has a few muscle cells will be able to control the contraction more precisely than a motor unit that has hundreds of muscle cells.

Structures of a Whole Skeletal Muscle

A skeletal muscle is made up of bundles of muscle cells held together with connective tissue. This fibrous connective tissue, called fascia, carries blood vessels and nerves into the muscle and mechanically transmits the force of the contraction from one end of the muscle to the other. The basic component of the muscle tissue bundle is the muscle cell, or muscle fiber. The cells are very fragile, but each one is wrapped in a connective tissue covering called endomysium (EN-doh-MAHY-see-um). Several cells and the nerve cells that supply them are bundled together to create a fascicle (FAS-sih-kul), which is wrapped with connective tissue called the perimysium. The fascicles, along with blood vessels, nerves, and muscle spindles (special sensory receptors of muscles that are discussed below in the nervous system section), are then bundled together by the epimysium, which is the connective tissue covering of the whole muscle. The epimysium blends into the tendons or aponeuroses, which attach the muscles to bones, cartilage, or other connective tissue coverings. The thickest part of a muscle that is primarily made of muscle cells and has a pinkish appearance is sometimes called the belly of the muscle. Tendons are very strong and thin and can easily anchor at transverse bony projections and joints to provide durability and save space. Once the small, delicate cells are wrapped in connective tissue and bundled together, a very strong and resilient structure is created. Figure 3-41 illustrates the structures that form a skeletal muscle.

Functions of the Muscles

The primary function of the muscular system is to create movement, but muscles also produce heat, support the skeleton, maintain posture, and provide some protection from external forces.

Movement

All muscle cells have the ability to contract, bringing the ends of the cell closer together. On a cellular scale, this movement is amplified by the many bundles of muscle cells to create movement of entire muscles. Cardiac and smooth muscles in the walls of organs squeeze contents out or push contents through organs or, in the case of blood vessels, change the diameter of the tube.

The main function of skeletal muscles is to move bones and sometimes to move connective tissue structures such as the lips. Most muscles attach indirectly to bone, meaning that their connective tissue covering continues past the muscle and blends into a tendon or aponeurosis, which then

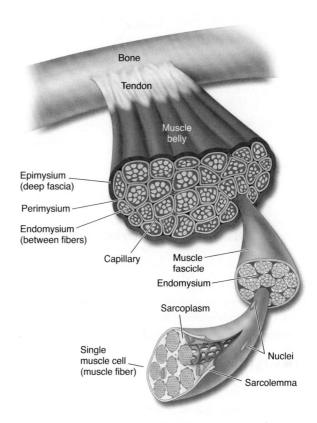

Figure 3-41. Structures of a skeletal muscle. (Reprinted with permission from McArdle WD, Katch FI, Katch VL. Exercise Physiology: Energy, Nutrition, and Human Performance. 5th ed. Baltimore: Lippincott Williams & Wilkins, 2001.)

attaches to the bone. If muscles attach directly to a bone, their connective tissue covering fuses with the connective tissue that covers the bone.

Each skeletal muscle has two kinds of attachments: origin and insertion. **The origin of a muscle is the attachment on the bone or connective tissue structure that is more stationary during muscle contraction. The insertion of a muscle is the point of attachment that moves most during contraction, often at the distal end.** All muscles have at least one of each of these two attachments. If muscle inserts into a bone, the bone will be pulled toward the origin of the contracting muscle. If a muscle inserts into a connective tissue structure, such as the lips, the lips will be pulled toward the origin of the contracting muscle (Fig. 3-42).

In addition to moving the skeleton and connective tissue structures, muscles also help move blood and lymph. Muscles become shorter and wider when they contract, which you see in a bodybuilder who strikes a pose. As the muscles contract, they constrict the blood and lymph vessels, squeezing the fluids out.

Heat Production

The core temperature of the body is maintained in a safe range of 96.8° to 98.6°F. Skeletal muscles release heat in the

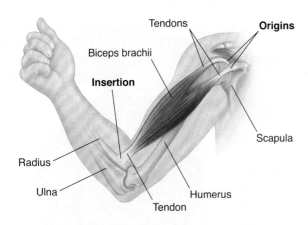

Figure 3-42. Muscle attachments: origin and insertion.

process of contraction, and the heat generated helps maintain the body's core temperature. Shivering, for example, involves the body making small, involuntary muscle contractions to release chemical energy or heat.

Skeletal Support

Skeletal muscles support and maintain posture by holding the body upright against gravity and by stabilizing joints. The skeleton is only a collection of bones, joints, cartilage, and ligaments. Even standing still, our muscles work continuously to hold the skeleton up in a balanced, stable position.

Protection

The muscles protect the structures underneath them. Our organs and bones would be much more vulnerable to trauma without the muscles surrounding them.

Effects of Massage on the Muscular System

Massage increases the nourishment and development of smooth, cardiac, and skeletal muscles by enhancing the delivery of oxygenated blood and removal of cellular waste.

The skeletal muscles and the surrounding soft tissue, which make up about half of our body weight, are the primary focus of massage therapy. In fact, sometimes massage is the best treatment for muscles, tendons, and fascia. It has been proven that massage can reduce tension by lengthening shortened muscles. It is highly effective at breaking the pain cycle by relieving muscular tension and increasing circulation. Inactive and paralyzed skeletal muscles benefit greatly from massage because it delivers oxygen and nutrients to muscle cells to keep them healthy.

Massage increases the excitability of muscles, making them more sensitive to nerve impulses. Faster reaction times, more effective movements, and better coordination can all result from massage.

Physical exertion is often followed by muscular fatigue, and massage is one of the most practical, beneficial treatments for muscular fatigue. By increasing nutrient delivery and waste removal from the muscles, massage minimizes the accumulation of chemicals that cause symptoms of muscular fatigue, such as lactic acid. Massage also maximizes healing.

> ### Alert
> *Massage techniques that are too aggressive may create fatigue-like symptoms or initiate a protective reflex contraction in the muscles.*

Manipulation of the muscles also produces heat, partly as a result of the increased circulation, partly because of increased chemical activity in muscle cells, and partly because of the heat generated when fascia is subjected to pressure. Muscle contractions produce heat as a byproduct of chemical reactions, and manipulation of the muscles increases these chemical reactions. Recall the thixotropic property of deep fascia, discussed earlier in the chapter. Without movement, fascia can thicken, contract, and become less pliable, restricting muscle movement and circulation within the muscles. Manipulation of the muscles deforms the fascia, which creates heat, similar to how bending a paperclip back and forth heats up the area being deformed. Because fascia and muscles are so intertwined, softened fascia can also restore muscular movement.

Nervous System

The nervous system serves as the body's communication and control center. **The nervous system regulates bodily processes to maintain homeostasis, keeping everything in the body in balance.** The nervous system receives stimuli, processes the information, and directs the body to respond to it. A stimulus is an irritant or something that can cause a response, and it can come from the inside of our bodies as well as the external environment. The nervous system is constantly monitoring these stimuli, integrating the input, and controlling the body to respond appropriately. When the nervous system is not functioning properly, the communication can break down or become inhibited, and the body's ability to carry out its normal functions is diminished. Simply, the body then cannot maintain homeostasis.

The nervous system is integral to muscle and soft tissue function, which is why massage therapists should understand its structures and functions. The tissues of the nervous system are organized into two separate divisions, called the central nervous system (CNS) and the peripheral nervous system (PNS). The CNS consists of the brain and spinal cord. The PNS is made up of all the nerve tissue outside the brain and spinal cord, including the cranial and spinal nerves.

Nervous System Tissue

The tissues of the nervous system include neurons, or nerve cells, and supportive cells called neuroglia. Individual neurons are organized in bundles with protective connective tissue wrappings. These bundles are called tracts, nerves, ganglia, and plexuses. Nerve tissue can be classified functionally by the direction of the nerve impulse, either toward or away from the CNS.

Neuron

The neuron, or nerve cell, is the basic unit of the nervous system (Fig. 3-43). The neuron has three main parts: the body, dendrites, and an axon. The body is the main portion of the neuron and contains the nucleus and other organelles that drive its functions. Dendrites are highly branched, tree-like fibers that start the communication path by receiving impulses from the external and internal environments and conducting that information toward the cell body along their plasma membranes. The axon is a long single fiber with branched ends that conducts impulses away from the cell body and takes the information to another structure, such as a muscle. Nerve cells are sometimes called nerve fibers because of their long axons and dendrites.

Some neurons have specialized Schwann cells strung along their axons and dendrites. These cells form a multilayered membrane of insulative tissue for the nerve cell called the myelin (MAHY-uh-lin) sheath. It protects and insulates nerves and allows nerve impulses to be transmitted very efficiently. The nuclei and cytoplasm of the Schwann cells are located on the outer surface of the myelin sheath, the neurilemma (NOO-rih-LEH-muh). Between the Schwann cells, along the neuron, are gaps called nodes of Ranvier (rahn-vee-AY), which are the active areas during nerve impulse transmission.

Figure 3-43. Structure of a neuron (nerve cell).

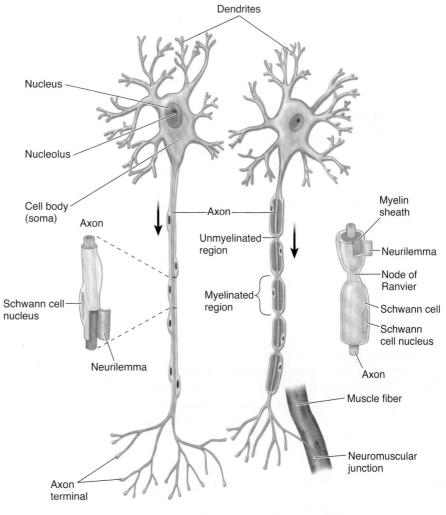

Unmyelinated fiber   **Myelinated fiber**

The neurilemma produces a chemical growth factor involved in a cellular repair mechanism for nervous tissues. Nerve cells are not regenerated on a regular basis, nor are they replaced upon damage. However, the axons and dendrites of injured nerve cells can regenerate from within the layers of neurilemma. This is a very slow process, and the tissue is not always functional once regenerated, but it gives hope to those with nerve injuries. The brain and spinal cord contain no Schwann cells, and repair of the brain or spinal cord is nearly impossible.

Neuroglia

The nerves are supported and connected with accessory cells called neuroglia. They come in five different forms (Fig. 3-44):

- Astrocytes—support and anchor nerve cells to blood capillaries

- Ependymal cells—line the cavities of the brain and spinal cord to help circulate the fluid that bathes and cushions the organs in those cavities

- Microglia—phagocytes that consume cellular debris

- Oligodendrocytes—fatty cells that wrap around nerves in the CNS to create the myelin sheath for insulation

- Schwann cells—form the myelin along a nerve cell in the PNS

Nerve Tissue Organization

In the CNS, neurons are collected together into bundles called nerve tracts. In the PNS, neuronal cell bodies are grouped together to form ganglia, and axons are grouped together to form a nerve.

The nerve has a structure similar to that of a muscle, with bundles of axons wrapped in connective tissue that are then bundled together with blood vessels in more connective tissue. Each neuron is wrapped with a connective tissue covering called an endoneurium (EN-doh-nur-ee-um). The neurons are grouped together in fascicles and wrapped in a perineurium (PAIR-ih-nur-ee-um). Several fascicles are grouped together, along with blood vessels, to form a nerve. The entire nerve is wrapped with a fibrous connective tissue covering called the epineurium (Fig. 3-45).

Nerve plexuses are large networks of intertwined nerves. The four main plexuses are the cervical, brachial, lumbar, and sacral, each serving a different region of the body (Fig. 3-46). These plexuses are important in massage therapy because they must be dealt with carefully to avoid damaging the nerve structures.

There are collections of individual nerve cell bodies in the PNS called ganglia (GAYNG-lee-uh). Even though they are part of the PNS, ganglia are located very close to the spinal cord, within the vertebral canal.

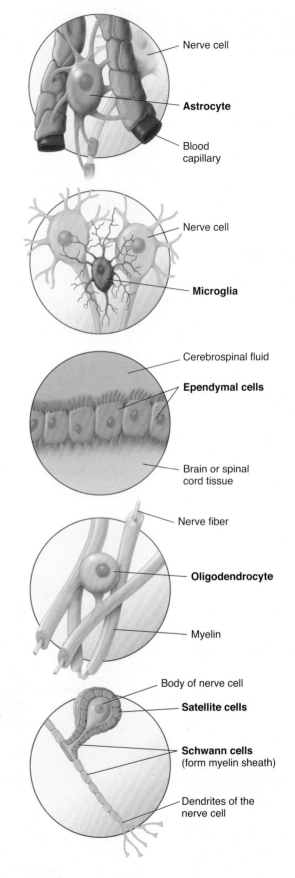

Figure 3-44. Forms of neuroglia.

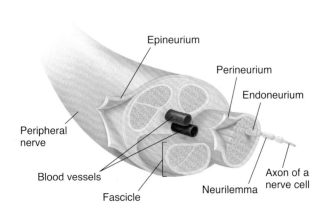

Figure 3-45. Structures of a nerve. (Reprinted with permission from Stedman's Medical Dictionary, 27th ed. Baltimore: Lippincott Williams & Wilkins, 2000.)

Classification by Function

There are many types of nerves that monitor, integrate, and respond to external and internal stimuli and changes occurring within the body. Functional classification of nerve cells separates them into two separate groups. **Sensory (afferent) neurons** receive sensory input and transmit that information to the CNS. **Motor (efferent) neurons** carry messages from the CNS to the muscle or organs that must react. Groups of sensory neurons form sensory nerves, and groups of motor neurons are called motor nerves. Most nerves, however, are mixed nerves, which have both sensory and motor neurons that carry information to and from the CNS.

Sensory Neurons

Sensory neurons are classified by their location, sensitivity, or structure. They send signals to the CNS in response to external or internal stimuli. **Proprioceptors** (PROH-pree-oh-SEP-torz) are sensory nerve cells sensitive to body position, muscle tone, and equilibrium. They are located in the muscles, tendons, joints, and inner ear. Exteroceptors respond to stimuli from the external environment, such as touch, pressure, temperature, smell, sight, and hearing. These are mostly found in the skin and near the surface of the body. Interoceptors, also called visceroceptors, detect stimuli such as pressure within the organs and blood vessels.

For a massage therapist, the proprioceptors and exteroceptors are the most important of all the sensory receptors. In the muscle, the muscle spindles are complex proprioceptors that are sensitive to the length of the muscle fibers and respond to changes in that length. Between the collagen fibers in tendons are Golgi (GOHL-jee) tendon organs that respond to tension within the tendon that results from muscle contraction (Fig. 3-47). Both muscle spindles and Golgi tendon organs provide information to the CNS regarding the length and tension of a muscle and its tendon(s).

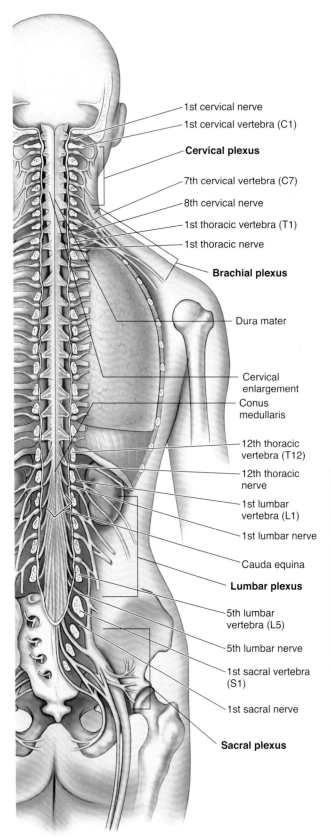

1st cervical nerve
1st cervical vertebra (C1)
Cervical plexus
7th cervical vertebra (C7)
8th cervical nerve
1st thoracic vertebra (T1)
1st thoracic nerve
Brachial plexus
Dura mater
Cervical enlargement
Conus medullaris
12th thoracic vertebra (T12)
12th thoracic nerve
1st lumbar vertebra (L1)
1st lumbar nerve
Cauda equina
Lumbar plexus
5th lumbar vertebra (L5)
5th lumbar nerve
1st sacral vertebra (S1)
1st sacral nerve
Sacral plexus

Figure 3-46. Nerve plexuses. (Reprinted with permission from Bear MF, Connors BW, Paradiso MA. Neuroscience: Exploring the Brain. 2nd ed. Baltimore: Lippincott Williams & Wilkins, 2001.)

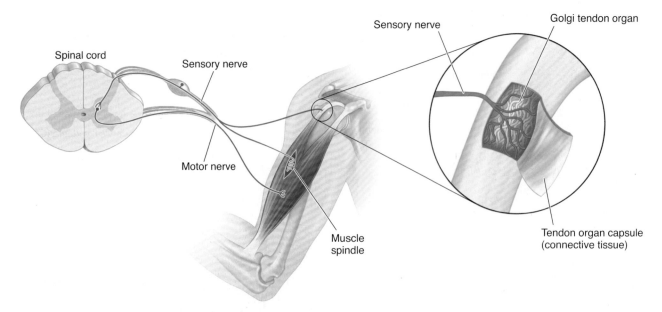

Figure 3-47. Muscle spindles and Golgi tendon organs.

Within a joint capsule are Ruffini end organs and Pacinian corpuscles. Both respond to pressure within a joint, essentially sensing the position of the joint by sensing different amounts of pressure at different places.

The muscle spindles and Golgi tendon organs respond as muscles move a joint through its range of motion, but joint proprioceptors are active when a joint is at the ends of its range. All of the proprioceptors act as a group to provide a sense of joint position, body position, effort, heaviness, and timing of movement. Input from the proprioceptors, along with input from other sensory organs such as the eyes and equilibrium sensors, is sometimes called a kinesthetic sense. Manipulating the muscle spindles and Golgi tendon

organs with advanced massage techniques can encourage muscles to shorten or lengthen. One of these techniques, appropriately called proprioceptive neuromuscular facilitation, is discussed in the Therapeutic Applications chapter.

The integument contains several different exteroceptors that constantly monitor our surroundings (Fig. 3-48). The closer these exteroceptors are to the surface of our skin, the more sensitive they are:

- Free nerve endings, also called nociceptors, located in the lower layer of the epidermis, detect pain and temperature.

Figure 3-48. Sensory receptors of the integument. (Reprinted with permission from Bear MF, Connors BW, Paradiso MA. Neuroscience: Exploring the Brain. 2nd ed. Baltimore: Lippincott Williams & Wilkins, 2001.)

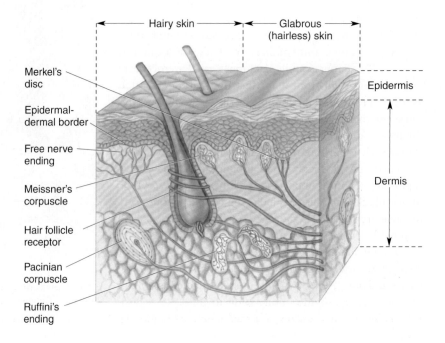

- Merkel cells, found in the lower layer of the epidermis, detect very light touch.
- Meissner's corpuscles, found in the upper part of the dermis in the lips, hands, feet, and genital organs, detect very light touch.
- Ruffini end organs, located in the dermis, detect heat and strong or continuous pressure.
- Pacinian corpuscles, found in the deep dermis, sense vibrations and deep pressure.

Motor Neurons

Motor neurons carry signals from the CNS to the muscles, creating a response that involves muscle contraction. The skeletal muscles can be effectors, or endpoints, for nervous signals, under voluntary control. The motor neurons can also control involuntary activity of the organs, glands, and smooth and cardiac muscle.

Mixed Nerves

Most of the nerves of the body are mixed nerves that contain both sensory and motor nerve cells. They can monitor for input, integrate the information received, and stimulate the body to respond to the input. The sciatic (sahy-AT-ik) nerve in the leg is an example of a mixed nerve that can receive and send information via individual neurons that run alongside each other.

Nerve Impulses

Nerve cells have two primary functions: irritability and conductivity. A neuron's irritability allows it to respond to a stimulus and translate that perception into a nerve impulse. Its conductivity allows the neuron to communicate that nerve impulse to another neuron, a muscle, or a gland.

Irritability

The neuron's irritability is the result of a chemical process of depolarization. There are several steps to creating a nerve impulse from a stimulus. Following is the series of events that takes place in response to a stimulus, such as a sharp thorn poking your finger:

1. Resting state—A nerve membrane at rest is in a polarized state, meaning that the positive and negative charges on either side of the membrane are not balanced. There are more sodium ions outside the neuron than there are potassium ions inside, creating an overall negative charge inside the membrane.

2. Excitation—When the thorn is perceived by a pain receptor, a neurotransmitter chemical is usually released to alter the permeability of the membrane.

3. Depolarization—The membrane becomes more permeable to sodium ions, and they diffuse into the cell, rushing from the high sodium concentration outside the cell to the lower sodium concentration inside. With the extra supply of sodium ions inside, the membrane becomes depolarized; that is, the negative and positive charges on either side of the membrane are balanced.

4. Repolarization—Almost as soon as the sodium has rushed in, the permeability of the membrane reverts, preventing any more sodium from entering. The cell membrane becomes more permeable to potassium, which quickly rushes out of the cell, restoring the positive charge outside the cell and the negative charge inside. The sodium–potassium pump uses ATP to move sodium ions out and potassium ions in to maintain sodium–potassium gradients necessary for the resting state.

This process is called the action potential, also known as the nerve impulse (Fig. 3-49). There is a threshold stimulus that acts as a switch for the impulse. If a stimulus is not strong enough and does not reach the threshold stimulus, the nerve impulse will not occur at all. Stimuli above the threshold stimulus will trigger the nerve impulse over the entire nerve cell. The permeability of the entire membrane spreads down the neuron, carrying the signal. This all-or-none response of whether there is an action potential or not means that either the whole nerve cell responds to the stimulus or it does not.

The PNS is equipped with Schwann cells that are strung like beads along the nerve cell. The Schwann cells insulate

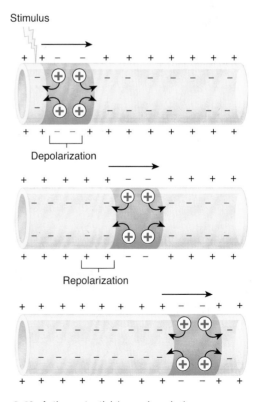

Figure 3-49. Action potential (nerve impulse).

the nerve membrane and in between the Schwann cells are gaps called nodes of Ranvier. The myelin provides insulation to the axon, like the plastic coating around electrical wires, preventing the nerve impulse from spreading out and short-circuiting. The nerve impulse is forced to jump from node to node instead of traveling along the entire surface of the membrane. By jumping over the Schwann cells, the impulse can travel much faster and transmission speed increases. The CNS does not have any Schwann cells, but it is equipped with oligodendrocytes that form the myelin sheath on some of the neurons that need insulation. The myelin insulation is especially helpful when there are hundreds of neurons transmitting hundreds of nerve impulses through one nerve.

Once the impulse reaches the end of the axon, it will send a signal to the next cell. There, the action potential may continue along the next cell or stimulate activity of a gland or organ.

Alcohol, cold temperature, continuous pressure, and anesthetics are some factors that can reduce the speed of the action potential. These factors either reduce the membrane's permeability to sodium or prevent oxygen and other nutrients from reaching the nerve. Without oxygen, cells suffer and eventually die.

Synaptic Transmission (Conductivity)

If the electrical impulse at the end of the axon is strong enough, the impulse will be conducted from one neuron to another neuron or an effector (muscle, organ, or gland). The impulses are conducted in a tiny but active gap called the synapse (SIHN-aps). The nerve cell that needs to transmit the impulse is called the presynaptic cell, and the cell that will receive the impulse is called the postsynaptic cell.

The electrical nerve impulse on the presynaptic cell triggers the axonal terminal to release a neurotransmitter chemical into the synapse. Approximately 30 different neurotransmitters are made in the brain and stored in vesicles at the axonal terminals all over the body. Some of the neurotransmitters are epinephrine (adrenaline), norepinephrine (noradrenaline), dopamine, serotonin, and acetylcholine. Acetylcholine, discussed in the muscular system section, is the neurotransmitter released at the neuromuscular junction. Once the vesicles release the neurotransmitter into the synapse, special receptor sites on the postsynaptic cell receive the neurotransmitters. The receptor site is activated and starts the action potential along the postsynaptic cell.

The synapse is designed such that the axon produces the neurotransmitters and the dendrites have specific receptor sites. In other words, a specific neurotransmitter must be received by the dendrite to complete the conduction. This design ensures a specific, one-way communication along the path (Fig. 3-50). Although most synapses are chemical (neurotransmitters and receptors), electrical synapses occur in cardiac or smooth muscle tissue where rhythmic, sequential muscle contractions are required.

Figure 3-50. Synapse. (Reprinted with permission from Bear MF, Connors BW, Paradiso MA. Neuroscience: Exploring the Brain. 2nd ed. Baltimore: Lippincott Williams & Wilkins, 2001.)

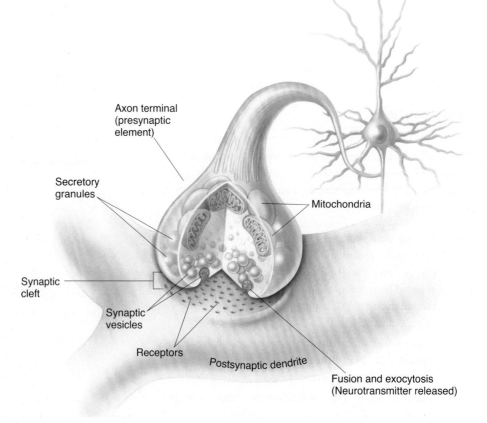

Axon terminal
(presynaptic
element)

Secretory
granules

Mitochondria

Synaptic
cleft

Synaptic
vesicles

Receptors

Postsynaptic dendrite

Fusion and exocytosis
(Neurotransmitter released)

Nervous System Organization

The nervous system is structurally organized in two distinct systems: the CNS and the PNS. The CNS consists of the brain and spinal cord. The PNS includes everything in the nervous system outside the brain and spinal cord: the nerves that exit the brain, called cranial nerves, and the nerves that exit the spinal cord, called spinal nerves.

Central Nervous System

The brain and the spinal cord are the structures that make up the CNS. This is the body's main control center for all of the body's functions, receiving sensory input from everywhere in the body, processing the information, and directing the body to make appropriate responses. Within the brain are four ventricles, or cavities, and outside the brain and spinal cord are three distinct layers of connective tissue coverings.

The Brain

The four main sections of the brain are the cerebrum (seh-REE-bruhm), the cerebellum (SAIR-eh-BEHL-uhm), the brainstem, and the diencephalon (DAHY-ehn-SEHF-uh-lahn) (Fig. 3-51).

The cerebrum is the largest portion, divided into two halves by a deep fissure called the longitudinal fissure. Each cerebral hemisphere is divided into four different sections,

called the parietal, occipital, temporal, and frontal lobes. The central fissure divides the brain into anterior and posterior sections, and just posterior to the central fissure is the parietal lobe. The parietal lobe receives information from the somatosensory receptors (touch, pressure, pain, temperature) and integrates information from all of the senses. The occipital lobe, the most posterior section of the cerebrum, processes visual input. The temporal lobe is located laterally and is responsible for hearing and the sense of smell. Anterior to the central fissure is the frontal lobe, which processes voluntary movement of our skeletal muscles, including speech. The cerebral hemispheres are connected by a mass of nervous tissue called the corpus callosum, which helps us coordinate movements that require the left and right side of our bodies to work together in activities such as crawling and walking.

The cerebellum is a cauliflower-like structure toward the back and base of the brain. It acts as the center for equilibrium and helps us maintain our balance. The cerebellum also controls coordination of skeletal muscles, maintains muscle tone, and allows movements to be fluid instead of jerky.

The brainstem, located at the central base of the brain, consists of the midbrain, pons, and medulla oblongata. The brainstem controls such activities as hearing, vision, breathing, sleep cycles, and organ activity.

The diencephalon sits above the brainstem, deep within the cerebrum, and includes the hypothalamus and thalamus. The hypothalamus plays a significant role in homeostasis. It regulates hunger, thirst, pain, sexual behavior, body temperature, and emotions. The activity of the thalamus is less specific, processing sensory input and redirecting it to the cerebrum.

The Spinal Cord

The spinal cord runs through the bony vertebral column, starting at the base of the brainstem and ending around the first or second lumbar vertebra. The spinal cord acts as a telegraph wire for sending signals to and from the brain. The inner core of the spinal cord is gray matter: nerve cell bodies without myelin covering. The outer periphery is white matter made of myelinated axons and dendrites (see Fig. 3-15).

Reflex Arcs

The spinal cord acts as the control center for reflexes, which are instantaneous, automatic responses that require very few nerve cells. The communication path allows the body to respond automatically and predictably to stimuli that are potentially dangerous. Reflex arcs are the specific nerve cell paths from stimulus to response, or receptor to effector. Receptors are located at the end of dendrites to detect stimuli. The information from a stimulus travels along a sensory neuron to the CNS. In the CNS, the impulses are

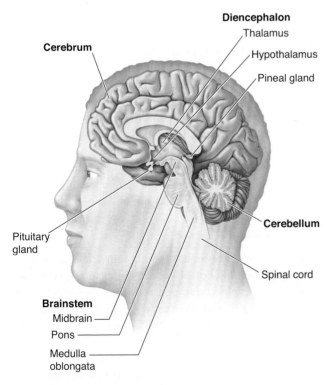

Diencephalon
Thalamus
Hypothalamus
Pineal gland

Cerebrum

Cerebellum

Pituitary gland

Spinal cord

Brainstem
Midbrain
Pons
Medulla oblongata

Figure 3-51. Brain.

coordinated and processed into an automatic, involuntary response. Once the response is determined, the motor neuron carries the signal away from the CNS to the effector. The effector is the muscle, organ, or gland that reacts or responds according to the information received. Motor reflexes, or somatic reflexes, activate skeletal muscles. Autonomic reflexes stimulate organs and glands to react. Figure 3-52 illustrates a reflex arc.

The simplest reflex arc only requires two neurons—one sensory and one motor. A nerve impulse travels along a sensory receptor to the spinal cord and back out to the effector along a motor neuron. Also called a spinal reflex, this reflex arc does not travel to the brain for coordination.

Stretch Reflexes

Stretch reflexes are protective muscle contractions that occur when the tissues are stretched too far and/or too fast. They prevent the muscle from being torn. The familiar test in which a doctor strikes a person's knee and the person responds with a kicking action is actually a stretch reflex that evaluates the patellar tendon. This tendon, found just inferior to the patella, is the tendon for the quadriceps femoris muscles that extend the knee joint and flex the hip joint. When the tendon is tapped, the muscle spindles in the quadriceps femoris sense that the muscle is being pulled too quickly. The proprioceptors send an impulse to the spinal cord, and the spinal cord sends an impulse back along a motor neuron to the quadriceps femoris, causing it to contract quickly in a protective mechanism. Stretch reflex

contraction of the quadriceps femoris quickly extends the knee with a kicking action.

Stretch reflexes come into play in massage therapy when you move a client's body. If a muscle is being stretched too fast and beyond its comfort zone, it can respond with a protective contraction that the client feels as a cramp. Therefore, always move the client's body carefully and knowledgeably to prevent protective muscle cramps.

Tendon Reflexes

Tendon reflexes occur when a muscle and its tendon are subjected to slow and gentle tension. The nerve impulse travels to the CNS, which determines that the muscle is not in danger of being torn and sends a nerve impulse that reflexively lengthens the muscle, allowing the stretch to go a bit further. Because the tendon reflex causes the opposite result from the stretch reflex, it is also important to a massage therapist. It can be used to encourage clients' tissues to stretch and create more space for circulation.

Protecting the body is the purpose of reflexes. When a stretch is potentially harmful to the muscle tissue, the body reflexively responds to the stretch with a contraction. A stretch that does not threaten the integrity of the tissues initiates the tendon reflex, which relaxes the muscle. The tendon reflex allows the connective tissue to stretch farther; the stretch reflex does not. For that reason, athletes can stretch more effectively by slowly and steadily increasing the stretch instead of by bouncing. Bouncing can induce the stretch reflex.

Flexor Reflexes

The flexor reflex, or withdrawal reflex, is another type of spinal reflex. The flexor reflex is activated usually in response to a harmful or painful stimulus, such as stepping on a tack or touching a hot pan. Unlike the stretch reflex that is activated by proprioceptors, the flexor reflex is activated by sensory receptors in the integument. The body uses three neurons to accomplish the safety mechanism of pulling away. A sensory neuron receives the input that is sent as an impulse to the spinal cord. There, an interneuron in the spinal cord transmits the impulse to a motor neuron. The impulse travels along the motor neuron to the appropriate muscles that must contract to move the body out of harm's way.

Ventricles

Enclosed inside the brain are four ventricles, or cavities. There are networks of blood capillaries in the ventricles that filter the blood and add cellular secretions to produce CSF. The fluid is constantly generated and circulated throughout the CNS to provide nutrients to and remove waste from the brain and spinal cord. It also acts as a cushion against impact and other trauma. The CSF eventually returns to the venous blood through the connective tissue covering of the brain.

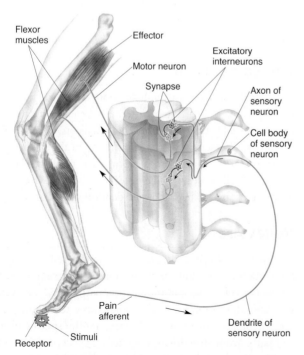

Figure 3-52. Reflex arc. (Reprinted with permission from Bear MF, Connors BW, Paradiso MA. Neuroscience: Exploring the Brain. 2nd ed. Baltimore: Lippincott Williams & Wilkins, 2001.)

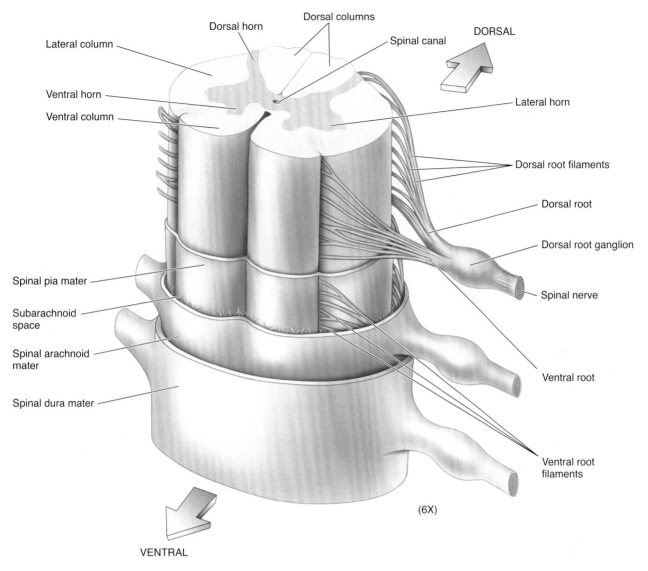

Figure 3-53. Meninges.

Meninges

The brain and spinal cord are supplied with three layers of connective tissue coverings called meninges (Fig. 3-53). The dura mater (DUHR-uh MAH-ter) is the toughest and outermost layer that provides a strong, protective covering for the structures of the CNS. The dura mater covering the spinal cord is sometimes referred to as the dural tube. The arachnoid mater (ah-RAK-noyd MAH-ter) is the middle layer with a structure like a spider web that allows CSF to flow through the meninges. The pia mater (PEE-ah MAH-ter) lies closest to the brain. It is delicate and carries most of the blood supply for the brain.

Peripheral Nervous System

The PNS consists of all the nerve tissue outside the CNS. Its function is to transmit information to and from the CNS. Again, nerves are made up of organized bundles containing nerve cells, connective tissue coverings, and blood vessels. The nerves that branch out from the brain are called cranial nerves, and the nerves that branch out from the spinal cord are called spinal nerves. Functionally, the PNS can be divided into the somatic and autonomic nervous systems. The somatic nervous system is responsible for voluntary skeletal muscle contractions. The autonomic nervous system (ANS) controls the involuntary smooth muscles of the organs, the cardiac muscles in the heart, and the activity of glands. The cranial and spinal nerves of the ANS are separated into the sympathetic and parasympathetic divisions, each with its own set of responses.

The PNS can be classified structurally, by the location of the nerves. There are cranial nerves, spinal nerves, and nerves in the extremities.

There are 12 pairs of cranial nerves originating from the brain (Fig. 3-54). The cranial nerves are identified by names

Figure 3-54. Cranial nerves.

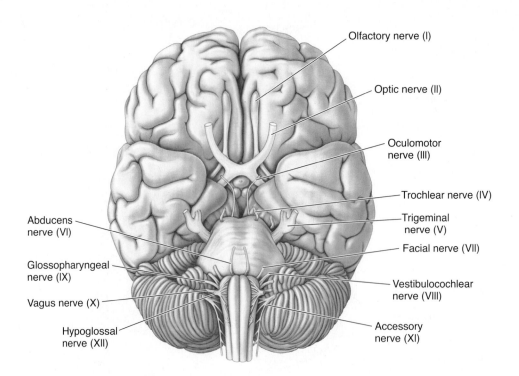

Olfactory nerve (I)

Optic nerve (II)

Oculomotor nerve (III)

Trochlear nerve (IV)

Trigeminal nerve (V)

Facial nerve (VII)

Vestibulocochlear nerve (VIII)

Accessory nerve (XI)

Abducens nerve (VI)

Glossopharyngeal nerve (IX)

Vagus nerve (X)

Hypoglossal nerve (XII)

and roman numerals, starting at the superior end. Most of them serve the head and neck region, but the vagus nerve (cranial nerve X) extends to the thoracic and abdominal cavities.

The 31 pairs of spinal nerves extend out from the spinal cord. They are identified according to where they exit the spinal cord, named for the closest vertebrae. For example, C8 exits the spinal cord just inferior to the seventh cervical vertebra (Fig. 3-55). Spinal nerves are mixed nerves, carrying sensory and motor neurons. Each spinal nerve is connected to the spinal cord by two roots. The dorsal root contains the sensory neurons that transmit nerve impulses to the spinal cord. The ventral root is made of the motor neurons that transmit the nerve impulses from the spinal cord out to the effectors.

Dermatomes are zones of the skin supplied by a specific spinal nerve root. The illustration in Figure 3-56 is an average representation of dermatomes, but the zones vary from person to person, and some dermatomes overlap. Massage therapists may encounter clients who suffer from a condition that affects one or more dermatomes.

The nerves in the extremities are located in the anterior and posterior arms and legs as shown in Figure 3-57. These are important for massage because they innervate the skeletal muscles of the body.

The PNS can also be classified by functions of the different tissues. The PNS is responsible for receiving sensory input and delivering nerve impulses that control bodily activities. The functions of the PNS can be separated into voluntary and involuntary activities. Voluntary activity is controlled by the somatic (soh-MAT-ik) nervous system. It serves all the skeletal muscles, allowing us to move muscles when we want to. Involuntary activities, including those of organs and glands, are controlled by the ANS.

Somatic Nervous System

The effectors of the somatic nervous system are our skeletal muscles, which are discussed in the section above on the muscular system. Recall that a motor unit is one motor neuron and all of the muscle cells that it controls. Precision movement is created by motor units with very few muscle cells. Strength is a function of the quantity of actin and myosin filaments within a muscle cell.

Neurological Memory

"Practice makes perfect," as the old saying goes. This is the basis for neurological memory. Repetition of a movement or holding the body's position in space reinforces the body's ability to produce that movement or position over time. The same activity, practiced over and over, creates a worn path in the brain and nervous system, sometimes called a nerve track. Very similar to a reflex arc, this figurative "groove" involves chemical and anatomical changes that reinforce learning. An association area of the brain handles the ability to remember movements and positions, but the nerve track promotes this ability. One theory of neurological memory suggests that the neurons that store the memories grow in size. Another theory is that the repetition increases the neuron's output of memory-enhancing proteins. The repetitions may also strengthen the connections between neurons, facilitating the transmission of impulses along a specific path.

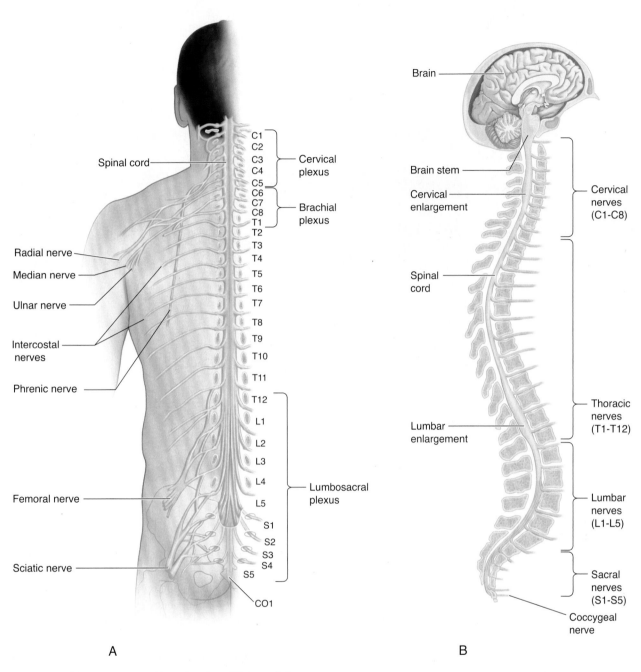

Figure 3-55. Spinal nerves. **(A)** Posterior view. **(B)** Lateral view.

The reinforcement of nerve tracks occurs with repetition, so repeating an activity correctly will reinforce the correct movement, and repeating an activity incorrectly will reinforce the incorrect movement. Unlearning an incorrect process and relearning it correctly is much more difficult than simply learning it properly from the beginning. For example, consider how children learn to hold a crayon or pencil. Those who learn to hold a pencil "incorrectly" will probably hold a pencil the same way for the rest of their lives despite efforts to hold it the "right" way. Once a nerve track is established, the body tends to respond predictably with the same

pattern, just like in a reflex response. Repatterning undesirable actions or behaviors requires effort and repetition of the desired action or behavior.

This concept is commonly seen in massage clients. When people get hurt, they tend to favor the injury and develop compensation patterns. Consider a person who stepped on a piece of glass and cut her foot. She might favor the injured foot with a limp or an abnormal posture, and her muscles and body will acquire a new "normal" position in space. The longer a client maintains the new position, the more the brain and nervous system reinforce the

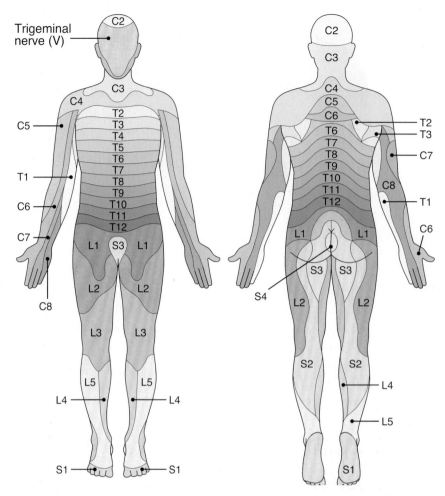

Figure 3-56. Dermatomes.

nerve track, and the more difficult it is for the client to return to the "normal" posture. Theoretically, a client who has an acute injury can return to a balanced posture more quickly than one who has allowed an injury to go untreated for months or years. Understanding this concept of neurological memory and educating your clients about it can help them understand that it may take more than one massage session to rid them of their aches and pains.

Autonomic Nervous System

The ANS controls the smooth muscles, cardiac muscles, organs, and glands, allowing them to function without our conscious effort. The ANS is divided into two systems that work together to maintain homeostasis: the sympathetic and parasympathetic divisions. When one of these two systems is too active or not active enough, homeostasis is disrupted, and the whole body suffers.

Sympathetic Nervous System
The sympathetic nervous system is the stimulatory division of the ANS. It is also known as the thoracolumbar division because it includes spinal nerves T1 through L2. It

activates the sympathetic response, sometimes called the fight or flight response, in which the body prepares for a stressful situation. Even a thought or perception of a threat can stimulate the sympathetic nervous system to release its neurotransmitters, including epinephrine (adrenaline) and norepinephrine (noradrenaline). When stimulated, the sympathetic nervous system affects many structures and organs, preparing them for an emergency situation. For example, the heart pumps faster to provide more oxygen, the skeletal muscles contract, the pupil of the eye dilates to allow more light in, the sweat glands are stimulated to perspire, and digestive activity slows down (Table 3-5).

Parasympathetic Nervous System
The parasympathetic nervous system is the relaxing, restorative division of the ANS. It is also known as the craniosacral (KRAY-nee-oh-SAY-kruhl) system because the motor pathways arise from the cranial nerves and sacral portions of the spinal nerves. The primary neurotransmitter of the parasympathetic nervous system is acetylcholine. When the parasympathetic nerves are triggered, the organs and glands have a response opposite to the sympathetic nervous response—the heart slows down, the

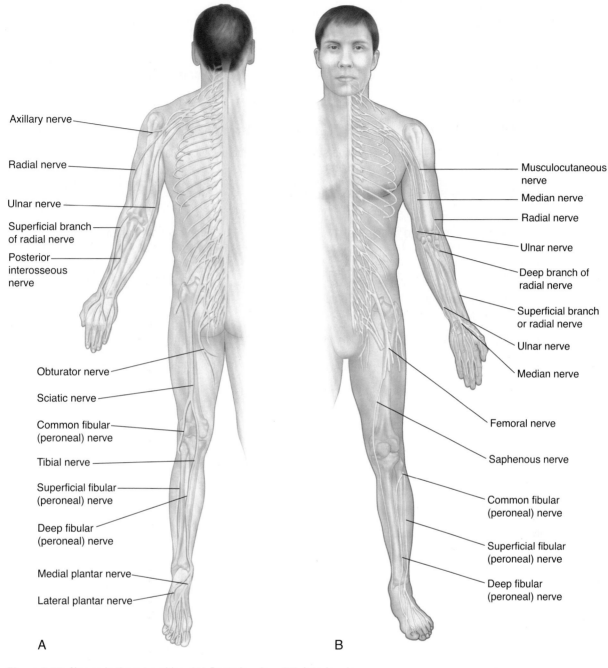

Axillary nerve

Radial nerve

Ulnar nerve

Superficial branch of radial nerve

Posterior interosseous nerve

Obturator nerve

Sciatic nerve

Common fibular (peroneal) nerve

Tibial nerve

Superficial fibular (peroneal) nerve

Deep fibular (peroneal) nerve

Medial plantar nerve

Lateral plantar nerve

A

Musculocutaneous nerve

Median nerve

Radial nerve

Ulnar nerve

Deep branch of radial nerve

Superficial branch or radial nerve

Ulnar nerve

Median nerve

Femoral nerve

Saphenous nerve

Common fibular (peroneal) nerve

Superficial fibular (peroneal) nerve

Deep fibular (peroneal) nerve

B

Figure 3-57. Nerves in the extremities. **(A)** Posterior view. **(B)** Anterior view.

skeletal muscles relax, the pupils constrict, sweat glands are not activated, and normal digestion occurs (Table 3-5). Typically, massage evokes the parasympathetic response, which is a relaxation response that encourages the body to "rest and digest."

These divisions of the nervous system work in balance. Too much stress or too much excitement can result in exhaustion. Likewise, too much rest or not enough activity has negative effects on the body. The body works best when structures and functions are balanced, including the activity of the ANS.

Functions of the Nervous System

There are three different responsibilities for the nervous system. Together, the functions of the nervous system help monitor input from both inside and outside the body and regulate the processes within our bodies to keep cellular metabolism in balance.

Monitor

The nervous system detects changes that occur within the body or outside the body. Sensory input of pain, pressure,

Table 3-5 Autonomic Nervous System Responses

Sympathetic	Effector	Parasympathetic
Dilation	Pupils of the eyes	Constriction
Inhibition	Digestive glands	Stimulation
Vasoconstriction	Blood supply to digestive system	Vasodilation
Decrease peristalsis	Smooth muscles of digestive system	Increase peristalsis
Increase strength and rate of contractions	Heart	Decrease strength and rate of contractions
Dilation	Bronchioles	Constriction
Stimulates epinephrine and norepinephrine release	Adrenal gland	None
Decrease activity	Kidneys	None
Relaxation	Urinary bladder	Contraction for urination
Release more glucose	Liver	None
Ejaculation	Penis	Erection
Vasodilation	Blood supply to skeletal muscles	None
Vasoconstriction	Blood supply to skin	None
Stimulates perspiration	Sweat glands in skin	None

and temperatures both inside and on the surface of our bodies are monitored by the nervous system. Monitoring our body positions in space so we know where we are and sensing scalding hot water on our skin are part of the nervous system's responsibilities.

Integrate

Once the nervous system has detected a change or has received sensory input, it processes the signal for an appropriate response. By monitoring body position, the nervous system can help us know if we are about to bump into something or fall over. When scalding hot water is detected on the skin, the nervous system knows that it is a dangerous situation that must be avoided. Conversely, when we receive a massage in a professional and safe environment, the sensory input is integrated by the nervous system to determine how much we will relax.

Respond

Finally, the nervous system takes the information it has detected and integrated and activates the appropriate

response, or motor output. Sometimes the nervous system activates a muscular contraction and other times it activates a gland to secrete hormones. Scalding hot water would cause the nervous system to respond with a motor output that contracts the muscles that can pull the body away from the hot water. In a frightening or emergency-type situation, the nervous system will activate the adrenal glands to release adrenaline and noradrenaline to prepare the body for impending physical exertion. A trusting and comfortable sensation during a massage can trigger the nervous system to send motor output signals to relax the skeletal muscles.

Effects of Massage on the Nervous System

All of the sensory input of your massage environment can affect the nervous system as well as the mental condition of the client, so be aware of your surroundings and be sensitive to client responses. Initial contact with the skin reflexively stimulates a sympathetic nervous response to prepare us for flight or fight in case the contact turns out to be a real or perceived threat. When the body has determined that the sustained touch does not pose any danger, it shifts the balance from a primarily sympathetic nervous response to a primarily parasympathetic response. Massage usually causes physiological changes associated with the parasympathetic nervous response of relaxation, changing the blood levels of several neurochemicals and hormones associated with pain:

- Increases dopamine (DOH-pah-meen)—a pain-relieving chemical involved in voluntary movement and clear thinking

- Increases endorphins (ehn-DOR-finz)—very strong pain-relieving chemicals that suppress all nerve functions to some degree

- Increases enkephalins (ehn-KEHF-uh-lihnz)—strong pain relievers involved in sensory integration

- Increases oxytocin (AHK-sih-TOH-sihn)—a chemical that increases the pain threshold, stimulates smooth muscle contractions, decreases sympathetic nervous response, and has sedative effects

- Increases serotonin (SAIR-uh-TOH-nihn)—a chemical that generally diminishes pain and appetite, regulates moods and sleep patterns, and stimulates smooth muscle contraction

- Decreases cortisol (KOR-tih-sohl)—a natural anti-inflammatory produced in response to stress that can accelerate the breakdown of tissues and prevent tissue repair, both of which can cause pain

- Decreases substance P—a neurotransmitter that triggers the pain response

Research has shown that massage can cause brain wave patterns of relaxation and alertness that were also associated with better performance on math computations.

Cardiovascular System

The cardiovascular system is a circulatory system that provides a link between the external environment and the internal fluid environment of the body by carrying nutrients and gases to all cells, tissues, organs, and organ systems and removing metabolic wastes. This exchange is necessary to maintain homeostasis within the body. Massage promotes the mechanical movement of fluids and thereby enhances the delivery of vital ingredients and removal of wastes.

In addition to the primary structures of the cardiovascular system (blood, blood vessels, and heart), the spleen, liver, bone marrow, and thymus gland also have circulatory functions, producing and storing blood components and differentiating immune cells.

Structures of the Cardiovascular System

The cardiovascular system consists of the blood, the blood vessels, the capillaries and the heart. These structures create separate pathways for blood, including the pulmonary circuit and the systemic circuit.

Blood

A single drop of blood contains about 10 million separate blood cells. Blood is a liquid connective tissue whose cells are suspended in an extracellular fluid matrix called plasma. Within the blood plasma are various components including RBCs, white blood cells, platelets, and proteins.

Blood Plasma

Plasma is a clear, straw-colored matrix that is similar in composition to cytosol. Mostly water, it also contains proteins, glucose, salts, vitamins, hormones, antibodies, and wastes. It acts as the transport system for delivering gases and nutrients throughout the body. Fibrinogen is a protein manufactured in the liver that resides in the plasma to help with hemostasis, the process of controlling blood loss and stopping blood flow. Alpha and beta globulins are plasma proteins that act as transport molecules for lipids and hormones; they are also made in the liver. Gamma globulins, or immunoglobulins, are antibodies made in the lymphoid tissues that float in the plasma and are one of the primary components of the immune system.

Erythrocytes

Erythrocytes (ee-RITH-roh-sahytz), also called red blood cells (RBCs), are biconcave, rounded structures with a central depression (Fig. 3-58). Erythrocytes are the only cells that

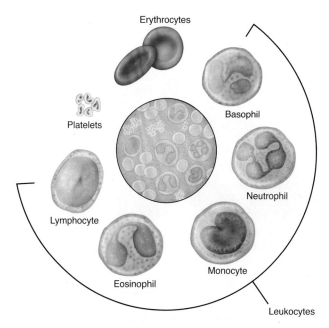

Figure 3-58. Erythrocytes, leukocytes, and platelets.

Erythrocytes

Platelets

Basophil

Neutrophil

Lymphocyte

Eosinophil

Monocyte

Leukocytes

do not have a nucleus. Instead, these cells are full of hemoglobin molecules that transport oxygen and buffer the pH of blood. Erythrocytes are enclosed by a highly permeable, elastic membrane that allows gases to diffuse through. Oxygen moves in and out of RBCs via diffusion. The high concentration of oxygen in the lungs causes oxygen to diffuse into the blood cells and onto the hemoglobin molecule. As the blood cells move through the body, oxygen diffuses out of the RBCs to tissues with lower concentrations of oxygen.

A tiny drop of blood contains over 5 million RBCs that circulate through the body 300,000 times in about 4 months before they break down and are actively destroyed by macrophages in the liver and spleen. Homeostasis is maintained via hematopoiesis in the red bone marrow, which generates approximately 3 million new RBCs each second.

Leukocytes

Leukocytes (LOO-koh-sahytz) are sometimes called white blood cells because they have a clear, colorless appearance (Fig. 3-58). They differ from erythrocytes because they are larger, they have a nucleus, they do not carry hemoglobin, and they have the special ability to squeeze through the cells in the capillary membranes to reside in the interstitial fluids (Fig. 3-59). There are five different kinds of leukocytes—neutrophils, basophils, eosinophils, lymphocytes, and monocytes—and they all function to defend the body against disease and foreign substances by destroying pathogens, which are bacteria, viruses, fungi, and other harmful agents that can cause disease.

A drop of blood only contains about 5,000 leukocytes, in contrast to 5 million erythrocytes. Leukocytes are produced by the bone marrow. They may circulate within the tissues for less than a day or reside in the tissues for months or years, depending on the severity of the infection or injury, serving as sentinels even in healthy tissues. In response to an injury or infection, leukocytes are produced at a higher rate and are much more abundant, so white blood cell counts can be useful tools for determining the presence of infection.

Platelets

Platelets, also called thrombocytes, are small, irregular, non-nucleated fragments of cells. Formed in the bone marrow as extensions of megakaryocytes that break off, these components are half the size of RBCs (Fig. 3-58). There are normally somewhere between 150,000 to 400,000 platelets in a drop of blood. Their main function is to aid in blood clotting, also known as hemostasis, and they can respond within 15 seconds to 2 minutes of the injury.

The Heart

The heart is the main structure of the cardiovascular system. It is about the size of a fist and is located between the lungs in the middle of the thoracic cavity. The heart has four separate chambers separated by muscle walls and valves. The two upper chambers are called atria (AY-tree-uh) and are encased by thin walls of cardiac muscle. The left and right atria are receiving chambers for incoming blood. The two ventricles have thicker walls and are located below the atria. The ventricles are the discharging chambers responsible for pumping blood from the heart to deliver it to the rest of the body (Fig. 3-60).

The myocardium, or cardiac muscle tissue, varies in thickness and is arranged in spiral bundles that wrap around the heart chambers. The spiral bundles contract with a wringing action that squeezes blood out of the chambers. Cardiac muscle tissue contracts spontaneously and independently and, unlike skeletal muscle, can contract even if all the nerve connections are severed. Cardiac muscle fibers contain electrical impulses that exchange charges back and forth to create a rhythmic contraction. These rhythmic contractions allow the heart to push approximately 6,000 quarts of blood through the body each day. The ANS controls the heart rate, which varies depending on the demands of the body for oxygen. The heart rate accelerates when the sympathetic nervous system is in control, and it decelerates under the parasympathetic response.

The valves in the heart are one-way gates that allow blood to flow in only one direction. Atrioventricular valves (AV valves) sit between the atrium and ventricle and are forced shut when the ventricles contract to prevent blood from leaking into the atria. The semilunar valves are located at the exits of the ventricles. When the ventricle contracts, the semilunar valves are forced open and allow blood to only flow out of the heart. When the ventricle relaxes, the

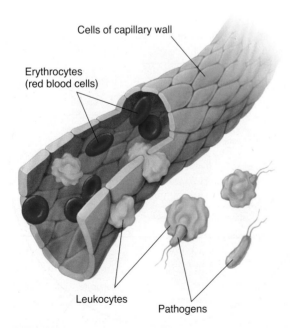

Cells of capillary wall

Erythrocytes
(red blood cells)

Leukocytes

Pathogens

Figure 3-59. Leukocytes passing through a membrane wall.

Figure 3-60. The heart and its chambers.

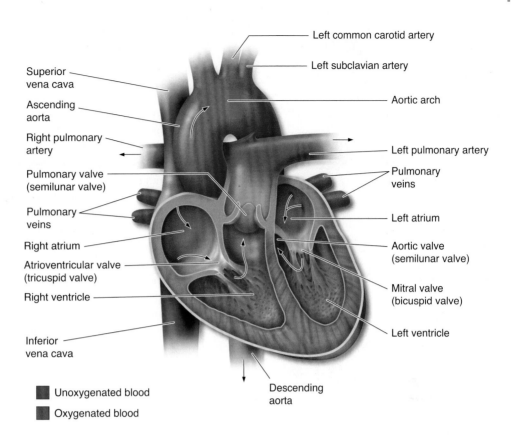

Superior vena cava

Ascending aorta

Right pulmonary artery

Pulmonary valve (semilunar valve)

Pulmonary veins

Right atrium

Atrioventricular valve (tricuspid valve)

Right ventricle

Inferior vena cava

Left common carotid artery

Left subclavian artery

Aortic arch

Left pulmonary artery

Pulmonary veins

Left atrium

Aortic valve (semilunar valve)

Mitral valve (bicuspid valve)

Left ventricle

Descending aorta

■ Unoxygenated blood

■ Oxygenated blood

semilunar valves prevent the blood from leaking back into the ventricles.

Blood follows a specific path through the heart:

1. Oxygen-depleted blood collects in the right atrium.

2. The right atrium contracts to push the blood through an AV valve into the right ventricle.

3. The ventricle, full of oxygen-depleted blood, contracts to push the blood through a semilunar valve into the pulmonary artery in the lungs.

4. The blood receives additional oxygen in the lungs and goes out through the pulmonary veins into the left atrium.

5. The left atrium contracts and forces oxygen-rich blood through an AV valve into the left ventricle.

6. The left ventricle contracts and forces oxygen-rich blood through a semilunar valve into the aorta, where it enters the arterial system and is delivered to the body.

Although there is a specific path, the left and right atria contract at the same time, and the left and right ventricles contract together.

Blood Vessels

The blood vessels transport blood from the heart to the rest of the body and back to the heart. The arteries, veins, and capillaries are collectively called the blood vessels. The largest blood vessel is the aorta (ay-OR-tuh), which measures about an inch across where it leaves the heart to transport oxygenated blood to the entire body. The smallest blood vessels are the capillaries, which are less than a tenth of a millimeter in diameter. Their small size limits the passage of molecules to a single file.

Arteries

An **artery** is a tube that carries blood away from the heart. The strong mechanical pumping force of the heart pushes the blood through the aorta and into its branches called arteries. As an artery travels further from the heart, it branches out, becoming smaller and thinner with distance. Arterioles are small arteries that are far from the heart, delivering the oxygenated blood to the capillaries. Figure 3-61 shows the arteries of the body. Gravity also helps the arteries move blood to different parts of the body. "Artery" is derived from the Greek word arteria, meaning air pipe. Originally, when they were discovered in corpses, the arteries were empty and assumed to transport air. Although it has since been determined that they carry blood, the name has not changed.

Arteries are constructed with three layers of tissues (Fig. 3-62). The interior layer, called the tunica intima or endothelium, is a layer of simple squamous epithelium that is very smooth and slippery. The middle layer, called the tunica media, is a layer of smooth muscle and elastic connective tissue. The smooth muscles keep the diameter of the

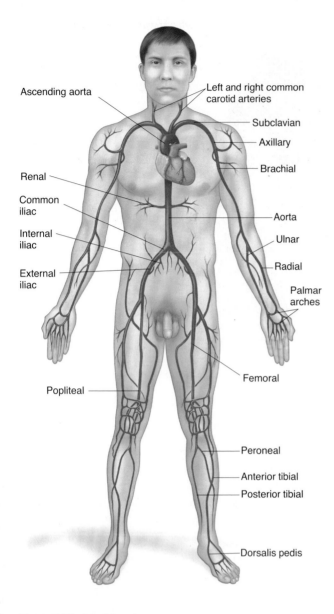

Ascending aorta

Left and right common
carotid arteries

Subclavian

Axillary

Brachial

Renal

Common
iliac

Aorta

Internal
iliac

Ulnar

External
iliac

Radial

Palmar
arches

Popliteal

Femoral

Peroneal

Anterior tibial

Posterior tibial

Dorsalis pedis

Figure 3-61. Arterial system.

arteries small, which increases the blood pressure the way a pinched water hose increases the water pressure. The outer layer of arteries is made of fibrous connective tissue called the tunica externa. It protects the arteries from damage and keeps the larger arteries from bursting as a result of the high blood pressure exerted by the force of the heart contraction.

Veins

Veins transport blood from the capillaries of the body back to the heart (Fig. 3-63). The smallest veins, called venules, receive the blood from the capillaries immediately after the blood has delivered its oxygen to and picked up carbon dioxide from the tissues, and immediately after the blood has picked up oxygen and dropped off carbon dioxide in the lungs. The largest veins are the superior vena cava and inferior vena cava, which are the last collection point of

deoxygenated blood before it goes into the heart. Much of the blood is moving against gravity, without the heart to pump it.

To compensate for the disadvantages and prevent blood from going the wrong direction, venous blood flow is aided by valves and skeletal muscle contractions. The valves are one-way gates that allow blood to flow in one direction only, similar to doors that only open outward. There are more valves in areas where blood typically must fight gravity to return to the heart, such as the legs. As the skeletal muscles contract, they squeeze the veins, and blood can only flow toward the heart. Figure 3-64 shows how the skeletal muscles work with the valves to encourage venous blood flow.

Veins are constructed with the same three layers as the arteries and are similar in size to the arteries but have thinner walls (see Fig. 3-62). The tunica media, or smooth muscle layer, is thinner and, as a result, the lumens of the veins are larger than those of arteries. The tunica externa of the veins is thinner because blood pressure is much lower in the veins, and they are not in danger of bursting.

Capillaries

Capillaries are the smallest, finest branches of the blood vessels where gases and fluids are exchanged. The capillary walls are composed of only one layer of cells and a basement membrane (Fig. 3-62). All transfers between blood and tissue cells occur at the capillary membranes via diffusion, osmosis, or filtration. Diffusion is a passive transport mechanism that allows molecules to pass through semipermeable membranes without assistance. Respiratory gases diffuse through the capillary walls and tissue cells. Osmosis allows water molecules, which are not fat soluble and cannot diffuse through the lipid bilayer, to use channel proteins to move through a membrane to balance concentrations on either side. Osmosis carries fluid from the interstitial spaces through the membrane and into the blood in the capillaries, where the concentration of solutes is higher. Filtration is the passive transport mechanism involving pressure gradients that takes water and dissolved substances through a membrane from a higher pressure to a lower pressure in an effort to balance concentrations on either side of the membrane. Filtration occurs in the kidneys (discussed later in this chapter) as well as at the arteriolar end of all capillaries.

Blood Circuits

The blood vessels can be separated into two separate pathways, called the pulmonary and systemic circuits. The pulmonary circuit takes blood to the lungs for gas exchange and returns it to the heart. The systemic circuit transports blood through the rest of the body.

Pulmonary Circuit

The pulmonary arteries carry deoxygenated blood from the right ventricle to the lungs. There, carbon dioxide

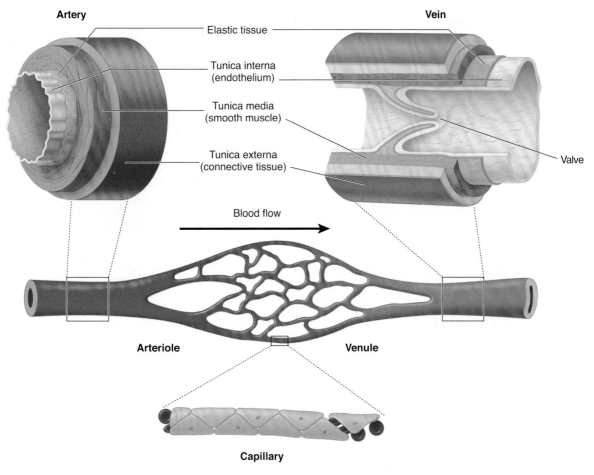

Figure 3-62. Comparison of arterial, venous, and capillary walls.

diffuses out of the blood and into the lungs, where it is exhaled into the external environment. Oxygen in the air we inhale diffuses from the lungs into the blood, and the pulmonary veins carry the oxygenated blood to the left atrium of the heart.

Systemic Circuit

The systemic arteries carry oxygenated blood to the capillaries throughout the body. Oxygen in the blood at the capillaries diffuses out into the tissues. Carbon dioxide diffuses from the tissues into the blood in the capillaries. The deoxygenated blood is then returned to the heart through the systemic veins.

Functions of the Cardiovascular System

The primary function of the cardiovascular system is to transport blood and all of its components. In addition to its important blood delivery service to all the cells of our bodies, the cardiovascular system has some other important functions. It carries cells that protect us from infection and diseases, provides immunity from disease, and prevents

blood loss. The cardiovascular system is also involved in regulating our core body temperature and maintaining the correct acidity of our blood, measured as pH.

Transportation

The cardiovascular system is the delivery system within the body. Using the blood as a transport mechanism, the cardiovascular system carries oxygen, carbon dioxide, hormones, and nutrients to and from all parts of the body. There is a certain pathway for taking blood from the heart to the lungs to pick up oxygen, a separate path that delivers oxygen-rich blood from the heart to the cells of the body, and yet another pathway for returning oxygen-deficient blood to the heart.

Protection

The cardiovascular system uses the blood to carry leukocytes, antibodies, and platelets throughout the body. The leukocytes (also called white blood cells), along with the antibodies, fight pathogens and destroy foreign substances. Their ability to protect us from infection and disease is called immunity.

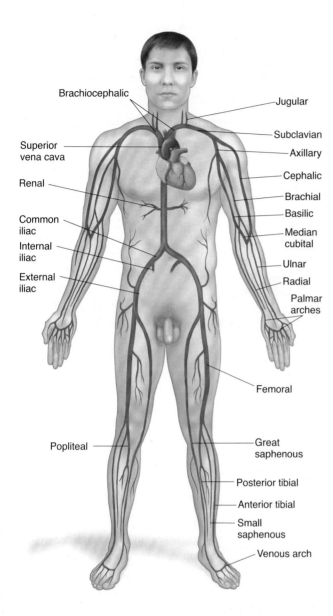

Figure 3-63. Venous system.

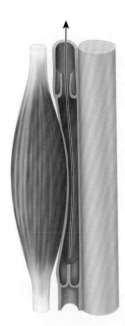

Figure 3-64. Skeletal muscle "pump" for venous blood flow. Skeletal muscle contraction squeezes the veins and their valves, causing venous blood to be forced through the one-way valves.

platelets are caught in the tangle, further reducing blood flow in the area. Leukocytes also get caught, which remove cellular debris and fight infection. As the platelet plug shrinks, the fibrin strands contract and pull the edges of the wound together to provide a framework for tissue repair.

Regulation

The cardiovascular system also helps maintain body temperature by constriction and dilation of the blood vessels. A thermostat in the brain maintains the body's normal temperature at approximately 98.6°F. When external temperatures, muscular exertion, or fever create excessive heat, vasodilation (dilation of the blood vessels) in the skin allows more warm blood to flow near the skin's surface, where heat can dissipate. Conversely, the vessels constrict (vasoconstriction) in the skin when the external environment is excessively cold, in an effort to preserve body heat. The brain needs blood to function properly and has priority over all other organs, regardless of the body's temperature or activity. In extreme situations, more blood will be sent to the brain and less to the rest of the body. Body heat is dissipated from the head, despite the body's core temperature. Thus, wearing a hat in colder temperatures helps keep fingers and toes warmer.

The acidity or alkalinity of a substance is measured as pH. Neutral pH, or pH balanced, indicates a substance that is neither acidic nor alkaline and has a pH of 7. When the pH is below 7, the solution is considered acidic, and above 7 it is considered basic, or alkaline. The interstitial fluids (also called extracellular fluids or tissue fluids) are kept at pH 7.4, which means that tissue fluids are slightly basic, or alkaline.

Platelets in the blood activate hemostasis, a clotting process that the body uses to automatically stop bleeding. By forming a blood clot, our bodies protect us from losing too much blood. When the clotting mechanism takes place on the integument, it forms a scab that protects us from having bacteria in the external environment enter the body through the open wound.

The mechanism of hemostasis starts when blood vessels within a tissue are injured and localized vasoconstriction occurs. Blood platelets accumulate and stick together. Once they adhere to each other, they release chemicals that attract more platelets to the area, and they clump together to form a platelet plug or clot to seal the hole in the blood vessel and slow the bleeding. Fibrinogen, a protein suspended in the blood, is converted into strands of fibrin, which tangle together at the injury site. As circulation continues, RBCs and

The blood has hemoglobin and plasma proteins that act as buffers, or chemicals that stabilize pH levels.

Effects of Massage on the Cardiovascular System

The effects of massage on the cardiovascular system are determined by where and how strokes are applied. Moderate pressure massage activates the parasympathetic nervous system, which means that the heart rate slows down, the force of contractions decreases, and blood pressure decreases. See Research Box 3.2. Percussive massage strokes initially cause the reflexive effect of vasoconstriction (blood vessel constriction) to reduce circulation to the area. Sustained percussion, however, can result in vasodilation (blood vessel dilation) in the area.

Mechanically, pressure on the blood vessels increases circulation. Capillaries with poor blood flow respond to this kind of mechanical pressure remarkably well and can then supply oxygenated blood to ischemic tissues. Massage increases the permeability of the capillary walls, enhancing the delivery of oxygen and nutrients as well as waste removal.

RESEARCH BOX 3-2

Massage and High Blood Pressure

High blood pressure is associated with elevated anxiety, stress and stress hormones, hostility, depression and catecholamines. Massage therapy and progressive muscle relaxation were evaluated as treatments for reducing blood pressure and these associated symptoms. Adults who had been diagnosed as hypertensive received ten 30 min massage sessions over five weeks or they were given progressive muscle relaxation instructions (control group). Sitting diastolic blood pressure decreased after the first and last massage therapy sessions and reclining diastolic blood pressure decreased from the first to the last day of the study. Although both groups reported less anxiety, only the massage therapy group reported less depression and hostility and showed decreased urinary and salivary stress hormone levels (cortisol). Massage therapy may be effective in reducing diastolic blood pressure and symptoms associated with hypertension.

Hernandez-Reif M, Field T, Krasnegor J, Hossain Z, Theakston H, Burman I. (2000). High blood pressure and associated symptoms were reduced by massage therapy. J Bodyw Mov Ther 2000;4:31–38.

Lymphatic System

The lymphatic system is similar to the cardiovascular system because of its many vessels, but it is not a true circulatory system. This branching network of lymph vessels is a one-way road that transports lymphatic fluid from all over the body and drains it into the bloodstream at a location near the heart. Although the cardiovascular system has the heart to push the blood through the blood vessels, the lymphatic system does not have a major pump. The lymphatic system of vessels and valves is able to function primarily via rhythmic contraction of the skeletal muscles and gravity. As the fluid is being moved toward the heart, it passes through several structures that filter out large and foreign particles so they do not enter the bloodstream. There are also structures of the lymphatic system that provide immunity by producing cells that destroy pathogens and other foreign particles.

Structures of the Lymphatic System

The lymphatic system includes the lymph, lymph vessels, lymph nodes, lymphatic organs including the spleen and thymus gland, and some lymph tissue in the intestine and tonsils.

Lymph

Remember that in the capillaries, blood plasma seeps through the capillaries to fill the interstitial space, or the space between cells. There, it acquires cellular debris and foreign substances that are eliminated by the surrounding cells. The interstitial fluid that is taken from all over the body into the lymphatic system is called **lymphatic fluid**, or **lymph**. The additional components of lymph include the lymphocytes, monocytes, proteins, and cellular waste.

Lymph Vessels

The interstitial fluids are first collected by the lymph capillaries throughout the body. The lymph capillaries join to form larger lymphatic vessels that carry the lymph back to the heart. The lymph from the upper right quadrant of the body exits the lymphatic system at the right lymphatic duct, which drains into the right subclavian vein. The lymph from the rest of the body drains out of the lymphatic system through the thoracic duct and into the left subclavian vein. The subclavian veins join together and empty lymph and deoxygenated blood into the heart (Fig. 3-65 illustrates the lymph vessels).

Lymph vessels have the same basic structure as veins but are smaller and more delicate. The vessels have valves to ensure lymph flows in one direction, and they have smooth muscles within their walls. The sections of the lymph vessels between the valves are called lymphangions, and the

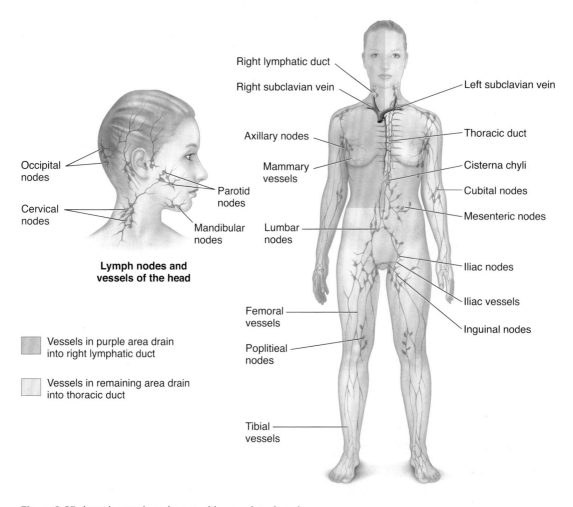

Right lymphatic duct

Right subclavian vein

Left subclavian vein

Axillary nodes

Thoracic duct

Mammary vessels

Cisterna chyli

Cubital nodes

Parotid nodes

Mesenteric nodes

Occipital nodes

Cervical nodes

Mandibular nodes

Lumbar nodes

Iliac nodes

Lymph nodes and vessels of the head

Iliac vessels

Femoral vessels

Inguinal nodes

Vessels in purple area drain into right lymphatic duct

Poplitieal nodes

Vessels in remaining area drain into thoracic duct

Tibial vessels

Figure 3-65. Lymph vessels and areas with many lymph nodes.

peristaltic contractions of the smooth muscles assist the flow of lymph very slightly. Being a one-way system without a mechanical pump behind it, the lymphatic system puts minimal pressure on the walls of the vessels, so the layers of muscle and fibrous connective tissue covering are thin. Like venous blood, much of the lymph travels against gravity. Skeletal muscle movements encourage lymph through the lymph vessels and valves, similar to the mechanism that encourages venous flow (see Fig. 3-64).

The flow of lymph through the vessels is also aided by the contraction of the diaphragm muscle during inspiration, which creates a vacuum-like suction that pulls blood and lymph upward and toward the heart. There are many lymph vessels in the central tendon of the diaphragm, so when it contracts, lymph is pushed through the one-way valves. Also, contraction of the diaphragm creates a vacuum in the thoracic cavity that pulls both lymph and venous blood through their respective vessels and one-way valves.

Lymph Nodes

Lymph nodes are oval, bean-shaped structures that house and produce lymphocytes and filter the lymphatic fluid.

Thousands of lymph nodes can be found in groups along the lymph vessels, and large concentrations of lymph nodes are found in the cervical, inguinal, and axillary regions (Fig. 3-65). Lymph nodes contain lots of macrophages and lymphocytes and have a structural framework of reticular connective tissue that creates a meshwork for filtering lymph. Pathogens and toxins in the lymph are destroyed or inactivated and filtered out with a series of fibrous traps. The clean lymphatic fluid flows out of the node and continues on its path toward the heart.

Lymph Organs and Tissues

The largest lymph organ is the spleen, which is approximately the size of the heart. The spleen produces lymphocytes, filters the blood, and removes old, worn-out erythrocytes from the blood. In the process of removing erythrocytes, iron is extracted for future use. The spleen also functions as a storage container for extra blood, releasing it when necessary. It acts as a conference center for immune cells and blood cells, providing a meeting place and activity center for them. Macrophages destroy foreign substances that have with chemical antigens on their surface that stimulate the immune response. Macrophages destroy foreign substances such as bacteria, pollen, and viruses that have antigens (proteins) on their surfaces that activate the immune response. To destroy antigenic cells and substances with antigenic proteins on them, the spleen has B cells that produce antibodies, proteins that recognize and bond to specific antigens. The antibodies coat the foreign substances, inactivating them or attracting macrophages to them. The process of inactivating foreign substances is called the immune response.

The thymus gland in children is located deep to the sternum, but as we age, the thymus gland shrinks and only a small amount of tissue remains in adults, superior to the heart. It is the site where some lymphocytes mature.

There are areas of clustered lymph tissue found in the tonsils and intestines. Tonsils are small masses of lymph tissue on either side of the soft palate at the back of the throat. These areas of moist epithelium are in contact with the external environment, so the tonsils help prevent bacteria and other pathogens from entering the throat. Some pathogens get past the tonsils and are able to get further into the gastrointestinal tract. If they get into the intestines, they are subjected to Peyer's patches, lymph tissue in the lining of the intestines, loaded with white blood cells that fight bacteria, viruses, and other microorganisms.

Functions of the Lymphatic System

The lymphatic system has transportation, immune, and homeostatic functions. The lymph vessels provide a roadway for lymph, which can carry nutrients as well as waste. The lymphatic system also provides immunity by producing cells that destroy foreign particles, pathogens, and toxins. Finally, the lymph vessels help maintain blood volume and blood pressure.

Transportation

Interstitial fluid, the fluid that surrounds our cells, contains chemicals and metabolic wastes that have been transported out of the cells. The lymphatic system is most commonly known for transporting "bad" things away from our tissues so they can be destroyed or removed from our bodies. However, there are some beneficial substances produced in the body that can only get to the bloodstream for delivery to the rest of the body by way of the lymph system. Fatty acids and vitamin A are end products of digestion found in the small intestine. From there, they are absorbed into the lymphatic system and eventually added to the bloodstream to nourish cells throughout the body.

Immunity

The lymphatic system helps us fight bacteria and other foreign substances. Leukocytes, or white blood cells, which are critical to immunity, are made in the bone marrow and are divided in the lymphatic tissue. The fluid that is drained from the interstitial spaces by the lymphatic system carries the leukocytes known as lymphocytes and monocytes. As the fluid is transported to the heart to be added to the blood, it is filtered in lymph nodes where antibodies and macrophages destroy or inactivate pathogens that cause illness.

Homeostasis

Once outside the cells, interstitial fluid can either diffuse back through the capillary walls into the blood or it can be drained via the lymphatic system. This is an important homeostatic mechanism for maintaining proper blood volume and blood pressure. If our blood volume or blood pressure is low, interstitial fluid will diffuse through the capillaries to be added to the blood. As a result, blood volume and blood pressure increase.

Effects of Massage on the Lymphatic System

Massage is especially beneficial to the lymphatic system. Because there are so many lymph vessels in the diaphragm muscle, massage therapists can utilize the diaphragm to increase lymphatic flow by asking clients to use deep breathing techniques.

Numerous lymph vessels travel through the superficial and deep fascia, and the mechanical pressure of massage strokes on these vessels increases the flow of lymph. Similarly, skeletal muscle contractions put pressure on the lymph vessels and pump lymph through the one-way valves. Joint movement and passive contractions applied during a massage activate this skeletal muscle pump, though not as effectively as active contractions.

Respiratory System

The respiratory system allows us to breathe, which is an activity controlled by the CNS. Awake or asleep, breathing continues as long as we are alive. The nervous system controls contractions of the diaphragm muscle, which pulls air into the respiratory system. In the lungs, oxygen diffuses from the air we breathe into the blood in the capillaries, and the circulatory system delivers the oxygen throughout the body. This is also where carbon dioxide is eliminated via exhalation.

Structures of the Respiratory System

The structures of the respiratory system include the nose, nasal cavity, pharynx (FAIR-inks), larynx, trachea (TRAY-kee-ah),

3 Body Systems

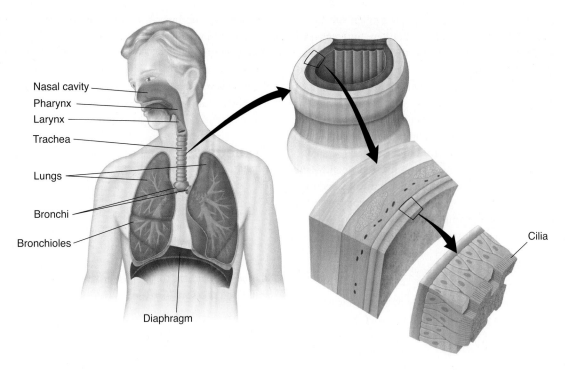

Figure 3-66. Respiratory system.

bronchi (BRAHN-kahy), bronchioles, alveoli (al-VEE-oh-lahy), and lungs (Fig. 3-66). These structures can be separated into two groups: the upper and lower respiratory tracts.

Upper Respiratory Tract

The upper respiratory tract includes the nose, nasal cavity, pharynx, larynx, and the upper part of the trachea. Cartilage, mucus, and ciliated cells are present in all of the structures of the upper respiratory tract. Cartilage maintains the shape of the structures to prevent the airway from collapsing and stopping air flow. The mucus traps foreign particles that are then swept toward the external environment by ciliated cells. The lungs are a good breeding ground for infection because they are moist and warm, so it is very important to have the cells that secrete mucus and the ciliated cells functioning properly.

Nose and Nasal Cavity

The first part of the respiratory tract to receive air from the external environment is the nose and the nasal cavity. The cartilage in the nose holds it open to allow air to enter easily. There, the mucous secretions moisten the air to keep the lungs from drying out. The capillaries lying just beneath the surface of the epithelium warm the air, again for the benefit of the delicate tissues of the lungs. There are olfactory cells within the nasal cavity that are the sensory receptors for smell.

Pharynx

As the incoming air leaves the nasal cavity, the air is received by the pharynx. The pharynx acts as a passageway for both the respiratory and digestive systems. Eustachian tubes connect the upper part of the pharynx to the middle ear, equalizing air pressure on either side of the ear's tympanic membrane. The pharyngeal tonsils, also called adenoids, are made of lymphatic tissue in the pharynx and are discussed in the lymphatic system section above. If the lymphatic activity is high enough, the tonsils can enlarge and the air passage can actually be obstructed.

Larynx

The larynx, or voice box, is made of cartilage and lies just inferior to the pharynx. The thyroid cartilage, commonly referred to as the Adam's apple, is part of the larynx. The epiglottis is a little structure in the larynx that prevents food from going down the airway. The vocal cords are connected to the larynx's cartilage, and as air moves by them, they vibrate and create sound.

Upper Trachea

The trachea is a tubelike structure that connects the larynx to the bronchi in the lungs. The trachea has cilia that sweep foreign particles caught in mucus up toward the external environment. These unwanted particles are coughed out, spat out, or swallowed.

Lower Respiratory Tract

The structures of the lower respiratory tract include the lower part of the trachea, the bronchi, bronchioles, alveoli, and lungs.

Lower Trachea

At the inferior end of the trachea, the airway splits into two separate paths. Rings of hyaline cartilage hold the trachea open, and mucus and cilia cooperate to remove foreign matter from the respiratory path.

Bronchi

The left and right branches of the airway following the trachea are called the bronchi. The bronchi enter the lungs and each of the bronchi branches into finer and finer airways. Bronchioles are the smallest airways inside the lungs and they do not contain any cartilage. Their walls are mostly made of smooth muscles that are controlled by the ANS. Although the air that reaches the bronchi is usually warm, moist, and particle-free, mucus and cilia are still present to sweep foreign particles out to the environment.

Alveoli

At the ends of the tiny bronchioles, air enters the pulmonary alveoli, which resemble clusters of grapes. They have thin walls of simple squamous epithelium that allow gases to be exchanged with the blood in the capillaries that wrap around them. Diffusion allows oxygen to move into the capillaries and carbon dioxide to move into the alveoli (Fig. 3-67). Surfactants are secreted by cells in the alveoli to reduce surface tension and allow the alveoli to expand without stress.

Lungs

The left and right lungs are separated by the section of the thoracic cavity that holds the heart and large blood vessels and is called the mediastinum (MEE-dee-ah-STAHY-num).

The tops of the lungs are just inferior to the clavicles and the bottoms of the lungs rest on the diaphragm. The lungs are enveloped in a serous membrane called the visceral pleura, and the thoracic cavity is lined with a serous membrane called the parietal pleura. The serous fluid that these membranes secrete provides lubrication to prevent friction between the two membranes and also helps keep the separate layers of membranes together. The concept is similar to how water between two layers of plastic wrap keeps the layers close together while allowing them to slip past each other easily.

Functions of the Respiratory System

The respiratory system moves air in and out of the lungs, which is also known as ventilation. In addition to ventilation, the respiratory system cooperates with the circulatory system to perform respiration, which provides oxygen to the body and removes carbon dioxide. Carbon dioxide removal is very important. People actually die faster from carbon dioxide accumulation than oxygen depletion.

The respiratory system also allows us to maintain the proper pH level for interstitial fluids and produce speech, and it provides body defenses by coughing and sneezing unwanted particles out of the airway.

Ventilation

Ventilation moves air in and out of the lungs, and respiration takes the carbon dioxide out of the body and brings

Figure 3-67. Alveoli and gas exchange.

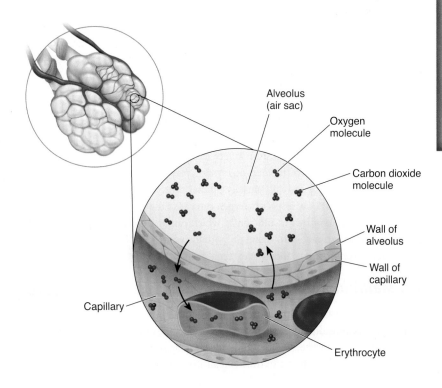

Alveolus (air sac)

Oxygen molecule

Carbon dioxide molecule

Wall of alveolus

Wall of capillary

Capillary

Erythrocyte

oxygen in. The gas exchange must occur in both directions to maintain homeostasis.

Inhalation

Inhalation, also known as inspiration, draws air into the lungs. It occurs as the diaphragm and external intercostal muscles contract. The floor of the thoracic cavity is pulled downward as a result of the diaphragm contraction, and the walls of the thoracic cavity are widened by the contraction of the external intercostals. The parietal pleural membranes are attached to the walls of the thoracic cavity and expand along with it, pulling air from the external environment into the respiratory pathway.

Exhalation

The ventilation process that moves air out of the lungs is called exhalation, or expiration. Normal exhalation is a passive process that mostly results from the relaxation of the diaphragm and external intercostals. Some activities require additional, forced exhalation, such as speaking, singing, or blowing. The internal intercostal muscles can be contracted to reduce the size of the thoracic cavity, and the abdominal muscles can be contracted to push the floor of the thoracic cavity upward.

Respiration

The exchange of oxygen and carbon dioxide that occurs in the respiratory system is called external respiration because the gas exchange occurs between our tissues and the external environment. As discussed above, internal respiration, or cellular respiration, occurs within the cells and tissues. Inhalation and exhalation are equally important for maintaining proper chemical levels in the blood. The respiratory and circulatory systems cooperate to provide a transport mechanism for the blood gas exchange.

The nervous system and chemical signals can trigger increased ventilation to provide more gas exchange via external respiration. The brain and motor nerves control the muscles that set the rate and depth of respiration. If you think about how we breathe when we cry, laugh, or exercise, you will see how emotions and physical activity affect our breathing patterns. Emotions are associated with chemicals produced in the brain, and those chemicals can stimulate or alter respiration.

The proprioceptors of the nervous system play an important part in respiratory activity. Muscle spindles sense tension in the muscle fibers. Low levels of oxygen can cause the respiratory muscles to contract insufficiently, which can be detected by the muscle spindles. To maintain homeostasis, the CNS will increase ventilation to increase external respiration.

pH Maintenance

The amount of carbon dioxide in the blood affects the pH. Too much carbon dioxide lowers the pH and makes blood more acidic than normal. Acidic fluids can destroy the cellular membrane and are harmful to the health of the cells and tissues. When the pH is too low, the body will try to raise the pH by increasing the breathing rate, exposing the lungs to more oxygen, getting rid of carbon dioxide, thus raising the proportion of oxygen levels in the tissues. When the pH is too high and the fluids are too basic, the body can respond by reducing respiratory activity to build up carbon dioxide and acidify the fluids. The cooperation between the respiratory and circulatory systems is an obvious example of how interdependent the body systems are from the cellular level all the way up to the organism level.

Speech Production

The larynx (LAIR-inks), or voice box, is part of the respiratory system where sounds can be created. Specifically, the vocal cords vibrate as air passes over them, creating sound. By combining movement of the tongue, lips, and cheeks and the speed of exhalation, we can control our voices to create precise sounds.

Body Defenses

There are some reflexive activities of the respiratory system that protect us from irritating objects in the airway. Irritation of the mucous membrane at the back of the throat or farther down the respiratory pathway can cause a cough, our body's attempt to eliminate unwanted material through the mouth. When the mucous membrane of the nasal passages is irritated, our body sneezes reflexively in an attempt to expel unwanted material through the nose.

Effects of Massage on the Respiratory System

The process of cellular respiration is enhanced by massage and manipulation of the tissues, partly as a result of the increased circulation. As muscles are massaged, the heat of friction and the oxidation of glycogen create additional amounts of carbon dioxide that the body has to expel to maintain homeostasis. We eliminate carbon dioxide by exhaling it through the lungs and can eliminate unusually high amounts by simply breathing deeply and more effectively. Furthermore, massage that lasts longer than 10 to 15 minutes activates the parasympathetic nervous response, which encourages slow, deep contractions of the diaphragm.

When excessive mucus accumulates in the respiratory tract, rhythmic tapotement can help loosen it and make it easier to cough out for relief from respiratory congestion.

Digestive System

The digestive system is the pathway for food from the moment it enters the mouth until it is eliminated at the anus. The nervous system sends motor signals to the structures of the digestive system to take the food we eat and transform it into a substance that can release the nutrients. The capillaries absorb the nutrients and deliver them throughout the body by way of the blood. The organ systems must work together for our bodies to function normally.

Structures of the Digestive System

The digestive system can be broken into two sets of structures: the alimentary canal and the accessory organs. The alimentary (AL-ih-MEN-tah-ree) canal is the passageway that includes the oral cavity, pharynx, esophagus, stomach, small intestine, and large intestine. The accessory digestive organs include the pancreas, liver, gallbladder, and salivary glands that produce chemicals necessary for digestion. Figure 3-68 shows the structures of the alimentary canal and the accessory digestive organs.

The Alimentary Canal

The alimentary canal, or digestive tract, is where food is broken down and eventually absorbed. It includes the oral cavity, pharynx, esophagus, stomach, small intestine, and large intestine. The canal is constructed of four layers, including the mucous membrane, submucosa, external muscle layer, and serous membrane. The deepest layer is the mucous membrane. It secretes mucus to lubricate the passage of food through the canal and secretes digestive enzymes to encourage the breakdown of food. Just outside the mucous membrane is the submucosa, which is a layer of connective tissue filled with blood vessels and lymph vessels. The external muscle layer is made of smooth muscle for most of the length of the canal, but the esophagus contains skeletal muscle. The outermost layer of the alimentary canal is fibrous connective tissue above the diaphragm, but below the diaphragm, most of the outer layer is a serous membrane called the visceral peritoneum.

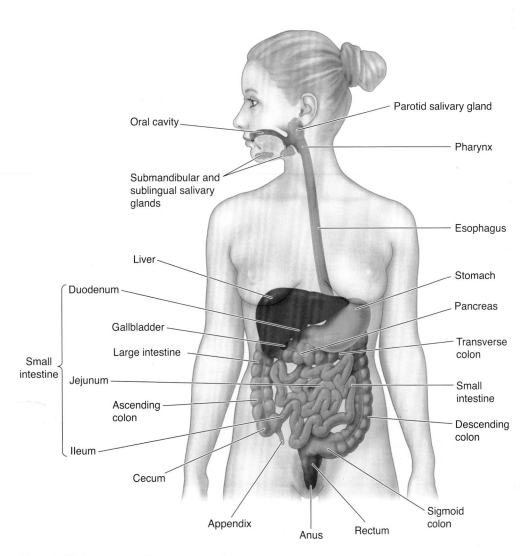

Figure 3-68. Structures of the digestive system.

Oral Cavity

The oral cavity contains the teeth and tongue, which begin the process of digestion. Teeth grind food into smaller pieces while the tongue circulates the food to make sure everything gets evenly chewed. The salivary glands are located below the tongue, above, below, and behind the TMJ. The saliva contains enzymes that chemically break down food even further.

Pharynx

The pharynx has overlapping layers of skeletal muscle whose fibers run perpendicular to each other. When these muscles rhythmically contract, they create peristalsis: wave-like contractions that move substances through a tube.

Esophagus

The esophagus is a tube that runs from the pharynx to the stomach, moving the food with peristaltic action.

Stomach

Once food reaches the stomach, it is stored and chemically broken down even further. The smooth muscles churn the food mechanically while gastric juice continues the chemical breakdown. The resulting chyme (KAHYM) exits the stomach.

Small Intestine

The chyme formed in the stomach then enters the small intestine, the major organ for absorption. Nutrients, water, and electrolytes are absorbed in the small intestine as the chyme passes through.

Large Intestine

The chyme leaves the small intestine and enters the large intestine, where more water and minerals are absorbed. Bacteria in the large intestine feed on fecal material and release gas as a byproduct. The remaining fiber and other indigestible wastes are eliminated at the exit of the large intestine, the anus.

Accessory Digestive Organs

The accessory organs of the digestive system include the pancreas, liver, gallbladder, and salivary glands. They secrete enzymes and hormones that are required for digestion. The pancreas also produces the hormones insulin and glucagon, which are critical for the regulation of blood sugar levels. The liver makes bile, which breaks fats into smaller pieces that are more easily digested, and it detoxifies and excretes wastes and toxins. Fats and glycogen for energy are stored in the liver, as are many vitamins, and iron for hemoglobin formation. The gallbladder is a small organ just below the liver that acts as a sort of holding tank for bile that is not being used. When the body must process large amounts of fat, the gallbladder releases bile to emulsify it. The salivary glands, located anterior to the ears (parotid glands), under the tongue (sublingual glands), and just under the lower jaw (submandibular glands), all produce saliva, which chemically breaks down starches, inhibits bacterial growth, and eases the processes of chewing and swallowing.

Functions of the Digestive System

Our digestive system is responsible for taking the food we consume and delivering the nutrients to the body. It does this by mechanically and chemically breaking down food, absorbing it, and eliminating the indigestible remains, all the while moving it through the digestive tract by propulsion and smooth muscle contractions called peristalsis.

Digestion

Digestion is the process of breaking food down by mechanical and chemical activity. When food enters the mouth, we chew it up and mechanically grind the food into smaller pieces. Saliva, secreted by three pairs of salivary glands and delivered to the oral cavity through ducts, contains a digestive enzyme that can chemically break down some foods. The stomach contains acids and enzymes to chemically break down food particles even more.

Several muscles are involved in the process of digestion. The process of chewing requires muscles to move the mandible, or lower jaw. The muscles of the tongue push food around the mouth to be chewed completely. Both skeletal and smooth muscles create peristalsis.

Absorption

Food that has been mechanically broken down into a substance called chyme can be chemically digested into absorbable nutrients. The nutrients are absorbed into the blood and lymph in the intestines. From there, the nutrients can be delivered throughout the body via the circulatory vessels.

Elimination

Because we cannot digest every component of food we eat, such as cellulose from plants, the digestive system eliminates the parts we cannot digest. The indigestible material, along with water and bacteria in the digestive tract, is called fecal matter. The fecal matter is propelled through the digestive tract and eliminated through the anus to the external environment, at which point it is called feces.

Peristalsis

The smooth muscles of the digestive tract, as discussed in the muscular system section, are layered structures capable of long, sustained contractions. The rhythmic contractions of the layers propel the contents of the digestive system through the digestive tract from oral cavity to anus.

Effects of Massage on the Digestive System

Massage generally stimulates cellular metabolism and increases the delivery of nutrients to cells and tissues. As the nutrients are used up, the body may recognize the need for more nutrients by triggering the appetite. Massage can mechanically push the indigestible waste through the intestines, but massage also evokes the parasympathetic nervous response that encourages digestive activity, so hunger can be a subtle reflexive effect of massage.

Urinary System

The urinary system is primarily responsible for forming and excreting urine; however, in doing so, it also performs many regulatory functions. There are nitrogen-based wastes produced during cellular metabolism that are only eliminated with the passive transport mechanism of filtration. Many of the harmful wastes are actively transported from the blood

to become part of the urine. The creatine phosphate mechanism for creating ATP in muscles generates some of the wastes that are removed by the kidneys, demonstrating the interdependence of the muscular system, circulatory system, and urinary system.

Structures of the Urinary System

The urinary system includes the kidneys, ureters, urinary bladder, and urethra (Fig. 3-69).

Kidneys

Our two kidneys are located against the posterior wall of the abdominal cavity, on either side of the spine, at the level of the superior lumbar vertebrae. Each kidney is the shape of a kidney bean and measures about 5 inches long, 2.5 inches wide, and 1 inch thick. These organs are suspended in the abdominal cavity by a fatty mass called the adipose capsule and a renal fascia, and are not well protected by bones, which is why they are such vulnerable organs. Losing weight too rapidly can reduce the size of the adipose capsule and change the position of the kidneys. If they shift inferiorly, the ureters can develop kinks, and eventually, if the urine cannot flow down to the urinary bladder, the urine can back up and damage the kidneys.

Figure 3-69. Structures of the urinary system.

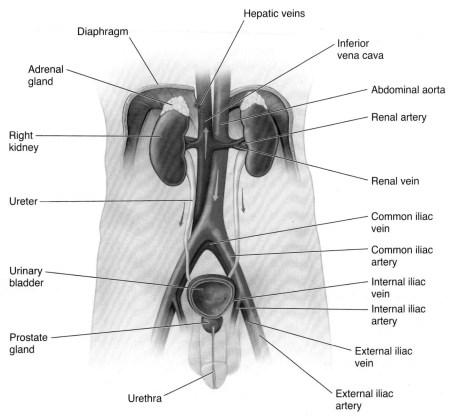

The functional part of the kidney is called the nephron, of which there are over a million in each kidney. They filter the blood; reabsorb needed water, ions, and nutrients from the filtered fluid; and secrete harmful substances from the blood into the nephron fluid and thus into the urine. Adequate amounts of water must be consumed for the urinary system to function properly.

Ureters

The ureters are tubes about 12 inches long and 0.25 inches in diameter that carry urine away from the kidneys. They have an inner lining of mucous membrane, but their outer walls are made of overlapping layers of smooth muscle and an outer connective tissue layer. Gravity and the peristaltic contractions of the ureters propel urine through the ureters toward the urinary bladder.

Urinary Bladder

The urinary bladder is a storage site for urine, located just behind the pubic symphysis. It is made of three layers of smooth muscle and has a mucous membrane lining of transitional epithelium. It can expand from its normal size of about 2 inches long to a distended size of about 5 inches long when full of urine.

Urethra

From the urinary bladder, the urethra carries urine to the exterior of the body for elimination, called urination. An involuntary smooth muscle sphincter at the exit of the urinary bladder closes the urethra when urine is being stored. There is also a voluntary skeletal muscle sphincter farther down the urethra that we control. When we contract the skeletal muscle sphincter, urine flow is stopped, and when we relax the sphincter, urine is excreted through the urethra to the external environment.

Functions of the Urinary System

The structures of the urinary system accomplish several tasks. They filter the blood to remove chemical wastes and excrete the wastes in the form of urine. The system regulates the volume of blood, pH of body fluids, and RBC formation in red bone marrow. The kidneys control blood volume (and thus blood pressure) by controlling how much water is lost in the urine.

Urine Formation

The urinary system goes through a series of steps to eliminate chemical wastes in the form of urine. First, the passive transport mechanism of filtration occurs in the capillaries that serve the kidneys. The blood traveling through the kidneys is under a high pressure that forces water and dissolved substances through the capillary walls. Second, the filtrate, or the solution that comes through the membrane, undergoes reabsorption. All of the dissolved material is not waste, so the body reabsorbs the substances that are useful, such as amino acids to build proteins, ions to use in cellular functions, glucose to use for creating ATP, and water to keep cells and tissues hydrated. Most of the substances must be actively or passively transported out of the kidney and back into the blood capillaries, but water passes through via osmosis. The third step of urine formation is secretion, which is how some additional ions, creatinine, and many drugs, such as penicillin, are removed.

Excretion

Once the urine has been produced, it is excreted from the body by the other structures of the urinary system. The urine travels from the kidneys through a pair of tubes called the ureters (YOO-rih-terz) to the urinary bladder. Urine is stored in the bladder temporarily, and is carried to the external environment through a tube called the urethra (yoo-REETH-rah).

Regulation

In the process of making urine, the complex structure and functions of the kidney also regulate blood volume, chemical content of blood, pH of body fluids, and RBC formation.

Blood Volume

The reabsorption activity of the kidney moves water from the kidney back into the blood capillaries via osmosis. The amount of water reabsorbed in the kidneys is a homeostatic mechanism that keeps the blood volume stable after water is lost through the skin as perspiration, out the lungs as water vapor, or out the digestive tract in the feces. The kidneys work at keeping blood volume constant despite widely changing patterns of fluid intake.

Chemical Balance

Once the blood has been filtered in the kidneys, the filtrate contains ions and other molecules that are necessary for cellular metabolism. Regulating the reabsorption of substances is another homeostatic mechanism for maintaining chemical balance in the blood and body fluids.

pH Balance

As mentioned in the cardiovascular system section, the pH of blood is normally kept at 7.4. The body constantly creates byproducts of cellular metabolism that affect pH levels, but homeostatic mechanisms maintain a stable pH in body fluids. The kidneys are the primary structures for regulating pH, although respiratory activity can also change pH levels. The kidneys can excrete bicarbonate ions and hydrogen ions, and can create and reabsorb bicarbonate ions to change the pH.

Red Blood Cell Formation

The kidneys are the primary structures that secrete erythropoietin, a hormone that stimulates RBC formation in the red marrow of bones. A small amount is present in the blood all the time, but when oxygen levels in blood are low, the kidneys secrete extra erythropoietin to increase the production of RBCs.

Effects of Massage on the Urinary System

The mechanical effects of massage result in more cellular and chemical waste to be excreted through the urine. Massage encourages smooth muscle contraction of the urinary bladder to eliminate more urine as a reflexive response of the parasympathetic nervous system to rest and digest.

Endocrine System

The endocrine system is a regulating control system of the body. It is made up of several ductless glands and some organs that are involved in other systems. Endocrine system hormones are secreted directly into the blood and circulate through the body. The hormones have specific effects on their target tissues to keep metabolic and developmental processes of the body functioning normally. They work both antagonistically and cooperatively to maintain homeostasis.

Structures of the Endocrine System

The major endocrine structures are the pituitary (pih-TOO-ih-tair-ee), thyroid (THAHY-royd), parathyroid, adrenal (a-DREE-nul), pineal (PAHY-nee-ahl), and thymus glands, as well as parts of the hypothalamus, pancreas, ovaries, testes, and placenta (Fig. 3-70).

Pituitary Gland

The pituitary gland is often called the master gland of the body (Fig. 3-71). Located at the base of the brain, it secretes six different hormones that stimulate other glands and organs to act. In addition to its six secretions, it stores and releases the two hormones secreted by the hypothalamus:

- Growth hormone (GH) primarily stimulates muscles and long bones to grow and regulates blood sugar.
- Prolactin (PRL) is similar to GH, but only activates milk production in the breasts.

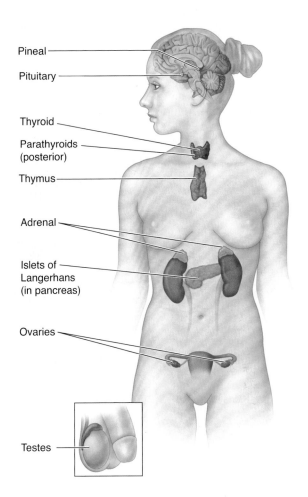

Figure 3-70. Structures of the endocrine system.

- Thyroid-stimulating hormone (TSH) regulates the thyroid gland.
- Adrenocorticotropic hormone (ACTH) regulates the adrenal gland.
- Follicle-stimulating hormone (FSH) promotes the maturation of eggs, the production of estrogen, and development of sperm production.
- Luteinizing hormone (LH) signals the ovary to release an egg and produce progesterone or the testes to produce testosterone.
- Oxytocin, secreted by the hypothalamus, stimulates contractions of the uterus and the milk "letdown" reflex of new mothers.
- Antidiuretic hormone (ADH), secreted by the hypothalamus, promotes water retention in the kidneys.

Thyroid Gland

The thyroid gland is slightly larger than the other glands and is located in the anterior neck area in two lobes on either side of the trachea. Its hormones, including

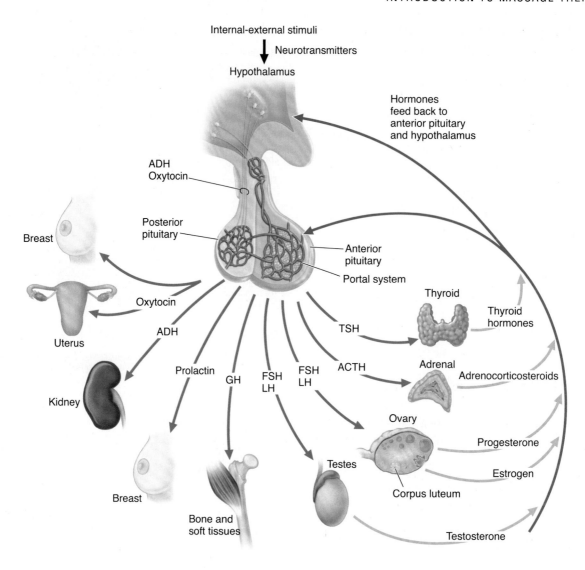

Figure 3-71. Pituitary gland activity.

thyroxin and triiodothyronine, regulate metabolism and reduce blood calcium levels by triggering calcium from the blood to be deposited in the bones. The thyroid requires iodine to produce its hormones; without enough dietary iodine, the thyroid overworks and becomes enlarged, creating a goiter. Since iodine was added to table salt, goiters are fairly rare.

Parathyroid Glands

There are at least four small, pea-shaped parathyroid glands that are usually embedded in the posterior wall of the thyroid. Their hormone, aptly called parathyroid hormone, increases calcium levels in the blood by triggering the bones to release calcium into the blood when calcium is needed. Parathyroid hormone also stimulates vitamin D synthesis (which stimulates the uptake of calcium in the intestine) and promotes calcium retention in the kidneys.

Adrenal Glands

The adrenal glands sit on the superior surface of the kidneys. The hormones they secrete include adrenal epinephrine (adrenaline), norepinephrine (noradrenaline), glucocorticoids, and mineralocorticoids. The adrenal hormones promote sodium and water conservation; they also help cope with long-term stress, reduce inflammation and edema, and reduce pain. In addition, adrenaline cooperates with the sympathetic nervous system to initiate the alarm response.

Pineal Gland

The tiny pineal gland hangs from the roof of the third ventricle in the brain and is responsible for producing melatonin. Although not proven, melatonin is commonly known to help the body recognize and move through sleep/wake cycles. When nerves in the eyes are exposed to light, the pineal gland is triggered to produce less melatonin. As night falls and environmental light diminishes, the pineal gland produces more melatonin.

Thymus Gland

The thymus gland, discussed in the lymphatic system section, is located posterior to the sternum and decreases in size as we get older. It produces thymosin, which triggers leukocytes to mature into T lymphocytes, special immune cells that help the body recognize foreign substances.

Other Endocrine Organs

Parts of the hypothalamus, pancreas, ovaries, testes, and placenta are considered components of the endocrine system because of their secretions.

The hypothalamus sits just above the pituitary gland and controls its hormone release, giving them a close, cooperative relationship. It produces ADH and oxytocin but immediately stores them in the pituitary gland. Once the hypothalamus stimulates the pituitary gland to release them, ADH causes the kidneys to reabsorb more water instead of excreting it in the urine, and oxytocin stimulates uterine contractions during childbirth and the initial milk letdown in the breasts.

The pancreas secretes glucagon and insulin, the hormones involved in metabolizing carbohydrates. Insulin is also very important in stimulating fat and protein synthesis. The ovaries produce the hormones estrogen and progesterone, and the testes produce testosterone. These hormones are responsible for sexual maturation and development.

The placenta develops in the uterus during pregnancy. It is the organ that serves as the intermediary between the mother and the fetus, made of tissue from both. It provides fetal nutrition, eliminates fetal wastes, and produces estrogen and progesterone. These hormones help maintain the pregnancy by preventing contractions that can cause miscarriage, and they prepare the mother's body for breastfeeding.

Effects of Massage on the Endocrine System

The glands of the endocrine system help maintain homeostasis via hormones and other chemicals secreted into the bloodstream. As massage increases circulation of blood and lymph, the effectiveness of the endocrine system is enhanced. Research has repeatedly shown that massage reduces levels of cortisol and epinephrine, stress-related hormones.

Reproductive System

The reproductive system is relatively inactive in humans until puberty; then the overall function is to produce offspring. The female reproductive system is slightly more complex than the male reproductive system, and the structures perform very different activities.

Structures of the Female Reproductive System

The many structures of the female reproductive system include the ovaries, uterine tubes (fallopian tubes), uterus, vagina, and mammary glands. The female reproductive organs are located in pelvis, except for the mammary glands, located in the breasts (Fig. 3-72).

Ovaries

The ovaries are the primary female sex organs that secrete the sex hormones estrogen and progesterone. Within the ovaries are immature egg cells that develop over time in response to sex hormones. LH, secreted by the pituitary gland, stimulates the ovaries to typically release one egg per menstrual cycle.

Fallopian Tubes

The fallopian tubes receive the eggs from the ovaries and transport the eggs to the uterus. Incidentally, fertilization usually occurs in the fallopian tubes. To transport the egg, the smooth muscles of the fallopian tubes use peristalsis to encourage the egg to move toward the uterus, and ciliated cells along the lining of the tubes rhythmically sweep toward the uterus.

Uterus

The uterus is the organ that serves as the incubator for the growing fetus. It is constructed with three layers. The inner layer is a lining of mucous membrane called the endometrium. The thick middle layer, the myometrium, is made of smooth muscle that expands to accommodate the growing fetus, and rhythmically contracts to deliver the baby. The outer layer of the uterus is a serous membrane called the perimetrium.

Vagina

The vagina is a muscular tube that connects the uterus to the external environment. It provides a pathway for sperm and becomes the infant's birth canal during delivery.

Mammary Glands

The mammary glands are modified sweat glands that produce milk and release it through the nipple to provide nourishment to the infant. Estrogen and progesterone promote breast development, PRL stimulates the initial production of milk, and oxytocin stimulates the continued production of milk as well as the release of the milk (letdown).

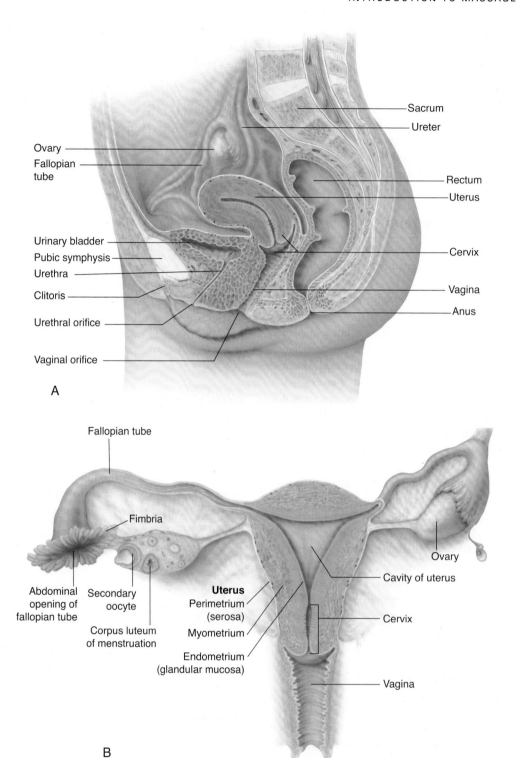

Figure 3-72. Structures of the female reproductive system. **(A)** Sagittal view (provided by the Anatomical Chart Co.) **(B)** Frontal view.

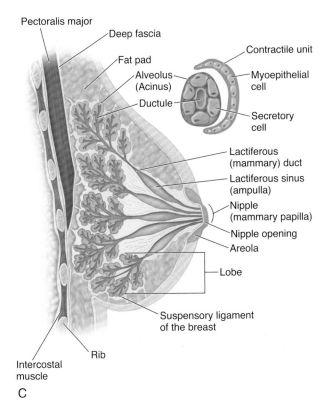

Figure 3-72. *(continued)* **(C)** Breast mammary gland.

Functions of the Female Reproductive System

The primary goal of the female reproductive system is to reproduce. To reach that goal, the system must produce sex hormones, produce and release ova (OH-vah), incubate the growing fetus in a safe nurturing environment, deliver the infant, and nourish the infant.

Sex Hormones

The hormones produced by the female reproductive system include estrogen and progesterone. They are released by the ovaries in varying amounts during the menstrual cycle. Estrogen promotes maturation of the eggs and helps prepare the uterus prior to implantation. Progesterone maximizes the ability of the uterus to maintain pregnancy by promoting blood vessel and gland formation in the uterine lining and inhibiting contractions of the uterus to prevent miscarriage. There are some physical changes that occur with the increased production of hormones during the teen years: the breasts enlarge, the reproductive organs enlarge, more body hair grows in the axillary and pubic areas, increased amounts of fat are deposited in the subcutaneous layer, the pelvis widens, and the menstrual cycle begins.

Ova

The eggs produced by the female reproductive system are referred to as ova. They start out as immature cells in the ovary and mature over time. Ovulation is the release of a mature egg from the ovary, stimulated by a hormone called luteinizing hormone.

Maternal Reproductive System Functions

Once an egg has been fertilized and has been implanted in the uterine lining, the female reproductive system is responsible for incubating the growing fetus in a safe, nurturing environment, delivering the baby, and nourishing the baby.

Delivering the baby, also called parturition or birth, is also a responsibility of the female reproductive system. During pregnancy, the smooth muscles of the uterus increase in size to expand with the growing fetus and to accomplish the delivery. In a normal pregnancy, the full-term fetus is squeezed out of the uterus by strong, smooth muscle contractions and through the vagina to the external environment. The smooth muscles work very hard to deliver the baby, and most women are encouraged to contract their abdominal muscles to reduce the size of the abdominal cavity and help push the baby out.

The mammary glands in the breasts are specialized sweat glands, as discussed in the integumentary system section. Once the baby is born, oxytocin stimulates the release of milk to feed the baby.

Structures of the Male Reproductive System

The male reproductive system includes the testes, ducts, accessory organs, and external genitalia (Fig. 3-73).

Testes

There are two testes, each about 1.5 inches long and 1 inch wide. Outside, they are encased in a fibrous connective tissue. Inside, they contain structures that form sperm and testosterone. The epididymis, where the sperm mature, is the beginning of the delivery system for the sperm, and it starts in the testes.

Ducts

Mature sperm travel through a series of ducts in their quest for an ovum:

1. Epididymis
2. Ductus deferens (vas deferens)
3. Urethra

Smooth muscles in the ducts propel the sperm toward the external environment with peristalsis.

Sagittal section

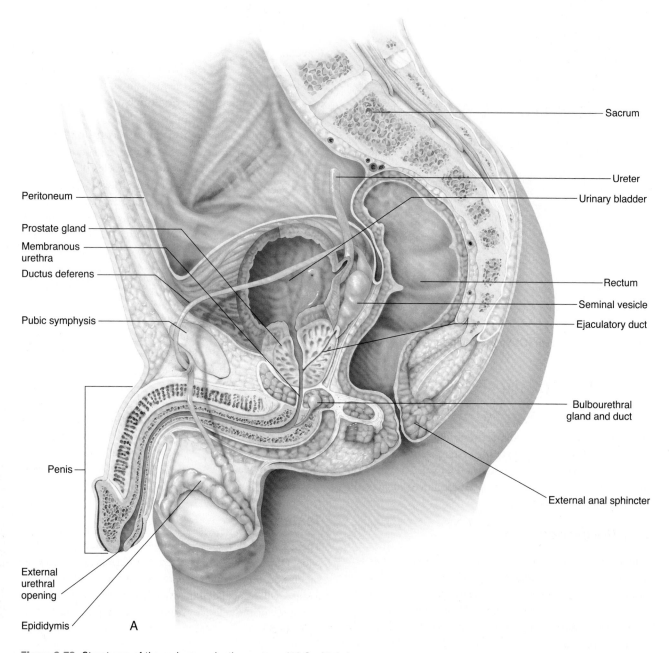

Sacrum

Ureter

Urinary bladder

Peritoneum

Prostate gland

Membranous
urethra

Ductus deferens

Rectum

Seminal vesicle

Ejaculatory duct

Pubic symphysis

Bulbourethral
gland and duct

Penis

External anal sphincter

External
urethral
opening

Epididymis   A

Figure 3-73. Structures of the male reproductive system. **(A)** Sagittal view.

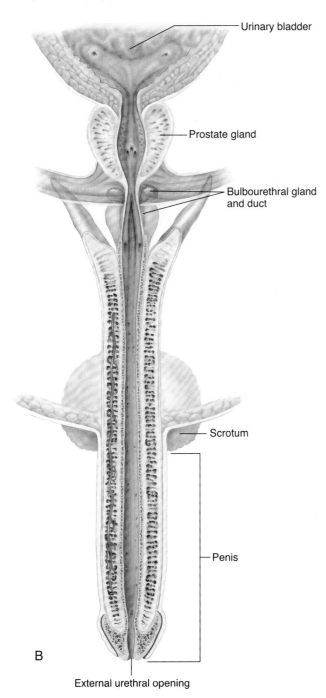

Figure 3-73. (*continued*) **(B)** Frontal view. (Assets provided by Anatomical Chart Co.)

Accessory Male Reproductive Organs

The accessory organs of the male reproductive system produce everything in the semen except the sperm. The seminal vesicles, bulbourethral glands, and prostate gland all secrete fluids containing sugar, vitamins, or enzymes. These components of semen nourish and activate the sperm as well as cleanse the urethra prior to sperm delivery. The prostate

gland wraps around the beginning part of the urethra. It has smooth muscle walls that contract during ejaculation, and the force of the contraction aids the expulsion of semen.

External Genitalia

The penis is an external genital organ that is responsible for urination and delivering sperm into the female reproductive tract. There are three areas of spongy tissue that fill with blood during sexual arousal and cause the penis to become erect. The parasympathetic nervous system can trigger erections unrelated to sexual stimulation.

The scrotum holds and protects the testes, maintaining their temperature below normal body temperature to avoid overheating the sperm. Muscles raise and lower the testes, as a protective mechanism; the wrinkled scrotal skin allows movement.

Functions of the Male Reproductive System

The functions of the male reproductive system are to produce the male sex hormone, produce sperm that can fertilize a female's egg, and deliver that sperm to the female.

Sex Hormone

Testosterone is the male sex hormone produced in the testes. It stimulates development and maturation of the male reproductive system, stimulates sperm production, and also results in some secondary sex characteristics of males. When testosterone production increases during the teen years, males undergo some physical changes that accompany their growth: the voice deepens, the bones thicken, skeletal muscles enlarge, and more body hair grows, especially in the axillary, facial, and pubic areas.

Sperm

Millions of immature sperm are produced daily in the testes, are pushed through the testes with peristaltic smooth muscle contractions, and arrive at the epididymis to mature. Mature sperm contain mitochondria to produce ATP, chemical energy. Each is equipped with a flagellum that it uses to propel itself through the ducts and into the female, which it can do only with energy from ATP.

Effects of Massage on the Reproductive Systems

Massage stimulates the parasympathetic nervous system, which increases circulation to the reproductive organs to better deliver nutrients and remove cellular waste. Massage also increases the production of oxytocin and serotonin, chemicals that regulate moods and stimulate smooth muscle contractions (as are found in the reproductive organs).

The resulting combination of increased blood flow and chemicals to the reproductive organs can unintentionally cause sexual arousal. Most massage schools teach students the physiologic responses that are responsible for sexual arousal so the students can be somewhat prepared for this kind of situation and know how to ethically and professionally manage the situation.

Special Senses

The special senses are not contained in a singular body system. Nonetheless, there are a variety of sensory systems that are important to massage therapy: proprioception, vision, hearing, smell, and taste.

Proprioception

The body's ability to recognize the location and position of all of its parts at any time is called proprioception. This sensory input is necessary for the body to move in a coordinated and safe manner. Proprioceptors, introduced earlier as part of the nervous system section, can be found in the muscles, tendons, joints, and inner ear. These sensory neurons convey information to the brain regarding body position, muscle tone, and equilibrium. Muscle spindles are proprioceptors located in the muscles that are specifically responsible for sensing the *length* of muscle fibers. Golgi tendon organs are specialized proprioceptors in the tendons that sense *tension* of the muscle fibers.

Vision

The vision system, or the eye, comprises the following primary structures:

- Cornea—the clear covering that protects the front of the eye
- Iris—the colored part of the eye
- Pupil—the hole in the center of the iris that dilates or constricts in response to light levels
- Lens—the clear, curved part of the eye behind the iris that focuses light onto the retina
- Retina—a light-sensitive layer of tissue lining the back of the eye that transmits the image to the brain
- Sclera—the white, outer layer of the eye
- Vitreous body—the spherical part of the eye behind the lens filled with a gel called vitreous humor
- Extrinsic muscles—muscles that move the eye in all directions

Hearing

The ear and its structures provide our sense of hearing. The ear consists of three sections: external ear, middle ear, internal ear.

The external ear includes the pinna (also called the auricle), the auditory canal, and the tympanic membrane (also called the eardrum).

The middle ear contains the auditory (eustachian) tube and three small bones called ossicles that amplify incoming sound waves. The ossicles are named for their shape: the malleus is similar to a hammer, the incus resembles an anvil, and the stapes is shaped like a stirrup.

The inner ear is mostly a bony labyrinth of canals that can be divided into three sections. The cochlea is located toward the front and is the hearing center of the ear. It contains the organ of Corti, which transmits sound waves to the brain. The vestibule is the next part of the ear, which responds to up-and-down changes in head position and gravity. The semicircular canals are the third portion of the inner ear, and they are sensitive to rotational movement of the head.

Smell

Our sense of smell is made possible by the olfactory membrane toward the roof of the nose. Olfactory cells, sensitive to chemicals, are located within the olfactory membrane. The axons of all of the olfactory cells come together to form the olfactory nerve, or cranial nerve I. The olfactory nerve passes through a thin sheet of bone and then comes in contact with the olfactory bulb. From there, the chemical signals are converted into electrical signals and pass down neurons, through the olfactory tract, and to the brain.

Taste

There are three types of papillae on the tongue that contain taste buds. Fungiform papillae, located near the front of the tongue, contain three to five taste buds each. Circumvallate papillae are found toward the back of the tongue, and each contains over 100 taste buds. Foliate papillae can be found along the sides of the tongue, and they also have over 100 taste buds apiece. Each taste bud has between 30 and 100 taste receptors that transmit information to the brain. Contrary to past teachings and popular belief, each taste receptor is sensitive to each of the five taste sensations: bitter, salty, sour, sweet, and umami.

Effects of Massage on the Special Senses

Massage impacts the special senses by invoking the parasympathetic nervous system response. The pupils constrict and hearing becomes more acute.

CHAPTER SUMMARY

Knowing the structures and functions of the body and knowing how massage can affect these structures can help you deliver safe and effective treatment. Massage affects the basic unit of life and, ultimately, the organism. It also gives you an opportunity to educate clients about how anatomical and physiological changes affect their health and well-being.

The main function of the skeletal muscles is to create movement, and restoration of the most functional movement is often the goal of massage therapy. Understanding the attachment points and actions of the muscles in this chapter is especially important because it means you know the structures you are manipulating, both to create benefit and avoid damage. Although massage focuses on the muscular system, massage therapy deals with the whole body. All of the body systems must cooperate for a person to function normally, and the interrelationships between the body systems are a critical part of the big picture of health. The effects of massage on the different body systems are outlined in Table 3-6.

Table 3-6 Effects of Massage on Different Body Systems

Integumentary System
- Mechanically warms the skin with friction
- Increases circulation of blood and lymph within the skin
- Stimulates sebaceous gland secretions, which make skin more supple and pliable
- Stimulates sweat production, which cools the body upon evaporation of sweat
- Breaks down fascial adhesions in the subcutaneous layer (superficial fascia) to restore circulation and movement to skin

Skeletal System
- Joint movement stimulates synovial fluid production, which cushions and lubricates synovial joints
- Increases the health of skeleton by enhancing circulation of blood and lymph to and from the bones

Muscular System
- Increases nutrition and development of muscles by enhancing circulation of blood and lymph to and from the muscles
- Increases the excitability of muscles, making them more sensitive to nerve impulses
- Increases heat in and around muscles to loosen fascia and restore movement and circulation to the muscles
- Decreases hypertonicity in muscles and tendons

Nervous System
- Increases production of dopamine, a pain-relieving chemical involved in voluntary movement and clear thinking
- Increases production of endorphins, strong pain-relieving chemicals
- Increases parasympathetic nervous system activation
- Increases production of enkephalins, strong pain relievers involved in sensory integration
- Increases secretion of oxytocin, a chemical that increases the pain threshold, stimulates smooth muscle contractions, decreases sympathetic nervous system activity, and has sedative effects
- Increases production of serotonin, which generally diminishes pain and appetite, regulates moods and sleep patterns, and stimulates smooth muscle contractions
- Decreases production of cortisol, a natural anti-inflammatory produced in response to stress that can accelerate tissue breakdown and prevent tissue repair
- Decreases substance P, a neurotransmitter that triggers the pain response

Cardiovascular System
- Increases circulation of blood in and around the area being addressed
- Reduces the symptoms of ischemia by increasing circulation to capillaries with poor blood flow
- Increases permeability of capillary walls, enhancing delivery of oxygen and nutrients
- Sustained percussion can cause vasodilation deep within the area being addressed to increase blood flow

Lymphatic System
- Increases circulation of lymph in and around the area being addressed
- Increases circulation of lymph to help the body fight germs
- Increases circulation of lymph, which increases removal of metabolic waste
- Reduces edema

continues on following page

Table 3-6 Effects of Massage on Different Body Systems *continued*

Respiratory System
• Encourages slow, deep contractions of the diaphragm, which helps remove carbon dioxide waste via the lungs
• Percussive techniques can relieve chest congestion by loosening mucus within lungs

Digestive System
• Enhances the digestive process reflexively by stimulating the parasympathetic nervous response
• Mechanically pushes indigestible waste through the intestines

Urinary System
• Increases cellular and chemical waste excreted via urine
• Encourages constriction of the smooth muscle of the urinary bladder to eliminate more urine as a reflexive response of the parasympathetic nervous system

Endocrine System
• Increases delivery of hormones and other chemicals as a result of increased circulation of blood
• Reduces levels of cortisol and epinephrine, stress-related hormones

Reproductive System
• Increases circulation to the reproductive organs
• Increases production of oxytocin and serotonin, which stimulate smooth muscle contractions
• Increases production of serotonin, which regulates moods

Special Senses
• Constricts the pupils

You may want to supplement this text with a book that is dedicated to anatomy and physiology for more thorough information. Countless anatomy and physiology texts are available in libraries and stores; some are listed in the suggested readings section at the end of the chapter.

CHAPTER EXERCISES

1. Define the following:

   Anatomy

   Homeostasis

   Muscle

   Muscle cell

   Nerve

   Neuron

   Osmosis

   Peristalsis

   Physiology

   Tissue

2. Describe where fascia can be found.

3. Define muscle origin and muscle insertion.

4. Identify at least 10 bony landmarks on yourself or a partner.

5. Name the five functions of the muscular system.

6. List the structures of a whole skeletal muscle.

7. Identify at least four functions of the integumentary system.

8. Compare and contrast the organization and bundled arrangements of the structures of a muscle, bone, and nerve.

9. Describe at least five of the body's parasympathetic nervous system responses.

10. Describe the difference between the stretch reflex and the tendon reflex.

11. Name at least five different kinds of sensory receptors.

12. Describe the similarities between the venous system and the lymphatic system.

13. Identify at least three effects of massage on the lymphatic system.

14. Describe at least three different functions of the respiratory system.

15. Name the five special senses.

SUGGESTED READINGS

Allen L. *Plain & Simple Guide to Therapeutic Massage & Bodywork Examinations*. 2nd ed. Baltimore: Lippincott Williams & Wilkins, 2010.

Ashton J, Cassel D. *Review for Therapeutic Massage & Bodywork Exams*. 3rd ed. Baltimore: Lippincott Williams & Wilkins, 2011.

Balch PA, Balch JF. *Prescription for Nutritional Healing*. New York: Avery, 2000.

Benjamin B, Borden G. *Listen to your Pain: The Active Person's Guide to Understanding, Identifying, and Treating Pain and Injury*. New York: Penguin Books, 1984.

Biel A. *Trail Guide to the Body*. Boulder, CO: Books of Discovery, 1997.

Buchholz D. *Heal Your Headache: The 1•2•3 Program for Taking Charge of your Pain*. New York: Workman Publishing, 2002.

Calais-Germain B. *Anatomy of Movement*. Seattle, WA: Eastland Press, 1993.

Chaitow L. *Fibromyalgia and Muscle Pain: Your Self-Treatment Guide*. London: Thorsons, 2001.

Chaitow L. *Fibromyalgia Syndrome: A Practitioner's Guide to Treatment*. London: Churchill Livingstone, 2000.

Chaitow L, Bradley D, Gilbert C. *Multidisciplinary Approaches to Breathing Pattern Disorders*. London: Churchill Livingstone, 2002.

Chikly B. *Silent Waves: Theory and Practice of Lymph Drainage Therapy: An Osteopathic Lymphatic Technique*. 2nd ed. Scottsdale, AZ: I.H.H. Publishing, 2004.

Clemente C. *Gray's Anatomy*. 30th ed. Philadelphia: Lippincott Williams & Wilkins, 1985.

Cohen BJ, Wood DL. *Memmler's Structure and Function of the Human Body*. 7th ed. Philadelphia: Lippincott Williams & Wilkins, 2000.

Cohen BJ, Wood DL. *Memmler's Structure and Function of the Human Body*. 9th ed. Philadelphia: Lippincott Williams & Wilkins, 2009.

Crowley LV, Abrams C. *Physiology*. Springhouse, PA: Springhouse Corporation, 1993.

Gray H, Lewis WH. *Anatomy of the Human Body*. 23rd ed. Philadelphia: Lea & Febiger, 1936.

Guinness AE, ed. *ABC's of the Human Body: A Family Answer Book*. Pleasantville, NY: Readers Digest Association, 1987.

Hendrickson T. *Massage for Orthopedic Conditions*. Philadelphia: Lippincott Williams & Wilkins, 2003.

Johnston CA. *Anatomy*. Springhouse, PA: Springhouse Corporation, 1993.

Kendall FP, McCreary EK, Provance PG. *Muscle Testing and Function*. 4th ed. Baltimore: Williams & Wilkins, 1993.

Lowe WW. *Functional Assessment in Massage Therapy*. 2nd ed. Corvallis, OR: Pacific Orthopedic Massage, 1995.

Fortin J. *Major Systems of the Body*. Milwaukee, WI: World Almanac Library, 2002.

Marieb EN. *Essentials of Human Anatomy and Physiology*. 5th ed. Menlo Park, CA: Benjamin/Cummings, 1997.

Mauskop A, Fox B. *What your Doctor May Not Tell You About Migraines: The Breakthrough Program that Can Help End Your Pain*. New York: Warner Books, 2001.

Melloni JL, Dox I, Melloni HP, Melloni BJ. *Melloni's Illustrated Review of Human Anatomy*. Philadelphia: JB Lippincott, 1988.

Moyer C, Rounds J, Hannum JW. A meta-analysis of massage therapy research. Psychol Bull 2004;130(1):3–18.

Northrup C. *Women's Bodies, Women's Wisdom*. New York: Bantam Books, 1998.

Paulino J, Griffith CJ. *The Headache Sourcebook*. New York: Contemporary Books/McGraw Hill, 2001.

Physicians' Desk Reference Pocket Guide to Prescription Drugs. 5th ed. New York: Pocket Books, 2002.

Persad RS. *Massage Therapy and Medications General Treatment Principles*. Toronto: Curties-Overzet, 2001.

Premkumar K. *Anatomy & Physiology: The Massage Connection*. 3rd ed. Baltimore: Lippincott Williams & Wilkins, 2012.

Rattray F, Ludwig L. *Clinical Massage Therapy: Understanding, Assessing and Treating over 70 Conditions*. Toronto: Talus, 2000.

Scanlon VC, Sanders T. *Essentials of Anatomy and Physiology*. 2nd ed. Philadelphia: FA Davis, 1991.

Sieg KW, Adams SP. *Illustrated Essentials of Musculoskeletal Anatomy*. 2nd ed. Gainesville, FL: Megabooks, 1985.

Sloane E. *Anatomy and Physiology: An Easy Learner*. Boston: Jones and Bartlett, 1994.

Starlanyl D, Copeland ME. *Fibromyalgia and Chronic Myofascial Pain: A Survival Manual*. 2nd ed. New York: New Harbinger Publications, 2001.

Takahashi T (editorial supervisor). *Atlas of the Human Body*. New York: HarperCollins, 1994.

Theodosakis MD, Adderly B, Fox B. *The Arthritis Cure*. New York: St. Martin's Press, 1997.

Travell JG, Simons DG. *Myofascial Pain and Dysfunction: The Trigger Point Manual*. Vol 1. Philadelphia: Lippincott Williams & Wilkins, 1983.

Travell JG, Simons DG. *Myofascial Pain and Dysfunction: The Trigger Point Manual*. Vol 2. Philadelphia: Lippincott Williams & Wilkins, 1992.

Utting, B. Lecture notes presented at: Utting School of Massage; 1994; Seattle, WA.

Watkins J. *Structure and Function of the Musculoskeletal System*. Champaign, IL: Human Kinetics, 1999.

Werner R. *A Massage Therapist's Guide to Pathology*. Baltimore: Lippincott Williams & Wilkins, 1998.

Willis MC. *Medical Terminology: The Language of Healthcare*. Baltimore: Lippincott Williams & Wilkins, 1996.

http://nccam.nih.gov/health/massage/massageintroduction.htm, accessed 9.5.11.

http://nccam.nih.gov/health/massage/massageintroduction.htm#funded, accessed 9.5.11.

http://users.rcn.com/jkimball.ma.ultranet/BiologyPages/T/Taste.html, accessed 8.29.11.

http://www.ahealthyme.com, accessed 3.5.06.

http://www.allaboutvision.com/resources/anatomy.htm, accessed 8.29.11.

http://www.bartleby.com/107/pages/page502.html, accessed 3.5.06.

http://www.cancer.gov, accessed 3.5.06.

http://www.cancer.org, accessed 3.10.06.

http://www.cdc.gov, accessed 3.5.06.

http://www.cell-biology.com, accessed 3.5.06.

http://www.dermnet.org.nz/index.html, accessed 3.5.06.

http://www.e-histology.net, accessed 3.5.06.

http://www.estrellamountain.edu/faculty/farabee/biobk/biobooktoc.html, accessed 3.5.06.

http://www.factmonster.com/ce6/sci/A0843878.html, accessed 3.5.06.

http://www.infoplease.com/ce6/sci/A0818305.html, accessed 3.5.06.

http://www.intelihealth.com/IH/ihtIH, accessed 3.5.06.

http://www.massagetherapyfoundation.org/research.html, accessed 9.5.11.

http://www.mayoclinic.com/invoke.cfm?objectid~43CB5F79-2B33-4F96-B7D06EC696826071, accessed 3.5.06.

http://www.mayoclinic.org/general-internal-medicine-rst/research.html, accessed 9.5.11.

http://www.medterms.com, accessed 8.29.11.

http://www6.miami.edu/touch-research/AdultMassage.html, accessed 9.5.11.

http://www.ncbi.nlm.nih.gov/books/NBK10812/, accessed 8.29.11.

http://www.nih.gov/icd/, accessed 3.5.06.

http://www.nlm.nih.gov/medlineplus/, accessed 3.5.06.

http://www.stlukeseye.com/anatomy/retina.html, accessed 8.29.11.

http://www.unomaha.edu/;swick/2740connectivetissue.html#ret, accessed 3.5.06.

http://www.uwstout.edu/faculty/moyerc/upload/MT-meta-analysis-PB2004.pdf, accessed 9.5.11.

http://www.webmd.com, accessed 3.5.06.

3 Body Systems

4

Kinesiology and Biomechanics

Objectives

Upon completion of this chapter, the student will be able to:

- Describe 10 directional terms
- Name the three main types of joints
- Demonstrate at least five pairs of antagonistic body movements on self or partner
- Demonstrate the difference between concentric and eccentric muscle contractions

- Describe the function of proprioceptors
- Name the three primary components of good body mechanics
- Demonstrate the asymmetric stance while leaning into a partner on the massage table
- List at least five ways to minimize your risk for injury

Key Terms

Anatomical position: Describes a person standing up, feet shoulder-width apart, arms at the sides, and palms facing forward.

Antagonist: A muscle that moves in opposition to the prime mover.

Asymmetric stance (also one-foot-forward stance): Standing position in which both feet are on the ground, shoulder-width apart, one foot is in front of the other, and the back foot is laterally rotated.

Biomechanics: The study of how movement of living creatures is affected by both internal and external factors.

Body mechanics: The efficient and effective use of your body when performing massage.

Concentric contraction: A muscle contraction in which the muscle shortens and the attachment sites of the muscle move closer together.

Deep: Refers to something farther from the surface of the skin, or deeper inside the body.

Distal: Refers to something that is farther away from the torso, toward the fingers or toes.

Eccentric contraction: A muscle contraction in which the distance between the muscle attachments increases and the muscle effectively gets longer.

Inferior (also caudad): Refers to something more toward the feet, or below.

Insertion of a muscle: The point of attachment that moves most during contraction, often at the distal end.

Joint: The mechanical structure where neighboring bones are attached, often with connective tissue and cartilage.

Kinesiology: The study of human movement.

Lateral: Refers to something farther away from the midline of the body

Medial: Refers to something closer to the midline of the body.

Origin of a muscle: The attachment on the bone or connective tissue structure that is more stationary during muscle contraction.

Prime mover (also agonist): The muscle that performs most of the intended movement.

Proprioceptor (PROH-pree-oh-SEP-tor): Sensory neuron responsible for detecting body position, muscle tone, and equilibrium.

Proximal: Describes something toward the attachment point of the limb to the body.

Range of motion (ROM): The end-to-end distance of a specific joint movement that is structurally possible.

Superficial: Refers to something closer to the surface of the skin.

Superior (also cephalad): Refers to something closer to a person's head, or above.

Symmetric stance (also parallel stance): Standing position in which both feet face forward about shoulder-width apart, hips face forward, and knees are bent.

Synergist: Assists the prime mover by contracting at the same time to facilitate more effective movement, also called an accessory muscle.

Now that you have a fundamental understanding of the structures and functions of the body systems, it is important to develop a working knowledge of how movement occurs in the body. Once you understand how the body moves, you will have the foundation to assess your client's movement patterns and design the appropriate treatment plan.

Kinesiology is the study of human movement. Biomechanics is the study of how the movement of living creatures is affected by both internal and external factors, such as neurological input, muscle–tendon interactions, gravity, and physical strain on the body. **Body mechanics** is the efficient and effective use of your body while performing massage. It is important to be concerned with body mechanics for two reasons. First, many clients have muscular and soft tissue pain and tension as a result of poor posture, restricted movement, or repetitive stress injuries (RSIs). Understanding how clients have developed their pain patterns allows you to help them prevent the development of pain patterns in the future. Ask clients about excessive or restricted movement patterns they encounter on a daily basis and how they move their body repetitively. Their answers will provide you with information about how the clients' bodies have compensated as a result of these movement patterns and give you clues for target areas for massage treatment. Second, in order to achieve longevity in your massage career, you must move your body in an efficient and effective manner to minimize the risk of discomfort, pain, or injury.

There is a lot of terminology in both kinesiology and body mechanics. Learning and using the terms comfortably is necessary to communicate accurately. The best way to learn a new skill is to learn the language from the beginning, so this chapter starts out with the terminology.

You will find yourself using this terminology regularly when communicating with clients and other healthcare professionals as well for keeping accurate and professional records. These terms are a large part of the language of massage.

Anatomical Position

The **anatomical position** of the body describes a person standing up on both feet, with the feet shoulder-width apart, arms at the sides, and palms facing forward (Fig. 4-1). The

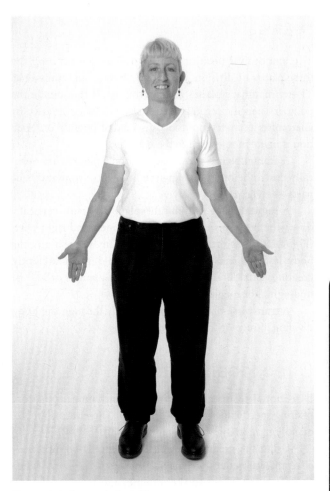

Figure 4-1. Anatomical position.

Anatomical Terminology

As a massage therapist you will make observations while looking at a client's body during assessment, treatment, and documentation. This makes it important for you to know the terminology for anatomical position, planes, directions, and body regions.

Figure 4-2. Planes of division.
(A) Frontal plane. **(B)** Sagittal plane.
(C) Transverse plane.

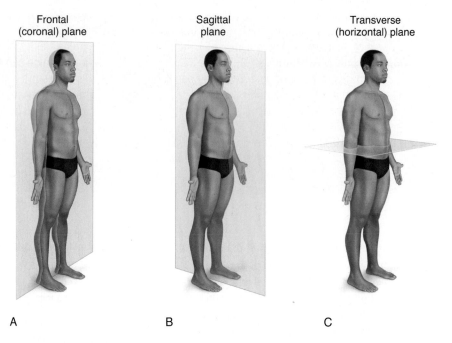

Frontal (coronal) plane

Sagittal plane

Transverse (horizontal) plane

A   B   C

anatomical position is used as a reference when describing the locations of structures on the body. When being evaluated for posture, clients stand in the anatomical position as a standard reference point for present and future observations.

Planes

The anatomical position is also used in determining the three planes of division: the sagittal, frontal, and transverse. These imaginary planes are like thin walls that divide the body or a specific organ into two parts, and they are used by anatomists as a reference tool. Any kind of physical observation is made in reference to these planes.

A frontal plane (also called a coronal plane) runs vertically down the body, dividing the body into front and back parts (see Fig. 4-2A).

A sagittal plane (SA-jih-tuhl) plane also runs vertically down the body, dividing the body into left and right parts (Fig. 4-2B). A sagittal plane can occur anywhere along the body, but if it runs exactly down the midline of the body, creating equal left and right halves, this plane is called the midsagittal or medial plane.

A transverse plane runs horizontally through the body, dividing it into top and bottom parts (Fig. 4-2C).

Directional Terms

Directional terms also refer to the anatomical position, offering specific locational information. These terms are frequently used in massage therapy (Fig. 4-3).

Using the medial plane as a reference, two directional terms are generated: medial and lateral. **Medial** refers to something closer to the midline, and lateral refers to

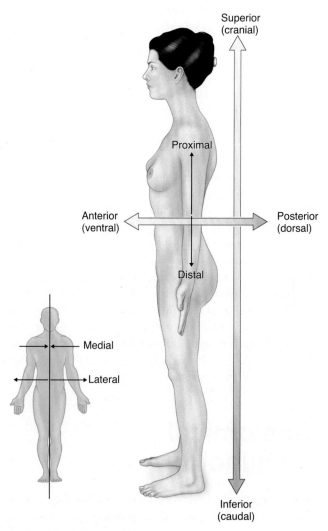

Figure 4-3. Directional terms.

something farther away from it. For instance, the ear is lateral to the eye because it is farther away from the midline.

Bilateral is a term that means two sides. In massage, bilateral refers to something on both sides of the body. A massage therapist's session notes might include a comment regarding bilateral temporomandibular joint (TMJ) pain, meaning that the client has pain on both sides of the jaw.

Conversely, unilateral refers to something on only one side of the body. Massage session notes that say a client has unilateral TMJ pain would suggest that jaw movement only hurts on one side.

The frontal plane is used as a reference for the terms anterior and posterior. Although these terms are preferred in massage therapy, the terms ventral and dorsal are sometimes used. Anterior (ventral) indicates something on the front side of the body or more toward the front. Posterior (dorsal) indicates something on the back side of the body or more toward the back. For example, the nose is anterior to the ear because it is more toward the front side of the body.

The transverse plane generates the terms superior and inferior. **Superior** (sometimes called cephalad) refers to something closer to a person's head, or above. **Inferior** (also called caudad) refers to something more toward the feet, or below. The knee is superior to the ankle because it is closer to the head.

Proximal and distal are terms that describe relative location on the extremities (limbs). **Proximal** describes something closer to the limb's attachment point on the body, and **distal** refers to something that is farther away from the torso, toward the fingers or toes. For example, the elbow is proximal to the wrist, and the wrist is distal to the elbow.

Superficial refers to something closer to the surface of the skin, and **deep** refers to something farther from the surface of the skin, or deeper inside the body. Superficial and deep are often used in massage therapy to describe the relative position of specific muscles in the body or to describe the depth to which the strokes are being applied. For example, the rhomboids are deep to the trapezius, and compression can access tissues that are too deep to reach with effleurage. Table 4-1 lists all the directional terms, definitions of each, and examples of their usage.

Body Regions

The body is divided into different regions for orientation purposes. The terminology is helpful when you want to refer to a general area of the body. Nearby landmarks are often used as identifiers for these body regions, as shown in Figure 4-4.

Table 4-1 Directional Terms

Term	Definition	Example
anterior (ventral)	pertaining to the front side or toward the front of the body	the nose is anterior to the ears
deep	more internal, deeper into the body	the lungs are deep to the ribs
distal	farther from the point of attachment or farther from the torso	the fingers are distal to the elbow
inferior (caudad)	located lower or toward the feet	the xiphoid process is inferior to the sternal notch
lateral[a]	farther away from the midline or toward the sides	the ear is lateral to the eye
medial[a]	closer to the midline or toward the middle of the body	the eye is medial to the ear
Posterior (dorsal)	pertaining to the back side or toward the back of the body	the spine is posterior to the sternum
proximal	closer to the point of attachment or closer to the torso	the knee is proximal to the ankle
superficial	closer to the surface of the skin	the epidermis is superficial to the muscles
superior (cephalad)	located higher or toward the head	the nose is superior to the navel

[a]Remember that the body must be in anatomical position (palms forward).

Kinesiology and Body Mechanics

4

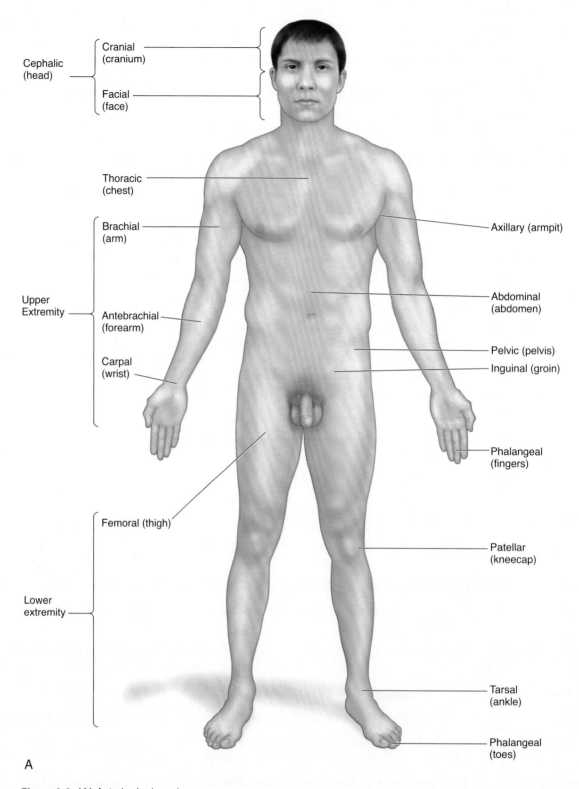

A

Figure 4-4. (A) Anterior body regions.

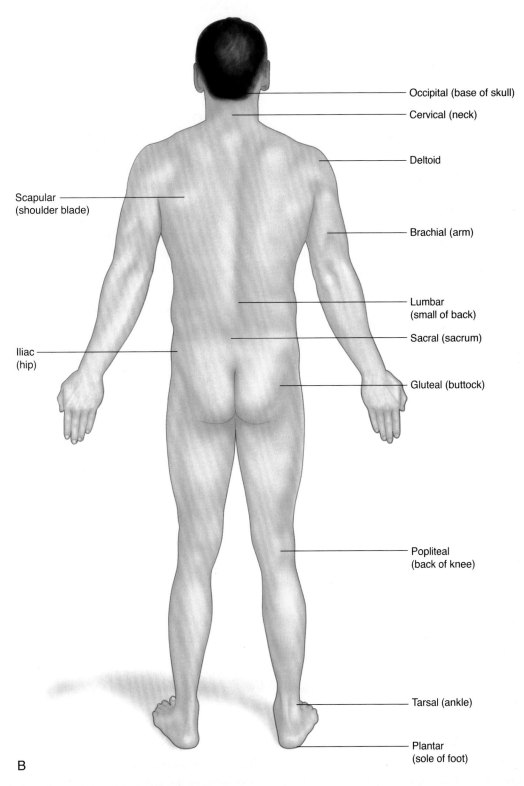

Occipital (base of skull)

Cervical (neck)

Deltoid

Scapular
(shoulder blade)

Brachial (arm)

Lumbar
(small of back)

Sacral (sacrum)

Iliac
(hip)

Gluteal (buttock)

Popliteal
(back of knee)

Tarsal (ankle)

Plantar
(sole of foot)

B

Figure 4-4. (*continued*) **(B)** Posterior body regions.

The anterior body regions (Fig. 4-4A) include:

- Cranial (KRAY-nee-uhl)
- Facial (FAY-shuhl)
- Thoracic (thoh-RASS-ik)
- Axillary (AK-sih-lair-ee)
- Brachial (BRAY-kee-uhl)
- Antebrachial (AN-tee-BRAY-kee-uhl)
- Carpal (CAR-puhl)
- Phalangeal (fuh-LAN-jee-uhl)
- Abdominal (ab-DOM-ih-nuhl)
- Pelvic (PEL-vik)
- Inguinal (IN-gwih-nuhl)
- Femoral (FEM-or-uhl)
- Patellar (pah-TEL-er)
- Tarsal (TAR-suhl)

The posterior body regions (Fig. 4-4B) include:

- Occipital (ok-SIP-ih-tuhl)
- Cervical (SER-vik-uhl)
- Deltoid (DEL-toyd)
- Scapular (SKAP-yoo-lahr)
- Brachial (BRAY-kee-uhl)
- Lumbar (LUM-bahr)
- Iliac (IL-ee-ak)
- Sacral (SAY-kruhl)

- Gluteal (GLOO-tee-uhl)
- Popliteal (pop-lih-TEE-uhl)
- Tarsal (TAR-suhl)
- Plantar (PLAN-tahr)

Incorporating Terminology into a Massage Session

If a client came to your office complaining that the inside of her right wrist was hurting, it could mean any number of things. The "inside" of the wrist could refer to the anterior side of the wrist or the medial side of the wrist, and the pain could be on the proximal or distal side of the carpals. If you were to note the client's complaint of pain in your massage session notes, you could use one of the following descriptions:

- Client complained of pain on the medial side of the right wrist, proximal to the carpals.
- Client complained of pain on the medial side of the right wrist, distal to the carpals.
- Client complained of pain on the anterior side of the right wrist, proximal to the carpals.
- Client complained of pain on the anterior side of the right wrist, distal to the carpals.

Proper terminology clarifies the situation and reduces the confusion. For the subsequent visit, any therapist could pick up the session notes and know which area was problematic.

Kinesiology

This section focuses on kinesiology, which is the study of human movement. You will explore arthrology (the study of the joints) as well as myology (the study of the muscles). The cooperation of the joints and muscles creates simple and complex body movements that are also described in this section.

Arthrology

A **joint** is the mechanical structure where neighboring bones are connected with connective tissue and cartilage. Joints are passive structures that primarily allow movement to occur between bones, but they also provide stability and shock absorption.

The attached ligaments and the soft tissue joint capsules limit movement at the joint, providing stabilization to the joint and the entire skeleton. By limiting movement, the ligaments keep the joint from moving into positions that can injure the bones, the muscles, or surrounding soft tissues. Joints also function as shock absorbers in the body. The articular cartilage and subchondral bone provide some shock absorption, and within synovial joints there is synovial fluid that absorbs shock.

Types of Joints

There are three main types of joints that can be classified according to the amount of movement that can occur at the joint or by the material found between the bones of the joint. The joints that are nearly immovable are called fibrous or synarthrotic (SIHN-ahr-THRAH-tik) joints. The joints that are slightly movable are cartilaginous or amphiarthrotic (AM-fee-ahr-THRAH-tik) joints. The joints that are freely movable are called synovial or diarthrotic (DAHY-ahr-THRAH-tik) joints (Table 4-2).

Table 4-2 Types of Joints

Type of Joint	Characteristics	Location	
Synarthrotic	Nearly immovable, fibrous	Skull sutures	
Amphiarthrotic	Slightly movable cartilaginous,	Pubis symphysis, between vertebrae	
Diarthrotic (synovial)	Freely movable, joint capsule with synovial fluid	Shoulder, hip, knee, elbow	
Ball-and-socket	Provides the greatest range of motion and allows movement in many directions (circumduction)	Glenohumeral joint (shoulder), acetabulum (hip joint)	
Condyloid	Allows movement in two planes (flexion, extension, lateral movement)	Metacarpophalangeal joints, between occiput and C1 (atlas)	

continues on following page

4 Kinesiology and Body Mechanics

Table 4-2 Types of Joints *continued*

Type of Joint	Characteristics	Location	
Gliding	Bones slide past each other (side to side movement)	Between carpals, between tarsals acromioclavicular joint	Carpals
Hinge	Allows movement in one plane (flexion, extension)	Elbow joint, knee joint, between phalanges	Humerus / Radius Ulna
Pivot	Allows rotational movement	Between C1 (atlas) and C2 (axis), between radius and ulna	Humerus / Radius Ulna
Saddle	Allows movement in many directions	Carpometacarpal joint of the thumb	Carpal / Metacarpal of thumb

Fibrous (Synarthrotic) Joints

Fibrous joints are made up of bones held together with fibrous connective tissue. These fibrous joints are functionally classified as synarthrotic, meaning very little, if any, movement occurs. The sutures of the skull (the cranium and the face) are examples of fibrous joints. While soft during infancy, these joints ossify as the child grows into adulthood, at which time there is very little movement that occurs at the sutures. Craniosacral therapy facilitates the movement of these joints, helping to restore homeostasis.

Understanding that bones are living tissue and remodel according to the stresses placed on them, it is simple to see how fibrous sutures are movable, even if only slightly.

Cartilaginous (Amphiarthrotic) Joints

Cartilaginous joints, true to their name, have cartilage between the bones. They are functionally classified as amphiarthrotic joints, indicating their ability to move slightly. The pubis symphysis and the joints between the vertebral bodies are examples of cartilaginous joints.

Synovial (Diarthrotic) Joints

The most prolific joints in the body are the synovial joints. The easy movement that occurs at these joints leads to their functional classification as diarthrotic joints. Synovial joints have several components:

- Articular cartilage—hyaline cartilage that covers the articular surfaces of the bones to reduce friction
- Bursae—synovial membrane–lined sacs full of synovial fluid that cushion the movement of tendons over bones (not present in all synovial joints)
- Joint capsule—a fibrous connective tissue sac that encloses the joint cavity
- Joint cavity—a space between the bones of the synovial joint that contains a lubricating, cushioning fluid
- Ligaments—fibrous connective tissue bands that hold the bones of the joint together and stabilize the joint
- Synovial membrane—the lining of the joint capsule that secretes synovial fluid, a thick, colorless, lubricating fluid similar in consistency to egg white

These freely movable joints are called synovial joints because the joint cavity is filled with synovial fluid. Produced in response to movement of the joint, synovial fluid provides lubrication for the joint, allowing free movement, and it also helps prevent injury to the hard structures involved in the movement. Examples of synovial joints include the knee, the shoulder, and the elbow.

There are six different types of synovial joints, grouped by their mechanical structure: gliding, hinge, pivot, condyloid (KAHN-dih-loyd), saddle, and ball-and-socket. Table 4-2 includes illustrations of these joints. The mechanical structure determines the kind of movement possible at a joint and the degree to which a joint can safely move, also known as its range of motion.

Gliding Joints

The bones of gliding joints have flattened sides that allow small amounts of sliding movement in a single plane between the bones. To demonstrate, put your hands flat on the table, thumbs touching, and slide your hands along each other while keeping your thumbs touching and your hands flat on the table. Gliding joints are found at the acromioclavicular joint; the interphalangeal, intercarpal, and intertarsal joints; and at the joints between superior and inferior vertebral facets. The joint is involved in body movements such as inversion and eversion of the ankle.

Hinge Joints

Hinge joints have a concave surface (a depression) on one bone, a convex surface (a rounded shape) on the other, and are held together with strong, collateral ligaments. The structure allows hinge joints to move in only one plane, very similar to the swing of a door. To visualize, think of a door hinge and how it can only open or close. The elbow, knee, fingers, and toes are examples of hinge joints that allow the body movements called flexion, commonly referred to as "bending," and extension, commonly called "straightening." The temporomandibular joint (TMJ) is a specialized hinge joint (see Box 4-1).

Pivot Joints

The pivot joints also fit together with matching surfaces, but one bone pivots within the annular (ring-shaped) ligament of the other bone. The resulting rotational movement occurs in a single plane in which one bone can pivot against the other. The proximal radioulnar pivot joint creates pronation and supination of the forearm. There is also a pivot joint between the atlas (C1) and axis (C2).

Condyloid Joints

The condyloid joint (also called the ellipsoid joint) is created from a convex, rounded, or oval projection at the end of one bone that fits into a concave surface on the other bone. The structure can rotate in two separate planes, allowing for body movements such as flexion, extension, adduction (movement of the bone toward the midline of the body), and abduction (movement away from the midline). The radiocarpal joint, metacarpophalangeal joints, and the joint between the occiput and the atlas are examples of condyloid joints.

Saddle Joints

Saddle joints have matching concave and convex surfaces, each shaped like a saddle. The structure allows for rotational movement in two planes. The carpometacarpal joint of the thumb and the calcaneocuboidal joint of the ankle are the only saddle joints, allowing flexion, extension, adduction, and abduction.

Ball-and-socket Joints

The ball-and-socket joint is made up of a large, spherical protrusion on one bone that fits into a cuplike cavity on the other. The ball-and-socket joints are multiaxial, meaning that rotational movement can occur in several different planes, and are therefore involved in many different body movements. Ball-and-socket joints include the shoulder and

BOX 4-1

The Temporomandibular Joint (TMJ)

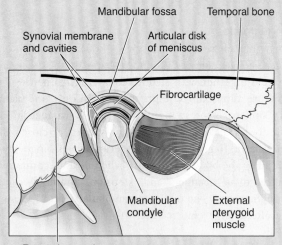

A Articular structures

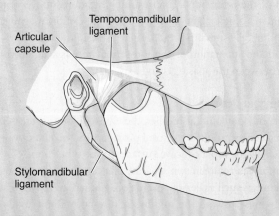

B Ligaments

The temporomandibular joint. **(A)** Articular structures. **(B)** Ligaments. (Reprinted with permission from Premkumar K. Anatomy & Physiology: The Massage Connection. 3rd ed. Philadelphia: Lippincott Williams & Wilkins, 2012.)

The TMJ comprises the joint and joint capsule between the temporal bone and the mandible of the jaw. It is a modified hinge joint that allows for elevation, depression, protraction, retraction, and lateral deviation of the mandible. Muscles of the TMJ are the major muscles involved in chewing: lateral pterygoid, temporalis, and masseter. Tightness in the TMJ muscles and forward head posture can create TMJ dysfunction. Massage techniques that relax these muscles may alleviate pain at this joint.

the hip, and are involved in flexion, extension, adduction, abduction, rotation (where a body part turns or pivots about its long axis), and circumduction (a combination of abduction, adduction, extension, and flexion that occurs in one continuous movement).

Range of Motion

Range of motion (ROM) is defined as the amount of movement that occurs at a joint. A normal ROM is the distance and direction that a joint can sustain without damage to surrounding tissues. The amount of movement is scientifically measured in degrees, and normal ranges are specific to each joint. Massage therapists tend to evaluate the movement more for quality and general quantity, without measuring degrees, to get information regarding the structures involved in a client's pain pattern.

Active ROM (AROM) requires a client to actively move her own joint, usually to demonstrate the quality and/or quantity of movement. AROM can provide information regarding condition of the muscles and tendons.

Passive ROM (PROM) requires the client to remain relaxed while the therapist moves the client's joint to determine quality and/or quantity of movement. PROM evaluations can provide information regarding the passive structures involved in the movement, such as ligaments and joints.

Resisted ROM, also called manual resistance, requires the client to actively attempt to move a joint while the therapist applies a small amount of resistance. These two counteracting forces result in an isometric contraction of the client's muscles that provides information about the condition of the client's soft tissue. More detailed information about ROM is covered in Chapter 7, Assessment.

Myology: The Study of Muscles

Skeletal muscles, introduced in Chapter 3, are the focus of massage therapy. To summarize, an entire skeletal muscle is made up of thousands of muscle cells bundled together in an organized fashion with connective tissue sheaths, and intertwined with blood vessels, nerves, and proprioceptors. The neuromuscular junctions are the points of communication between the nervous system and muscular system, but the muscles cannot contract without energy in the form of adenosine triphosphate. Muscular contraction, a form of mechanical work, can be classified according to muscular work and the resulting movement. Joint movements, or movements of the joints of the skeleton, are accomplished with muscular work. The different kinds of joints are discussed in the arthrology section above, and the muscles responsible for those movements are discussed in this section. **Muscles have many functions: they contract and work together to move the skeleton, they can stabilize parts of the body to help other muscles create the appropriate movement, and they can work against each other to balance movements.**

Skeletal Muscle Contraction

Skeletal muscles require nerve impulses and energy in order to contract. In Chapter 3, we discussed the way a nerve impulse is transmitted from the nervous system to the muscular system at the neuromuscular junction. Once the nerve signal arrives at the muscle, there must be sufficient energy to activate muscle contraction. The body can generate the necessary energy in different ways, and the mechanism utilized at the time is the one that best fits the body's resources and immediate needs.

Nerve Supply to Muscles

A nerve impulse starts out at the central nervous system (CNS) and is quickly transmitted out to the muscles to activate a contraction. The first major detour from the brain and spinal cord is through one of the intertwined, complex nerve plexuses (see Fig. 3-46):

- Cervical plexus—includes C1–C4 nerves, and innervates muscles of the head, neck, and diaphragm

- Brachial plexus—includes C5–C8 and T1 nerves, and innervates the muscles of the upper extremities

- Lumbar plexus—includes L1–L4 nerves, and innervates the abdominals, thigh flexors, knee extensors, and hip adductors

- Sacral plexus—includes L4, L5, and S1–4 nerves, and innervates the gluteal muscles, hamstrings, and several leg and foot muscles

The individual nerves that carry impulses to particular muscles can be located in the special muscle section and plates at the end of this chapter.

Once the impulse has been diverted along the appropriate nerve plexus, it travels down the appropriate nerve, eventually arriving at the neuromuscular junction.

Neuromuscular Junction

The very end of the motor neuron is called the axonal terminal. The microscopic gap between the axonal terminal and the muscle cell is called the synaptic cleft. This collection of structures where the nervous system and the muscular system communicate is called the neuromuscular junction. When the nerve impulse reaches the axonal terminal, a chemical is released into the synaptic cleft and received by the muscle cell. The chemicals trigger the muscle to contract.

Energy Requirements for Muscle Contraction

Muscle contraction requires energy. This energy can only be provided by a chemical called adenosine triphosphate (ATP), which is created in our bodies naturally. Muscles store their own ATP, but only enough for about 1 to 2 seconds of contraction, so it must be regenerated constantly. ATP is created in three ways: direct phosphorylation, the anaerobic mechanism (without oxygen), and the aerobic mechanism (with oxygen). Figure 4-5 illustrates the three mechanisms for regenerating ATP for muscle contraction.

Direct Phosphorylation

During strenuous exercise, our bodies use the ATP stored in muscles in addition to all three mechanisms of creating ATP.

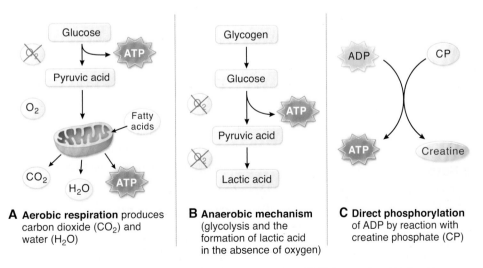

A Aerobic respiration produces carbon dioxide (CO_2) and water (H_2O)

B Anaerobic mechanism (glycolysis and the formation of lactic acid in the absence of oxygen)

C Direct phosphorylation of ADP by reaction with creatine phosphate (CP)

Figure 4-5. Mechanisms for generating adenosine triphosphate (ATP) in muscles. **(A)** Aerobic respiration produces carbon dioxide and water. **(B)** Anaerobic mechanism (glycolysis and the formation of lactic acid in the absence of oxygen). **(C)** Direct phosphorylation of adenosine diphosphate (ADP) by reaction with CP.

At first, the cell can use the stored ATP to contract. As stored ATP is being used up, additional ATP molecules can be generated via direct phosphorylation, the quickest mechanism for creating ATP. In this process, creatine phosphate (CP) stored only in muscle cells transfers a phosphate group to nearby adenosine diphosphate (ADP) molecules to create ATP. See Figure 4-5A. The disadvantage of this mechanism is that CP is depleted just as fast as ATP is created, and when it is gone, the muscle must generate ATP another way.

Anaerobic Cellular Respiration

The anaerobic process takes over after direct phosphorylation. When the oxygen in the muscle cells has been used for other cellular metabolic processes, the body enters a state of oxygen debt. The muscles can still produce ATP even during oxygen debt by using the anaerobic respiration mechanism. In the absence of oxygen, a glucose molecule can be broken down through the process of glycolysis to produce ATP, allowing the muscle to contract. The process is faster than aerobic respiration, but it is not very efficient—only two ATP molecules are generated from each molecule of glucose. See Figure 4-5B.

A side effect of anaerobic respiration is lactic acid production. Recent research strongly suggests that lactic acid is not involved in muscle fatigue nor muscle soreness. Muscle soreness is likely the result of microtears in the muscle. In fact, lactic acid can be converted back into pyruvate to be used in aerobic respiration in the muscle cells and used as a source of energy. A small amount of the lactic acid in the muscles is carried to the liver via the blood, where it is converted back to glucose with energy from ATP.

Muscle fatigue in endurance activity occurs when all available glycogen is consumed, the mental component of exhaustion comes into play, blood supply may be insufficient, and muscles may not respond as quickly or strongly as they had been. True muscle fatigue, however, occurs when the muscle cannot contract at all because of a lack of calcium ions in the sarcoplasm. With prolonged muscle activity, calcium leaks out through the calcium channels in the sarcolemma that are normally closed. Insufficient levels of calcium result in the inability to sustain muscle contraction. In this instance, true muscle fatigue is exhibited when athletes wobble and collapse toward the end of extreme endurance events.

Aerobic Cellular Respiration

Aerobic cellular respiration uses ATP to break down glucose and generate more ATP. See Figure 4-5C. There are three separate stages of aerobic respiration, including glycolysis, the Krebs citric acid cycle, and the electron transport system. Glycolysis, the process of breaking down glucose, is actually an anaerobic process that can occur in the presence of oxygen but does not require oxygen. What makes the three-step process an aerobic one is the fact that mitochondria are required to generate the ATP this way, and they require oxygen. Although it is the slowest method for generating ATP, it is also the most efficient.

The term "aerobic exercise" reflects the aerobic respiration process of generating ATP in the muscles, where moderate movement can be done for an extended period of time without needing to breathe heavily (acquire additional oxygen) following the activity.

Proprioceptors

Muscle contraction is controlled on a more refined level by the proprioceptors of the nervous system. **Proprioceptors** (PROH-pree-oh-SEP-torz) are sensory nerve cells that respond to body position, muscle tone, and equilibrium.

Muscle spindles are complex proprioceptors found in the muscles that are sensitive to the length of the muscle fibers and respond to changes in that length. Golgi (GOHL-jee) tendon organs are proprioceptors found between the collagen fibers in tendons that respond to muscle tension at the tendon (see Fig. 4-6). Together, the muscle spindles and Golgi tendon organs provide information to the CNS regarding the length and tension of a muscle and its tendon(s).

Proprioceptors within a joint capsule are Ruffini end organs and Pacinian corpuscles. Both respond to pressure within a joint, essentially sensing the position of the joint by sensing different amounts of pressure at different places.

The muscle spindles and Golgi tendon organs respond as muscles move a joint through its ROM, but joint proprioceptors are active when a joint is at the ends of its range. All of the proprioceptors act as a group to provide a sense of joint position, body position, effort, heaviness, and timing of movement; together, this is sometimes called a kinesthetic sense.

Manipulating the muscle spindles and Golgi tendon organs with advanced massage techniques can encourage muscles to shorten or lengthen. One of these techniques, appropriately called proprioceptive neuromuscular facilitation, is discussed in Chapter 10, Therapeutic Applications.

Types of Muscle Fibers

Each muscle has a combination of slow-twitch fibers and fast-twitch fibers that determines the endurance and speed of that muscle's contractions. The ratio of the fibers varies from muscle to muscle and person to person, depending on the person's physical activity and genetics.

Slow-twitch Fibers

Slow-twitch fibers (also called Type I fibers) are smaller in size than the fast-twitch fibers. They are red due to their rich blood supply and higher iron content, and rely on aerobic cellular respiration for energy. See Figure 4-7. They are slow to contract and are not very powerful, but they can remain

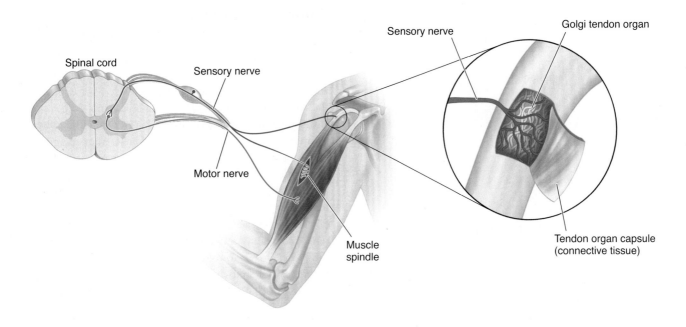

Figure 4-6. Muscle spindles and Golgi tendon organs.

contracted for long periods of time. Slow-twitch fibers are more prevalent in muscles that need to sustain contraction over long periods of time, such as the erector spinae, the postural muscles of the back.

Fast-twitch Fibers

There are two kinds of fast-twitch fibers (Fig. 4-7). Type IIa are pink and are slightly larger than the slow-twitch fibers. Type IIx are the largest fibers, and since they do not have a blood supply, they appear white. Fast-twitch fibers contract

quickly and powerfully in short bursts, utilizing the anaerobic respiration mechanism. The powerful muscles in the arms and legs tend to have a higher proportion of fast-twitch fibers.

Skeletal Muscle Activity

In Chapter 3, we discussed the two kinds of attachments of skeletal muscles: the **origin** is where a muscle attaches to a bone or connective tissue structure that is generally

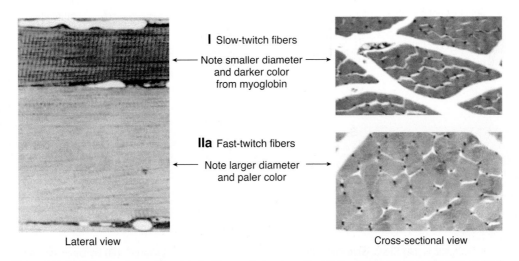

Figure 4-7. Muscle fiber types. (Reprinted with permission from Cael C. Functional Anatomy, Musculoskeletal Anatomy, Kinesiology, and Palpation for Manual Therapists. Philadelphia: Lippincott Williams & Wilkins, 2010.)

Kinesiology and Body Mechanics

4

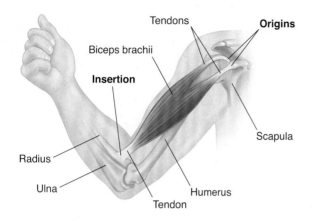

Figure 4-8. Muscle attachments: origin and insertion.

stationary, and the insertion is the attachment that moves most during normal contraction, often at the distal end (Fig. 4-8). This simple description for origin and insertion becomes a little more complicated when learning about muscle activity because contraction of a skeletal muscle may or may not result in movement. If no movement is produced when the muscle contracts, it is considered a static contraction. If some kind of movement results from the muscle contraction, it is called a dynamic contraction.

Significant increases or decreases in muscle activity impact the condition of the muscles, sometimes to the point that the health of the muscle is affected. Restrictions and dysfunctions in the ability of a muscle to perform normal contractions are the main focus of therapeutic massage, with the goal being restoration of the client's maximum functional muscle contraction.

Static Contractions

Static contractions, also called isometric contractions, do not produce movement of bones or body parts. In this situation, a muscle contracts, exerting force on its attachments, but the attachments do not move. See Figure 4-9A. Microscopically, the cross bridges attach, but the myofilaments do not slide closer together. Instead of producing movement and heat, isometric contractions only create heat. Squeezing your knees together and clenching your jaw are examples of isometric contractions.

Muscle tone is another example of static contraction. In a healthy, awake person, every skeletal muscle is in a state of partial contraction called muscle tone. The nervous system is constantly sending signals to approximately 10% of the muscle's cells to remain contracted, so the muscle cells within a whole muscle take turns being contracted to avoid fatigue. Muscle tone is especially important for maintaining posture or joint position. When people speak of "good muscle tone," they are referring to muscles that appear healthy and firm, not necessarily the partial contractions that hold our bodies upright.

Dynamic Contractions

Dynamic contractions, also called isotonic contractions, result in some kind of body movement as the muscle attachments get closer together or farther apart. Dynamic contractions can be either concentric or eccentric.

In concentric contractions, the myofilaments slide together, the muscle shortens, and the attachment sites of the muscle move closer together (Fig. 4-9B). Examples of concentric contractions include finger flexion and knee flexion.

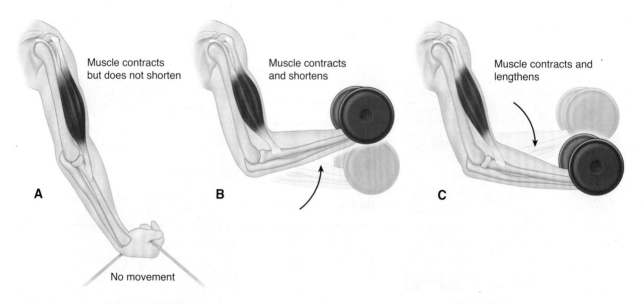

Figure 4-9. Types of contractions. **(A)** Static, **isometric**—the muscle contracts but does not shorten. **(B)** Dynamic, **concentric**—the muscle shortens as it contracts. **(C)** Dynamic, **eccentric**—the muscle lengthens as it contracts. (Reprinted with permission from Cael C. Functional Anatomy, Musculoskeletal Anatomy, Kinesiology, and Palpation for Manual Therapists. Philadelphia: Lippincott Williams & Wilkins, 2010.)

Eccentric contractions involve muscle contractions in which the muscle attachments move farther apart, effectively lengthening the muscle (Fig. 4-9C). Eccentric contractions are often used to resist gravity or slow down some kind of movement. For example, slowly lowering a pitcher of water onto a table utilizes muscle contractions to hold the pitcher's weight against gravity while the pitcher is being lowered. The muscles are contracting, but are also being lengthened.

Extreme Conditions of Muscle Activity

The deterioration of a muscle due to inactivity is called atrophy. When a muscle is inactive for a long period of time either by choice or as a result of nerve damage, the health of the muscle tissue deteriorates. The inactive muscle requires less energy, so its demand for oxygen and nutrition decreases. Consequently, circulation to the muscle diminishes, and a downward spiral ensues. The filaments within the muscle cells deteriorate, the muscle cells get smaller, and the size and strength of the entire muscle decrease.

Hypertrophy occurs when a muscle becomes enlarged as a result of forceful and repetitive activity. The number of muscle cells remains the same, but the length and diameter of the existing muscle cells increase because the number of myofilaments within the muscle cell increases.

Tetany is a sustained and forceful muscle contraction that occurs when nerve impulses arrive at the muscle so frequently that the muscle has no opportunity to relax at all. Sustained tetany eventually results in muscle fatigue, and the muscle is unable to hold a contraction.

Muscle Movement and Coordination

Individual muscles cooperate in conjunction with each other to create movement. Muscles can act as prime movers, synergists, fixators (also called stabilizers or supports), and antagonists. Each plays a role in the creation of body movement or stabilization of the body during movement, and any one muscle can fill any one of the roles at different times, depending on the movement.

Prime movers, also called agonists, are muscles that perform most of the intended movement. The main role of the prime mover is to contract the muscle. For example, in elbow extension, the triceps brachii muscle is the prime mover. **Synergists**, also known as accessory muscles, help the prime mover by contracting at the same time to facilitate more effective movement. The anconeus muscle is a synergist for triceps brachii in elbow extension. Special synergists called fixators, also called stabilizers or supports, hold a joint or another part of the body steady while the prime mover contracts. If the arm were behind the body during elbow extension, the teres minor muscle might act as a fixator to hold the arm back. **Antagonists** are muscles that move

in opposition to the prime mover. One of the antagonistic muscles to the triceps brachii is the biceps brachii, which flexes the elbow.

Skeletal muscles all have one or more antagonists. Typically located on the opposite side of the bone from the prime mover, the antagonist lengthens while the prime mover contracts. Remember, muscles can only pull, not push. **For movement to occur, antagonists must lengthen while the prime mover and synergists contract.**

Generally, when the nervous system stimulates the prime mover to contract, it also reflexively inhibits the antagonist, allowing it to relax and lengthen in order for the prime mover do its work. Figure 4-10 illustrates this concept in elbow flexion with the biceps brachii and triceps brachii muscles.

In addition to maintaining balance in the body, antagonists can slow the action of a prime mover. In Figure 4-10, for example, the triceps brachii acts as a counterbalance for the biceps brachii. The act of throwing a bowling ball is an example of the deltoid muscle acting as an antagonist to both gravity and some of the pectoralis major muscles, slowing the downward movement of the entire arm and preventing the arm from dropping like a dead weight.

A more complex example of prime movers and antagonists is the rotator cuff. The rotator cuff is a group of four muscles that surround the shoulder joint: supraspinatus, infraspinatus, teres minor, and subscapularis. The rotator cuff muscles cooperate to move the humerus in a large circle, in the ROM called circumduction. The individual muscles,

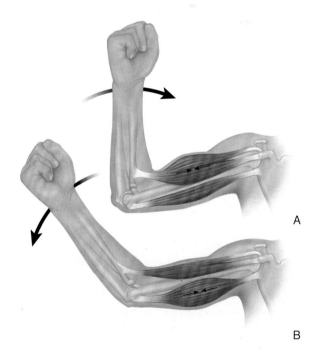

A

B

Figure 4-10. Biceps brachii muscle in elbow flexion. **(A)** Elbow flexion: prime mover, biceps brachii; antagonist, triceps brachii. **(B)** Elbow extension: prime mover, triceps brachii; antagonist, biceps brachii.

however, can be antagonists to each other, as in the case of the infraspinatus and subscapularis. During medial rotation of the humerus, the subscapularis is the prime mover and the infraspinatus is the antagonist. In other words, for the humerus to move into medial rotation, the infraspinatus must lengthen while the subscapularis contracts.

Overdeveloping only one of two muscles with antagonistic actions can cause awkward movements and abnormal body positions. For example, if a body builder overdevelops the biceps brachii in comparison to the antagonistic triceps brachii, the arm will remain slightly bent as it hangs down in a relaxed resting position.

Effects of Exercise on Muscles

Generally, aerobic exercise involves at least 15 minutes of continuous, moderate muscle activity. Regular aerobic exercise does not increase the size of muscle cells, but it does increase the number of mitochondria within a muscle cell and thus the endurance of the muscle. Remember, the mitochondria are the powerhouses of the cell that generate ATP. When the body experiences regular exercise, muscle cells store greater amounts of oxygen and ATP to be prepared for the next period of exercise.

Resistance exercises involve muscles being tasked during physical activity with additional resistance such as weights or elastic bands. The movements can be static or dynamic, either preventing or allowing movement to occur. As a result of resistance activity, the muscle cells increase their numbers of mitochondria and also increase the number of myofilaments within each muscle cell. The increased numbers of actin and myosin filaments increases the diameter of the muscle cell and ultimately increases the diameter and strength of the entire muscle.

Effects of Stretching on Muscles

People commonly associate exercise and stretching. Stretching is the elastic elongation of the soft tissues such as muscles, tendons, fascia, ligaments, and joint capsules. The purpose of stretching is to lengthen and relax contracted soft tissues to improve flexibility and mobility and allow the body to rebalance itself. Stretching is most effective when the tissues are warm, particularly because the tissues are more elastic and pliable when warm. Conversely, cold muscles and soft tissues are less elastic, more resistant to stretching, and may be more prone to injury. Thus, it is more effective and safer to stretch after having performed some physical activity that increases circulation to the target muscles. When you recommend clients stretch as a form of self-care, it is important that they know to warm their muscles and soft tissues via exercise, a hot pack, shower, or bath before performing their stretches.

Body Movements

The joints allow the body to move when the muscles contract and pull the bones. We have identified the different types of synovial joints and the types of movements that can occur at those joints, as well as the different types of muscle contractions and ways the muscles cooperate to produce coordinated, balanced body movement. In this section, we combine the arthrology with the myology to discuss the many body movements that are created by one or more joint movements and many different muscles. For instance, the shoulder area is not only capable of movement at the glenohumeral joint but is also capable of movements of the scapula bone. Many body movements, most of them occurring at joints, are illustrated in Table 4-3:

- Flexion—the "bending" movement that decreases the angle of a joint

- Extension—the "straightening" or "arching" movement that increases the angle of a joint

- Adduction—movement toward the midline of the body

- Abduction—movement away from the midline of the body

- Rotation—any movement that involves rotation around an axis

- Circumduction—a combination of abduction, adduction, extension, and flexion that occurs in one continuous movement. For example, drawing a circle in the air while keeping your arm straight is circumduction of the shoulder.

- Horizontal adduction—movement of the arm toward the midline of the body in the horizontal plane

- Horizontal abduction—movement of the arm away from the midline of the body in the horizontal plane

- Elevation—an upward or superior movement of the scapula or mandible

- Depression—downward or inferior movement of the scapula or mandible

- Protraction—forward or anterior movement of the scapula or mandible

- Retraction—posterior or recoiling movement of the scapula or mandible

- Upward rotation—a rotation of the scapula, moving the inferior angle of the scapula laterally and superiorly

- Downward rotation—a rotation of the scapula, moving the inferior angle of the scapula medially and inferiorly

- Inversion of the foot (supination)—movement of the sole of the foot toward the midline of the body

- Eversion of the foot (pronation)—movement of the sole of the foot away from the midline of the body

Table 4-3 Body Movements

Movement	Description	Movement	Description
Extension	**Increases the angle at a joint**		
Spine extension		Finger extension	
Neck extension		Knee extension	
Shoulder extension		Hip extension	
Elbow extension		**Flexion**	**Decreases the angle at a joint**
		Spine flexion	
Wrist extension		Neck flexion	
Thumb extension		Shoulder flexion	

continues on following page

Table 4-3 Body Movements *continued*

Movement	Description	Movement	Description
Elbow flexion		**Lateral flexion** Lateral flexion of the spine	**Curves the spine to the left or to the right**
Wrist flexion		Lateral flexion of the neck	
Thumb flexion		**Dorsiflexion** Dorsiflexion	**Lifts the toes of the foot superiorly and lowers the heel**
Finger flexion	 Finger flexion	**Plantarflexion** Plantarflexion	**Lowers the toes of the foot and raises the heel**
Hip flexion	 Hip flexion	**Hyperextension** Hyperextension of the spine	**Joint is extended past anatomical position**
Knee flexion		Hyperextension of the neck	

continues on following page

Table 4-3 Body Movements *continued*

Movement	Description	Movement	Description
Pronation Pronation of the forearm	**Turns the palm of the hand down**	Ankle abduction	
Supination Supination of the forearm	**Turns the hand palm up**	**Adduction (commonly clarified as A-D-duction)** Shoulder adduction	**Takes a structure toward the body or brings fingers together**
Abduction (commonly clarified as A-B-duction) Shoulder abduction	**Takes a structure away from the body or separates fingers**	Wrist adduction	
Wrist abduction		Thumb adduction	
Thumb abduction		Finger adduction	
Finger abduction		Hip adduction	
Hip abduction		Ankle adduction	

continues on following page

Table 4-3 Body Movements *continued*

Movement	Description	Movement	Description
Eversion Eversion	**Turns the sole of the foot laterally, combining dorsiflexion and abduction**	**Opposition** Thumb opposition	**Movement of the thumb toward the "pinkie finger"**
Inversion Inversion	**Turns the sole of the foot medially, combining plantarflexion and adduction**	**Rotation** Spine rotation	**A twisting or turning of a bone along its own axis**
Lateral deviation Mandible	**The body part moves laterally**	Neck rotation	
Circumduction Shoulder circumduction	**A fluid circular movement that combines flexion, extension, abduction and adduction**	Lateral rotation of the humerus	
Hip circumduction		Medial rotation of the humerus	
Lateral rotation of the femur		Elevation of the pelvis	

continues on following page

Table 4-3 Body Movements *continued*

Movement	Description	Movement	Description
Medial rotation of the femur		**Protraction**	**Moves the mandible or scapula anteriorly**
		Protraction of the mandible	
Depression	**Opens the jaw or lowers the entire scapula**	Protraction of the scapula	
Depression of the mandible			
Depression of the scapula		**Retraction**	**Moves the mandible or scapula posteriorly**
		Retraction of the mandible	
Elevation	**Closes the jaw or lifts the entire scapula or femur**		
Elevation of the mandible		Retraction of the scapula	
Elevation of the scapula			
Inhalation	**Expands and lifts the bony thorax**	**Exhalation**	**Contracts and lowers the bony thorax**
Inhalation		Exhalation	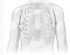

- Dorsiflexion—movement of the toes and foot superiorly, toward the body
- Plantarflexion—movement of the toes and foot inferiorly, away from the body
- Lateral flexion—lateral movement of the spine away from the midline
- Pronation—turning the palm of the hand downward
- Supination—turning the palm of the hand upward, as in holding a bowl of soup

Terminology is important when referring to movement. For example, "bending the arm" is an unclear statement because "the arm" includes dozens of bones and joints. A more accurate description is flexion of the elbow. Likewise, "straightening the leg" is a description of knee extension, and "straightening the back" is the act of extending the spine. Practice using the scientific terms so you are comfortable using them in professional communication and documentation.

Body Movement Pairs

Functionally, when a muscle concentrically contracts, its antagonist relaxes. For every movement, there is an antagonistic movement that takes the body in the opposite direction. These body movement pairs are as follows:

- Flexion and extension
- Abduction and adduction
- Lateral flexion to the left and lateral flexion to the right
- Lateral rotation and medial rotation
- Plantarflexion and dorsiflexion
- Inversion and eversion
- Elevation and depression
- Protraction and retraction
- Pronation and supination
- Inhalation and exhalation

Although most people do not realize it, inhalation and exhalation involve skeletal muscle contractions. When a person inhales normally, or breathes in, the diaphragm muscle contracts to increase the volume of the chest cavity and pull

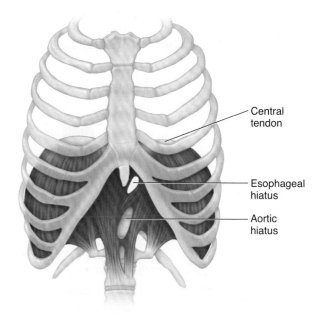

Figure 4-11. Diaphragm muscle.

Central tendon

Esophageal hiatus

Aortic hiatus

air into the respiratory tract. Exhalation occurs primarily when the diaphragm muscle relaxes (Fig. 4-11). External and internal intercostals can expand and contract the rib cage during heavy breathing, and accessory muscles can also be involved in these movements.

Knowing these pairs of opposite movements will be helpful in assessing your client as well as determining the best course of treatment.

Massage therapists should know the major joints of the body, the normal movements for each of those joints, and which muscles provide those movements. (See the special muscle section and plates at the end of this chapter.) The dynamic contractions of skeletal muscles are responsible for creating joint movements, some of which are specific to a particular joint or bone. Recognizing a client's limited ROM in a joint is critical to avoid hurting the client. Knowing how muscles should be functioning at a particular joint and whether a client's pain is triggered by the concentric or eccentric contraction of a muscle helps you make the initial assessment and determine subsequent treatment.

Biomechanics

Biomechanics studies the mechanics of movement and how movement is affected by internal and external factors including gravity, muscle–tendon interactions, neurological input, and physical strain. The basic concepts of biomechanics applied to massage therapy is a practice we call body

mechanics, and it will help you use your body effectively and efficiently to avoid developing your own pain patterns, injuries, and fatigue. As you learn and practice your strokes and techniques, monitor your body to make sure that you establish good body movement habits and that you are keeping your body relaxed and comfortable. Body awareness is key. If you learn how to apply strokes carefully and efficiently at the beginning of your career, good body mechanics will become second nature.

Alert

Holding and moving your body inefficiently during a massage session can lead to fatigue, increased discomfort, pain, and injury.

Due to the repetitive nature of the work, massage therapists tend to develop injuries and pain patterns in certain areas of the body. Not all therapists suffer from pain and injury, though, and with good body mechanics, body awareness, and mindful injury prevention, you can enjoy a long and injury-free massage therapy career.

Components of Good Body Mechanics

Critical components of good body mechanics include efficient structural alignment of your body, proper stance, and ergonomics. The body should move fluidly, using gravity and the movement of the whole body to deliver the massage instead of using the muscles of the shoulders, arms, hands, fingers, and thumbs. Movement of the body as a whole improves the fluidity and rhythm of the massage.

Maximizing the amount of pressure and minimizing your muscular work while giving a massage is very important. Efficient structural alignment will help accomplish both. When your body is aligned efficiently, your physical work and the resulting stresses and strains are distributed throughout the body rather than being concentrated on one or two specific joints. Maintaining efficient structural alignment during a massage can be achieved with the proper stance. The symmetric and asymmetric stances are stable and balanced, providing good structural alignment for applying strokes as well as manipulating clients on the massage table. Stable, balanced structures are much more efficient than unstable, unbalanced structures. You can increase your stability by keeping your center of gravity low with bent knees. You can increase your balance by holding most of your weight on one foot while using the other foot for balance.

An equally important concept that can facilitate good body mechanics is ergonomics, which is the applied science of adapting the workplace to maximize efficiency and safety. In massage therapy, we apply ergonomics by ensuring that your equipment is properly adjusted and easily accessible, and that the environment is arranged efficiently and with everyone's safety in mind.

Efficient Structural Alignment

You need to maintain efficient alignment of your body to protect your muscles and joints from excessive stress and strain that can result in pain and injury. Consider the alignment of the skeleton in a standing posture. The body is relaxed and comfortable, and the stresses of gravity are dispersed among the weight-bearing joints. Maintaining a similar postural alignment while practicing massage is the first step toward good body mechanics. Keeping your body relaxed is more comfortable for you as well as the clients. Using relaxed wrists and hands to apply massage strokes actually feels more comfortable to clients than using tight, tense wrists and hands.

Efficient structural alignment consists of keeping the spine neutral (no flexion or extension), stacking the joints of the arm delivering the pressure, and stacking the joints of the leg you put your weight on. The muscles and joints complicate the task of keeping that structural alignment because the skeleton has a tendency to move at the joints. It takes some practice to achieve and maintain efficient structural alignment during massage, but it is well worth it for the energy it will conserve and the muscle strain you will avoid. Figure 4-12 illustrates inefficient structural alignment.

Leaning

Massage therapists have to apply strokes with varying amounts of pressure as well as lift and manipulate the client's body. One of the keys to generating power and establishing stability behind your massage work is to use your body as a rigid structure that takes advantage of gravity for applying pressure during a massage stroke. Leaning

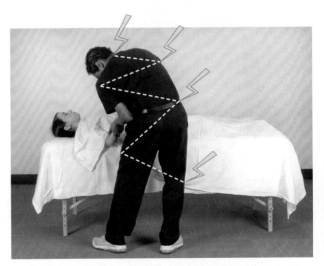

Figure 4-12. Inefficient structural alignment causes unnecessary muscle strain for the therapist. (Reprinted with permission from Frye B. Body Mechanics for Manual Therapists: A Functional Approach to Self-Care. Philadelphia: Lippincott Williams & Wilkins, 2010.)

into the stroke uses the weight, strength, and stability of your whole body to let gravity do some of the work. Your body uses mostly the postural muscles to maintain the leaning position, requiring little additional effort or energy to provide pressure on the client. Pushing, on the other hand, takes a lot more of your energy because you use the mechanical strength of your muscles to do the work.

Leaning allows you to apply appropriate pressure with minimal stress on your muscles and joints. If you have ever tried to push a heavy piece of furniture across the floor, your natural instincts probably led you to lean into the furniture with your arms straight, and your feet in a staggered position. You do not need to use those kinds of forces for massage, but the example shows how to maximize the work you do, with the least physical exertion. Leaning into the client's body with proper body mechanics creates a more fluid technique than pushing, is less tiring, and feels better to the client. Not only does it feel better to clients, it offers them a sort of safety net by increasing your sensitivity to their soft tissues. If a client's body is resisting additional pressure, sometimes it twitches or jumps or tenses up nearby muscles. When you lean on clients, you are better able to feel the tissues resist. Therapists who push are less likely to feel the resistance and are more apt to push beyond the client's tolerance, possibly hurting the client. The slow application of pressure that occurs with a lean allows the tissue to take more pressure without damage.

Lifting

Massage therapists do a fair amount of lifting during a massage. Draping, undraping, and passive joint movements generally require that you lift different parts of the client's body, and it is especially important to use good body mechanics for lifting. Structural alignment is as important for lifting as it is for leaning:

- Keep the body part you are lifting close to your body.
- Keep a neutral spine.
- Use your leg muscles to push into the lift rather than your back or shoulder muscles to move the body part.
- Use both hands to lift when you can.

In the interest of your own well-being, you can politely ask clients to help you by saying, "Could you lift your leg just a bit so I can slip this sheet underneath it?" Most clients are more than willing to help, and some even lift their limbs without a request, just to be helpful. You can injure yourself lifting clients, regardless of the weight of the body part, if you use improper body mechanics (Figure 4-13).

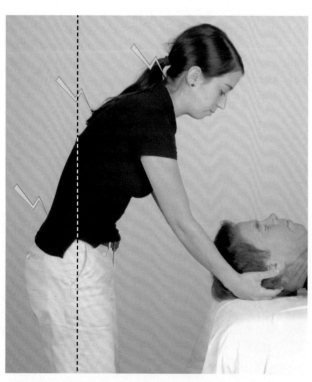

Figure 4-13. Improper body mechanics during lifting creates unnecessary muscle strain on the therapist's neck and back. (Reprinted with permission from Frye B. Body Mechanics for Manual Therapists: A Functional Approach to Self-Care. Philadelphia: Lippincott Williams & Wilkins, 2010.)

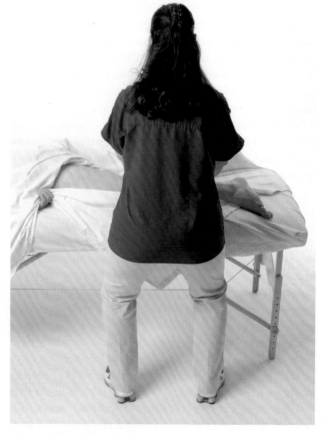

Figure 4-14. Symmetric stance.

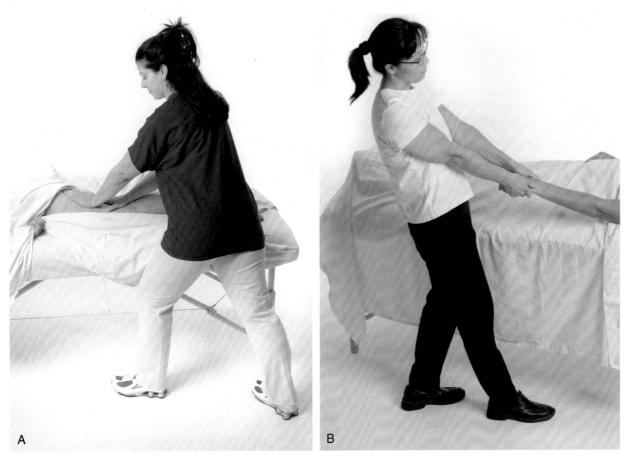

Figure 4-15. Asymmetric stance. **(A)** Asymmetric lean. **(B)** Asymmetric pull.

Symmetric Stance

The **symmetric stance**, also called the parallel stance, has both feet facing forward about shoulder-width apart, hips facing forward, knees bent. In this position, your body is symmetrical (the same on both sides) while facing your work (Fig. 4-14). This stance is good for performing light strokes that travel only a few inches along the client's body and when the stroke travels directly transversely, across the client's body.

Asymmetric Stance

The **asymmetric stance**, also called the one-foot-forward stance, has one foot in front of the other, the front foot facing the work, the back foot laterally rotated. The hips face the work, the feet are about shoulder-width apart, the front knee is flexed, and the back knee is extended. Your weight is primarily supported by your back foot and the client's body at the contact point, and the front foot is used more for balance than support (Fig. 4-15A). This asymmetric stance is most often used in massage therapy because it provides the best leverage for strokes that require a lot of pressure and makes it easier to move around the table throughout the massage.

The asymmetric stance can also be used for pulling. If you maintain structural alignment, your own weight does

the pulling rather than your muscles. Simply grasp your client's arm or hand, relax your elbows and shoulders, and lean backward (Fig. 4-15B).

The asymmetric stance offers more leverage than the symmetric stance. In terms of body mechanics, you can apply more pressure with the same amount of exertion if you lean from your back foot than if you flex at the hips and lean from your waist. Try to keep your ears, shoulders, hips, and back heel in a straight line. It minimizes unnecessary stress on your body and maximizes the pressure you can apply. You can use the steps in Box 4-2 to take an asymmetric position next to a client on the massage table.

An open, asymmetric stance allows you to maintain the head-to-heel line as long as you are an appropriate distance away from the table. Typically, therapists keep their front foot less than 10 inches away from the table, but this is a general distance that is adjusted for different strokes and different applications. Standing too close to or too far from the table compromises the head-to-heel line.

Once you get comfortable with the stances, the following guidelines can help you establish an efficient asymmetric alignment for applying most massage strokes (Fig. 4-16):

- Use the back foot to support your weight.
- Use the front foot for balance.

BOX 4-2

Taking an Asymmetric Stance Next to a Client on a Massage Table

1. Stand about 6 inches away from the middle of the massage table, with your head, hips, and toes all facing the center of the table.

2. Spread your feet shoulder-width apart.

3. Turn toward the client's head by pivoting on your toes. Your toes, hips, and face will all be facing your client's head, at an angle to the massage table, with one foot in front of the other.

4. Take a half step backward with your back foot to spread your feet apart. You may want to laterally rotate your back leg for stability.

5. Place the hand that is contralateral to (on the opposite side of) your back foot on the client's shoulder.

6. Lean on the client's shoulder and lift your weight off your front foot to rest your weight on the client's body and the floor under your back foot.

7. Place your other hand on the client for balance.

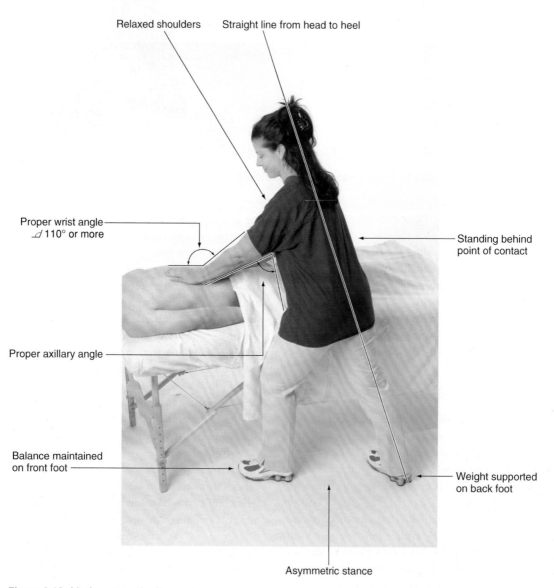

Figure 4-16. Ideal asymmetric alignment.

- Use the hand that is contralateral to the back foot to apply the stroke (use the right hand if the left foot is in back) to avoid twisting at the waist.
- Keep your ears, shoulders, hips, and the heel of your back foot in a line as much as possible.
- Point your front foot and hips toward your work instead of twisting at the waist.
- The wrist angle, between the posterior surface of the hand and the forearm, should be no less than 110°.
- The axillary angle, or the angle between your humerus and the side of your body, should not exceed 90°.
- Position yourself behind your work instead of on top of it.

Try to keep the axillary angle of about 90°, keeping your arm about perpendicular to your body, to help you achieve efficient alignment. When the angle is less than 90° or your arm is too close to your body, you may be applying pressure from an angle that puts undue and unsafe stresses on your glenohumeral joint. When the angle exceeds 90° or your arm is too far away from your body, you have to use your muscles to hold your body up, creating additional muscle strain and increasing the possibility of pain or injury. To maintain this angle while performing a long stroke that travels some distance along the client's body, you have to walk slowly and smoothly with the stroke (Fig. 4-17).

Your wrist should remain relaxed, and the angle between the posterior surface of the hand and the forearm should not be less than about 110° (see Fig. 4-16). Try this: actively extend your wrist and notice the limit of the extension. That position is as far as you want to push your wrist when applying strokes. When the angle is less than that, the structures running through the carpal tunnel are compressed.

It is safer for clients if the pressure of your stroke is delivered at an oblique angle or from a somewhat sideways direction instead of directly perpendicular to the client's tissues. When pressure comes from an angle, clients can roll away from pressure that is painful or uncomfortable, giving them a sense of control over the session. When the pressure comes from directly behind the contact point where the massage stroke is applied to their skin, clients cannot roll away. Besides, in order to apply pressure directly into the client's tissues rather than at an angle, you would need to be standing on top of the client in order to maintain good body mechanics.

Ergonomics

Ergonomics adapts the workspace to maximize a person's productivity, well-being, and safety. The components of ergonomics in a massage practice include equipment and workspace design.

Equipment

Massage equipment is not standard. There are different sizes and shapes of massage tables, some of them at a fixed height and others that are manually or electrically adjustable. Stools may or may not have wheels or adjustable heights. In order to maintain good body mechanics, the height of the table or, more importantly, the height of the client's body on the table is critical. The general rule is to make sure that the top of the table is about at the middle of your index finger or the middle of your thigh, but that is only a general starting point (Fig. 4-18). It is important

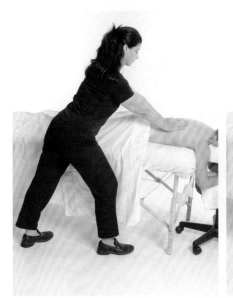
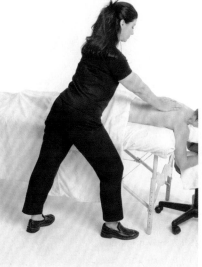
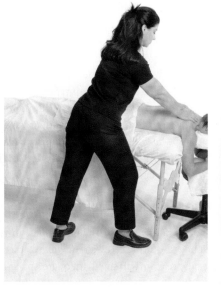

Figure 4-17. Walking with stroke.

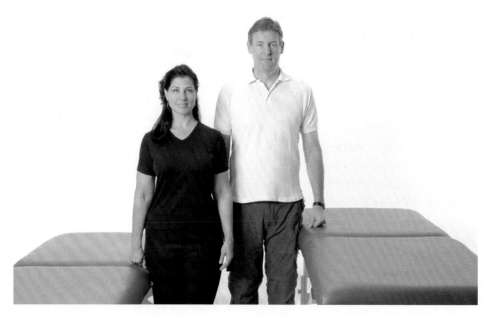

Figure 4-18. Proper table height.

to take your own body type into consideration with the table height. If you have a long torso and short legs or you have a short torso and long legs, you will need to adjust the table to ensure your body remains in alignment as you perform massage. If your table is too high, you may feel neck and shoulder tension, discomfort, or pain, symptoms that suggest you are elevating your shoulders while giving massages. Conversely, if your table is too low, you may feel tension or pain in your low back, suggesting that you are bending at the waist while treating clients.

You may need to adjust the height of your table for different clients. The body of a very thin client can be a foot lower than the body of a very thick client, and these differences will affect your body mechanics significantly. When the client's body is at the right height, you can use your body with ease, and the massage can flow smoothly. If your massage table is not adjustable, you will have to adjust your stance in an effort to maintain good body mechanics.

Sitting on a chair or stool uses less energy than standing, and there are times during the massage that you can sit in a chair and still maintain good body mechanics. Any time you work on a client's head, hands, or feet, it may be better to sit down (Fig. 4-19). Chairs and stools with wheels are especially easy to use, because you can easily move them around with your feet while your hands maintain contact with your client's body.

Workspace Design

The arrangement of the equipment in your massage workspace should take efficiency as well as safety into consideration. You will need adequate space around the table to maintain good body mechanics, to move easily around the table, and to make sure your clients can maneuver in the room without bumping into anything, tripping over

anything, or getting hurt. There should be enough floor space around your massage table so you can use an asymmetric stance and lean into your client without stepping on anything or running into a wall. If you do not have enough room around the table, your tendency will be to stand too

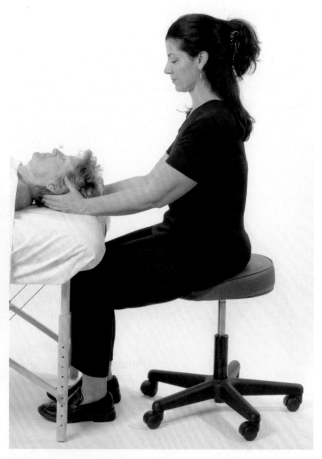

Figure 4-19. Sitting on a chair to conserve energy.

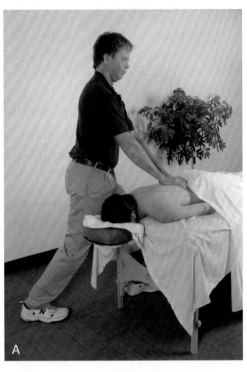

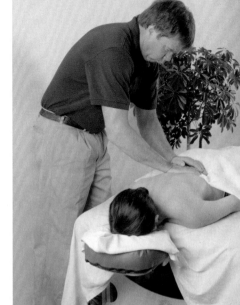

Figure 4-20. **(A)** Adequate workspace allows for efficient structural alignment. **(B)** Inadequate workspace results in compromised body mechanics. (Reprinted with permission from Frye B. Body Mechanics for Manual Therapists: A Functional Approach to Self-Care. Philadelphia: Lippincott Williams & Wilkins, 2010.)

close to your client's body and apply the pressure with muscular work or lose the proper alignment of your body and endanger your joints. You should also take the size and shape of your own body into account. For example, if you are very tall you may need more space around the table than if you are shorter. In general, you should have at least 3 feet of space around your table to be able to move freely during the session. Figure 4-20 illustrates the difference between adequate and inadequate workspace.

Body Awareness

It will be helpful to incorporate body awareness as you learn massage, paying attention to your body's positions, movements, and sensations during a massage session. Make sure that you establish good body movement habits and that you keep your body relaxed and comfortable. For example, massage therapists tend to shrug their shoulders when they are first learning massage as well as when they are fatigued. The result is usually tight and sore shoulders by the end of the day. If you pay attention to your body, you will notice the improper position of your shoulders and can relax and drop your shoulders before pain and tension set in.

Breathing is an important component of body awareness you might not have considered. Curiously enough, massage students tend to hold their breath when they are first learning. It may seem obvious, but it is important to keep breathing while doing massage. The muscles need oxygen to generate energy. You may occasionally want to utilize deep breathing to increase circulation and decrease muscle tension. There is more information about breathing and an exercise for learning how to breathe from the diaphragm in Chapter 9, Massage Strokes and Flow.

You may want to incorporate a body mechanics "check" at opportune points throughout the massage, perhaps when you hold up the sheet to allow clients to turn over or when you redrape a particular area of the body. You can practice body awareness by periodically asking yourself questions while you give a massage:

- Am I using my whole body?
- Is there a straight line formed by my head, hips, and back foot?
- Are my hips and front foot facing my work?
- Are my wrists, hands, and shoulders relaxed?
- Are any of my joints hyperextended?
- Am I breathing?
- Does my body hurt anywhere?

There is no doubt that at some point in your career you will experience some pain and discomfort, either in a massage session or as the result of performing several massages over time; increased body awareness will help you make the necessary adjustments to minimize your chance of injury.

Improper Body Mechanics

Your ability to deliver strength, pressure, and control are compromised by poor structural alignment. Worse yet, inefficient alignment can lead to injury. Massage involves a lot of repetitive movements and compression, both of which are stressful on the joints. A vicious circle of bad body mechanics begins as bad body mechanics lead to fatigue, fatigue often exacerbates bad body mechanics, and so on.

The hands, fingers, thumbs, and wrists are used extensively in massage. Although the hands are the first things that come to mind when you think about giving a massage, the rest of your body supports your hands in the application of a stroke or technique. One massage performed with poor body mechanics may not cause much harm, but after several massages a day over months and years, bad body mechanics will undoubtedly cause trouble. You can develop chronic pain, injuries, and other uncomfortable symptoms in your hands, fingers, thumbs, wrists, shoulders, neck, back, and low back. In severe cases, these conditions can end your career. This section points out how improper body mechanics can develop into pain patterns, and how you can minimize the risk of injury.

Injury

Massage puts undue stress on the muscles and joints even when you do use good body mechanics. Essentially, the body is not designed to perform repetitive motions for an extended period, which is what occurs in massage therapy. RSIs result when specific body movements are repeated enough to stress the involved structures to the point of damage. Several areas of the body are prone to pain patterns, possible reasons for which are described below:

- Neck and shoulders
  - The table may be too high.
  - You may be pushing instead of leaning.
- Wrist and hands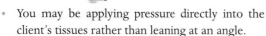
  - You may be applying pressure directly into the client's tissues rather than leaning at an angle.
  - You may be using your fingers and thumbs to squeeze and knead more than necessary.
  - You may not be stacking the joints of your fingers and thumb when applying strokes.
- Back
  - You may be bending and/or overreaching.
  - You may be lifting with improper alignment.

- Knees
  - You may be hyperextending (locking) your knees.
  - You may be twisting, leaving toes pointed in one direction while the hips point in another direction.
- Ankles and feet
  - You may be standing too much.
  - You may need shoes that are more supportive.

A sudden increase in your workload or decrease in the amount of rest you take between massage sessions can also develop pain patterns. For example, your massage practice suddenly jumps from 3 to 5 clients a week to 10 clients per week. This large influx of clients is financially appealing, but you will do yourself a long-term favor by pacing yourself and scheduling these clients over a 2-week period.

Repetitive motions impact the musculotendinous unit as muscles repeatedly exert strain on their tendons. Symptoms of inflammation, mild-to-severe discomfort or pain, decreased strength, and decreased ROM can result. Examples of specific musculotendinous injuries include muscle strain, tendinitis, or tenosynovitis (inflammation of the tendon sheath) in the shoulder, forearm, hands, fingers, or thumbs.

Nerve compression impairs nerve function and results in symptoms such as burning, tingling, pins and needles (paresthesia), and radiating pain. A couple of nerve compression injuries are carpal tunnel syndrome and thoracic outlet syndrome. Briefly, the carpal tunnel is created by the carpals of the wrist forming a passageway for blood vessels, tendons, and the median nerve, which serves the thumb and first two fingers. Excessive, sustained pressure on the carpal tunnel can negatively affect the structures running through it, eventually becoming a nerve compression injury called carpal tunnel syndrome. Thoracic outlet syndrome is a similar nerve compression injury resulting from restricted and tight soft tissues that compress the brachial plexus, which serves the shoulder, forearm, and hand.

Injury Prevention

Now that you recognize the possibility of developing your own pain patterns by practicing massage, you can appreciate how important it is to take care of your body. If you do not keep your muscles healthy with sufficient exercise, water consumption, stretching, and massage, your body will be more susceptible to injury and fatigue. Massage is a physically demanding career that requires strength and flexibility. Strength will help you perform massage strokes, lift clients, and assist clients who need help getting on and off the table. Since massage involves a lot of muscular activity on your part, it is wise to stretch before and between massage sessions to keep your soft tissues flexible. Remember to:

- Breathe deeply.
- Relax.

- Stretch slowly to avoid the stretch reflex.
- Hold the stretch for at least 10 seconds to trigger the tendon reflex, which comfortably enhances the stretch.

If massage is going to be your career, you may want to consider strength training, yoga, tai chi, or stretching on a regular basis as part of your self-care regimen. Self-care for the massage therapist, including examples of stretches, is covered in more detail in Chapter 13, Professional Massage Practice.

Along with developing strength and flexibility, it is also a good idea to develop your cardiovascular system to increase your endurance, which you can incorporate into your self-care regimen. Endurance is not necessary to perform one massage, but as you increase your practice to multiple massages each day and more than 10 a week, you will need endurance to sustain your practice. If your endurance is low, you may get tired easily, your body mechanics may suffer, and you may be more likely to suffer an injury.

The following are guidelines to help you with injury prevention:

- Consistently use all the components of good body mechanics.
- Rest your body and your hands by scheduling clients a minimum of 15 minutes apart.
- Stretch before and after massage sessions.
- Use the proper table height.
- Make sure you have plenty of room to move around the table.

- Use a variety of techniques in your massage sessions.
- Be cautious with applications of sustained pressure.
- Increase your own physical fitness and endurance.
- Get plenty of sleep and rest.

If you notice any soreness, aches, fatigue, pain, burning, numbness, tingling or loss of function, or signs of inflammation including redness, heat, or swelling, you must try to figure out what is causing the symptoms and make the appropriate changes to your structural alignment, techniques, equipment, or schedule. You may want to visit a healthcare professional for evaluation and treatment. **Do not risk your career by tolerating pain and injury.**

CHAPTER SUMMARY

Body mechanics are best learned in a classroom with an instructor to help you, but the concepts outlined in this chapter can serve as reminders outside the classroom. There are differing thoughts and opinions about which stances are best for minimizing stress on your body and maximizing your energy to practice massage. As you learn and practice massage, your body awareness can guide you to the stances and positions that are most comfortable and do not create discomfort or pain in your body. To start, just choose a stance, relax your body, and begin to work. If you feel muscle tension developing or you start feeling fatigued at any point during a massage, change your position or change your technique. You must raise your body awareness and develop good body mechanics as you learn the strokes and flow of massage so you can build a successful practice without damaging your body.

SPECIAL MUSCLE SECTION

Action Movement	Muscle	Origin	Insertion (bone that is moved is CAPITALIZED)	Nerve (spinal segment nerve numbers)	Plate(s)
SHOULDER					
Elevation	Levator scapula	Transverse processes of C1–C4	Medial border of SCAPULA	Cervical & dorsal scapular (C3,4,5)	Plate 4-1
	Rhomboid major	C7, T1–5	Medial border of SCAPULA	Dorsal scapular (C4,5)	Plate 4-1
	Trapezius (upper)	Occiput, ligamentum nuchae	Lateral end of clavicle, lateral spine of SCAPULA	Accessory (C2,3,4)	Plate 4-1
Depression	Serratus anterior	Outer surfaces of ribs 8–10	Anterior surface of medial border of SCAPULA	Long thoracic (C5,6,7)	Plate 4-2
	Subclavius	Junction of first rib and costal cartilage	Inferior surface of CLAVICLE	Branch of brachial plexus (C5,6)	Plate 4-3
	Trapezius (lower)	T4–12	Root of spine of SCAPULA	Accessory (C3,4)	Plate 4-1
Protraction	Serratus anterior	Outer surfaces of ribs 8–10	Anterior surface of medial border of SCAPULA	Long thoracic (C5,6,7)	Plate 4-2
Retraction	Rhomboid major	C7, T1–5	Medial border of SCAPULA	Dorsal scapular (C4,5)	Plate 4-1
	Trapezius (middle)	Ligamentum nuchae, C7-T4	Spine of SCAPULA	Accessory (C3,4)	Plate 4-1
Upward Rotation	Serratus anterior	Outer surfaces of ribs 8–10	Anterior surface of medial border of SCAPULA	Long thoracic (C5,6,7)	Plate 4-2
	Trapezius (lower)	T4–12	Root of spine of SCAPULA	Accessory (C3,4)	Plate 4-1
	Trapezius (upper)	Occiput, ligamentum nuchae	Lateral end of clavicle, lateral spine of SCAPULA	Accessory (C2,3,4)	Plate 4-1
Downward Rotation	Levator scapula	Transverse processes of C1–C4	Medial border of SCAPULA	Cervical & dorsal scapular (C3,4,5)	Plate 4-1
	Pectoralis minor	Anterior surface of ribs 3,4,5	Coracoid process of SCAPULA	Lateral pectoral (C5,6,7)	Plate 4-3
	Rhomboid major	C7, T1–5	Medial border of SCAPULA	Dorsal scapular(C4,5)	Plate 4-1
Forward Rotation	Pectoralis minor	Anterior surface of ribs 3,4,5	Coracoid process of SCAPULA	Lateral pectoral (C5,6,7)	Plate 4-3
Flexion	Coracobrachialis	Coracoid process of scapula	Medial side of middle of HUMERUS	Musculocutaneous (C5,6,7)	Plate 4-4
	Deltoid (anterior)	Lateral third of clavicle	Deltoid tuberosity of HUMERUS	Axillary (C5,6)	Plate 4-3
	Pectoralis major	Medial clavicle, sternum, costal cartilages of ribs 2–6	Greater tubercle of HUMERUS	Lateral and medial pectoral (C7,C8,T1)	Plate 4-3
Accessory Muscles/Assist Flexion	Biceps brachii	Long head: supraglenoid tubercle of scapula Short head: coracoid process of scapula	Tuberosity of RADIUS	Musculocutaneous (C5,6)	Plate 4-4
	Subscapularis	Subscapular fossa on anterior scapula	Lesser tubercle of HUMERUS	Subscapular (C5,6,7)	Plate 4-2

(continued)

SPECIAL MUSCLE SECTION (*Continued*)

Action Movement	Muscle	Origin	Insertion (bone that is moved is CAPITALIZED)	Nerve (spinal segment nerve numbers)	Plate(s)
SHOULDER *(continued)*					
Extension	Deltoid (posterior)	Spine of scapula	Deltoid tuberosity of HUMERUS	Axillary (C5,6)	Plate 4-3
	Latissimus dorsi	Thoracolumbar fascia, iliac crest, inferior angle of scapula, spinous processes of T7-S3)	Bicipital groove of HUMERUS	Thoracodorsal, brachial plexus (C6,7,8)	Plate 4-1
	Teres major	Lower third of scapula	Bicipital groove of HUMERUS	Upper and lower scapular (C5,6)	Plate 4-1
Accessory Muscles/Assist Flexion	Triceps brachii	Long head: infraglenoid tubercle of scapula lateral head: upper third of posterior humerus medial head: distal half of humerus	Olecranon process of ULNA	Radial (C6,7,8)	Plate 4-4, Plate 4-8
Abduction	Deltoid	Anterior: lateral third of clavicle middle: lateral acromion posterior: spine of scapula	Deltoid tuberosity of HUMERUS	Axillary (C5,6)	Plate 4-3
	Supraspinatus	Supraspinous fossa of scapula	Greater tubercle of HUMERUS	Suprascapular (C5,6)	Plate 4-5
Accessory Muscles/Assist Abduction	Biceps brachii (long head)	Supraglenoid tubercle of scapula	Tuberosity of RADIUS	Musculocutaneous (C5,6)	Plate 4-4
	Infraspinatus	Infraspinous fossa of scapula	Greater tubercle of HUMERUS	Suprascapular (C5,6)	Plate 4-5
Adduction	Latissimus dorsi	Thoracolumbar fascia, iliac crest, inferior angle of scapula, spinous processes of T7-S3)	Bicipital groove of HUMERUS	Thoracodorsal, brachial plexus (C6,7,8)	Plate 4-1
	Pectoralis major	Medial clavicle, sternum, costal cartilages of ribs 2–6	Greater tubercle of HUMERUS	Lateral and medial pectoral (C7,C8,T1)	Plate 4-3
	Teres major	Lower third of scapula	Bicipital groove of HUMERUS	Upper and lower scapular (C5,6)	Plate 4-1
Accessory Muscles/Assist Adduction	Biceps brachii (short head)	Coracoid process of scapula	Tuberosity of RADIUS	Musculocutaneous (C5,6)	Plate 4-4
	Coracobrachialis	Coracoid process of scapula	Middle of medial HUMERUS	Musculocutaneous (C5,6,7)	Plate 4-4
	Teres minor	Upper axillary border of scapula	Greater tubercle of HUMERUS	Axillary (C5,6)	Plate 4-5
Lateral Rotation	Deltoid (posterior)	Spine of scapula	Deltoid tuberosity of HUMERUS	Axillary (C5,6)	Plate 4-3
	Infraspinatus	Infraspinous fossa of scapula	Greater tubercle of HUMERUS	Suprascapular (C5,6)	Plate 4-5
	Teres minor	Upper axillary border of scapula	Greater tubercle of HUMERUS	Axillary (C5,6)	Plate 4-5

(continued)

SPECIAL MUSCLE SECTION (*Continued*)

Action Movement	Muscle	Origin	Insertion (bone that is moved is CAPITALIZED)	Nerve (spinal segment nerve numbers)	Plate(s)
SHOULDER *(continued)*					
Medial Rotation	Anterior deltoid	Lateral third of clavicle	Deltoid tuberosity of HUMERUS	Axillary (C5,6)	Plate 4-3
	Latissimus dorsi	Thoracolumbar fascia, iliac crest, inferior angle of scapula, spinous processes of T7-S3)	Bicipital groove of HUMERUS	Thoracodorsal, brachial plexus (C6,7,8)	Plate 4-1
	Pectoralis major	Medial clavicle, sternum, costal cartilages of ribs 2–6	Greater tubercle of HUMERUS	Lateral and medial pectoral (C7,C8,T1)	Plate 4-3
	Subscapularis	Subscapular fossa (anterior surface of scapula)	Lesser tubercle of HUMERUS	Subscapular (C5,6,7)	Plate 4-5
	Teres major	Lower third of scapula	Bicipital groove of HUMERUS	Upper and lower scapular (C5,6)	Plate 4-1
ELBOW					
Flexion	Biceps brachii	Long head: supraglenoid tubercle of scapula Short head: coracoid process of scapula	Tuberosity of RADIUS	Musculocutaneous (C5,6)	Plate 4-6
	Brachialis	Distal half of anterior humerus	Proximal tuberosity of ULNA	Musculocutaneous (C5,6,7)	Plate 4-7
	Brachioradialis	Lateral, distal humerus	Styloid process, distal end of RADIUS	Radial (C5,6)	Plate 4-7
Extension	Triceps brachii	Long head: infraglenoid tubercle of scapula lateral head: upper third of posterior humerus medial head: distal half of humerus	Olecranon process of ULNA	Radial (C6,7,8)	Plate 4-8
Assist Extension/ Accessory Muscles	Anconeus	Lateral epicondyle of humerus	Olecranon process of ULNA	Radial (C7,8)	Plate 4-7
Pronation	Pronator quadratus	Anterior, distal ulna	Anterior, distal RADIUS	Median (C6,7)	Plate 4-6
	Pronator teres	Medial epicondyle of humerus, coronoid process of ulna	Middle of lateral RADIUS	Median (C6,7)	Plate 4-6
Assist pronation/ Accessory muscles	Anconeus	Lateral epicondyle of humerus	Olecranon process of ULNA	Radial (C7,8)	Plate 4-7
	Brachioradialis	Lateral, distal humerus	Styloid process, distal end of RADIUS	Radial (C5,6)	Plate 4-7
Supination	Biceps brachii	Long head: supraglenoid tubercle of scapula Short head: coracoid process of scapula	Tuberosity of RADIUS	Musculocutaneous (C5,6)	Plate 4-6
	Supinator	Lateral epicondyle of humerus; proximal, posterior end of ulna	Anterior, proximal third of RADIUS	Radial (C6)	Plate 4-6

(continued)

SPECIAL MUSCLE SECTION (*Continued*)

Action Movement	Muscle	Origin	Insertion (bone that is moved is CAPITALIZED)	Nerve (spinal segment nerve numbers)	Plate(s)
WRIST					
Flexion	Flexor carpi radialis	Medial epicondyle of humerus	Bases of 2nd and 3rd METACARPALS	Median (C6,7)	Plate 4-6
	Flexor carpi ulnaris	Lateral epicondyle of humerus	Base of 5th METACARPAL	Ulnar (C7,8)	Plate 4-6
	Palmaris longus	Medial epicondyle of humerus	Palmar aponeurosis, anterior flexor retinaculum at PALM	Median (C7,8)	Plate 4-6
Extension	Extensor carpi radialis brevis	Lateral epicondyle of humerus	Base of 3rd METACARPAL	Radial (C7,8)	Plate 4-9
	Extensor carpi radialis longus	Lateral supracondylar ride of humerus	Dorsal 2nd METACARPAL	Radial (C7,8)	Plate 4-9
	Extensor carpi ulnaris	Lateral epicondyle of humerus, posterior border of ulna	Base of 5th METACARPAL	Radial (C7,8)	Plate 4-9
Abduction	Extensor carpi radialis brevis	Lateral epicondyle of humerus	Base of 3rd METACARPAL	Radial (C7,8)	Plate 4-9
	Extensor carpi radialis longus	Lateral supracondylar ride of humerus	Dorsal 2nd METACARPAL	Radial (C7,8)	Plate 4-9
	Flexor carpi radialis	Medial epicondyle of humerus	Bases of 2nd and 3rd METACARPALS	Median (C6,7)	Plate 4-6
Adduction	Extensor carpi ulnaris	Lateral epicondyle of humerus, posterior border of ulna	Base of 5th METACARPAL	Radial (C7,8)	Plate 4-9
	Flexor carpi ulnaris	Lateral epicondyle of humerus	Base of 5th METACARPAL	Ulnar (C7,8)	Plate 4-6
FINGERS					
Flexion	Flexor digitorum profundus				Plate 4-6
	Flexor digitorum superficialis				Plate 4-6
Extension	Extensor digiti minimi				Plate 4-10
	Extensor digitorum				Plate 4-10
	Extensor indices				Plate 4-9
Abduction	Abductor digiti minimi				Plate 4-11
	Abductor pollicis longus				Plate 4-10
	Flexor digiti minimi				Plate 4-11
	Interossei				Plate 4-12
	Lumbricals				Plate 4-12
	Opponens digiti minimi				Not pictured

(continued)

Kinesiology and Body Mechanics

4

SPECIAL MUSCLE SECTION (*Continued*)

Action Movement	Muscle	Origin	Insertion (bone that is moved is CAPITALIZED)	Nerve (spinal segment nerve numbers)	Plate(s)
FINGERS *(continued)*					
Adduction *(continued)*	Dorsal interosseous				Plate 4-12
	Palmar interosseous				Plate 4-12
THUMB					
Adduction	Adductor pollicis				Plate 4-12
Flexion	Flexor pollicis brevis				Plate 4-11
	Flexor pollicis longus				Plate 4-12
Extension	Extensor pollicis brevis				Plate 4-10
	Extensor pollicis longus				Plate 4-9
Opposition	Opponens pollicis				Plate 4-11
Abduction	Abductor pollicis brevis				Plate 4-11
HIP					
Flexion	Gluteus medius	External iliac fossa	Lateral, greater trochanter of FEMUR	Superior gluteal (L5,S1)	Plate 4-13
	Gluteus minimus	External iliac fossa (anterior to gluteus medius)	Greater trochanter of FEMUR	Superior gluteal (L5,S1)	Plate 4-13
	Gracilis	Inferior pubis	Medial, upper TIBIA	Obturator (L2,3,4)	Plate 4-15, 4-16
	Iliacus	Iliac fossa, lateral sacrum	Greater psoas tendon, lesser trochanter of FEMUR	Femoral (L2,3)	Plate 4-14
	Pectineus	Lateral pubis	Lesser trochanter and posterior FEMUR	Obturator/sacral plexus (L2,3,4)	Plate 4-15, 4-16
	Psoas major	T12, L1–4	Lesser trochanter of FEMUR	Lumbar plexus (L1,2,3)	Plate 4-14
	Rectus femoris	Anterior, inferior iliac spine	Patellar tendon into tuberosity of TIBIA	Femoral (L2,3,4)	Plate 4-15
	Sartorius	ASIS	Superior medial TIBIA	Femoral (L2,3,4)	Plate 4-15, 4-16
	Tensor fascia latae	Iliac crest, ASIS	Iliotibial band into TIBIA and FIBULA	Superior gluteal (L4,5,S1)	Plate 4-17
Extension	Adductor magnus	Ramus of pubis, ramus of ischium, ischial tuberosity	Linea aspera and adductor tubercle of FEMUR	Sacral plexus (L4,5,S1,2,3)	Plate 4-15, 4-16
	Biceps femoris	Ischial tuberosity, posterior femoral shaft	Head of FIBULA	Peroneal and sciatic (L4,5,S1,2)	Plate 4-17
	Gluteus maximus	Upper outer ilium, sacrum, coccyx	Iliotibial band, posterior FEMUR	Inferior gluteal (L5,S1,2)	Plate 4-13
	Gluteus minimus	External iliac fossa (anterior to gluteus medius)	Greater trochanter of FEMUR	Superior gluteal (L5,S1)	Plate 4-13

(continued)

SPECIAL MUSCLE SECTION (*Continued*)

Action Movement	Muscle	Origin	Insertion (bone that is moved is CAPITALIZED)	Nerve (spinal segment nerve numbers)	Plate(s)
HIP *(continued)*					
Extension *(continued)*	Semi-membranosus	Lateral ischial tuberosity	Medial condyle of TIBIA	Sciatic (L4,5,S1,2,3)	Plate 4-17
	Semitendinosus	Ischial tuberosity	Upper, medial TIBIA near tibial tuberosity	Sciatic (L4,5,S1,2,3)	Plate 4-17
Abduction	Gemellus inferior	Upper ischial tuberosity	Medial greater trochanter of FEMUR	Sacral plexus (L4,5,S1,2,3)	Plate 4-13
	Gemellus superior	Spine of ischium	Medial greater trochanter of FEMUR	Sacral plexus (L4,5,S1,2,3)	Plate 4-13
	Gluteus maximus	Upper outer ilium, sacrum, coccyx	Iliotibial band, posterior FEMUR	Inferior gluteal (L5,S1,2)	Plate 4-13
	Gluteus medius	External iliac fossa	Lateral, greater trochanter of FEMUR	Superior gluteal (L5,S1)	Plate 4-13
	Gluteus minimus	External iliac fossa (anterior to gluteus medius)	Greater trochanter of FEMUR	Superior gluteal (L5,S1)	Plate 4-13
	Obturator externus	External margin of obturator foramen, obturator membrane	Medial greater trochanter of FEMUR	Sacral plexus (L4,5,S1,2,3)	Plate 4-13
	Obturator internus	Internal margin of obturator foramen, obturator membrane	Medial greater trochanter of FEMUR	Sacral plexus (L4,5,S1,2,3)	Plate 4-17
	Piriformis	Anterior sacrum, ilium near posterior iliac spine	Greater trochanter of FEMUR	Sacral plexus (L4,5,S1,2,3)	Plate 4-13, 4-17
	Sartorius	ASIS	Superior medial TIBIA	Femoral (L2,3,4)	Plate 4-15, 4-16
	Tensor fascia latae	Iliac crest, ASIS	Iliotibial band into TIBIA and FIBULA	Superior gluteal (L4,5,S1)	Plate 4-17
Adduction	Adductor brevis	Medial ramus of pubis	Linea aspera of FEMUR	Sacral plexus (L4,5,S1,2,3)	Plate 4-15, 4-16
	Adductor longus	Anterior pubis	Linea aspera of FEMUR	Sacral plexus (L4,5,S1,2,3)	Plate 4-15, 4-16
	Adductor magnus	Ramus of pubis, ramus of ischium, ischial tuberosity	Linea aspera and adductor tubercle of FEMUR	Sacral plexus (L4,5,S1,2,3)	Plate 4-15, 4-16
	Biceps femoris	Ischial tuberosity, posterior femoral shaft	Head of FIBULA	Peroneal and sciatic (L4,5,S1,2)	Plate 4-17
	Gluteus maximus	Upper outer ilium, sacrum, coccyx	Iliotibial band, posterior FEMUR	Inferior gluteal (L5,S1,2)	Plate 4-13
	Gracilis	Inferior pubis	Medial, upper TIBIA	Obturator (L2,3,4)	Plate 4-15, 4-16
	Iliacus	Iliac fossa, lateral sacrum	Greater psoas tendon, lesser trochanter of FEMUR	Femoral (L2,3)	Plate 4-14
	Pectineus	Lateral pubis	Lesser trochanter and posterior FEMUR	Obturator/sacral plexus (L2,3,4)	Plate 4-15, 4-16
	Psoas major	T12, L1–4	Lesser trochanter of FEMUR	Lumbar plexus (L1,2,3)	Plate 4-14

(continued)

4   Kinesiology and Body Mechanics

SPECIAL MUSCLE SECTION (*Continued*)

Action Movement	Muscle	Origin	Insertion (bone that is moved is CAPITALIZED)	Nerve (spinal segment nerve numbers)	Plate(s)
HIP *(continued)*					
Medial Rotation	Gluteus medius	External iliac fossa	Lateral, greater trochanter of FEMUR	Superior gluteal (L5,S1)	Plate 4-13
	Gluteus minimus	External iliac fossa (anterior to gluteus medius)	Greater trochanter of FEMUR	Superior gluteal (L5,S1)	Plate 4-13
	Tensor fascia latae	Iliac crest, ASIS	Iliotibial band into TIBIA and FIBULA	Superior gluteal (L4,5,S1)	Plate 4-17
Lateral rotation	Adductor brevis	Medial ramus of pubis	Linea aspera of FEMUR	Sacral plexus (L4,5,S1,2,3)	Plate 4-15, 4-16
	Adductor longus	Anterior pubis	Linea aspera of FEMUR	Sacral plexus (L4,5,S1,2,3)	Plate 4-15, 4-16
	Adductor magnus	Ramus of pubis, ramus of ischium, ischial tuberosity	Linea aspera and adductor tubercle of FEMUR	Sacral plexus (L4,5,S1,2,3)	Plate 4-15, 4-16
	Biceps femoris	Ischial tuberosity, posterior femoral shaft	Head of FIBULA	Peroneal and sciatic (L4,5,S1,2)	Plate 4-17
	Gemellus inferior	Upper ischial tuberosity	Medial greater trochanter of FEMUR	Sacral plexus (L4,5,S1,2,3)	Plate 4-13
	Gemellus superior	Spine of ischium	Medial greater trochanter of FEMUR	Sacral plexus (L4,5,S1,2,3)	Plate 4-13
	Gluteus maximus	Upper outer ilium, sacrum, coccyx	Iliotibial band, posterior FEMUR	Inferior gluteal (L5,S1,2)	Plate 4-13
	Obturator externus	External margin of obturator foramen, obturator membrane	Medial greater trochanter of FEMUR	Sacral plexus (L4,5,S1,2,3)	Plate 4-13
	Obturator internus	Internal margin of obturator foramen, obturator membrane	Medial greater trochanter of FEMUR	Sacral plexus (L4,5,S1,2,3)	Plate 4-17
	Piriformis	Anterior sacrum, ilium near posterior iliac spine	Greater trochanter of FEMUR	Sacral plexus (L4,5,S1,2,3)	Plate 4-13, 4-17
	Quadratus femoris	Upper, lateral ischial tuberosity	Posterior greater trochanter of FEMUR	Sacral plexus (L4,5,S1,2,3)	Plate 4-13
KNEE					
Flexion	Biceps femoris	Ischial tuberosity, posterior femoral shaft	Head of FIBULA	Peroneal and sciatic (L4,5,S1,2)	Plate 4-17
	Gastrocnemius	Femoral condyles	Achilles tendon into CALCANEUS	Tibial (S1,2)	Plate 4-20
	Gracilis	Inferior pubis	Medial, upper TIBIA	Obturator (L2,3,4)	Plate 4-15, 4-16
	Popliteus	Lateral femoral condyle	Posterior, medial shaft of TIBIA	Tibial (S1,2)	Plate 4-20
	Sartorius	ASIS	Superior medial TIBIA	Femoral (L2,3,4)	Plate 4-15, 4-16
	Semi-membranosus	Lateral ischial tuberosity	Medial condyle of TIBIA	Sciatic (L4,5,S1,2,3)	Plate 4-17
	Semitendinosus	Ischial tuberosity	Upper, medial TIBIA near tibial tuberosity	Sciatic (L4,5,S1,2,3)	Plate 4-17
Extension	Rectus femoris	Anterior, inferior iliac spine	Patellar tendon into tuberosity	Femoral (L2,3,4)	Plate 4-15

(continued)

SPECIAL MUSCLE SECTION (*Continued*)

Action Movement	Muscle	Origin	Insertion (bone that is moved is CAPITALIZED)	Nerve (spinal segment nerve numbers)	Plate(s)
KNEE (*continued*)					
Extension (*continued*)	Tensor fascia latae	Iliac crest, ASIS	Iliotibial band into TIBIA and FIBULA	Superior gluteal (L4,5,S1)	Plate 4-17
	Vastus intermedius	Anterior, upper 2/3 of femur	Patellar tendon into TIBIA	Femoral (L2,3,4)	Plate 4-15
	Vastus lateralis	Lateral, upper femur	Patellar tendon into TIBIA	Femoral (L2,3,4)	Plate 4-15
	Vastus medialis	Medial femur	Patellar tendon into TIBIA	Femoral (L2,3,4)	Plate 4-15
Medial rotation	Gracilis	Inferior pubis	Medial, upper TIBIA	Obturator (L2,3,4)	Plate 4-15, 4-16
	Popliteus	Lateral femoral condyle	Posterior, medial shaft of TIBIA	Tibial (S1,2)	Plate 4-20
	Sartorius	ASIS	Superior medial TIBIA	Femoral (L2,3,4)	Plate 4-15,4-16
	Semi-membranosus	Lateral ischial tuberosity	Medial condyle of TIBIA	Sciatic (L4,5,S1,2,3)	Plate 4-17
	Semitendinosus	Ischial tuberosity	Upper, medial TIBIA near tibial tuberosity	Sciatic (L4,5,S1,2,3)	Plate 4-17
Lateral rotation	Biceps femoris	Ischial tuberosity, posterior femoral shaft	Head of FIBULA	Peroneal and sciatic (L4,5,S1,2)	Plate 4-17
	Gluteus maximus	Upper outer ilium, sacrum, coccyx	Iliotibial band, posterior FEMUR	Inferior gluteal (L5,S1,2)	Plate 4-13
	Tensor fascia latae	Iliac crest, ASIS	Iliotibial band into TIBIA and FIBULA	Superior gluteal (L4,5,S1)	Plate 4-17
ANKLE/ FOOT					
Dorsiflexion	Extensor digitorum longus	Medial, upper 3/4 of fibula and lateral condyle of tibia	Dorsal aponeurosis of middle and distal PHALANGES	Deep peroneal (L5,S1)	Plate 4-19
	Extensor hallucis longus	Middle of fibula	Dorsal distal PHALANX of big toe	Deep peroneal (L5,S1)	Plate 4-18
	Peroneus tertius	Inferior fibula	METATARSAL V	Peroneal (L4,5,S1,2)	Plate 4-19
	Tibialis anterior	Lateral condyle and shaft of tibia	Base of METATARSAL I	Deep peroneal (L4,5)	Plate 4-18
Plantarflexion	Flexor digitorum longus	Posterior, middle half of tibia	Distal PHALANGES II-V	Tibial (S2,3)	Plate 4-19, 4-20
	Flexor hallucis longus	Lower, posterior 2/3 of fibula	Bottom of distal PHALANX I	Tibial (S2,3)	Plate 4-19, 4-20
	Gastrocnemius	Femoral condyles	Achilles tendon into CALCANEUS	Tibial (S1,2)	Plate 4-20
	Peroneus brevis	Inferior, lateral fibula	Base of METATARSAL V	Peroneal (L4,5,S1,2)	Plate 4-21
	Peroneus longus	Lateral head of fibula	Base of METATARSAL I	Peroneal (L4,5,S1,2)	Plate 4-21
	Soleus	Proximal tibia and fibula	Achilles tendon into CALCANEUS	Peroneal (L4,5,S1,2,3)	Plate 4-20
	Tibialis posterior	Tibia and fibula	TARSALS and METATARSALS	Tibial (L4,5,S1,2,3)	Plate 4-20
Eversion (pronation / Abduction)	Extensor digitorum longus	Medial, upper 3/4 of fibula and lateral condyle of tibia	Dorsal aponeurosis of middle and distal PHALANGES	Deep peroneal (L5,S1)	Plate 4-19
	Peroneus brevis	Inferior, lateral fibula	Base of METATARSAL V	Peroneal (L4,5,S1,2)	Plate 4-21

(continued)

SPECIAL MUSCLE SECTION (*Continued*)

Action Movement	Muscle	Origin	Insertion (bone that is moved is CAPITALIZED)	Nerve (spinal segment nerve numbers)	Plate(s)
ANKLE/ FOOT *(continued)*					
Eversion (pronation / Abduction) *(continued)*	Peroneus longus	Lateral head of fibula	Base of METATARSAL I	Peroneal (L4,5,S1,2)	Plate 4-21
	Peroneus tertius	Inferior fibula	METATARSAL V	Peroneal (L4,5,S1,2)	Plate 4-21
Inversion (suppination / adduction)	Extensor hallucis longus	Middle of fibula	Dorsal distal PHALANX of big toe	Deep peroneal (L5,S1)	Plate 4-18
	Flexor digitorum longus	Posterior, middle half of tibia	Distal PHALANGES II-V	Tibial (S2,3)	Plate 4-19
	Flexor hallucis longus	Lower, posterior 2/3 of fibula	Bottom of distal PHALANX I	Tibial (S2,3)	Plate 4-19
	Gastrocnemius	Femoral condyles	Achilles tendon into CALCANEUS	Tibial (S1,2)	Plate 4-20
	Soleus	Proximal tibia and fibula	Achilles tendon into CALCANEUS	Peroneal (L4,5,S1,2,3)	Plate 4-20
	Tibialis anterior	Lateral condyle and shaft of tibia	Base of METATARSAL I	Deep peroneal (L4,5)	Plate 4-18
	Tibialis posterior	Tibia and fibula	TARSALS and METATARSALS	Tibial (L4,5,S1,2,3)	Plate 4-20
	Foot muscles, dorsal view				Plate 4-22
	Foot muscles, plantar view				Plate 4-23
SPINE/THORAX					
Flexion	External obliques	Inferior ribs 5–12	Anterior ILIAC crest, linea alba	Intercostal (T7–12, L1)	Plate 4-24
	Internal obliques	Anterior iliac crest	Inferior RIBS 10–12, linea alba, PUBIS	Intercostal (T7–12, L1)	Plate 4-24
	Rectus abdominis	Pubic crest and pubic symphysis	Costal cartilages (RIBS), xiphoid process of STERNUM	Intercostal (T5–12)	Plate 4-24
Extension	Erector spinae group (iliocostalis, longissimus, spinalis)	Large group, multiple origins, from thoracolumbar aponeurosis, ribs, spinous processes of vertebrae	Insertions are superior to the origins, ranging from the posterior RIBS to the mastoid process of the TEMPORAL bone and OCCIPUT	Spinal nerves (T1–12, L1–5, S1–3)	Plate 4-27
	Multifidi	Articular processes C4–C7, transverse processes T1–12, posterior sacrum, posterior iliac spine	Spine of VERTEBRA superior to origin, from one to three vertebrae higher	All spinal nerves (C1-S4)	Plate 4-27
	Rotatores	Transverse processes C1-L5	Lamina of VERTEBRA directly superior to origin	Spinal nerves (C1-S4)	Plate 4-27
Lateral flexion / Hip elevation	External obliques	Inferior ribs 5–12	Anterior ILIAC crest, linea alba	Intercostal (T7–12, L1)	Plate 4-24
	Internal obliques	Anterior iliac crest	Inferior RIBS 10–12, linea alba, PUBIS	Intercostal (T7–12, L1)	Plate 4-24
	Quadratus lumborum	Thoracolumbar aponeurosis, iliac crest	Twelfth RIB, VERTEBRAE L1–4	Lumbar plexus (T12,L1,2,3)	Plate 4-24

(continued)

SPECIAL MUSCLE SECTION (*Continued*)

Action Movement	Muscle	Origin	Insertion (bone that is moved is CAPITALIZED)	Nerve (spinal segment nerve numbers)	Plate(s)
SPINE/THORAX *(continued)*					
Rotation	External obliques	Inferior ribs 5–12	Anterior ILIAC crest, linea alba	Intercostal (T7–12, L1)	Plate 4-24
	Internal obliques	Anterior iliac crest	Inferior RIBS 10–12, linea alba, PUBIS	Intercostal (T7–12, L1)	Plate 4-24
	Multifidi	Articular processes C4–C7, transverse processes T1–12, posterior sacrum, posterior iliac spine	Spine of VERTEBRA superior to origin, from one to three vertebrae higher	All spinal nerves (C1–S4)	Plate 4-27
	Rotatores	Transverse processes C1-L5	Lamina of VERTEBRA directly superior to origin	Spinal nerves (C1–S4)	Plate 4-27
MUSCLES OF RESPIRATION					
Exhalation	External obliques	Inferior ribs 5–12	Anterior ILIAC crest, linea alba	Intercostal (T7–12, L1)	Plate 4-24
	Internal intercostals (posterior)	Lower border of ribs, costal cartilage	Upper border of RIB and costal cartilage just inferior to origin	Intercostal (T1–12)	Plate 4-26
	Internal obliques	Anterior iliac crest	Inferior RIBS 10–12, linea alba, PUBIS	Intercostal (T7–12, L1)	Plate 4-24
	Rectus abdominis	Pubic crest and pubic symphysis	Costal cartilages (RIBS), xiphoid process of STERNUM	Intercostal (T5–12)	Plate 4-24
	Transversus abdominis	Thoracolumbar aponeurosis, iliac crest	Abdominal aponeurosis, pubis, linea alba	Intercostal (T7–12,L1)	Plate 4-24
Inhalation	Diaphragm	Ribs 7–12, costal cartilages, xiphoid process, L1–3	Central tendon of DIAPHRAGM	Phrenic (C3,4,5)	Plate 4-26
	External intercostals	Lower border of ribs	Upper border of RIB just inferior to origin	Intercostal (T1–12)	Plate 4-26
	Internal intercostals (anterior)	Lower border of ribs, costal cartilage	Upper border of RIB and costal cartilage just inferior to origin	Intercostal (T1–12)	Plate 4-26
	Scalenus anterior	Transverse processes C2–5	First RIB	Cervical plexus (C1–7, T1)	Plate 4-28
	Scalenus medius	Transverse processes of C1–6	First RIB	Cervical plexus (C1–7,T1)	Plate 4-28
	Scalenus posterior	Transverse processes of C4–6	Second RIB	Cervical plexus (C1–7,T1)	Plate 4-28
NECK					
Extension	Erector spinae group (iliocostalis, longissimus, spinalis)	Large group, multiple origins, from thoracolumbar aponeurosis, ribs, spinous processes of vertebrae	Insertions are superior to the origins, ranging from the posterior RIBS to the mastoid process of the TEMPORAL bone and OCCIPUT	Spinal nerves (T1–12, L1–5, S1–3)	Plate 4-27
	Levator scapulae	Transverse processes C1–4	Vertebral border of superior SCAPULA	Scapular (C4,5)	Plate 4-34

(continued)

SPECIAL MUSCLE SECTION (*Continued*)

Action Movement	Muscle	Origin	Insertion (bone that is moved is CAPITALIZED)	Nerve (spinal segment nerve numbers)	Plate(s)
NECK *(continued)*					
Extension *(continued)*	Multifidi	Articular processes C4–C7, transverse processes T1–12, posterior sacrum, posterior iliac spine	Spine of VERTEBRA superior to origin, from one to three vertebrae higher	All spinal nerves (C1-S4)	Plate 4-34
	Rotatores	Transverse processes C1-L5	Lamina of VERTEBRA directly superior to origin	Spinal nerves (C1-S4)	Plate 4-34
	Semispinalis	Transverse processes C4-T6	OCCIPUT, spinous processes VERTEBRAE C2–6	Cervical, thoracic (C4,5,6)	Plate 4-33
	Splenius capitis	Spinous processes of C7-T3	Mastoid process of TEMPORAL bone	Cervical (C3–5)	Plate 4-33
	Splenius cervicis	Spinous processes T3–6	Transverse processes of VERTEBRAE C2–4	Cervical (C4–6)	Plate 4-33
	Trapezius (upper)	Occiput, ligamentum nuchae	Lateral end of clavicle, lateral spine of SCAPULA	Accessory (C2,3,4)	Plate 4-33
Flexion	Scalenes	Transverse processes C2–7	First and second RIBS	Cervical plexus (C1–7, T1)	Plate 4-28
	Sternocleido-mastoid	Sternal head, medial clavicle	Mastoid process of TEMOPORAL bone, OCCIPUT	Accessory (C2,3)	Plate 4-30, 4-31
Lateral flexion	Levator scapulae	Transverse processes C1–4	Vertebral border of superior SCAPULA	Scapular (C4,5)	Plate 4-34
	Sternocleido-mastoid	Sternal head, medial clavicle	Mastoid process of TEMPORAL bone, OCCIPUT	Accessory (C2,3)	Plate 4-30, 4-31
	Trapezius (upper)	Occiput, ligamentum nuchae	Lateral end of clavicle, lateral spine of SCAPULA	Accessory (C2,3,4)	Plate 4-33
Rotation	Levator scapulae	Transverse processes C1–4	Vertebral border of superior SCAPULA	Scapular (C4,5)	Plate 4-34
	Multifidi	Articular processes C4–C7, transverse processes T1–12, posterior sacrum, posterior iliac spine	Spine of VERTEBRA superior to origin, from one to three vertebrae higher	All spinal nerves (C1-S4)	Plate 4-34
	Rotatores	Transverse processes C1-L5	Lamina of VERTEBRA directly superior to origin	Spinal nerves (C1-S4)	Plate 4-34
	Sternocleido-mastoid	Sternal head, medial clavicle	Mastoid process of TEMOPORAL bone, OCCIPUT	Accessory (C2,3)	Plate 4-30, 4-31
	Trapezius (upper)	Occiput, ligamentum nuchae	Lateral end of clavicle, lateral spine of SCAPULA	Accessory (C2,3,4)	Plate 4-33
	Deep neck muscles				Plate 4-32
TEMPOROMANDIBULAR JOINT					
Elevation (closes the jaw)	Temporalis	Lateral temporal bone	Coronoid process and anterior ramus of MANDIBLE	Trigeminal (cranial V)	Plate 4-29
	Masseter	Zygomatic arch	Angle and lateral surface of MANDIBLE	Trigeminal (cranial V)	Plate 4-29
	Medial pterygoid	Medial pterygoid plate	TMJ capsule, condyle of MANDIBLE	Trigeminal (cranial V)	Plate 4-29

(continued)

SPECIAL MUSCLE SECTION (*Continued*)

Action Movement	Muscle	Origin	Insertion (bone that is moved is CAPITALIZED)	Nerve (spinal segment nerve numbers)	Plate(s)
TEMPOROMANDIBULAR JOINT *(continued)*					
Depression (opens the jaw)	Platysma	Fascia of superior thorax	Lower border of MANDIBLE, fascia around chin	Facial (cranial VII)	Plate 4-31
	Lateral pterygoid	Lateral pterygoid plate	Angle of MANDIBLE	Trigeminal (cranial V)	Plate 4-29
Accessory muscles/Assist depression	Suprahyoids (digastric, genio-hyoid, myohyoid, stylohyoid)	Inferior mandible, mas-toid process, styloid pro-cess of temporal bone	HYOID bone	Facial (cranial VII)	Plate 4-35
Protraction	Lateral pterygoid	Lateral pterygoid plate	Angle of MANDIBLE	Trigeminal (cranial V)	Plate 4-29
	Medial pterygoid	Medial pterygoid plate	TMJ capsule, condyle of MANDIBLE	Trigeminal (cranial V)	Plate 4-29
	Masseter	Zygomatic arch	Angle and lateral surface of MANDIBLE	Trigeminal (cranial V)	Plate 4-29
Retraction	Temporalis	Lateral temporal bone	Coronoid process and anterior ramus of MANDIBLE	Trigeminal (cranial V)	Plate 4-29
Lateral deviation	Masseter	Zygomatic arch	Angle and lateral surface of MANDIBLE	Trigeminal (cranial V)	Plate 4-29
	Lateral pterygoid	Lateral pterygoid plate	Angle of MANDIBLE	Trigeminal (cranial V)	Plate 4-29

Kinesiology and Body Mechanics

4

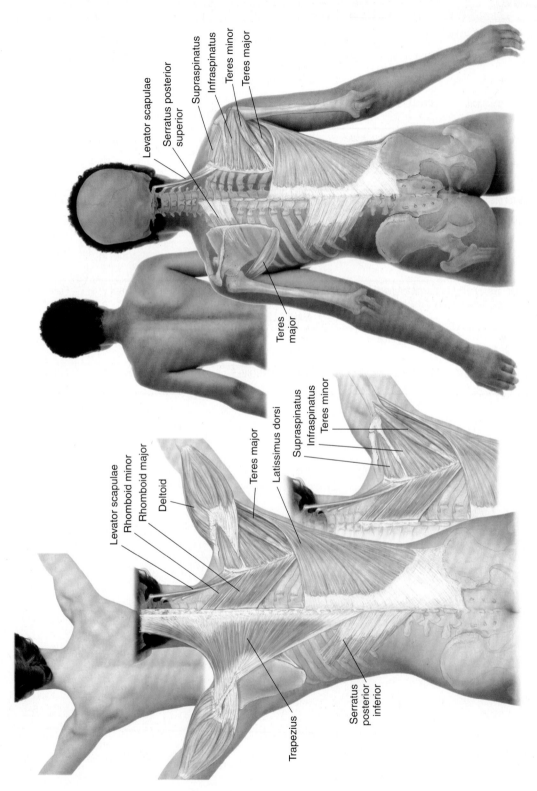

Plate 4-1

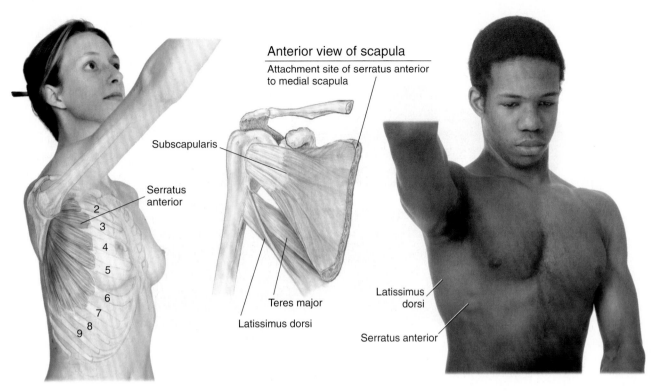

Anterior view of scapula

Attachment site of serratus anterior to medial scapula

Subscapularis

Serratus anterior

2
3
4
5
6
7
8
9

Teres major

Latissimus dorsi

Latissimus dorsi

Serratus anterior

Plate 4-2

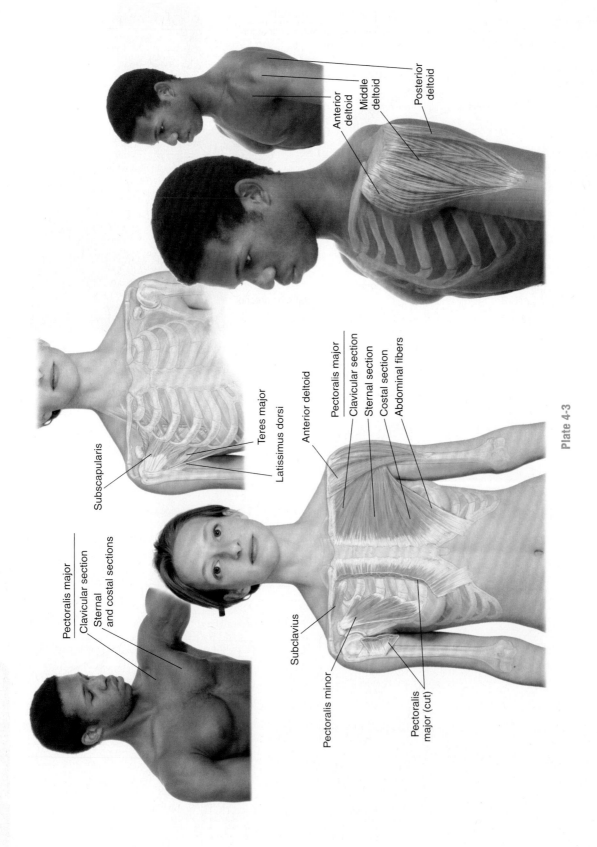

Anterior deltoid

Middle deltoid

Posterior deltoid

Subscapularis

Teres major

Latissimus dorsi

Anterior deltoid

Pectoralis major
Clavicular section
Sternal section
Costal section
Abdominal fibers

Pectoralis major
Clavicular section
Sternal and costal sections

Subclavius

Pectoralis minor

Pectoralis major (cut)

Plate 4-3

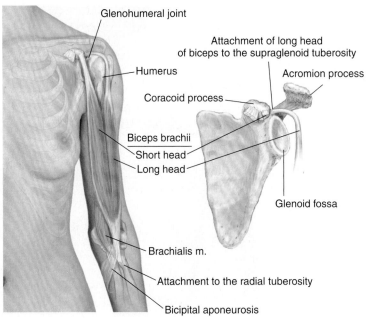

Glenohumeral joint

Attachment of long head
of biceps to the supraglenoid tuberosity

Humerus

Acromion process

Coracoid process

Biceps brachii

Short head

Long head

Glenoid fossa

Brachialis m.

Attachment to the radial tuberosity

Bicipital aponeurosis

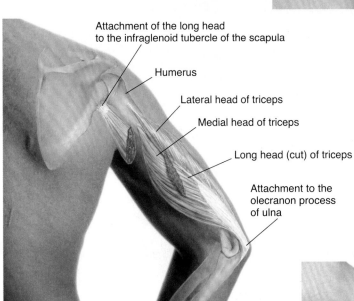

Attachment of the long head
to the infraglenoid tubercle of the scapula

Humerus

Lateral head of triceps

Medial head of triceps

Long head (cut) of triceps

Attachment to the
olecranon process
of ulna

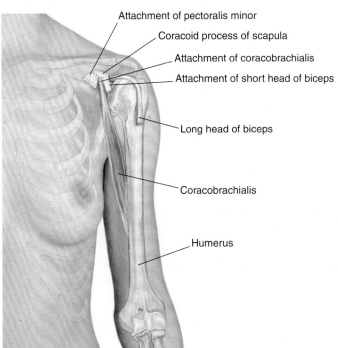

Attachment of pectoralis minor

Coracoid process of scapula

Attachment of coracobrachialis

Attachment of short head of biceps

Long head of biceps

Coracobrachialis

Humerus

Plate 4-4

Kinesiology and Body Mechanics

4

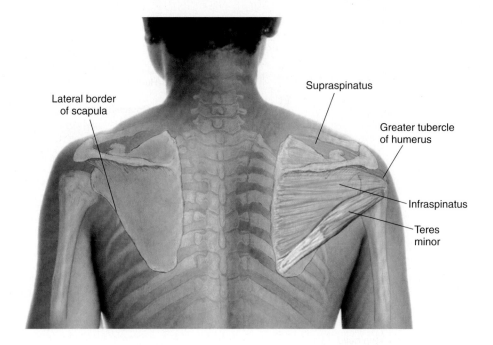

Lateral border of scapula

Supraspinatus

Greater tubercle of humerus

Infraspinatus

Teres minor

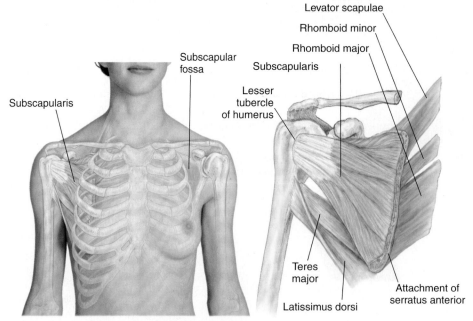

Subscapularis

Subscapular fossa

Lesser tubercle of humerus

Subscapularis

Levator scapulae

Rhomboid minor

Rhomboid major

Teres major

Latissimus dorsi

Attachment of serratus anterior

Plate 4-5

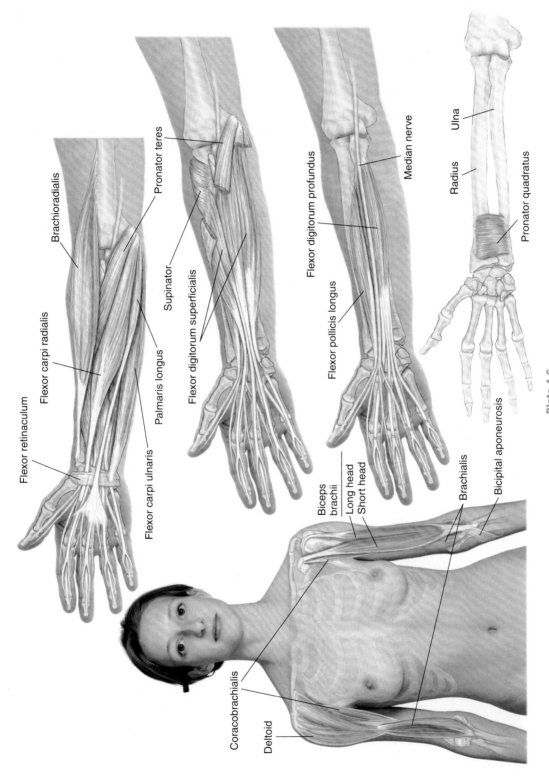

Brachioradialis

Pronator teres

Flexor carpi radialis

Supinator

Flexor retinaculum

Palmaris longus

Flexor digitorum superficialis

Flexor carpi ulnaris

Flexor digitorum profundus

Median nerve

Flexor pollicis longus

Ulna

Radius

Pronator quadratus

Plate 4-6

Biceps brachii — Long head, Short head

Brachialis

Bicipital aponeurosis

Coracobrachialis

Deltoid

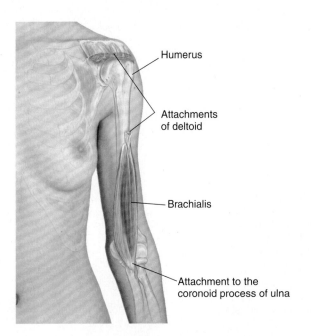

Humerus

Attachments
of deltoid

Brachialis

Attachment to the
coronoid process of ulna

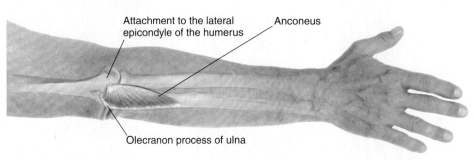

Attachment to the lateral
epicondyle of the humerus

Anconeus

Olecranon process of ulna

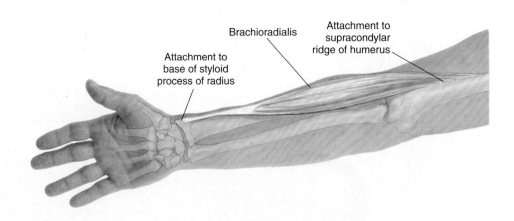

Brachioradialis

Attachment to
supracondylar
ridge of humerus

Attachment to
base of styloid
process of radius

Plate 4-7

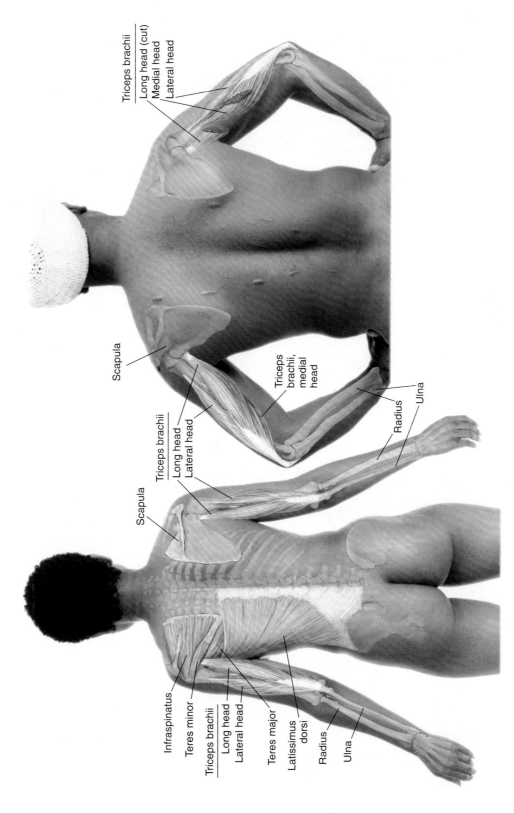

Triceps brachii (cut)
Long head
Medial head
Lateral head

Scapula

Triceps brachii, medial head

Triceps brachii
Long head
Lateral head

Scapula

Radius

Ulna

Infraspinatus

Teres minor

Triceps brachii
Long head
Lateral head

Teres major

Latissimus dorsi

Radius

Ulna

Plate 4-8

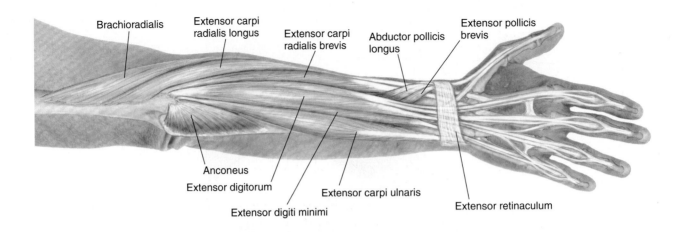

Brachioradialis

Extensor carpi radialis longus

Extensor carpi radialis brevis

Abductor pollicis longus

Extensor pollicis brevis

Anconeus

Extensor digitorum

Extensor digiti minimi

Extensor carpi ulnaris

Extensor retinaculum

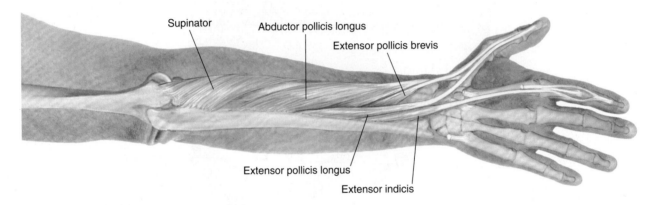

Supinator

Abductor pollicis longus

Extensor pollicis brevis

Extensor pollicis longus

Extensor indicis

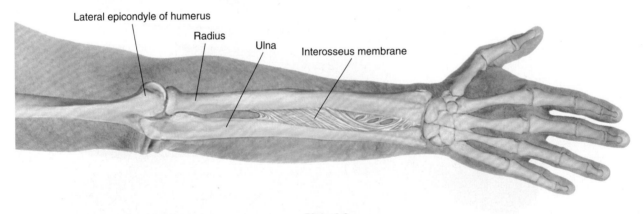

Lateral epicondyle of humerus

Radius

Ulna

Interosseus membrane

Plate 4-9

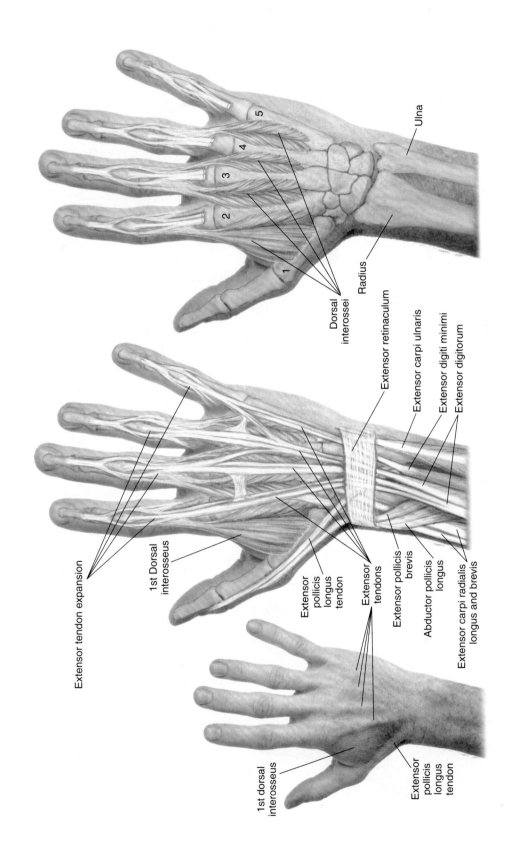

Ulna

Radius

Dorsal interossei

Extensor retinaculum

Extensor carpi ulnaris

Extensor digiti minimi

Extensor digitorum

Extensor tendon expansion

1st Dorsal interosseus

Extensor pollicis longus tendon

Extensor tendons

Extensor pollicis brevis

Abductor pollicis longus

Extensor carpi radialis longus and brevis

1st dorsal interosseus

Extensor pollicis longus tendon

Plate 4-10

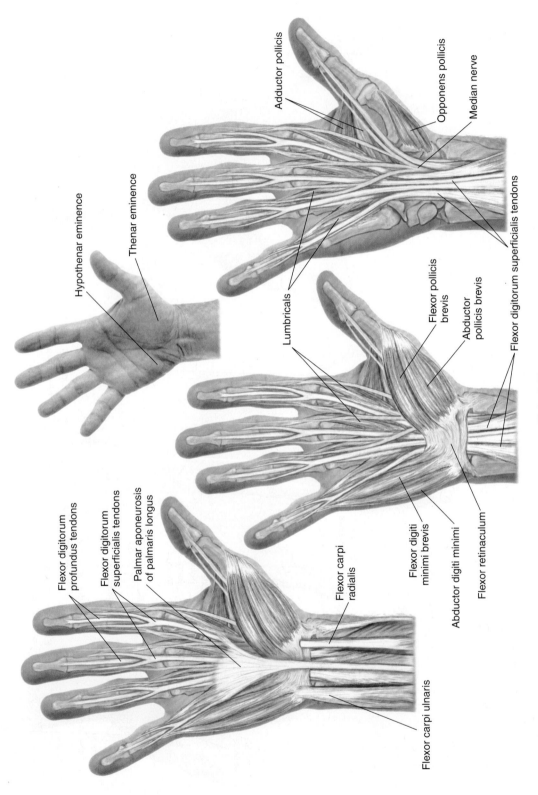

Adductor pollicis

Opponens pollicis

Median nerve

Hypothenar eminence

Thenar eminence

Lumbricals

Flexor pollicis brevis

Abductor pollicis brevis

Flexor digitorum superficialis tendons

Flexor digitorum profundus tendons

Flexor digitorum superficialis tendons

Palmar aponeurosis of palmaris longus

Flexor carpi radialis

Flexor digiti minimi brevis

Abductor digiti minimi

Flexor retinaculum

Flexor carpi ulnaris

Plate 4-11

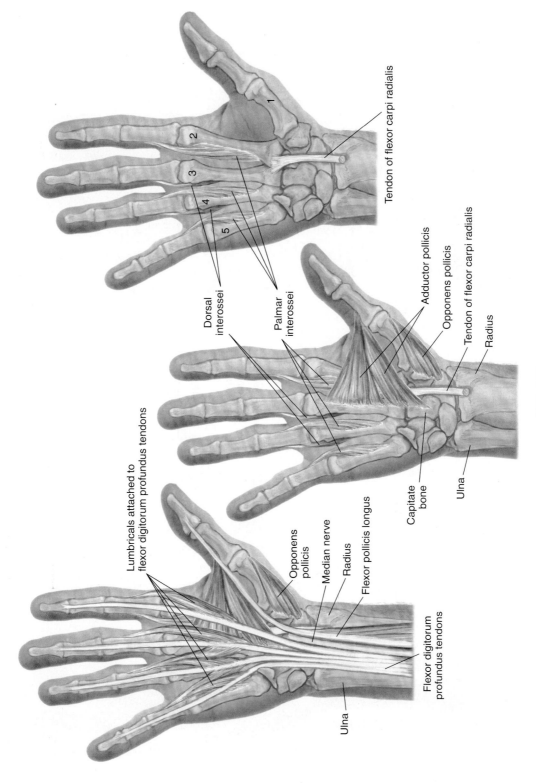

Tendon of flexor carpi radialis

Dorsal interossei

Palmar interossei

Adductor pollicis

Opponens pollicis

Tendon of flexor carpi radialis

Radius

Capitate bone

Ulna

Lumbricals attached to flexor digitorum profundus tendons

Opponens pollicis

Median nerve

Radius

Flexor pollicis longus

Flexor digitorum profundus tendons

Ulna

Plate 4-12

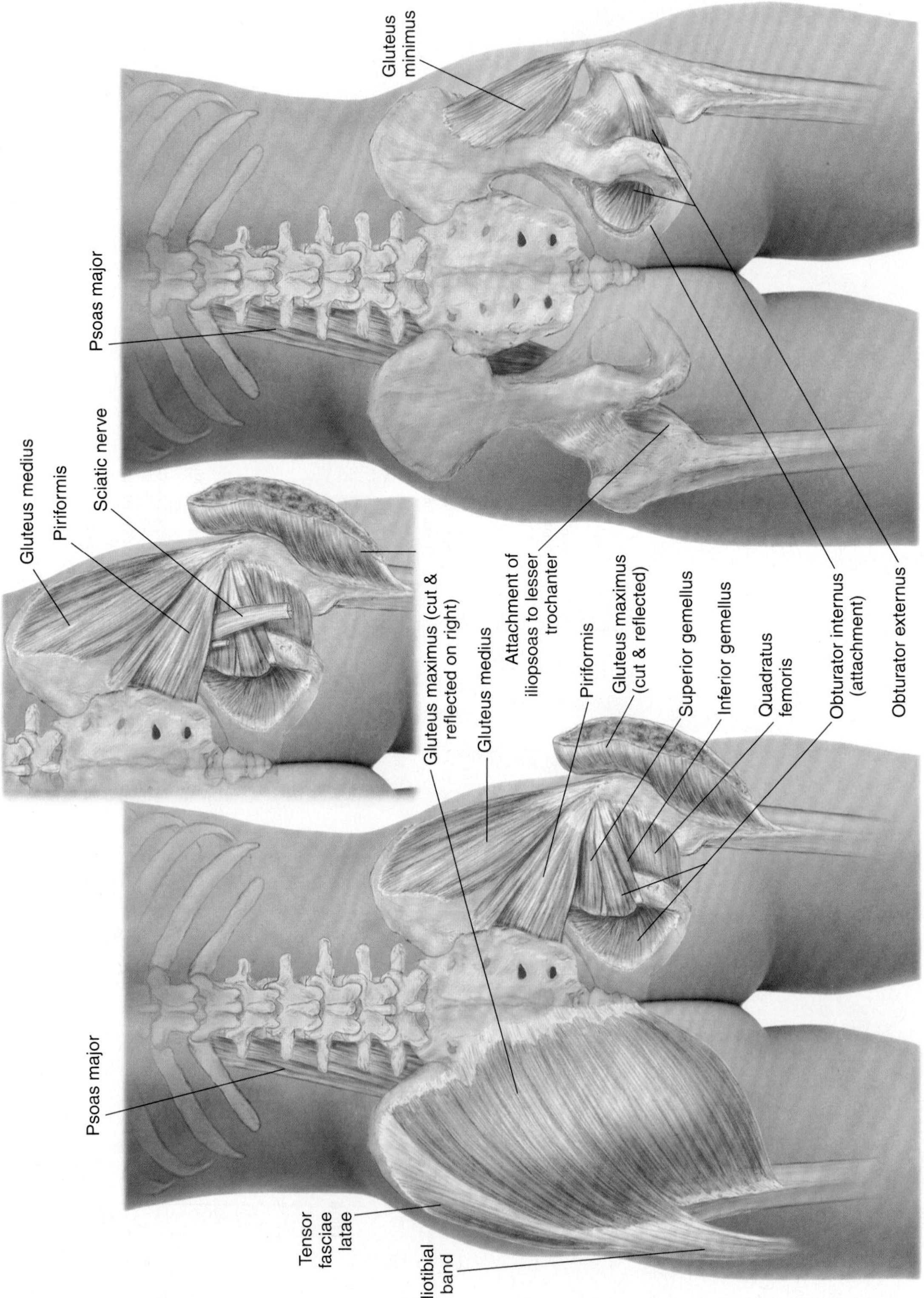

Gluteus minimus

Psoas major

Gluteus medius
Piriformis
Sciatic nerve

Gluteus maximus (cut & reflected on right)
Gluteus medius
Attachment of iliopsoas to lesser trochanter
Piriformis
Gluteus maximus (cut & reflected)
Superior gemellus
Inferior gemellus
Quadratus femoris
Obturator internus (attachment)
Obturator externus

Psoas major

Tensor fasciae latae

Iliotibial band

Plate 4-13

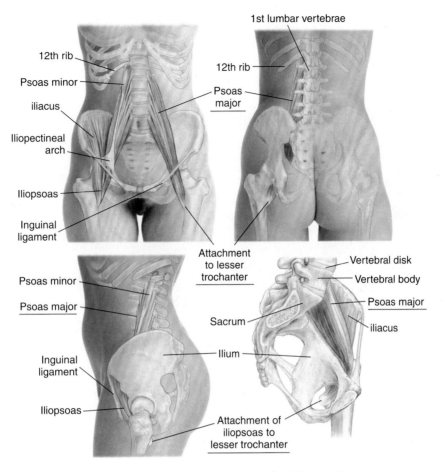

1st lumbar vertebrae

12th rib

Psoas minor

iliacus

Iliopectineal arch

Iliopsoas

Inguinal ligament

12th rib

Psoas major

Attachment to lesser trochanter

Psoas minor

Psoas major

Inguinal ligament

Iliopsoas

Vertebral disk

Vertebral body

Psoas major

iliacus

Sacrum

Ilium

Attachment of iliopsoas to lesser trochanter

Sagittal section

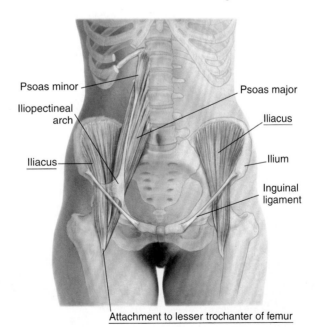

Psoas minor

Iliopectineal arch

Iliacus

Psoas major

Iliacus

Ilium

Inguinal ligament

Attachment to lesser trochanter of femur

Plate 4-14

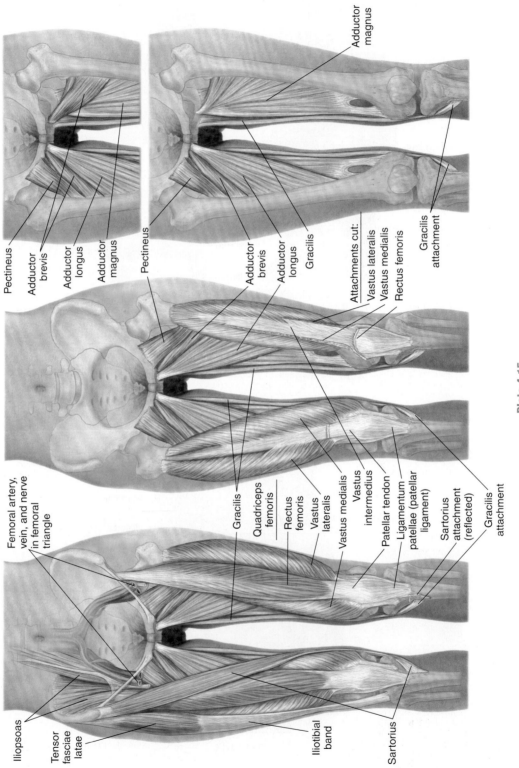

Pectineus

Adductor brevis

Adductor longus

Adductor magnus

Pectineus

Adductor brevis

Adductor longus

Gracilis

Attachments cut:
Vastus lateralis
Vastus medialis
Rectus femoris

Gracilis attachment

Adductor magnus

Femoral artery, vein, and nerve in femoral triangle

Gracilis

Quadriceps femoris
Rectus femoris
Vastus lateralis

Vastus medialis

Vastus intermedius

Patellar tendon

Ligamentum patellae (patellar ligament)

Sartorius attachment (reflected)

Gracilis attachment

Iliopsoas

Tensor fasciae latae

Iliotibial band

Sartorius

Plate 4-15

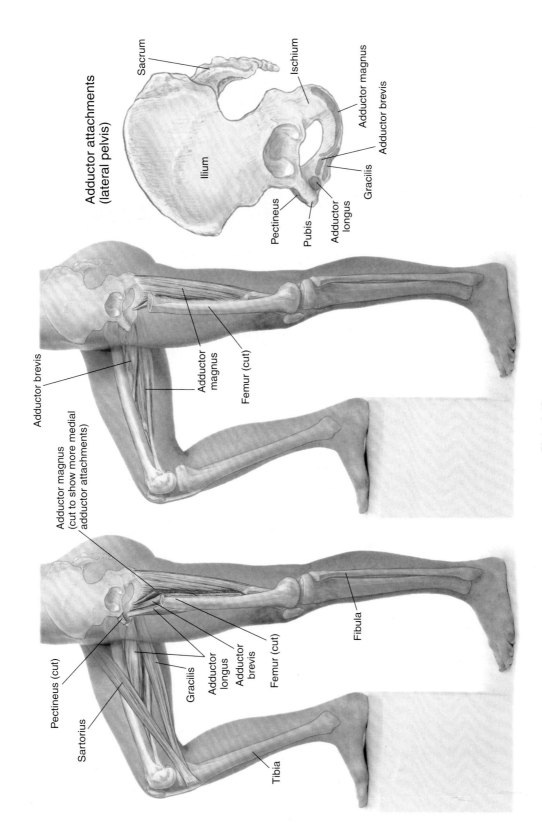

Adductor attachments
(lateral pelvis)

Sacrum

Ischium

Adductor magnus

Adductor brevis

Adductor longus

Gracilis

Pubis

Pectineus

Ilium

Adductor brevis

Adductor magnus

Femur (cut)

Adductor magnus
(cut to show more medial
adductor attachments)

Pectineus (cut)

Sartorius

Gracilis

Adductor longus

Adductor brevis

Femur (cut)

Fibula

Tibia

Plate 4-16

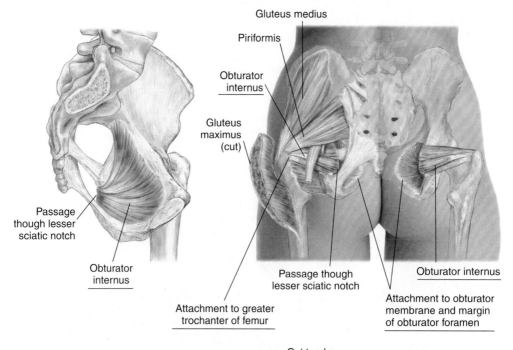

Gluteus medius

Piriformis

Obturator internus

Gluteus maximus (cut)

Passage though lesser sciatic notch

Obturator internus

Passage though lesser sciatic notch

Obturator internus

Attachment to greater trochanter of femur

Attachment to obturator membrane and margin of obturator foramen

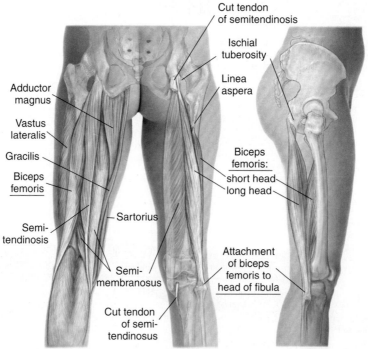

Cut tendon of semitendinosis

Ischial tuberosity

Linea aspera

Adductor magnus

Vastus lateralis

Gracilis

Biceps femoris

Semi-tendinosis

Sartorius

Semi-membranosus

Biceps femoris:
short head
long head

Attachment of biceps femoris to head of fibula

Cut tendon of semi-tendinosus

Plate 4-17

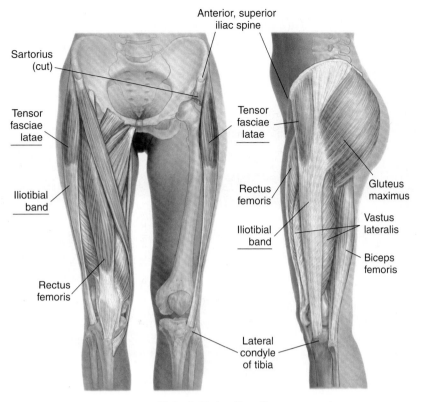

Plate 4-17 *(continued)*

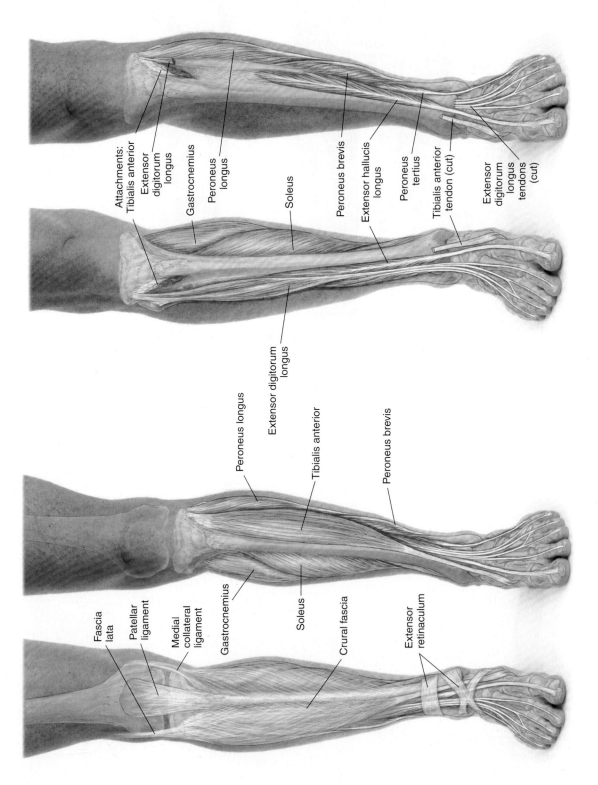

Attachments:
Tibialis anterior
Extensor digitorum longus
Gastrocnemius
Peroneus longus
Soleus
Peroneus brevis
Extensor hallucis longus
Peroneus tertius
Tibialis anterior tendon (cut)
Extensor digitorum longus tendons (cut)

Peroneus longus
Extensor digitorum longus
Tibialis anterior
Peroneus brevis

Fascia lata
Patellar ligament
Medial collateral ligament
Gastrocnemius
Soleus
Crural fascia
Extensor retinaculum

Plate 4-18

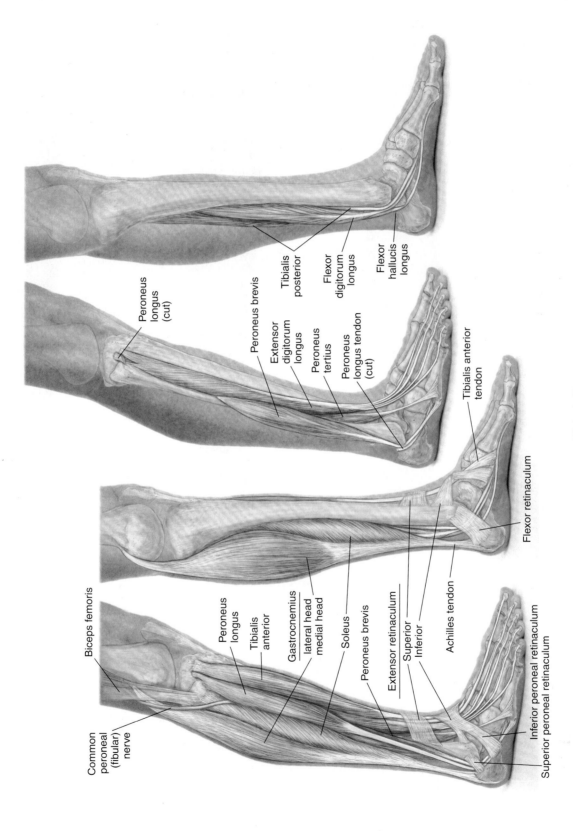

Peroneus longus (cut)

Peroneus brevis

Extensor digitorum longus

Peroneus tertius

Peroneus longus tendon (cut)

Tibialis posterior

Flexor digitorum longus

Flexor hallucis longus

Tibialis anterior tendon

Flexor retinaculum

Biceps femoris

Common peroneal (fibular) nerve

Peroneus longus

Tibialis anterior

Gastrocnemius
lateral head
medial head

Soleus

Peroneus brevis

Extensor retinaculum
Superior
Inferior

Achilles tendon

Inferior peroneal retinaculum

Superior peroneal retinaculum

Plate 4-19

4   Kinesiology and Body Mechanics

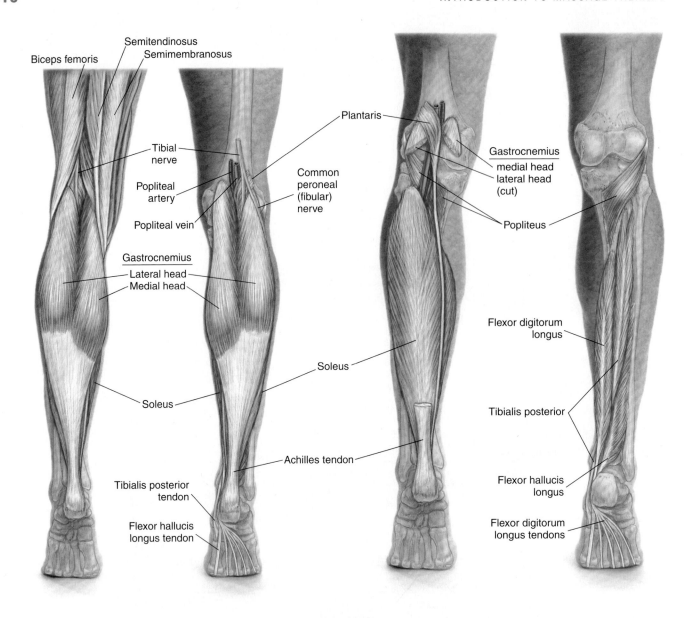

Biceps femoris
Semitendinosus
Semimembranosus
Tibial nerve
Popliteal artery
Popliteal vein
Gastrocnemius
Lateral head
Medial head
Soleus
Tibialis posterior tendon
Flexor hallucis longus tendon
Common peroneal (fibular) nerve
Soleus
Achilles tendon
Plantaris
Gastrocnemius
medial head
lateral head (cut)
Popliteus
Flexor digitorum longus
Tibialis posterior
Flexor hallucis longus
Flexor digitorum longus tendons

Plate 4-20

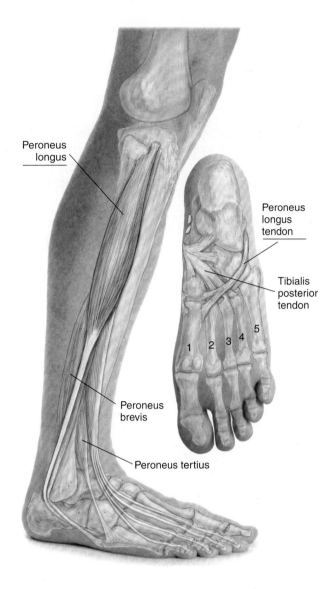

Peroneus
longus

Peroneus
longus
tendon

Tibialis
posterior
tendon

1 2 3 4 5

Peroneus
brevis

Peroneus tertius

Plate 4-21

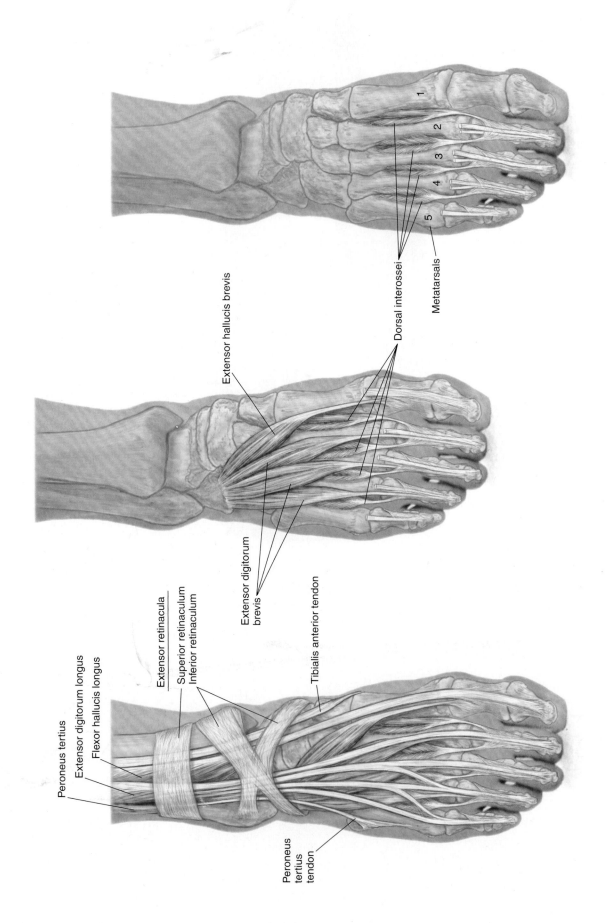

Extensor hallucis brevis

Dorsal interossei

Metatarsals

1
2
3
4
5

Extensor digitorum brevis

Peroneus tertius
Extensor digitorum longus
Flexor hallucis longus

Extensor retinacula
Superior retinaculum
Inferior retinaculum

Tibialis anterior tendon

Peroneus tertius tendon

Plate 4-22

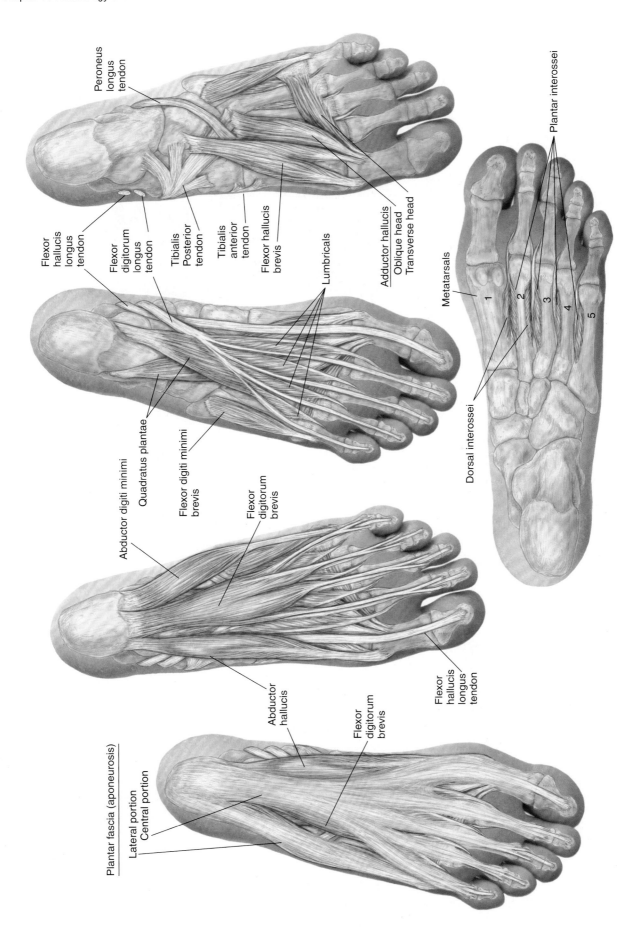

Peroneus longus tendon

Flexor hallucis longus tendon

Flexor digitorum longus tendon

Tibialis Posterior tendon

Tibialis anterior tendon

Flexor hallucis brevis

Lumbricals

Adductor hallucis
Oblique head
Transverse head

Plantar interossei

Metatarsals

1
2
3
4
5

Dorsal interossei

Abductor digiti minimi

Quadratus plantae

Flexor digiti minimi brevis

Flexor digitorum brevis

Abductor hallucis

Flexor digitorum brevis

Flexor hallucis longus tendon

Plantar fascia (aponeurosis)
Lateral portion
Central portion

Abductor hallucis

Flexor digitorum brevis

Plate 4-23

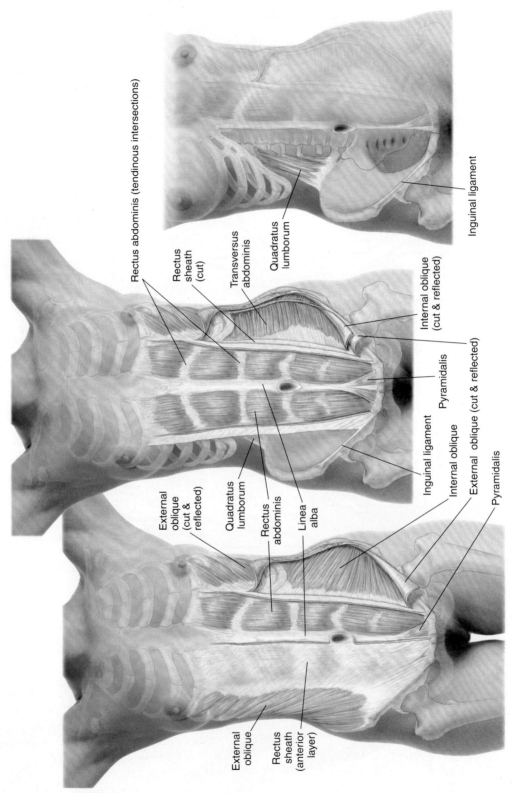

Rectus abdominis (tendinous intersections)

Rectus sheath (cut)

Transversus abdominis

Quadratus lumborum

Inguinal ligament

Internal oblique (cut & reflected)

Pyramidalis

Inguinal ligament

Internal oblique

External oblique (cut & reflected)

Pyramidalis

External oblique (cut & reflected)

Quadratus lumborum

Rectus abdominis

Linea alba

External oblique

Rectus sheath (anterior layer)

Plate 4-24

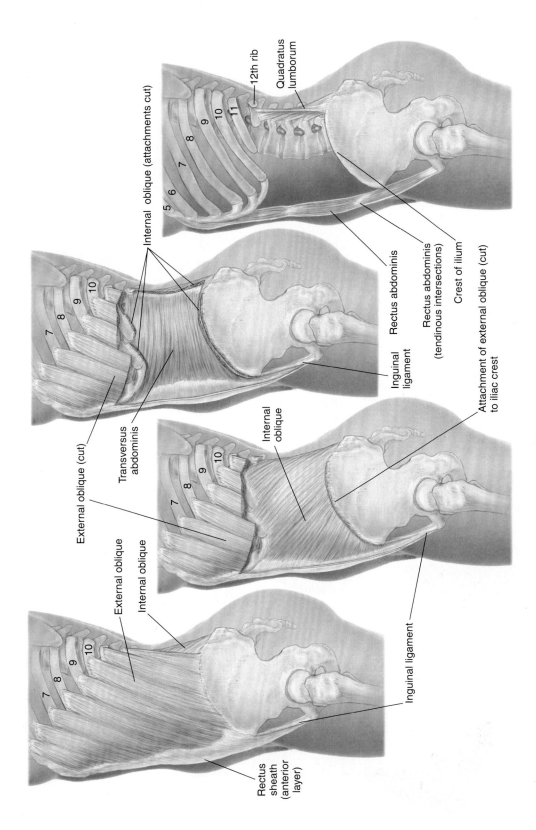

12th rib

Quadratus lumborum

Internal oblique (attachments cut)

5 6 7 8 9 10 11

Rectus abdominis

Rectus abdominis (tendinous intersections)

Crest of ilium

Attachment of external oblique (cut) to iliac crest

Inguinal ligament

Internal oblique

7 8 9 10

External oblique (cut)

Transversus abdominis

External oblique

Internal oblique

7 8 9 10

Inguinal ligament

7 8 9 10

Rectus sheath (anterior layer)

Plate 4-25

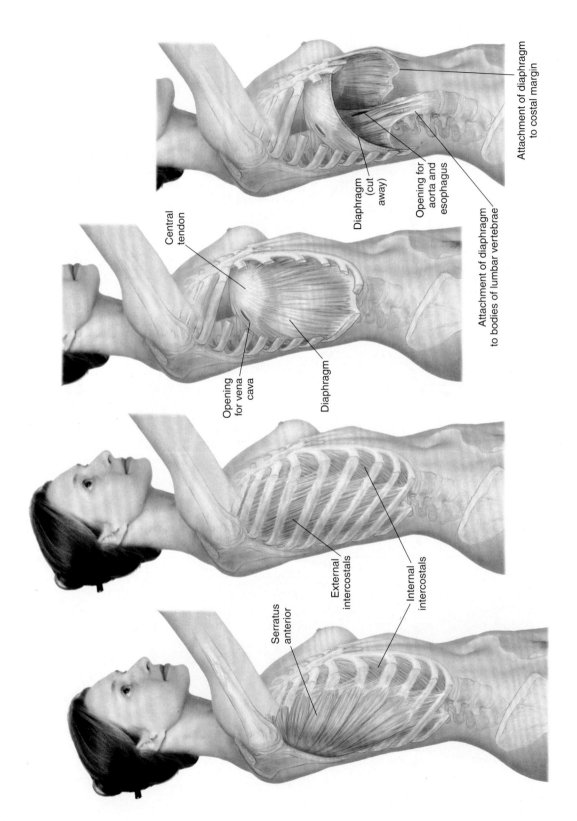

Attachment of diaphragm to costal margin

Attachment of diaphragm to bodies of lumbar vertebrae

Diaphragm (cut away)

Opening for aorta and esophagus

Central tendon

Opening for vena cava

Diaphragm

External intercostals

Internal intercostals

Serratus anterior

Plate 4-26

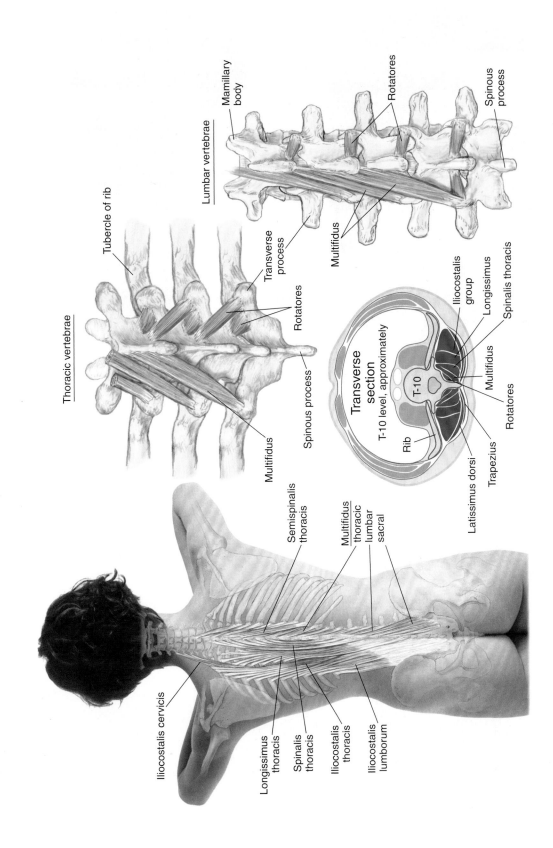

Mamillary body

Rotatores

Spinous process

Lumbar vertebrae

Multifidus

Tubercle of rib

Transverse process

Rotatores

Thoracic vertebrae

Multifidus

Spinous process

Transverse section
T-10 level, approximately

Iliocostalis group

Longissimus

Spinalis thoracis

Multifidus

Rotatores

T-10

Rib

Latissimus dorsi

Trapezius

Semispinalis thoracis

Multifidus
thoracic
lumbar
sacral

Iliocostalis cervicis

Longissimus thoracis

Spinalis thoracis

Iliocostalis thoracis

Iliocostalis lumborum

Plate 4-27

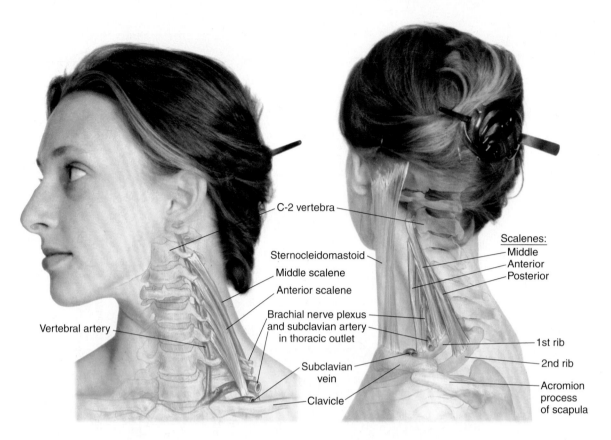

C-2 vertebra

Sternocleidomastoid

Middle scalene

Anterior scalene

Brachial nerve plexus
and subclavian artery
in thoracic outlet

Vertebral artery

Subclavian
vein

Clavicle

Scalenes:
Middle
Anterior
Posterior

1st rib

2nd rib

Acromion
process
of scapula

Plate 4-28

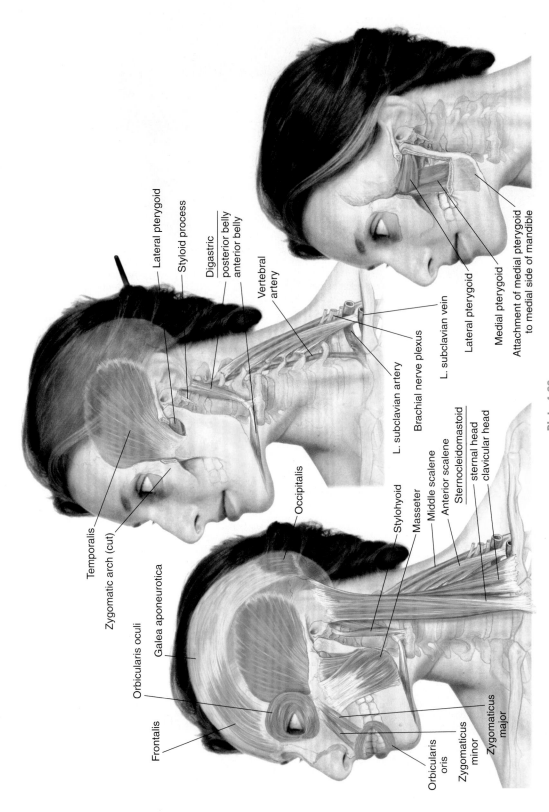

Lateral pterygoid

Styloid process

Digastric
posterior belly
anterior belly

Vertebral artery

Attachment of medial pterygoid to medial side of mandible

Medial pterygoid

Lateral pterygoid

L. subclavian vein

Brachial nerve plexus

L. subclavian artery

Temporalis

Zygomatic arch (cut)

Occipitalis

Stylohyoid

Masseter

Middle scalene

Anterior scalene

Sternocleidomastoid
sternal head
clavicular head

Orbicularis oculi

Galea aponeurotica

Frontalis

Orbicularis oris

Zygomaticus minor

Zygomaticus major

Plate 4-29

4 Kinesiology and Body Mechanics

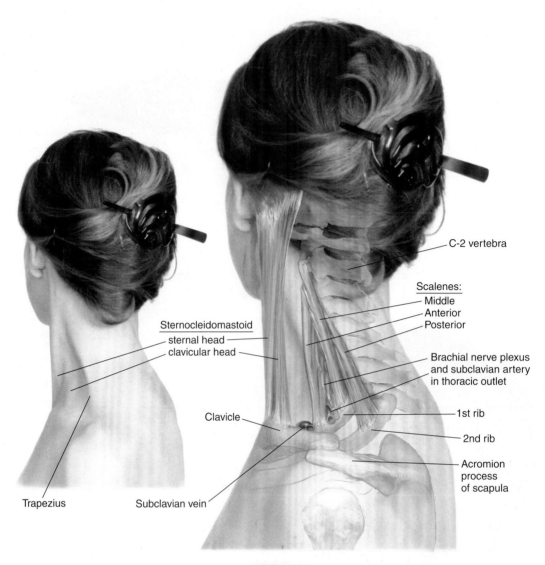

C-2 vertebra

Scalenes:
Middle
Anterior
Posterior

Sternocleidomastoid
sternal head
clavicular head

Brachial nerve plexus
and subclavian artery
in thoracic outlet

1st rib

2nd rib

Clavicle

Acromion
process
of scapula

Trapezius

Subclavian vein

Plate 4-30

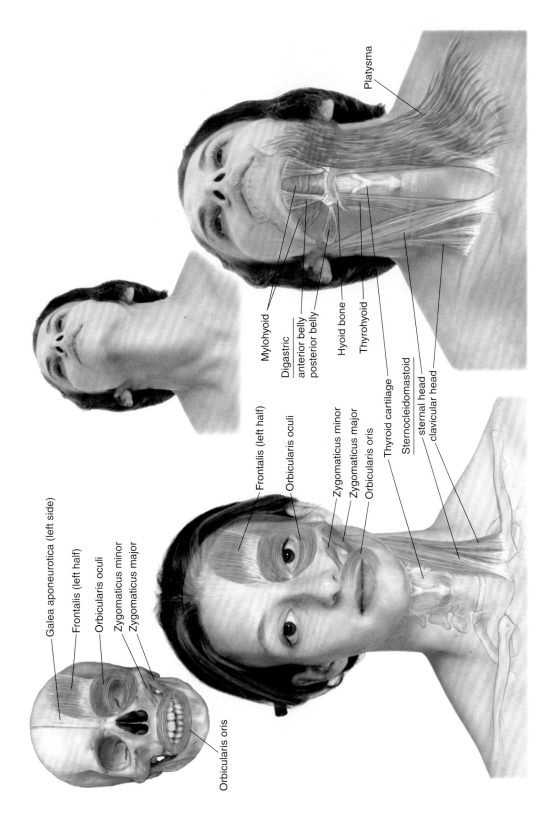

Galea aponeurotica (left side)
Frontalis (left half)
Orbicularis oculi
Zygomaticus minor
Zygomaticus major

Orbicularis oris

Frontalis (left half)
Orbicularis oculi

Zygomaticus minor
Zygomaticus major
Orbicularis oris

Thyroid cartilage
Sternocleidomastoid
sternal head
clavicular head

Mylohyoid
Digastric
anterior belly
posterior belly

Hyoid bone
Thyrohyoid

Platysma

Plate 4-31

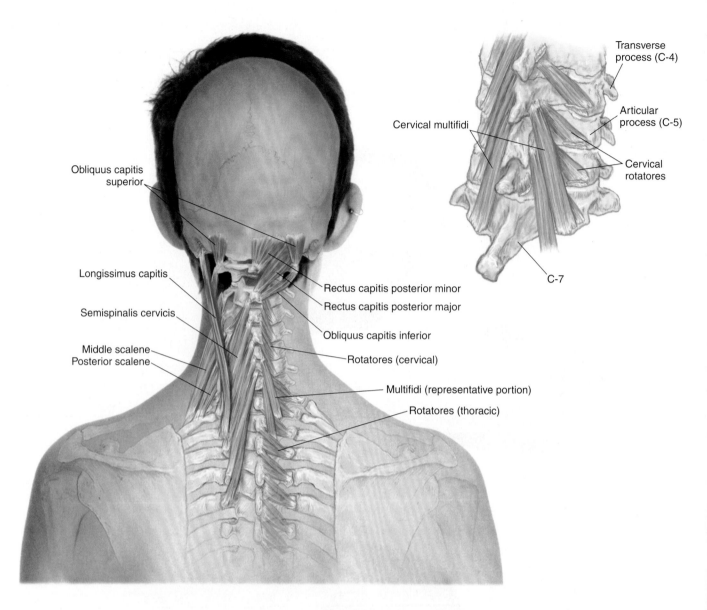

Transverse process (C-4)

Articular process (C-5)

Cervical multifidi

Cervical rotatores

C-7

Obliquus capitis superior

Longissimus capitis

Semispinalis cervicis

Middle scalene
Posterior scalene

Rectus capitis posterior minor
Rectus capitis posterior major

Obliquus capitis inferior

Rotatores (cervical)

Multifidi (representative portion)

Rotatores (thoracic)

Plate 4-32

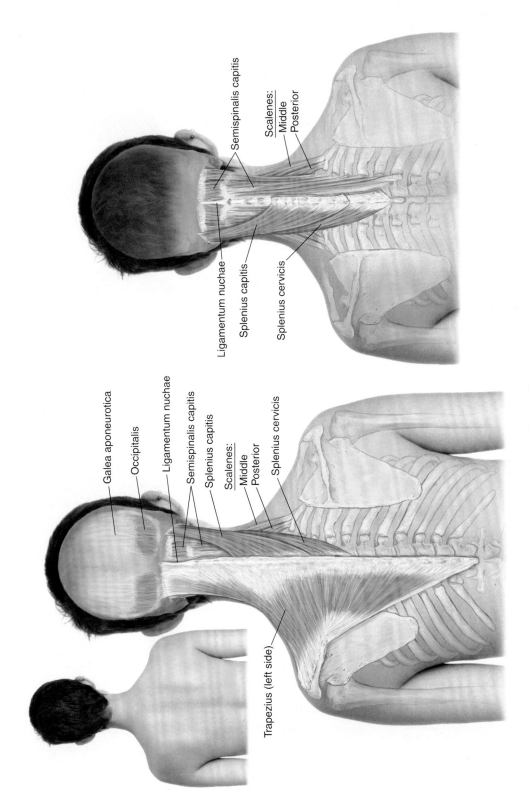

Semispinalis capitis

Scalenes:
Middle
Posterior

Ligamentum nuchae

Splenius capitis

Splenius cervicis

Galea aponeurotica

Occipitalis

Ligamentum nuchae

Semispinalis capitis

Splenius capitis

Scalenes:
Middle
Posterior

Splenius cervicis

Trapezius (left side)

Plate 4-33

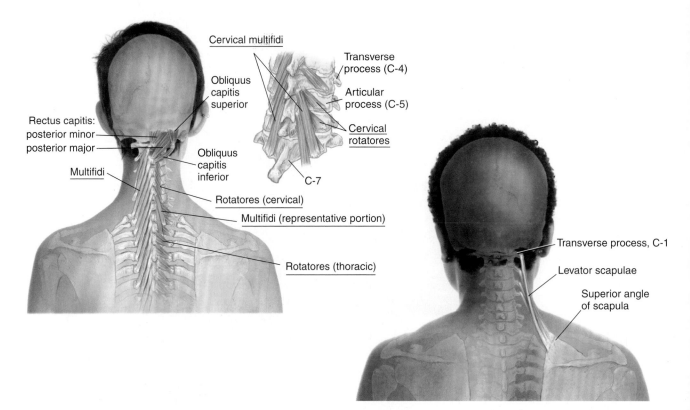

Cervical multifidi

Transverse process (C-4)

Articular process (C-5)

Obliquus capitis superior

Cervical rotatores

Rectus capitis:
posterior minor
posterior major

Obliquus capitis inferior

Multifidi

C-7

Rotatores (cervical)

Multifidi (representative portion)

Rotatores (thoracic)

Transverse process, C-1

Levator scapulae

Superior angle of scapula

Plate 4-34

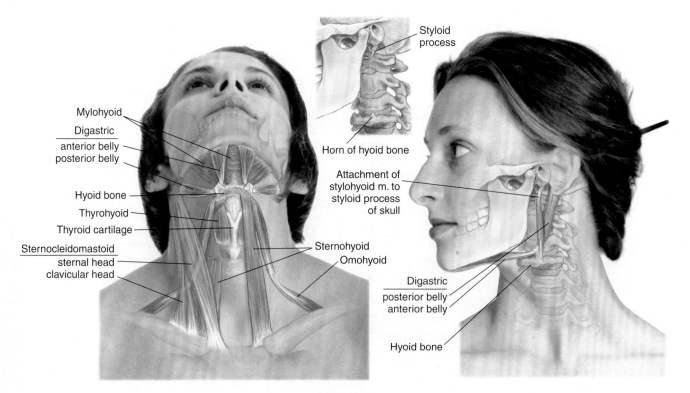

Styloid process

Mylohyoid

Digastric
anterior belly
posterior belly

Horn of hyoid bone

Hyoid bone

Attachment of stylohyoid m. to styloid process of skull

Thyrohyoid

Thyroid cartilage

Sternocleidomastoid
sternal head
clavicular head

Sternohyoid

Omohyoid

Digastric
posterior belly
anterior belly

Hyoid bone

Plate 4-35

CHAPTER EXERCISES

1. Define the following terms:

   - Anatomical position
   - Axillary angle
   - Biomechanics
   - Body mechanics
   - Concentric muscle contraction
   - Eccentric muscle contraction
   - Kinesiology
   - Prime mover
   - Synergist
   - Antagonist
   - Fixator

2. Demonstrate the following body movements:

   - Flexion of the elbow
   - Extension of the knee
   - Lateral flexion of the spine
   - Medial rotation of the humerus
   - Abduction of the femur
   - Circumduction of the hip
   - Dorsiflexion of the ankle
   - Supination of the hand
   - Lateral deviation of the mandible
   - Elevation of the scapula

3. List at least five components of a synovial joint.

4. Describe static and dynamic muscle contractions.

5. Identify and describe the three methods of generating energy in muscles.

6. Name the three components of good body mechanics.

7. Practice walking with your stroke. Ask a partner to lie prone on the massage table, and put your relaxed hand on his or her lumbar region. Move the stroke toward the partner's head without changing your axillary angle by walking with the stroke.

8. Familiarize yourself with the proper wrist position. Perform active wrist extension, and notice the limit of the ROM. Rest your hand on a desktop, tabletop, or massage table, and lean on that hand. Without moving your feet or your hand, slowly shift your weight so your shoulders move closer to the tabletop and are eventually positioned directly over your hand, and then shift in the opposite direction, away from the tabletop. Notice your wrist angle, axillary angle, and the stress on your shoulder joint as your body moves too close and too far away from your contact hand.

9. Practice efficient alignment with a partner. Lean on a variety of objects of different heights, and try to maintain the head-to-heel line using the asymmetric stance. You can try leaning on the seat of a chair, the top of a massage table, a doorknob, a windowsill, or a bookshelf.

10. Practice using relaxed wrists and hands. Ask a partner to rest his or her arm on the desktop, tabletop, or massage table. First, clench your hand into a tight fist and use your tightened forearm to lean on your partner's arm for a few seconds. Then, relax your arm, wrist, and hand and lean on your partner's arm a second time. Ask your partner for feedback regarding how the two pressures differ, which one was more comfortable, and whether or not one hurt.

SUGGESTED READINGS

Aslani M. *Massage for Beginners*. New York: Carroll & Brown, 1997.

Bruder L. Navigating the pathway to phenomenal touch: 10 steps to transform your massage. *Massage Magazine* 2002; (96): 74–82.

Cael C. *Functional Anatomy, Musculoskeletal Anatomy, Kinesiology, and Palpation for Manual Therapists*. Baltimore: Lippincott, Williams & Wilkins, 2010.

Frye B. *Body Mechanics for Manual Therapists: A Functional Approach to Self-Care*. Baltimore: Lippincott, Williams and Wilkins, 2010.

Greene L, Goggins RW. *Save Your Hands: The Complete Guide to Injury Prevention and Ergonomics for Manual Therapists*. Coconut Creek, FL: Body of Works Books, 2008.

Latchaw M, Egstrom G. *Human Movement with Concepts Applied to Children's Movement Activities*. Englewood Cliffs, NJ: Prentice-Hall, 1969.

Lidell L, Thomas S, Cooke CB, et al. *The Book of Massage*. New York: Simon & Schuster, 1984.

Lindsey R, Jones BJ, Whitley A. *Body Mechanics, Posture, Figure and Fitness*. 4th ed. Dubuque, IA: Wm. C. Brown, 1979.

Maxwell-Hudson C. *Complete Massage*. New York: Dorling Kindersley, 2001.

Moorcroft C. *Myology and Kinesiology for Massage Therapists*. Baltimore: Lippincott, Williams & Wilkins, 2012.

Muscolino J. *Kinesiology: The Skeletal System and Muscle Function*. 2nd ed. St. Louis: Mosby, 2011.

Nordin M, Frankel VH. *Basic Biomechanics of the Musculoskeletal System*. 3rd ed. Baltimore: Lippincott, Williams & Wilkins, 2001.

Premkumar K. *Anatomy & Physiology: The Massage Connection*. 3rd ed. Baltimore: Lippincott Williams & Wilkins, 2012.

Rattray F, Ludwig L. *Clinical Massage Therapy: Understanding, Assessing and Treating over 70 Conditions*. Toronto: Talus Incorporated, 2000.

Seedor MM. *Body Mechanics and Patient Positioning*. New York: Teachers College Press, 1977.

Souriau P. *The Aesthetics of Movement*. Souriau M, trans-ed. Amherst, MA: The University of Massachusetts Press, 1983.

Trager M, Hamond C. *Movement as a Way to Agelessness: A Guide to Trager Mentastics*. Barrytown, NY: Station Hill Press, 1995. http://www.exrx.net/Lists/Articulations.html, accessed 12.6.11.The 12 Body Systems

5

Pathology and Pharmacology

Objectives

Upon completion of this chapter, the student will be able to:

- Define pathology and describe how it relates to massage therapy
- Define pharmacology and describe how it pertains to massage therapy
- List at least three classes of pharmaceuticals
- Describe the difference between an indication and a contraindication
- Describe the difference between a local and a systemic contraindication

Key Terms

Acute: Refers to a condition that has developed very quickly and severely, or has a short duration.

Chronic: Refers to a condition that has persisted for a long time, develops slowly, or recurs.

Contraindication: A situation or condition in which massage could worsen the condition.

Etiology: The study of the source or cause of disease.

Indication: A condition for which massage could be beneficial and is recommended.

Local contraindication: A situation in which massage would be considered therapeutic except in a localized area, whereby using massage could cause further harm.

Pathology: The study of disease processes or of any deviation from a normal, healthy condition.

Pharmacology: The study of the preparation, mechanisms, applications, and effects of medications.

Subacute: The period from about 3 days to 3 weeks after a condition started.

Systemic contraindication: A condition or situation in which massage should be avoided altogether.

Pathology is the study of disease processes or any deviation from a normal, healthy condition. For massage therapy in particular, pathology is the study of disease or dysfunction to determine whether or not massage is contraindicated.

Pathological conditions are often treated with medications to alleviate their symptoms or treat their cause. Pharmacology (fahr-muh-KAH-loh-jee) is the science of the preparation, mechanisms, application, and effects of these medications.

Massage can affect pathological conditions as well as the effects of medications. This chapter guides you through the process of assessing the appropriateness of massage; you may need to consult more expanded resources on pathology and medications. See Suggested Readings and web sites at the end of this chapter for more information.

Pathology

This chapter covers some common pathological conditions and body conditions massage therapists encounter in their practice. Some conditions that upset the body's homeostasis are considered precursors to, or symptoms of, a disease process. For example, increased muscle tension in and of itself is not necessarily pathological, but it is sometimes a precursor to, or symptom of, fibromyalgia, a chronic muscular pain condition.

Diseases have different causes, signs, and symptoms. Etiology is the study of the source or cause of disease, which may point to heredity, infection, autoimmunity, trauma, or aging. Signs and symptoms of a disease are the subjective and objective indicators that lead to a diagnosis of a pathological condition or disease.

Pathological conditions can be characterized by the length of time they have persisted or how suddenly they presented. The stages of healing may vary depending on the severity and depth of the injury or condition and the individual's capacity for healing:

- Acute—refers to a condition that developed quickly and severely, or has a short duration
- Subacute—the period from about 3 days to 3 weeks after a condition started
- Chronic—refers to a condition that develops slowly, recurs, or persists for a long time

A contraindication for massage is a situation or condition for which massage should be avoided because it could worsen the condition. Some conditions are considered local contraindications, meaning that massage should be avoided only in the affected area. For example, massage is appropriate for someone who has a bruise, but the bruise itself is a local contraindication and should be avoided. There are also systemic contraindications, which are health conditions in which massage should be avoided altogether because massage could aggravate the condition or spread the disease. Any time fever is present, as in the acute stages of a cold, massage is systemically contraindicated.

Conversely, an indication is a condition for which massage would be beneficial or recommended. If you question whether massage should or should not be applied, withhold massage treatment until the appropriate healthcare professional can examine and diagnose the condition. **Remember the rule: when in doubt, refer out.** It is not within your scope of practice as a massage therapist to diagnose or prescribe, so suggesting a client see another healthcare professional must be done sensitively and carefully. Use a gentle approach when bringing awareness to a possible symptom or condition and explain that a more thorough examination is prudent. If the client asks you about a condition that you think may require a diagnosis, you can simply say, "I cannot diagnose any medical conditions, but massage may not be helpful. I recommend that you see your healthcare professional for further evaluation before we continue treatment." However, if you happen to notice a condition or a set of symptoms that may require a diagnosis, you can carefully encourage the client to recognize and discuss the symptoms. Once the client is aware of the symptoms or condition, you could suggest that a professional diagnosis may put his or her mind at rest. Referring clients out for conditions reinforces a client-centered philosophy.

Each condition presented in this chapter includes a brief description, some symptoms that can help identify it, and an explanation of whether massage is commonly indicated (recommended) or contraindicated (inappropriate). Additionally, there are "In Brief" boxes offering snapshots of conditions so you can quickly see the risks and benefits of massage therapy.

Pharmacology

Pharmacology is the study of the preparation, mechanisms, applications and effects of medications. Common medications and treatments for symptoms or conditions identified in this chapter are mentioned because a client may be using them when they come for massage treatment. They are mentioned as information only. These treatments and medications are prescribed by other healthcare professionals, not massage therapists. In this text, a healthcare professional is a practitioner who can diagnose and prescribe, such as a medical doctor (MD), osteopathic doctor (DO), nurse practitioner (NP), or chiropractor (DC).

Alert

Diagnosing and prescribing are not in the massage therapist's scope of practice.

Generally, if a medication is taken internally and is delivered through the bloodstream, massage techniques such as effleurage and pétrissage, which increase blood flow, may increase the effect of the medication in the body. It is always good to know about the client's health and treatment regimens that may be affected by massage.

Thousands of medications are prescribed for various symptoms and pathological conditions. Many of them can be categorized into major groupings or classifications of medications by their purpose and the mechanism that makes them work. Because medications are so common, you should be aware of basic drug classifications and how such drugs may interact with massage. Intentionally or not, massage can amplify or reduce the effect of a medication, and it can relieve side effects of some medications. The *Physicians' Desk Reference* (PDR) is a yearly publication that compiles the drug manufacturers and drug products as well as indications and contraindications for their use. A PDR is a good reference to have so you can look up specific drug names and identify possible contraindications for massage. Additionally, there are excellent resources specific to massage: *Pharmacology for Massage Therapy and Massage Therapy and Medications* (see Suggested Readings). If you do not have a reference book or are not sure whether massage is contraindicated when a client is taking a particular medication, you should consult with the client's healthcare professional.

Following are some common drug classifications, their indications, how the medications work, implications for massage, and their common names. **It is important to note that these change as new drugs are introduced and old ones are removed from the market—this requires you to research the most recent and accurate information regarding medications.**

Anti-inflammatory Drugs/ Analgesics

Inflammation is the body's response to different kinds of irritants, including bacteria, exposure to extreme temperatures, chemicals, hormonal changes, autoimmune activity, or a physical injury. Generally characterized by heat, redness, swelling, itching, and pain, inflammation may be reduced with various anti-inflammatory medications. When clients are taking an anti-inflammatory and/or analgesic medication, you want to be careful with massage techniques

that require that the client monitor pain levels, such as positional release, because the medication sometimes reduces the client's perception of pain and pressure.

Alert

Any massage techniques that create therapeutic inflammation, such as deep transverse friction, should be avoided.

Common classifications and names are:

- Salicylates—relieve pain, reduce fever, reduce swelling and joint stiffness (aspirin, buffered aspirin, Anacin, Bayer, Bufferin)
- Acetaminophen—relieve pain, reduce fever (Tylenol, Panadol, Tempra)
- Non-steroidal anti-inflammatory drugs—relieve inflammation, joint stiffness, swelling, and some can reduce fever (ibuprofen: Advil, Motrin, Nuprin; Relafen; Aleve; Lodine)
- Corticosteroids—steroidal anti-inflammatories that reduce redness, swelling, itching (cortisone, hydrocortisone, methylprednisolone, prednisone, Aristocort, Cortastat, Liquid Pred, Solu-Medrol, Sterapred)
- Narcotic—relieve pain and some suppress cough (codeine, hydrocodone, morphine, oxycodone, Demerol, Darvon, OxyContin)
- Combination medications—relieve pain and some reduce swelling or fever (Excedrin Extra-Strength combines acetaminophen, salicylates, and caffeine; Darvocet, Lortab, and Percocet combine narcotics with acetaminophen)

Muscle Relaxants

Muscle relaxants reduce the chemical activity responsible for communication between the nervous system and the muscular system. As a result, the muscles receive fewer signals to contract. They are prescribed to reduce muscular tension and acute muscular spasm resulting from injury or anxiety. While taking muscle relaxants, clients may feel weak and tired, often with reduced sensitivity to pain. Massage techniques that require clients to monitor pain levels, such as positional release, direct pressure, or friction, should be used with caution or avoided altogether depending on how the client is feeling after sustaining an injury.

Common classifications and names are:

- Centrally acting skeletal muscle relaxants—Flexeril, Skelaxin, Valium, Soma
- Peripherally acting skeletal muscle relaxants—Dantrium

Anti-anxiety Medications

Anti-anxiety medications are prescribed to manage or alter the sympathetic nervous system response. Suppression of the central nervous system (CNS) may result in side effects such as dizziness, poor coordination, forgetfulness, confusion, and depression. With the client's diminished ability to monitor changes that occur during massage, it is important to make adjustments accordingly. Additionally, the client's ability to move after a massage may be hindered and dizziness is likely, so encourage your client to use caution when sitting up and getting off the massage table.

Common classifications and names are:

- Barbiturates—amobarbital (Amytal), phenobarbital (Luminal)
- Benzodiazepines—alprazolam (Xanax), diazepam (Valium), lorazepam (Ativan), triazolam (Halcion)
- Buspirone—buspirone hydrochloride (BuSpar)

Antidepressants

Many kinds of antidepressants are prescribed to minimize or eliminate depression, and sometimes to relieve pain or to help people stop smoking. Usually, antidepressants change the chemistry of the nervous system by increasing the production of certain chemicals or blocking specific chemical pathways. These medications sometimes cause constipation, a side effect that can be relieved with massage. Since massage increases the levels of some of the critical brain chemicals involved in depression, be aware that the client may have an abnormal reaction to the medication, and use massage in cooperation with the prescribing healthcare professional. Common classifications and names are:

- Tricyclics—nortriptyline (Alti-Nortriptyline), amitriptyline (Elavil), imipramine (Apo-Imipramine)
- Monoamine oxidase inhibitors—isocarboxazid (Marplan), phenelzine (Nardil), tranylcypromine (Parnate)
- Selective serotonin reuptake inhibitors (SSRIs)—fluoxetine (Prozac, Sarafem), sertraline (Zoloft), paroxetine (Paxil), escitalopram (Lexapro), citalopram (Celexa)
- Other antidepressants—nefazodone (Serzone), bupropion (Wellbutrin), venlafaxine (Effexor)

Cardiovascular Disease Management

Drugs used to manage cardiovascular disease affect the body via the dilation of blood vessels or by diminishing the sympathetic nervous system response. When a client is taking one of these medications, the massage may cause the client to feel more fatigued, sluggish, and/or dizzy afterward. Make clients aware that this may occur and caution them to sit up and get off the table slowly once the massage session is over. Most common classifications and names are:

- Antilipemics (for high cholesterol)—cholesterol synthesis inhibitors (Lipitor, Zocor, Mevacor, Pravachol), fibric acid derivatives (Tricor, Lopid), bile-sequestering drugs (Colestid, Prevalite)
- Antianginal drugs (for angina)—beta-adrenergic antianginals (beta blockers: Inderal, Toprol XL, Betaloc, Lopressor, Tenormin, Corgard), calcium channel blockers (Norvasc, Cardene, Calan, Procardia, Cardizem), nitrates (Nitrodisc, Nitrostat, Cedocard, Monoket)
- Antihypertensive drugs (for hypertension)—sympatholytic drugs (Cardura, Tenex, Dopamet, Hytrin), vasodilating drugs (Hyperstat, Nu-Hydral, Nitropress), angiotensin-converting enzyme inhibitors (Accupril, Monopril, Vasotec, Lotensin)
- Diuretics (for hypertension and water retention)—thiazide and thiazide-like diuretics (Lozol, Lozide, Naturetin, Renese), loop diuretics (Lasix, Bumex), potassium-sparing diuretics (Spiractin, Inspra)

Anti-infectives

Antimicrobial drugs are used to treat infections by disrupting chemical processes within the offending microorganisms. Anti-infectives sometimes have gastrointestinal side effects, and massage may be able to reduce those symptoms. While the client's body is fighting infection, with or without the aid of antibiotics, the immune system is compromised. During that time, it is important to avoid overstressing the body. Keeping the client's best interest in mind, use gentler massage techniques to minimize the mechanical and reflexive effects of massage. Most common classifications and names are:

- Antibacterial drugs (fight bacterial infections)—penicillins (Augmentin, Wymox, Cloxapen, Ticillin), cephalosporins (Keflex, Declor, Cefzil, Vantin, Rocephin), tetracyclines (Declomycin, Monodox, Vibramycin), macrolides (erythromycin: Erythrocin, Diomycin), vancomycin (Vancocin), aminoglycosides (streptomycin, tobramycin), fluoroquinolones (Cipro, Levaquin, Maxaquin), sulfonamides (Bactrim, Sulfatrim), nitrofurantoin (Furadantin, Macrobid)
- Antiviral drugs (fight viral infections)—antiherpesvirus drugs (Zovirax, Famvir, Valtrex), influenza drugs

(oseltamivir: Tamiflu; zanamivir: Relenza; rimantadine: Flumadine)

- Antimycotic drugs (fight fungal infections)—amphotericin B (Amphotec, Fungizone), fluconazole (Diflucan), ketoconazole (Nizoral)

Antihistamines

Chemicals called histamines are released when the body goes through an allergic response. Histamines cause capillaries to leak extra fluids, resulting in swelling and itching. In some cases, they can even cause contractions of involuntary muscles such as the bronchi, restricting or preventing the essential process of breathing. Antihistamines block the effects of histamines (the prefix, anti-, means against), decrease blood vessel dilation and permeability, decrease nerve sensitivity in the skin, and reduce the itching and swelling associated with allergies. Common side effects of antihistamines are drowsiness, anxiety, dizziness, and lethargy as well as distorted or masked reactions to the massage. You must be aware of these effects and educate your clients so your clients know what to expect. Common classifications and names are:

- Ethanolamines—clemastine fumarate (Tavist, Dayhist), dimenhydrinate (Dramamine), diphenhydramine hydrochloride (Benadryl, Hydramine)
- Alkylamines—brompheniramine maleate (Dimetapp), chlorpheniramine maleate (Chlor-Trimeton)
- Piperidines—cetirizine (Zyrtec), desloratadine (Clarinex), fexofenadine hydrochloride (Allegra, Allegra-D), loratadine (Alavert, Claritin)

Most medications are taken orally, but some are applied topically or are injected. Be careful to avoid areas that are being treated with topical medications or the area immediately surrounding the injection site. Not only are those areas possibly undergoing some sort of infection/healing process that presents a local contraindication, massage can interfere with the absorption or you can accidentally transfer some of the medication onto your own body.

Any area that has received topical applications or injections of medication should be avoided for up to 24 hours afterward, depending on the drug and the condition being treated.

Anticoagulant Therapy

Clients who are taking anticoagulants such as warfarin (Coumadin) or anisindione (Miradon) currently have or are at risk for blood clots.

Any anticoagulant ("anti-clotting agent" or "blood thinner") presents a systemic contraindication for massage that requires the prescribing healthcare professional's clearance before proceeding with massage.

The parasympathetic nervous system response to massage may be enhanced by medications. Be aware that clients taking medication may feel especially weak or tired following a massage. Be available to help clients sit up and get off the table if they need assistance, and make sure that they are alert and awake enough to get home safely.

Pathology, Pharmacology, and Massage

The following section identifies each body system, lists some pathologies (abnormal conditions) associated with that system, notes some of the related pharmacological treatments, and discusses if or when massage is indicated.

Abnormal Conditions of Cells and Tissues

There are some abnormal conditions of cells and tissues of the body that you may see in your massage practice.

Cancer

Although cancer occurs in different body systems, all over the body, it starts at the cellular level when normal body cells undergo a mutation (genetic change) and start replicating at

abnormally high rates. A mass of these cells is called a tumor. A solid tumor occurring in the cells is a carcinoma, whereas one that occurs in muscular or connective tissue is a sarcoma. Cancer in the blood and lymph does not typically result in a solid tumor and is referred to as hematologic cancer or more specifically, leukemia, myeloma, and lymphoma. If the mutated cells travel to another place in the body, they can encourage the growth of a tumor where they settle.

Massage is locally contraindicated at the site of the tumor or tumors.

The American Cancer Society's web site (www.cancer.org) lists some known carcinogens, including:

- Alcoholic beverages
- Arsenic
- Asbestos

- Hepatitis B virus, hepatitis C virus, human immuno-deficiency virus type 1
- Estrogens, estrogen therapy
- Genetics/heredity
- Formaldehyde
- Lifestyle factors such as excessive weight and lack of physical activity
- Radiation from x-rays and gamma rays
- Radon
- Solar radiation
- Sunlamp or sunbed exposure
- Tobacco chewing and smoking

Although there are a number of specific causes and risk factors for cancer, these conditions do not always result in cancer. For example, radiation is a known carcinogen (substance or agent that causes cancer), but everyone who has been exposed to radiation does not develop cancer. Cancer must be diagnosed by a qualified professional, so clients who have cancer are likely under a doctor's care. Treatments can include surgery, radiation therapy, chemotherapy, radiofrequency thermal ablation, bone marrow transplant, hormone treatment, cryotherapy (freezing the cancerous cells), and many other developing and experimental therapies. It has not been proven that massage is specifically beneficial for cancer, and some people still feel that massage may make the condition worse. **Massage can be very beneficial in helping clients cope with pain, stress, fatigue and sleep loss, high blood pressure, nausea, loss of appetite, and the feelings of isolation and fear or anxiety that accompany cancer and the side effects of cancer treatments.**

Plantar Fasciitis

The plantar fascia is a band of connective tissue that stretches along the base of the foot between the calcaneus (heel) and the distal ends of the metatarsals. Plantar fasciitis (PF) is a painful condition of the plantar fascia that can result when it is repeatedly microscopically injured from overuse or stress (see Plantar Fasciitis in Brief). People suffering from PF generally feel more discomfort upon getting out of bed in the morning or after the foot has been immobile for a period of time. The pain often diminishes when the foot warms up. The most tender spot is on the sole of the foot, just anterior to the calcaneus. It is common to see a bone spur on the anterior edge of the calcaneus in x-rays of people who have PF, but it is not clear whether the bone spur caused or was caused by the fascial pain. There are varying opinions as to whether this is an inflammatory or degenerative condition, so treatments are understandably different. **Massage is beneficial for PF. By reducing muscle tension, especially in the deep calf muscles of the lower leg, increasing** circulation, and softening and stretching the collagen fibers in the fascia, massage can reduce the discomfort of PF as well as help the condition heal.

Integumentary (Skin) Conditions

Because massage therapists have so much contact with the skin, they may see or feel a change in a client's skin before the client does. If the skin is compromised in any way, as happens with a scratch or cut, it cannot function effectively as a protective barrier. Avoid any area of skin that has a wound or abnormality as a local contraindication for massage because there could be an increased possibility of infection. If you suspect a condition is more serious, refer the client to a healthcare professional for further evaluation. All treatments other than massage are mentioned below because clients may already be using them when they come to you for massage therapy.

Open Wounds or Sores

An open wound or sore is any injury to the skin that breaks the surface and leaves it open for bacteria to enter and possible infection to occur. Types of open wounds or sores include incisions (cuts), lacerations (rips and tears), abrasions (scrapes), fissures (cracks), vesicles (blisters), pustules (pus-filled vesicles), and ulcers (open sores with dead tissue). You can recognize

---

Plantar Fasciitis in Brief

Pronunciation: PLAN-tar fah-she-Y-tis

What is it?
Plantar fasciitis (PF) is a condition caused by repeated microscopic injury to the plantar fascia of the foot.

How is it recognized?
PF is acutely painful after prolonged immobility. Then the pain recedes when the foot is warmed up, but comes back with extended use. It feels sharp and bruise like, usually at the anterior calcaneus.

Massage risks and benefits
Risks: If the plantar fascia is acutely inflamed (which is unlikely), local deep massage should be delayed. Massage to the plantar fascia for a client who has recently had a cortisone injection may increase the risk of rupture.
Benefits: Massage can help release tension in deep calf muscles that put strain on the plantar fascia; it can also help to affect the quality of scar tissue at the site of the injury.

these conditions by the presence of blood or other fluid leaking out, or a crust or scab at the site of the injury.

Massage is locally contraindicated for the affected area. If the client has a related systemic condition such as diabetes, massage is a systemic contraindication unless you obtain medical clearance from the client's healthcare professional.

Typically, open wounds are covered with a bandage and treated with topical medications that often contain antibiotics, analgesics, or antihistamines.

Acne Vulgaris

Acne vulgaris, commonly known as acne, is a bacterial infection of the oil (sebaceous) glands that can be influenced by hormones, bacterial activity, stress, and liver congestion resulting from a high-fat diet, smoking, drugs (medications), and chemical pollutants (see Acne Vulgaris in Brief). Acne is commonly recognized as raised, white or black and sometimes reddened, inflamed pimples often found on the face, neck, and upper back.

Massage is locally contraindicated for acne because it can increase the possibility of spreading infection, and the lubricant can make acne worse.

Treatment for acne may include topical or oral medications, depending on the severity of the condition.

Superficial Scar Tissue

Superficial scar tissue is new tissue growth that occurs during the acute stage of an injury to the skin (see Scar Tissue in

Acne Vulgaris in Brief

Pronunciation: AK-ne vul-GAR-is

What is it?
Acne vulgaris is a condition of sebaceous glands usually found on the face, neck, and upper back. It is closely associated with adolescence, but often persists well into adulthood.

How is it recognized?
Acne looks like raised, inflamed bumps or pustules on the skin, sometimes with white or black tips.

Massage risks and benefits
Risks: Acne locally contraindicates massage because of the risk of infection, causing pain, and exacerbating the symptoms with the application of an oily lubricant.
Benefits: A client with acne can receive massage elsewhere on the body, and enjoy the same

Scar Tissue in Brief

What is it?
Scar tissue is new tissue that grows after an injury, infection, or surgery. It can grow in any kind of tissue, but this discussion is limited to scar tissue that affects any layer of the skin.

How is it recognized?
Deeply scarred skin may lack pigmentation, hair follicles, and sweat glands.

Massage risks and benefits
Risks: Skin that is injured and not yet healed obviously contraindicates massage at least locally, both because of pain and the risk of infection.
Benefits: Skin that is intact but scarred, even if the scar tissue has not fully matured, may benefit from the enhanced local circulation and mobilization provided by careful massage.

Brief). It is made of randomly structured, dense, fibrous tissue that has a decreased blood supply, may have decreased sensory neurons, and has no hair follicles or pigmentation (Fig. 5-1).

Massage is locally contraindicated during the acute stage of a skin injury because bacteria could enter any break or tear in the skin.

Once the scar has formed, massage on and around the scar tissue can increase the speed of healing by increasing circulation to the area, which minimizes fascial restriction and increases mobility of the tissue. You should be aware that the scar tissue may have reduced sensation, and you will need to be especially sensitive to the client's feedback. **In the subacute and chronic stages of a skin injury, massage is indicated and can be very beneficial.**

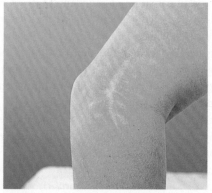

Figure 5-1. Scar tissue. (Reprinted with permission from Weber J, Kelley J. Health Assessment in Nursing. 2nd ed. Philadelphia: Lippincott Williams & Wilkins, 2003.)

Soft tissue work is the recommended treatment for superficial scar tissue and may be initially applied by a physical therapist or a massage therapist.

Fungal Infections

Fungal infections are contagious conditions of the skin that can be caused by several types of fungi and result in lesions called tinea (see Fungal Infections in Brief). Fungal infections are recognized as red, circular lesions and itchy patches that thrive in warm, moist places. Touching or scratching the lesions will spread the infection. Examples include ringworm and athlete's foot.

> Massage is locally contraindicated if the area is small and minimal lesions are present such as in the feet in athlete's foot. If the affected area is large, massage is systemically contraindicated until the infection is healed.

In the case of athlete's foot with no blisters, you may be safe to work on the client's feet through the sheet. Use your discretion and remember, when in doubt, do not touch.

Treatment for this condition usually includes topical fungicides and/or oral medications.

Fungal Infections in Brief

What are they?
Fungal infections of human skin, also called mycoses, are caused by fungi called dermatophytes. The characteristic lesions caused by dermatophytes are called tinea. Several types of dermatophytes cause tinea in different areas; lesions are typically named by location.

How are they recognized?
Most tinea lesions begin as one reddened circular itchy patch. Scratching the lesions spreads the fungi to other parts of the body. As the lesions grow, they tend to clear in the middle and keep a raised scaly red ring around the edges. Athlete's foot, another type of mycosis, produces oozing blisters and cracking between the toes. Fungal infections of toenails or fingernails produce thickened, pitted, discolored nails that may detach.

Massage risks and benefits
Risks: Most fungal infections locally contraindicate massage in all stages.
Benefits: Massage has no particular positive impact on fungal infections, but if the affected areas are very limited, such as only the feet or a small, covered lesion on the body, then massage may be administered elsewhere for general benefit. A client who has fully recovered from a fungal infection can enjoy the same benefits from massage as the rest of the population.

Skeletal System Conditions

The mechanical design of the joints enforces limits on a joint's range of motion, as does the condition of soft tissue structures surrounding the area. Tight muscles, injured tendons and ligaments, and abnormalities in other connective tissue structures generally create dysfunction and compensation patterns in the movement of the bones and joints of the skeleton. Generally, if the muscles and soft tissue are brought back into balance, then the bones and joints may return to, or more easily retain, their most functional alignment. All treatments other than massage are typically prescribed by a healthcare professional. Again, it is not in the massage therapist's scope of practice to diagnose or prescribe. The treatments below are mentioned because clients may already be using one or more of the following treatments when they come to you for massage therapy.

Postural Deviations

Postural deviations are overdeveloped or abnormal curves in the spine (see Postural Deviations in Brief). In the thoracic section, an overdeveloped curve is a hunched posture and is called kyphosis. Someone with an excessive lumbar

Postural Deviations in Brief

What are they?
Postural deviations are overdeveloped thoracic or lumbar curves (hyperkyphosis and hyperlordosis, respectively), or a lateral curve, possibly with a twist, in the spine (scoliosis, rotoscoliosis).

How are they recognized?
Extreme curvatures are easily visible, although radiography is used to pinpoint exactly where the problems begin and end.

Massage risks and benefits
Risks: Extreme postural deviations are sometimes connected to serious underlying diseases that influence the growth patterns of bone and soft tissues. Severe compression of the rib cage may lead to respiratory or cardiac impairment, along with a risk of pneumonia sand rib fragility.
Benefits: As long as underlying factors are addressed and bodywork is well tolerated, massage may have a powerfully positive effect on postural deviations, helping to balance soft tissue stress and improve alignment, efficiency of posture, and ease of movement.

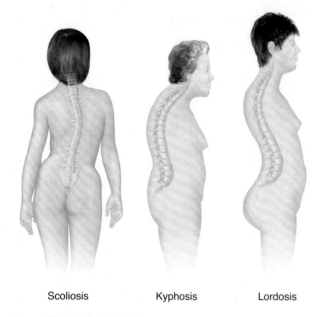

Scoliosis   Kyphosis   Lordosis

Figure 5-2. Postural deviations.

curvature, or lordosis, often stands with "locked" knees and a protruding pelvis. When the spine curves from side to side instead of running vertically, the condition is called S- or C-curve scoliosis (Fig. 5-2). These curves can have functional or structural causes. Functional postural deviations occur when the soft tissue structures, muscles, tendons, and ligaments pull the spine out of alignment. Structural deviations are congenital, meaning that the person was born with the bones already in the deviated formation, or result from untreated functional conditions that may have been caused by an injury. Deviations can be recognized by the extreme visible curves apparent by visual or palpable assessment. X-ray images can detect minor curves, but these tests are ordered

by a healthcare professional such as a DC, DO, NP, or MD. **Massage is indicated for reducing the chronically lengthened and shortened muscle and soft tissue tension and pain of scoliosis, but massage will not make the bones realign.**

Treatment for postural deviation may include physical therapy for exercises, chiropractic care for relieving pressure in the spine, and more dramatically, braces or surgical rods for severe scoliosis.

Fractures

A fracture is any type of cracked or broken bone (Fig. 5-3). A fracture is usually accompanied by increased pain and decreased function at the joint closest to the injury. Some conditions mask the symptoms of a fracture, such as a sprained ankle ligament or shin splints, but a healthcare professional can officially diagnose a fracture using an x-ray or bone scan.

Massage is locally contraindicated during the acute stage of a fracture, but massage to the rest of the body will enhance circulation and encourage healing.

Treatment for fractures includes immobilization, casting, and in more severe injuries surgery to repair the fractured bone(s) with pins or plates. **Several days after a bone has been fractured, massage can be beneficial for healing and is locally indicated.** Specifically, massage that focuses on lymphatic drainage can help increase circulation and reduce inflammation in the area of injury.

Sprains

A sprain refers to an injured ligament (see Sprains in Brief). Ligaments connect bone to bone and stabilize joints. Sprains occur when ligaments are suddenly overstretched or torn

Figure 5-3. Types of fractures.

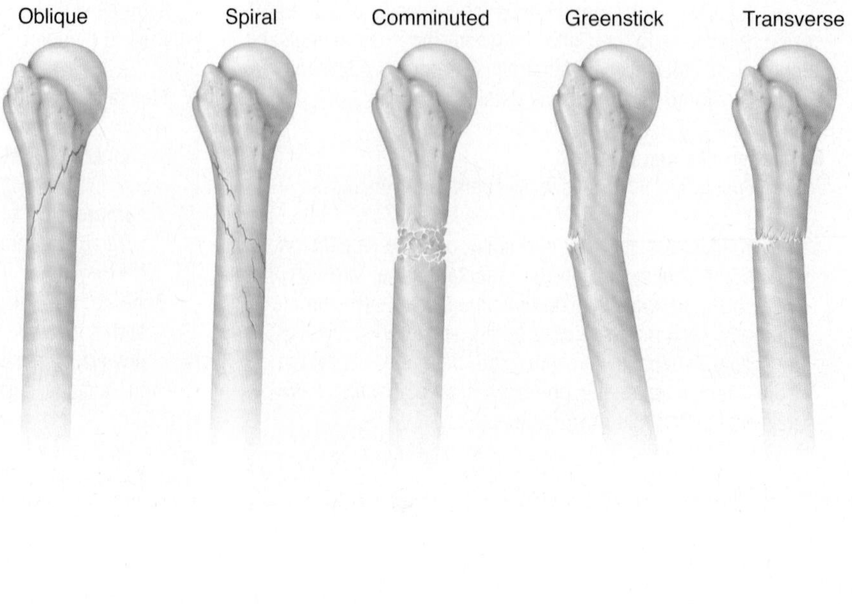

Oblique   Spiral   Comminuted   Greenstick   Transverse

Sprains in Brief

What are they?
Sprains are injured ligaments. Injuries can range in severity from a few traumatized fibers to a complete rupture.

How are they recognized?
In the acute stage, pain, redness, heat, swelling, and loss of joint function are evident. Later, these symptoms are less extreme, although perhaps not entirely absent. Passive stretching of the affected ligament is painful until all inflammation has subsided.

Massage risks and benefits
Risks: Acutely inflamed sprains locally contraindicate intrusive work until the inflammation has subsided, but lymphatic work to decrease edema may be safe and appropriate. Sprains can sometimes mask symptoms of minor fractures; if symptoms are not significantly relieved within a few days, this possibility should be pursued with a medical professional.
Benefits: Damaged ligaments that are not acutely inflamed respond well to specific massage along with passive stretching and full use within pain tolerance.

because of trauma or an exceeded range of motion. When torn, their ability to maintain the stability of the joint is compromised. In the acute stage (24 to 72 hours), the symptoms include pain, redness, heat, swelling, and decreased mobility at the affected joint. Swelling, in particular, is a part of the body's healing mechanism, limiting movement to prevent further injury. These symptoms decrease as healing progresses; however, pain remains during all stages. Sometimes sprains cover up the symptoms of a fracture. If you suspect this, you should refer the client to a healthcare professional to rule out fracture prior to massage treatment. A severe sprain may be medically diagnosed as a rupture or separation of the ligament from the bone.

Massage is locally contraindicated during the acute stage of a severe sprain except for lymphatic drainage to aid the swelling, but the client's entire body will benefit from the relaxing and restorative qualities of massage therapy.

Treatment for sprains includes immobilization via a splint or support bandage, ice and compression to reduce swelling, and elevation to keep excess lymphatic fluid from accumulating in the injured area. **Massage is indicated in the subacute stage, when it can enhance healing and decrease swelling and adhesion as well as create helpful scar tissue and restore range of motion to the affected joint.**

Gentle and limited ranges of movement may help reduce scar tissue formation, but the client may need physical therapy or other professional medical treatments prescribed.

Osteoarthritis

Osteoarthritis literally means inflammation of the bone and joint (see Osteoarthritis in Brief). More specifically, it is a condition that occurs when repetitive wear and tear of synovial joint structures result in irritation and inflammation. Fingers, thumbs, knees, and hips are common joints affected in this condition. **Massage therapists may develop this condition over time because of repetitive use of fingers and thumbs.** Clients with this condition complain of stiffness and pain in the affected joints that may be accompanied by signs of inflammation such as redness and heat. Occasionally, muscles around the affected joint will become tense, effectively "splinting" the area to decrease mobility. Chronic muscle tension can result in the formation of trigger points (TrPs) in the muscle, which are explained in the section on muscular system conditions.

Massage is locally contraindicated in the acute stage of osteoarthritis when inflammation is present.

Treatment for osteoarthritis may include pain or anti-inflammatory or COX-2 inhibitor medications, steroid injections, nutritional supplements such as glucosamine and chondroitin, or dietary modifications. **Massage is indicated**

Osteoarthritis in Brief

Pronunciation: os-te-o-arth-RY-tis

What is it?
Osteoarthritis is joint inflammation brought about by wear and tear causing cumulative damage to articular cartilage.

How is it recognized?
Affected joints are stiff, painful, and occasionally palpably inflamed. Bony deformation may be easily visible or palpable. Osteoarthritis most often affects knees, hips, and distal joints of the fingers.

Massage risks and benefits
Risks: Acutely inflamed arthritis (which isn't typical) at least locally contraindicates massage that may promote local fluid flow and exacerbate inflammation.
Benefits: Full body and specific massage for painful joints can reduce stiffness and pain, and improve the quality of life for people with osteoarthritis, even though it is unlikely to contribute to any internal joint repair process.

in the subacute and later stages of osteoarthritis to relieve pain and stiffness as well as to increase joint mobility. Massage can also help treat TrPs in the surrounding muscles and tight muscles and soft tissue that are splinting the joint, reduce pain, and encourage relaxation.

Muscular System Conditions

There are many indications for massage therapy for clients with muscle or movement dysfunction. Abnormal posture is often accompanied by muscles that are out of balance. When one muscle of a pair of antagonistic muscles is hypertonic, they are considered out of balance. The hypertonic muscle pulls the joint into an abnormal resting position and the body must compensate for the imbalance. Muscles that get out of balance are in a less than optimal state or have a reduced functional activity. Any deviation from normal, healthy function or movement indicates that a muscle or series of muscle groups have abnormal stresses placed on them. One goal of massage therapy is to bring the muscles and surrounding soft tissue back into balance to create the most functional movement for the client. You should understand muscular system symptoms, conditions, or states of dysfunction. All treatments other than massage are typically prescribed by the client's healthcare professionals who can diagnose and prescribe within their scope of practice. Again, it is not in the massage therapist's scope of practice to diagnose or prescribe, but these treatments are mentioned because clients may already be using one or more of the following treatments when they come to you for massage therapy.

Hypertonic Muscles

Muscles that are too tight are referred to as hypertonic, meaning that they have contracted and have not completely relaxed. Exercise, for example, puts muscles through repetitive contractions, and when the exercise is finished, the muscles may not "remember" their original resting length. Because they are so used to contracting, they may assume a new, shorter resting length and are considered hypertonic. When muscles are hypertonic, circulation within them is reduced, so they receive less oxygen than they need, a condition called ischemia (iss-KEE-mee-ah). The symptoms can include pain, discomfort, restrictions in functional movement, and compensation patterns. This is an interconnected pattern commonly called the pain–spasm cycle (Fig. 5-4).

1. Pain causes a person to tense up, resulting in hypertonicity.
2. Hypertonicity causes ischemia.

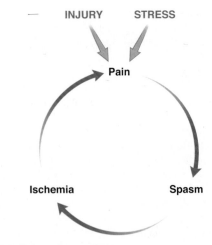

Figure 5-4. Pain–spasm cycle.

3. Ischemia causes pain.
4. Pain causes hypertonicity, and the pattern repeats.

Massage is beneficial for all of the symptoms of hypertonic muscles, including pain, the shortened muscle length, and ischemia. Therapeutic techniques can be used to reflexively trigger the muscles to lengthen. People commonly treat hypertonic muscles with or without a professional diagnosis by using ice packs or heat packs, soaking in hot tubs, analgesics (pain relievers), muscle relaxants, and self-massage. Pain relievers can be helpful because they can break the pain–spasm cycle by reducing pain, which allows more movement of the muscle, which increases the circulation to the muscle. Ice is also very helpful because in addition to its analgesic properties that break the pain cycle, the homeostatic mechanism of our body will flood the area with warm blood to maintain a stable core body temperature. Circulation increases healing.

Muscle Spasms and Cramps

Muscle spasms and cramps occur when a skeletal muscle contracts involuntarily and does not relax immediately (see Spasms, Cramps in Brief). Spasms are low-grade, long-lasting muscle contractions that result in decreased movement at the related joint and can last for weeks. A cramp is a spasm that is accompanied by visibly shortened muscle fibers and intense pain. Spasms and cramps are caused by ischemia (decreased oxygen), muscle splinting after an injury, and low levels of calcium and magnesium in the blood.

Massage to the muscle bellies is contraindicated in the acute stage of a muscle spasm to prevent further injury; however, it is acceptable to manipulate the tendons of that muscle and the antagonistic muscles to reflexively relax the affected muscle.

Reflexive massage techniques are covered in the Therapeutic Applications chapter.

Spasms, Cramps in Brief

What are they?
Spasms and cramps are involuntary contractions of skeletal muscle. Spasms are considered to be low-grade, long-lasting contractions, while cramps are short-lived, very acute contractions.

How are they recognized?
Cramps are extremely painful, with visible shortening of muscle fibers. Long-term spasms are painful and may cause inefficient movement but may not have acute symptoms.

Massage risks and benefits
Risks: Muscles in acute, painful contraction do not invite rigorous massage on the belly; this may be more irritating or even damaging than not. Some underlying pathologies may cause muscle cramping; these must be ruled out or accommodated if this is a frequent event.

Benefits: Stretching along with massage at attachment sites of contracting muscles are often effective strategies for reducing tone. Muscles that have been in involuntary contraction respond well to massage, which can reduce residual pain and clean up chemical wastes.

Myofascial Pain Syndrome in Brief

MY-o-fash-al pane SIN-drome

What is it?
Myofascial pain syndrome (MPS) is a collection of signs and symptoms associated with the development of myofascial trigger points (TrPs) in muscles.

How is it recognized?
MPS is recognized mainly by the TrPs that arise in predictable locations in affected muscles. Active TrPs create hard painful knots or taut bands; the pain may refer to distant locations. Latent TrPs may not generate pain unless they are irritated.

Massage risks and benefits
Risks: The only risk massage has for clients with MPS is that overtreatment could leave them sore. This condition involves pain-sensitizing chemicals that must be addressed in addition to reducing tone at and around TrPs.

Benefits: MPS indicates massage, which can interrupt the cycles that promote painful TrPs and help to mitigate the causes of pain and soreness that accompany these phenomena.

In the subacute and chronic stages of a muscle spasm, massage is indicated because it can decrease pain and hypertonicity as well as increase circulation, resulting in more oxygen and nutrients delivered to and removal of waste from the area. This helps break the pain–spasm cycle. Sometimes spasms are referred to as muscle guarding or splinting. In this phenomenon, the body responds to pain by holding a muscle contraction to minimize movement in an attempt to protect an area from further injury.

Massage is locally contraindicated for situations of splinting or protective guarding.

As part of the body's own healing mechanism, splinting serves an important purpose, and if the muscles that are acting as splints are relaxed, further injury could result. Treatment for spasms is commonly used with or without a professional diagnosis or prescription and may include heat packs, ice packs, analgesics, muscle relaxants, self-massage, and nutritional supplements such as calcium, magnesium, and potassium.

Trigger Points (Myofascial Pain Syndrome)

TrPs are spasms that occur at the motor end unit, or the point of communication between nerve cells and muscle cells, which result in painful knots or taut bands within the tissue (see Myofascial Pain Syndrome in Brief). When very few muscle cells are in spasm, they become hyperirritable and refer pain to another part of the body because of the neuron involvement. There are several factors that contribute to the formation of TrPs:

- Decreased circulation to a hypertonic muscle
- Insufficient hydration of the muscle cells and tissues, which creates homeostatic imbalance that can affect the action potential
- Mechanical stress on a muscle caused by bony misalignments or excessive pressure from a purse or backpack strap
- Inadequate sleep, which can overwork the sympathetic nervous system to stay alert
- Increased stress, which can also affect homeostasis with overactivity of the sympathetic nervous system

TrPs are not pathological, but can be a symptom of a pathological condition. For example, TrPs are often a symptom of fibromyalgia, a chronic muscle pain condition. **Massage is indicated for TrPs to relieve them and allow the muscle to relax as well as to increase circulation to the muscle tissue.** All treatments other than massage are typically prescribed by the client's healthcare professional, whose scope of practice includes prescription. Again, it is not in the massage therapist's scope of practice to diagnose or prescribe. Treatment may include heat packs, ice packs, injections of pain medication, oral pain medication, and muscle relaxants. These treatments are only mentioned because clients may already be using one or more of the treatments when they come to you for massage therapy.

Fibromyalgia

Fibromyalgia is a chronic muscle pain syndrome that also may be referred to as fibrositis, myofibrositis, or fibromyositis (see Fibromyalgia in Brief). A syndrome is diagnosed when a client has a certain set of symptoms. Fibromyalgia is characterized by neuroendocrine and sleep disruption as well as tender points in the muscles and soft tissue. The American College of Rheumatology has determined diagnostic criteria for fibromyalgia: at least 3 months of symptoms at the same level in intensity; at least 11 of 19 mapped tender points (diffuse pain elicited from digital pressure of about 4 kg); active tender points must be distributed all over, located in each quadrant of the body; fatigue; waking up unrefreshed; and memory and/or cognitive problems. See Fig. 5-5 for a map of the fibromyalgia tender points.

Fibromyalgia symptoms can come and go, so a person might have 11 tender points one day but only 8 tender points

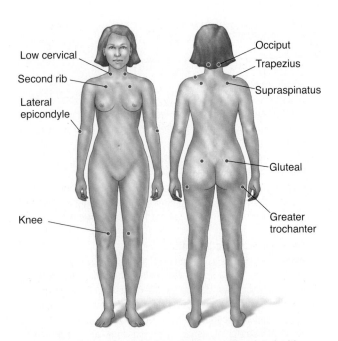

Figure 5-5. Fibromyalgia tender points map. (Reprinted with permission from Werner R. A Massage Therapist's Guide to Pathology. 5th ed. Baltimore: Lippincott Williams & Wilkins, 2013.)

on another day. While specialists or researchers may still use tender points, the amount of pressure a doctor needed to apply to the points was too subjective for repeatability, so an alternative set of guidelines has been developed for doctors to use in general practice.

Pain is the predominant symptom in this condition, present in the muscles and soft tissues to varying degrees. The soft tissue hypersensitivity can elicit pain with any kind of movement or light touch. Typically, the higher the stress level and the more compromised the internal healing environment, the more hypersensitive the client and client's tissues are. Any time you treat clients with fibromyalgia, you should carefully consider their stress level and internal healing environment, which may affect their pain tolerance. **Massage is indicated for fibromyalgia as long as you do not overtreat the client.** Due to the increased sensitivity to pain, decreased circulation to the muscles, tender points, and TrPs, sometimes massage can create more stress on the body and worsen the condition. There is a fine line between appropriate treatment and overtreatment. Over time, you will easily detect changes in the muscles and surrounding soft tissue through palpation in a massage and will be able to apply the appropriate treatment. **Less is often more** when treating this particular condition, which can be managed by using less pressure or treatments of shorter duration.

All treatments other than massage are typically prescribed by the client's healthcare professional and are only mentioned to make you aware of what your clients may

---

Fibromyalgia in Brief

Pronunciation: fy-bro-my-AL-je-ah

What is it?
Fibromyalgia syndrome (FMS) is a chronic pain syndrome involving neuroendocrine disruption, sleep disorders, and the development of a predictable pattern of tender points in muscles and other soft tissues.

How is it recognized?
FMS is diagnosed when other diseases have been ruled out, and when 11 active tender points are found distributed among all quadrants of the body, along with fatigue, morning stiffness, and poor quality sleep.

Massage risks and benefits
Risks: FMS patients tend to be hypersensitive and easy to overtreat. Care must be taken to stay within their tolerance for pain and adaptability.
Benefits: Fibromyalgia indicates massage, which can help reduce pain, improve sleep, and otherwise add to quality of life.

bring into your treatment room to know whether you need to adjust the treatment. With fibromyalgia, people tend to respond differently to the same treatment, but ice may increase symptoms and should generally be avoided. Treatments for this condition may include pain, sleep, and/ or antidepressant medications and muscle relaxants as well as changes in nutritional habits, nutritional supplementation, exercise, stretching, acupuncture, and anything to reduce the client's stress level, which includes massage.

Muscle Strain

A muscle strain involves torn muscle tissue and is characterized by mild-to-severe localized pain, stiffness, and inflammation (heat, redness, and swelling) (see Strains in Brief). Inflammation increases with the severity of the injury. Resisted movement, in which the client is moving against a counterforce, and stretching will also elicit pain in a strained muscle. A muscle that undergoes excessive stretch or excessive contraction can suffer a muscle strain.

Massage is locally contraindicated during the acute and subacute periods following a muscle strain. If the strain is determined by a physician to be very severe, such as a rupture of the entire muscle, massage is locally contraindicated until the physician has determined that the muscle has healed.

The body starts the healing process in the acute phase of a muscle strain by depositing a dense network of collagen fibers at the injury site in random arrangements. Because this network is not aligned with the muscle fibers,

the surrounding layers of tissue cannot slip past each other as easily, and the layers have a tendency to stick to each other and create fascial adhesions. Thus, gentle movement is beneficial for a healing muscle strain because it prevents the buildup of fascial adhesions. Even so, the client should be cautious about exerting the injured muscle during the subacute period because the new collagen fiber network lacks strength and the risk of reinjury is higher. Once the adhesions have settled in and bound tissue layers together are left untreated, scar tissue will form (Fig. 5-6).

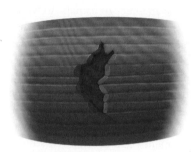

A Injured muscle tissue

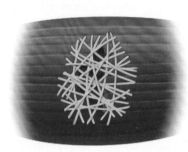

B Random arrangement of deposited scar tissue

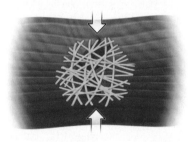

C Structural weak spot

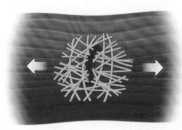

D New injury at site of scar tissue

Figure 5-6. Muscle tissue injury.

Strains in Brief

What are they?
Strains are injuries to muscles involving torn fibers.

How are they recognized?
Pain, stiffness, and occasionally palpable heat and swelling are all signs of muscle strain. Pain may be exacerbated by passive stretching or resisted contraction of the affected muscle.

Massage risks and benefits
Risks: Rigorous massage to an acute muscle injury may exacerbate inflammation and tissue damage.
Benefits: Massage after the acute stage of inflammation has passed can powerfully influence the production of useful scar tissue, reduce adhesions and edema, and reestablish range of motion.

Massage is indicated for muscle strains to help break up adhesions and scar tissue, to reduce edema (swelling), and to restore range of motion to the joint nearest the strain.

Strains are often self-diagnosed, but should be medically diagnosed in order for you, as a massage therapist, to avoid working on a contraindicated condition.

Treatment for strains can include ice or heat, medications to reduce inflammation, analgesics, and muscle relaxants if muscle guarding occurs with the injury.

Tendinopathy

A tendinopathy is an injury or damage to tendons and their fascial sheaths (see Tendinopathies in Brief). Tendinitis is the most common injury you may see as a massage therapist. Specifically, tendinitis involves injury and inflammation of the tendon, usually at the union of the muscle and tendon (musculotendinous juncture) or where the tendon attaches to the bone (tenoperiosteal juncture). Tendons have a limited blood supply that is further compromised by compression, repetitive movements, and constant twisting. In the acute stage, tendinitis is recognizable by pain, stiffness, and inflammation as well as decreased movement. In the subacute stage, adhesions begin to form from a random collagen matrix.

Tendinopathies in Brief

Pronunciation: ten-dih-NOP-ath-ez

What are they?
Tendinopathies are injuries or damage to tendons and their fascial sheaths. While it is possible for these injuries to involve acute inflammation (as indicated in the traditional terms tendinitis or tenosynovitis), most long-term tendon injuries are related to collagen degeneration rather than inflammation. The term for this condition is tendinosis.

How are they recognized?
Pain and loss of range of motion are often present with tendinopathies. Pain is exacerbated by resisted exercise of the damaged muscle–tendon unit. Damage to the tenosynovial sheath may also create pain, resistance to movement, and crepitus: a grinding texture as the tendon moves through its fascial covering.

Massage risks and benefits
Risks: Tendinopathies with true inflammation are rare, but when they occur, bodywork is best delayed until the acute phase is complete. An exception to this is lymphatic work, which may help to limit some of the negative aspects of swelling.
Benefits: Most tendinopathies indicate massage, which aims to help improve the quality

Although massage is locally contraindicated in the acute stage, systemic massage is indicated.

Treatments for tendinitis may include ice, heat, rest or inactivity of the affected tendon, pain medication, anti-inflammatory medications, or applications of ultrasound. Local massage is indicated in the subacute stage to increase circulation to the surrounding tissues, reduce edema, break up fascial adhesions or scar tissue, and reestablish range of motion to the joint affected.

Nervous System Conditions

Massage affects the nervous system in several ways, depending on the technique and the speed of its application. If the goal is to stimulate the client's system, you could apply techniques using a faster pace to evoke the sympathetic nervous response. Conversely, if the goal is to relax the body, the techniques could be applied more slowly to evoke the parasympathetic nervous response. Specific massage applications using the nervous system to facilitate muscular changes are discussed in the Therapeutic Applications chapter. Many conditions can affect the nervous system and its components. If the client is experiencing burning, tingling, paresthesia (pins and needles), radiating numbness, or a similar sensation, nerves may be involved.

Endangerment Sites

Endangerment sites are places on the body where nerves and blood vessels are not well protected by muscles or bones. These sites are not pathological conditions, but you should be aware of their locations.

Continuous, direct, or heavy pressure or pounding on any of the endangerment sites may cause damage and is contraindicated.

Massage techniques applied at these sites should include light pressure or should be avoided altogether (see Fig. 5-7).

Sciatica

Sciatica (sahy-AT-ik-uh) is inflammation of the sciatic nerve. It is characterized by aching or cramping sensations and/or shooting or burning pain in the buttocks and down the leg into the foot. Sometimes the discomfort is accompanied by tingling, reduced sensation or numbness, paresthesia (pins and needles sensation), and even loss of function. True sciatica involves irritation to the sciatic nerve near its root at

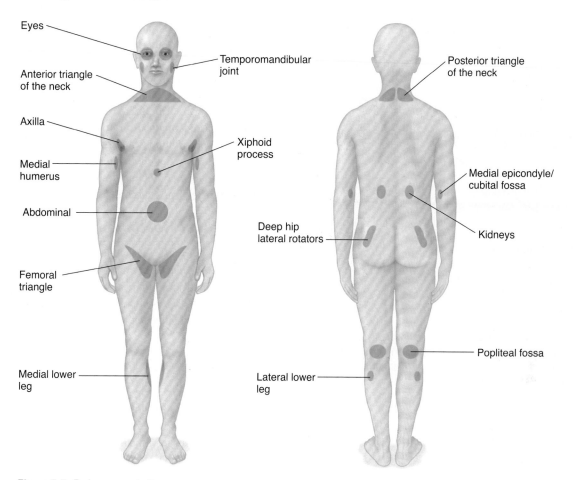

Figure 5-7. Endangerment sites.

the spinal cord, which may be caused by more serious pathology. Spinal cord or nerve root impingement should be examined and diagnosed by a healthcare professional. The nervous system is not within the massage therapy scope of practice, and treating a nerve root is inappropriate.

Massage is locally contraindicated for true sciatica that stems from the spinal cord or nerve root.

The symptoms of sciatica can also be caused by irritation or inflammation of the sciatic nerve because of muscular impingement by a tight piriformis muscle, one of the deep hip rotator muscles near the ischium. **Massage is indicated for sciatic nerve irritation if there is a muscular cause because it can relax the problematic muscle tissue and relieve the pressure on the nerve.** Many clients come in with self-diagnosed sciatica, but without a professional diagnosis, you cannot determine where the nerve is being affected. As mentioned above, massage is locally contraindicated for true sciatica, but that does not rule out massage of the deep hip rotator muscles. Therefore, you can attempt massage on the deep hip rotators to see if it relieves the discomfort at all. If massage does not decrease the symptoms, the client may have nerve root or spinal cord irritation, and you should

refer such clients to their healthcare professional for further evaluation.

Treatment for sciatica may include muscle relaxants, pain medication, physical therapy, traction, cortisone injections to reduce inflammation, chiropractic or osteopathic adjustment, or surgery in more severe cases.

Headaches

A headache is pain in the head and neck region that can be classified as muscular (tension), vascular (congestion or spasm and dilation), or traction–inflammatory (pathological); it can also be due to nerve irritation or chemical imbalances (see Headaches in Brief). Headaches can have a sudden or gradual onset, and the pain can be on one or both sides of the head and neck. It is not within the massage therapy scope of practice to diagnose or prescribe, so all treatments mentioned, other than massage, are typically self-administered or prescribed by healthcare professionals who can prescribe treatments within their scope of practice. These treatments are mentioned because clients may already be using them when they come for a massage. You should always ask if the client has any health issues or is using treatments that may be affected by massage.

Headaches in Brief

What are they?
Headaches are pain caused by any number of factors. Muscular tension, nerve irritation, vascular spasm and dilation, and chemical imbalances can all contribute to headache. They can sometimes indicate a serious underlying disorder.

How are they recognized?
Headache pain can range from being mild to debilitating; it can involve the whole head or be isolated to a particular area; it can be described as dull, aching, or sharp, electrical and agonizing.

Massage risks and benefits
Risks: Headaches due to infection or central nervous system injury contraindicate massage. Many clients with migraine avoid massage and other stimulus during a headache, but might pursue it as a way to reduce frequency or intensity when the condition is not acute.
Benefits: Tension-type headaches, which are the most common variety of headaches, often respond beautifully to massage, which can address both stress and the mechanical imbalances in muscle tension that are so often involved.

Tension Headaches

Tension headaches are the most common type of headache, caused by muscular tension or hypertonic muscles. Some of the muscles often involved with tension headaches include the sternocleidomastoid, suboccipitals, masseter (jaw muscle), and neck extensors (splenius cervicis and splenius capitis). Tension and TrPs in these muscles refer pain into the head and contribute to tension headaches. The pain typically occurs bilaterally (both sides) in the head and neck region. **Massage is indicated for tension headaches at all stages.**

There are numerous self-treatments for tension headaches, but doctors may prescribe ice to reduce pain and muscular spasm, pain and/or anti-inflammatory medication, muscle relaxants, or nutritional supplements such as magnesium and feverfew.

Vascular Headaches

Vascular headaches, also known as congestion headaches, are related to increased blood flow within the vessels in the cranium. Vasodilation can put pressure on the nerves, and pressure on nerves causes pain and discomfort. They are often associated with unilateral (one-sided) throbbing or stabbing pain, but the symptoms can also occur bilaterally.

Massage is indicated in the subacute stage of vascular headaches. This type of headache may require diagnostic testing such as magnetic resonance imaging or computed tomography scan to rule out underlying pathology.

Once pathology has been ruled out, professionally prescribed drug treatments may include pain medication, anti-inflammatory medication, muscle relaxants, SSRIs, or tricyclic antidepressants. Other than drug therapy, doctors sometimes identify the client's nutritional sensitivities and use stress management techniques such as acupuncture, biofeedback, exercise, and massage.

Pathological Headaches

As a massage therapist, you will not likely see a client with a pathological headache because they are caused by serious underlying conditions such as tumors, aneurysm, or CNS infection and are diagnosed and treated by a healthcare professional. These headaches are very severe and often last for days.

Massage is systemically contraindicated for pathological headaches.

Treatment for pathological headaches is always determined and supervised by the client's healthcare professional and may require surgery and/or hospitalization.

Thoracic Outlet Syndrome

Thoracic outlet syndrome (TOS) is impingement of the brachial plexus nerve bundle and the blood vessels going to and from the arm (see Thoracic Outlet Syndrome in Brief). As mentioned with fibromyalgia, a syndrome is diagnosed when a client has a collection of specific symptoms that is not a true pathological condition. Tight muscles, cervical or rib misalignment, atrophied muscles, a herniated intervertebral disk, or spondylosis (a bone spur at the nerve root) are some of the causes of this condition. TOS is characterized by paresthesia (pins and needles), tingling, shooting pain, weakness, numbness, feeling of fullness, and possible discoloration due to diminished circulation. **Massage is indicated for TOS if the impingement is caused by muscle tightness or spasm.**

If the client's TOS is related to anything other than muscular tension, massage will be locally contraindicated at the problematic area.

If the symptoms do not diminish with massage, impingement may be due to another cause and such clients should be referred to their healthcare professional to get a diagnosis and treatment plan.

Professionally prescribed treatments for TOS that clients may be using will vary, depending on the cause that has been professionally diagnosed.

Thoracic Outlet Syndrome in Brief

Pronunciation: thor-AS-ik OUT-let SIN-drome

What is it?
Thoracic outlet syndrome (TOS) is a collection of signs and symptoms brought about by occlusion of nerve and blood supply to the arm.

How is it recognized?
Depending on what structures are compressed, TOS shows shooting pains, weakness, numbness, and paresthesia (pins and needles) along with a feeling of fullness and possible discoloration of the affected hand and arm from impaired circulation.

Massage risks and benefits
Risks: Care must be taken not to exacerbate pressure on delicate structures, either with massage or with positioning on the table. Outside of this limitation, massage has no specific risks for clients with TOS.
Benefits: Massage that works to create space for unimpeded blood and nerve impulse flow can have a profound positive impact on TOS. If the problem arises from structural anomalies, massage may not make much difference beyond temporary symptomatic relief. Muscular imbalances must be addressed from multiple dimensions and directions to achieve lasting change.

Stress

One of the main reasons that people visit their healthcare practitioner is stress or its various side effects such as anxiety, depression, sleep disruption, or compromised immune function. According to Hans Selye, the man who developed the concept of stress around 1930, stress is defined as "the non-specific response of the body to any demand, whether it is caused by, or results in, pleasant or unpleasant conditions." He clarifies the difference between eustress (from the Greek root "eu" for good) and distress (from the Latin root for bad), and explains that the body itself responds similarly to eustress and distress, but that the person's attitude and emotions that accompany the stressors determine whether damage is caused to the body.

Stressors can be one or a combination of physiological or emotional factors including physical injury, pain, illness, pathology, environmental changes (temperatures, humidity, pollution), excessive stimulation from food or medication, or changes in emotional circumstances and/or states, as well as real or perceived physical or emotional threats. The body's response to a prolonged stressor is a mechanism Selye called the "general adaptation syndrome" (GAS). There are three phases of GAS:

1. The alarm reaction—the immediate fight or flight response when a stressor has been detected

2. Adaptation and resistance—the body defends itself against the stressor, and initial alarm symptoms subside or disappear as the stressor goes away or is accepted as nonthreatening

3. Exhaustion—after prolonged exposure to the stressor, the energy required for adaptation is depleted, resulting in fatigue and other symptoms of illness

Since Selye first introduced GAS to the scientific world, endless amounts of research have been performed on the neurochemistry and physiology of stress.

The body responds to stress by releasing chemicals that trigger physiological changes that help the body cope with the stressor. When the body is working efficiently and effectively, the chemicals released are completely metabolized by the body during the sympathetic nervous response, and once the stressor is no longer present, the body returns to the parasympathetic state. Sometimes the body responds inefficiently to stressors by producing too many chemicals, resulting in an inappropriate physiological response. For example, the body may not be able to respond quickly enough to a stressor, or the sympathetic nervous response may be extended for an unnecessarily long time.

Massage is indicated for the reduction of stress and the facilitation of the restoration of homeostasis. Mechanically, any basic massage techniques applied slowly and rhythmically will effectively reduce stress to the body. Reflexively, massage can combat stress by promoting the parasympathetic nervous system response, which has a restorative effect on the body.

Alert
Even though massage can affect a person's emotional state, it is out of your scope of practice to treat client's emotional issues. If you suspect clients may need professional help in this area, refer them to the appropriate healthcare professional.

Cardiovascular System Conditions

As massage therapy mechanically increases circulation, it increases the delivery of oxygen to and the removal of waste from the cells and tissues. Without oxygen, cells do not thrive and eventually die. Once the cell dies, it is destroyed and its remains are eliminated. The ends of the capillaries are very small structures and allow only small molecules to pass through. Larger particles may get caught in the very fine branches, essentially causing capillary congestion. As fragments of dead cells block the ends of the capillaries, they become less effective as transport membranes. Oxygen, other gases, and nutrients cannot get through the obstructed capillaries easily. This condition only compounds itself: the congested capillaries do not allow oxygen to pass through, the lack of oxygen causes cells to die, those cells add to the congestion, and so on. Eventually, this situation causes pain. Medically, this condition is called ischemia. Because massage mechanically enhances the circulatory system, it can alleviate ischemia by relaxing the muscles and creating more space between the muscle cells, which restores blood flow and provides better oxygen delivery and waste removal, which leads to better healing.

Increased circulation is a key to healing. Because massage techniques can mechanically enhance blood flow, they also enhance the body's healing mechanism. The healing mechanism begins when tissues are damaged:

1. Vasodilation is automatically activated to flood the injured tissues with oxygenated blood, creating additional heat and redness.

2. As the area becomes enlarged with increased blood flow, inflammation occurs.

3. The capillary walls then become thinner, allowing water to seep from the plasma, through the capillary walls, and into surrounding tissues.

4. The resultant edema, or swelling, puts extra pressure on the nerves, causing pain.

5. Once the swelling occurs, blood flow slows down and leukocytes pass through the capillaries to the injured tissues. They clean up the area, send out chemical signals to attract more leukocytes, and kill bacteria that may have entered the tissue.

6. After inflammation subsides, other healing mechanisms take place. Sometimes tissues are regenerated or scar tissue is formed to replace tissue that cannot be regenerated.

The speed of healing varies with age, health, nutrition, emotional and environmental stressors, and self-care.

Generally, massage in the acute stage (24 to 72 hours) of tissue injury should be avoided while the tissue healing process is beginning.

In the subacute stage of tissue injury and beyond, massage can increase tissue health via increased capillary transport of nutrition, may reduce emotional stress, and can be an effective element of self-care. Cardiovascular system conditions can be local or systemic. All treatments other than massage are typically prescribed by healthcare professionals who can do so within their scope of practice. Again, it is not in the massage therapist's scope of practice to diagnose or prescribe.

Bruise

A bruise (contusion) is a broken capillary or multiple capillaries in a localized area from which red blood cells seep out into the tissue, resulting from an injury such as a bump or fall. Bruises begin with, and can be recognized by, the black and bluish color that develops from deoxygenated hemoglobin molecules that cannot be resupplied with oxygen. Eventually, this hemoglobin degrades and byproducts of the breakdown give the bruise a green and yellowish color. Generally, the healing mechanism works well and should not be disturbed.

A bruise is a local contraindication for massage therapy because the injured tissue is already in the process of being repaired by the body.

Varicose Veins

Varicose veins are damaged and distended veins with internal valve damage (see Varicose Veins in Brief). Without the valves to prevent backflow of blood, the deoxygenated blood pools at the last valve that is functional. Varicose veins are often found in the legs, where the blood is moving against

Varicose Veins in Brief

Pronunciation: VARE-ih-kose vanez

What are they?
Varicose veins are distended veins, usually in the legs, caused by venous insufficiency and retrograde blood flow.

How are they recognized?
Varicose veins are ropy, bluish, elevated veins that twist and turn out of their usual course. They are most common in branches of the great saphenous veins on the medial side of the calf, although they are also found on the posterior aspects of the calf and thigh. Varicose veins can also develop at other locations, in which case they have other names.

Massage risks and benefits
Risks: Extreme varicose veins, especially with compromised skin, contraindicate any massage that might disrupt or irritate them. Milder varicose veins locally contraindicate deep specific work, but are safe for superficial massage as long as the skin is healthy. It is important to note that people with varicose veins are at increased risk for deep vein thrombosis, so massage therapists need to be knowledgeable about both conditions.
Benefits: Massage is unlikely to change or improve varicose veins. As long as they are accommodated, clients with varicose veins can enjoy the same benefits from bodywork as the rest of the population.

Hypertension in Brief

Pronunciation: hy-per-TEN-shun

What is it?
Hypertension is the technical name for high blood pressure.

How is it recognized?
High blood pressure is usually silent. The only way to identify it is by taking several blood pressure readings over time.

Massage risks and benefits
Risks: High blood pressure that accompanies other cardiovascular disease suggests that the client may have trouble adapting to changing environments, and bodywork must be adjusted accordingly. Medications that manage hypertension may also require some accommodation.
Benefits: For borderline or mild high blood pressure, massage may be a useful tool in healthcare management.

Edema in Brief

Pronunciation: eh-DEE-mah

What is it?
Edema is retention of interstitial fluid due to electrolyte or protein imbalances, or because of mechanical obstruction in the circulatory or lymphatic systems.

How is it recognized?
Edematous tissue is puffy or boggy in early stages. It may become hard (indurated) if it is not resolved quickly. The area may be hot if associated with local infection, or quite cool if local circulation is impaired.

Massage risks and benefits
Risks: Most forms of edema contraindicate massage, especially when the tissue is indurated or nonresilient. In these situations, a chemical imbalance or physical obstruction must be resolved before most types of bodywork are safe.
Benefits: Acute edema that is not related to infection may be appropriate for lymphatic types of massage. Subacute or postacute musculoskeletal injuries may be edematous and respond well to various bodywork approaches.

gravity most of the time, and are recognized by their bluish, ropey, and elevated appearance. Deep, specific massage techniques should be avoided over varicose veins, but whole-body, superficial massage is indicated.

Doctors sometimes treat varicose veins with support hose, elastic bandages, elevation of the legs, injections of chemicals into the affected vein to shut it down, or surgical removal.

Lymphatic and Immune System Conditions

Because massage therapy mechanically increases the movement of lymph, it can enhance the health of a body and the healing process.

High Blood Pressure (Hypertension)

High blood pressure, or hypertension, is a condition in which the blood inside the blood vessels is pushing harder than average on the walls of the blood vessels (see Hypertension in Brief). Typically, the presence and severity of hypertension is diagnosed by an MD, and the client may be taking some type of medication for this condition.

In severe cases of high blood pressure, massage is systemically contraindicated until clients get their healthcare professional's approval for receiving massage treatment.

For mild cases of high blood pressure, massage is indicated to reduce physical stress and encourage the parasympathetic response within the body. When clients come to you for massage therapy, their doctors may have prescribed blood pressure medications or dietary changes such as reduction of salt or fat intake.

Edema

Edema is a lymphatic condition that occurs when excess fluid is retained between the cells (see Edema in brief). It is characterized by puffy and swollen tissue in an area where fluid is retained. **When edema is related to immobility, inactivity, or musculoskeletal injury, massage is indicated.** It can help return the lymphatic fluid to the heart by increasing the client's circulation.

Massage is systemically contraindicated for edema in the cases where a doctor has diagnosed a specific pathological condition because massage can potentially make the condition and the resulting edema worse.

Medical prescriptions for edema with an underlying pathological cause include diuretic medications that reduce the blood volume in the body by causing it to excrete more water via urine.

Fever

The normal body temperature is 98.6°F, which can vary by a couple of degrees, depending on the person and the time of day. In most adults, fever is the body's immune system response that raises the body's core temperature above 100°F when measuring orally, or above 101°F when measuring a rectal or ear temperature (see Fever in brief). Children have a fever when their rectal temperature is 100.4°F or higher. Usually as the result of a bacterial or viral infection, the body elevates its core temperature (brings on fever) to help destroy the invading bacteria or virus. Increased body temperature stimulates leukocyte production, prevents bacterial and viral growth by limiting the liver's release of iron, stimulates antiviral agent (interferon) production, increases the heart rate to circulate more leukocytes, and speeds up chemical reactions and cell wall permeability. The disadvantage of fever is the accompanying discomfort. In the case of high fever involving temperatures over 104°F, complications may arise. Blood chemistry falls out of balance, and dehydration and brain damage are possible.

During a fever, massage that requires an adaptive response is strictly contraindicated because the body is going through an acute healing process. Reflexive or very light massage, however, may help a client with a fever sleep better.

Respiratory System Conditions

There are infectious and noninfectious respiratory conditions you may encounter in your office. To maintain the most sanitary environment for you and your clients, your goal is to prevent the spread of pathogens, so be particularly aware of clients who cough and sneeze, and make sure you thoroughly disinfect surfaces that may have been contaminated: doorknobs, chairs, desktops, etc.

The Common Cold

The common cold is a viral infection of the upper respiratory tract (see Common Cold in Brief). It may be characterized by mild fever, headache, sore throat, postnasal drip, congestion, and coughing.

Massage is contraindicated in the acute stage (24 to 72 hours) of a cold, or if fever is present.

Massage is indicated for a cold in the subacute stage (after 72 hours).

Although many people self-prescribe for the common cold, healthcare professionals also prescribe treatments including rest, increased fluid intake, antihistamine medications, decongestants, and cough suppressants.

Sinusitis

Sinusitis is a condition of inflamed paranasal sinuses (see Sinusitis in Brief). Infectious cases can be caused by a number of pathogens and noninfectious cases can result from allergies or physical obstructions.

In the acute stage of an infectious case of sinusitis, massage is systemically contraindicated.

In chronic and noninfectious cases of sinusitis, clients can receive massage, but you should be aware of their comfort. Some client may not feel comfortable in the face cradle or in the prone position. **Massage is appropriate for chronic and noninfectious cases of sinusitis, as long as the client is comfortable.**

Treatment for sinusitis ranges from simply raising the humidity of the air and increasing water intake, to over-the-counter decongestants, to prescription-strength corticosteroids and antibiotics.

Sinusitis in Brief

Pronunciation: sy-nus-I-tis

What is it?
Sinusitis is inflammation of the paranasal sinuses from infection, allergies, or physical obstruction.

How is it recognized?
Signs and symptoms include headaches; tenderness over the affected area; runny or congested nose; facial or tooth pain; headache; fatigue; and, if it's related to an infection, thick, opaque mucus, fever, and chills.

Massage risks and benefits
Risks: Acute sinus infections contraindicate any bodywork that could exacerbate symptoms. If the client has fever, chills, and other signs of systemic infection, it is best to delay any rigorous massage until this has passed. A client with a tendency toward inflamed sinuses may have problems lying flat on a table, especially, face down. It is important to be able to make accommodations for this problem.
Benefits: Very gentle massage around the face, as long as no infection is present, may help the sinuses to drain, and for sinus pain to diminish. A client with inflamed sinuses who does not have an infection can benefit from bodywork as long as he or she is comfortable on the table.

Asthma

Asthma is a chronic obstructive pulmonary disease that occurs when the smooth muscles of the bronchial tubes constrict and their membranes are inflamed and have produced excessive mucus (see Asthma in Brief). The result is an asthma attack, which is marked by coughing, wheezing, and difficulty breathing, especially exhaling. Clients who have asthma have typically been diagnosed by a health professional and know how to treat their symptoms.

Massage is contraindicated for clients who are in the midst of an asthma attack.

Clients who live with asthma may have hypertonic muscles of respiration, including the scalenes, intercostals, and diaphragm. **Massage is beneficial for clients who have asthma, but because they may be hypersensitive to scents and oils, you should have lubricants available that are hypoallergenic.**

Treatment for asthma requires patients to raise awareness of their condition and try to avoid the stimuli that trigger attacks. Steroids and bronchodilators are sometimes prescribed to reduce inflammation and open up the bronchioles.

Asthma in Brief

Pronunciation: AZ-muh

What is it?
Asthma is the result of airway inflammation, intermittent airflow obstruction, and bronchial hyperresponsiveness.

How is it recognized?
Asthma attacks are sporadic episodes involving coughing, wheezing, and difficulty with breathing, especially exhaling.

Massage risks and benefits
Risks: A client in the midst of an acute asthma attack is not a good candidate for massage. It is important to prepare the session room for clients with a tendency toward asthma by avoiding scents, candles, and essential oils that might exacerbate symptoms, and by using a hypoallergenic lubricant.
Benefits: Clients with asthma or other breathing problems, who are not in the midst of an acute episode, typically have extremely tight breathing muscles: the diaphragm, intercostals, and scalenes can benefit from any work that improves their efficiency.

Digestive System Conditions

Stress evokes a sympathetic nervous system response, which slows digestive activity. Clients who suffer from gastrointestinal conditions may or may not be under the care of a healthcare professional, so you need to know when to refer a client to a doctor for a diagnosis and treatment as well as be aware of some of the more common conditions and how to deliver safe and effective massage.

Irritable Bowel Syndrome

Spastic colon, mucus colitis, and functional bowel syndrome are other names for irritable bowel syndrome (IBS) (see Irritable Bowel Syndrome in Brief). Although symptoms vary with individuals, most clients with IBS will have irregular bowel activity, suffering from both constipation and diarrhea, abdominal bloating, and intestinal cramping. Stress and anxiety often cause symptoms of IBS, and sometimes diet can aggravate the condition. **Massage can benefit clients with IBS as long as their symptoms are not aggravated with bodywork.**

Peptic Ulcers

Peptic ulcers, commonly known as ulcers, are open sores in the esophagus, stomach, and duodenum that are resistant to healing due to physical irritation or ineffective healing processes (see Peptic Ulcers in Brief). Accompanied by burning

---

Peptic Ulcers in Brief

Pronunciation: PEP-tik UL-surz

What are they?
Ulcers are sores that for various reasons don't heal normally; they remain open and vulnerable to infection. Peptic ulcers occur on the inner surfaces of the esophagus, stomach, or duodenum.

How are they recognized?
The symptoms of peptic ulcers include general burning or gnawing abdominal pain between meals that is relieved by taking antacids or eating. Other symptoms include bloating, burping, gas, and vomiting after meals.

Massage risks and benefits
Risks: Specific or intrusive work on the abdomen may exacerbate symptoms of peptic ulcers. Also, because massage tends to stimulate digestive activity, clients may want to time their massage sessions around their eating schedule.
Benefits: Massage has no direct impact on peptic ulcers, but the overall parasympathetic effect that usually accompanies bodywork may be a positive experience for a person who struggles with this condition.

---

pain in the stomach or chest that is sometimes eased by eating, other symptoms include abdominal bloating, burping, or vomiting after meals.

Massage that involves mechanical manipulation or pressure is locally contraindicated for peptic ulcers.

This condition is diagnosed by a healthcare professional who may prescribe antibiotics and other chemicals that reduce acid production. Some types of ulcers do not respond to medications and instead respond better when medications that damage the stomach lining are simply avoided. **Massage can be beneficial for clients with peptic ulcers because it reduces stress, increases circulation of blood and lymph, and aids healing, as long as the abdomen is avoided.**

Endocrine System Conditions

Most people with endocrine system conditions can receive massage safely and can benefit from it, but it is best to work cooperatively with the primary healthcare professional. Just as massage can increase the circulation of endocrine system secretions, it can also increase the delivery of medications clients may be taking for endocrine conditions.

Irritable Bowel Syndrome in Brief

What is it?
Irritable bowel syndrome (IBS) is a collection of signs and symptoms that indicate a problem with colon function. Symptoms are aggravated by stress and diet.

How is it recognized?
The symptoms of IBS include abdominal pain along with constipation or diarrhea (or alternating between the two); bloating or abdominal distension; and a sensation of incomplete emptying with defecation.

Massage risks and benefits
Risks: Massage poses no specific risks for clients with IBS as long as they are comfortable receiving bodywork.
Benefits: If the experience of touch feels safe to a client with IBS, massage can be a powerful aid to someone whose digestive comfort is related to stress.

Diabetes Mellitus

One of the most common endocrine system conditions you will encounter in your practice is diabetes mellitus (see Diabetes Mellitus in Brief). When the body is unable to properly metabolize sugars (such as glucose) due to low levels of insulin or ineffective insulin receptor sites, blood sugar rises. Some of the excess sugars can be eliminated in the urine without trouble, but as the blood sugar rises to an abnormally high level (hyperglycemia), excess water is pulled from the body's cells to eliminate the extra sugars. Symptoms often include frequent urination, excessive thirst, and elevated appetite as well as weight loss, nausea, and vomiting. Because the body is unable to metabolize glucose, which is the most efficient cellular fuel, the body turns to stored fat and proteins such as muscle tissue. The problem with burning muscle tissue for fuel is that there is a lot of cellular waste that can cause complications such as cardiovascular disease, edema, ulcers and amputations, kidney disease, impaired vision or blindness, and neuropathy. Hyperglycemia can also cause ketoacidosis, a condition in which the pH balance of the blood becomes too acidic. Prolonged ketoacidosis can lead to diabetic shock, coma, and even death.

The most common kinds of diabetes are type 1 and type 2. Type 1 diabetics must measure their blood sugar levels regularly and take insulin to metabolize sugars and keep their blood sugar in a safe range. If they take too much insulin, their blood sugar can drop too low (hypoglycemia) and lead to insulin shock, an emergency condition characterized by confusion, weakness, and dizziness. Type 2 diabetes, sometimes called adult-onset diabetes, is usually manageable with proper diet and exercise, but some type 2 diabetics have to supplement with insulin. **Massage is generally safe for diabetic clients who have good circulation and healthy tissues. Because massage may reduce blood sugar, diabetic clients should not receive massage shortly after taking insulin.** Just in case a diabetic client starts acting confused, weak, or dizzy (signs of hypoglycemia), it is a good idea to have snacks available that are high in sugar such as candy or fruit juice.

Diabetes Mellitus in Brief

Pronunciation: di-ah-BE-tez meh-LY-tus

What is it?
Diabetes is a group of metabolic disorders characterized by problems with glucose metabolism.

How is it recognized?
Early symptoms of diabetes include frequent urination, thirst, and increased appetite along with weight loss, nausea, and vomiting. These symptoms can be subtle enough that the first indicators of disease are the complications it can cause: neuropathy, impaired vision, kidney dysfunction, or other problems.

Massage risks and benefits
Risks: If the circulatory and urinary systems are impaired, a client with diabetes may have limited capacity to adapt to the changes that rigorous massage demands. Advanced disease can result in skin damage and ulcers, especially to the legs and feet; these are cautions for bodywork as well. Numbness associated with diabetic neuropathy can interfere with a client's ability to give accurate feedback about pain and pressure. And massage has been seen to drop blood sugar; clients may experience hypoglycemia if they have a massage and supplement insulin without adequate food.

Benefits: A client with well-managed diabetes and no contraindicating complications can enjoy the same benefits from massage as the rest of the population, with the caveat that massage may temporarily cause a drop in blood sugar, so the client and therapist should anticipate that possibility.

Breast Cancer in Brief

What is it?
Breast cancer is the growth of malignant tumor cells in breast tissue. These cells can invade skin and nearby muscles and bones. If they invade lymph nodes, they can metastasize to the rest of the body.

How is it recognized?
The first sign of breast cancer is a small painless lump or thickening in the breast tissue or near the axilla. The lump may be too small to palpate, but may show on a mammogram. Later the skin may change texture, the nipple may change shape, and discharge may occur.

Massage risks and benefits
Risks: Breast cancer patients undergo treatments that are extremely taxing on general health as well as on physical and emotional well-being. Ports or other surgical equipment may be present. Further, this cancer can invade the skeleton, leading to unstable and easily fractured bones. Any bodywork in this context must respect all these challenges.

Benefits: As long as the challenges of both breast cancer and its treatments are accommodated, massage can be a wonderful, supportive, important coping mechanism for many patients.

Reproductive System Conditions

Massage mechanically increases circulation to help maintain the health of reproductive organs. Massage can provide some relief from symptoms by reducing the stress level and by increasing circulation. Because relaxation massage induces a parasympathetic nervous response, all of the parasympathetic effects can occur, including penile erection.

Breast Cancer

Breast cancer is malignant tumor growth in the breast tissue that may spread to the skin, muscles, lymph nodes, and the rest of the body (see Breast Cancer in Brief). Although men are also diagnosed with breast cancer, most cases occur in women. Breast cancer is characterized by a small, often painless lump or thickening of the breast tissue and can be detected by breast self-exams and mammograms. **According to the American Cancer Society, early detection of breast cancer through breast self-exams, clinical breast exams, and mammograms is critical to reducing the breast cancer death rate.**

Massage for cancer patients can be controversial. The treating physician should be included in the decision to include massage as part of the client's healthcare regimen, and many physicians will advise against massage.

 If you massage a client with cancer, local contraindications include any areas that are affected by edema, surgery, soreness, or numbness. With breast cancer patients, the lymph nodes, especially in the axillary area, should be avoided.

Massage can help cancer patients feel better and can encourage homeostasis, but again, discuss massage treatment with the client's physician. Clients who have lost their hair because of chemotherapy treatment may especially enjoy having their scalps massaged. Medical treatment for breast cancer may include surgery, radiation treatment or chemotherapy to reduce the growth of the tumor(s), and hormone therapy.

Prostate Cancer

Prostate cancer occurs when malignant tumor cells grow in the prostate gland, and may spread to the bones or lymph nodes nearby (see Prostate Cancer in Brief). A diagnosis is officially made by an MD and symptoms include urination problems in the early stages and blood in the urine, painful ejaculation, and bone pain in the later stages. **Massage may be indicated for prostate cancer, but only if approved by the client's healthcare professional.**

Prostate Cancer in Brief

Pronunciation: PROS-tate KAN-ser

What is it?
Prostate cancer is the growth of malignant cells in the prostate gland, which may metastasize, usually to nearby bones or into pelvic or inguinal lymph nodes.

How is it recognized?
The symptoms of prostate cancer include problems with urination: weak stream, frequency, urgency, nocturia, all arising from constriction of the urethra. Later symptoms include blood in the urine, painful ejaculation, and persistent bone pain.

Massage risks and benefits
Risks: Massage for prostate cancer patients, as with all cancer patients, must be gauged to the constitutional health and resilience of the client. Accommodations for both the disease, which may lead to bone damage, and for the treatments, which can involve anything from chemotherapy to radiation to surgery, must be individualized for each client.
Benefits: As with all cancer patients, massage that respects both the disease and the challenges presented by treatment can be an effective strategy for managing pain, insomnia, depression, anxiety, and many other complications related to this challenging disorder.

Treatments prescribed by the doctor may include radiation or chemotherapy, which may reduce the growth of the tumor, or hormone therapy.

Pregnancy

While pregnancy is not a dysfunction or pathological condition, it is a special condition of the reproductive system that you, as a massage therapist, must understand. During pregnancy, a woman's body undergoes many hormonal, chemical, and physical changes that require special attention during a massage. Pregnant women often suffer nausea and vomiting during the early stages of pregnancy. As the body constantly changes shape and balance, the proprioceptors constantly provide different information regarding muscle tension and position. The pregnant woman cannot "get used to" a balanced posture and can feel clumsy or uncoordinated. Additionally, ligaments are hormonally triggered to loosen up toward the end of pregnancy, destabilizing the pelvis. The fetus can put pressure on circulatory structures, causing complications, and the size and weight of the baby can make almost any position uncomfortable.

In an uncomplicated pregnancy, massage is indicated with specific considerations for each trimester. More specific information regarding pregnancy is covered in the Special Populations chapter.

Conditions of the Special Senses

The special senses include proprioception, vision, hearing, smell, and taste. The abnormal conditions affecting the special senses do not typically have specific contraindications, but the therapist may need to pay special attention to the needs of these clients. Massage is generally safe for clients who suffer from conditions of the special senses.

Clients who are deaf or blind will require special attention from the therapist to ensure a safe, relaxing, and comfortable massage experience. Clients with compromised proprioception may need the therapist to offer a stabilizing hand to keep from falling or injuring themselves, such as when they are getting on and off the table or turning over during a massage session.

CHAPTER SUMMARY

Having a fundamental understanding of pathology and pharmacology is important for you as a massage therapist. It will help you know when a massage as well as a certain technique/s are indicated and contraindicated for a particular client within the context of any given session. Keeping the rule, "when in doubt, don't," should always be in the forefront of your mind as you make decisions regarding each individual massage session. Additionally, consulting the In Brief boxes in this chapter or a pathology text specific to massage will help you decide how to approach and what techniques to include or exclude in a certain massage session. Having this decision-making process will help best serve your client's unique massage needs.

CHAPTER EXERCISES

1. Define the following terms and explain why it is important for a massage therapist to know them:

   a. Pathology
   b. Etiology
   c. Pharmacology

2. Describe the following phases of pathological conditions:

   a. Acute
   b. Subacute
   c. Chronic

3. Identify at least five pathological conditions for which massage is indicated.

4. Give five examples of local contraindications and two examples of systemic contraindications.

5. Describe the pain–spasm cycle.

6. Define "trigger points" and identify at least three contributing factors to their formation.

7. Explain the general adaptation syndrome (GAS) mechanism as it relates to prolonged stress.

8. Describe the difference between sprain and strain.

9. Explain why a fever is contraindicated for massage therapy.

10. Describe the benefits of massage therapy in the subacute and chronic stages of a muscle spasm.

SUGGESTED READINGS

Ashton J, Cassel D. *Review for Therapeutic Massage & Bodywork Exams.* Philadelphia: Lippincott Williams & Wilkins, 2011.

Balch PA, Balch JF. *Prescription for Nutritional Healing.* New York: Avery, 2000.

Benjamin B, Borden G. *Listen to your Pain, The Active Person's Guide to Understanding and Identifying and Treating Pain and Injury.* New York: Penguin Books, 1984.

Biel A. *Trail Guide to the Body.* Boulder, CO: Books of Discovery, 1997.

Buchholz D. *Heal Your Headache: The 1•2•3 Program for Taking Charge of your Pain.* New York: Workman Publishing, 2002.

Calais-Germain B. *Anatomy of Movement.* Seattle, WA: Eastland Press, 1993.

Chaitow L. *Fibromyalgia and Muscle Pain: Your Self-Treatment Guide.* London: Thorsons, 2001.

Chaitow L. *Fibromyalgia Syndrome: A Practitioner's Guide to Treatment.* London: Churchill Livingstone, 2000.

Chaitow L, Bradley D, Gilbert C. *Multidisciplinary Approaches to Breathing Pattern Disorders.* London: Churchill Livingstone, 2002.

Clemente C. *Gray's Anatomy.* 30th ed. Philadelphia: Lippincott Williams & Wilkins, 1985.

Cohen BJ, Wood DL. *Memmler's Structure and Function of the Human Body.* 9th ed. Philadelphia: Lippincott Williams & Wilkins, 2009.

Crowley LV, Abrams C. *Physiology.* Springhouse, PA: Springhouse Corporation, 1993.

Gray H, Lewis WH. *Anatomy of the Human Body.* 23rd ed. Philadelphia: Lea & Febiger, 1936.

Guinness AE, ed. *ABC's of the Human Body, A Family Answer Book.* Pleasantville, NY: Readers Digest Association, 1987.

Hendrickson T. *Massage for Orthopedic Conditions.* Philadelphia: Lippincott Williams & Wilkins, 2003.

Kendall FP, McCreary EK, Provance PG. *Muscle Testing and Function.* 4th ed. Baltimore: Williams & Wilkins, 1993.

Lowe WW. *Functional Assessment in Massage Therapy.* 2nd ed. Corvallis, OR: Pacific Orthopedic Massage, 1995.

Marieb EN. *Essentials of Human Anatomy and Physiology.* 5th ed. Menlo Park, CA: Benjamin/Cummings, 1997.

Mauskop A, Fox B. *What your Doctor May Not Tell You About Migraines: The Breakthrough Program that Can Help End Your Pain.* New York: Warner Books, 2001.

Melloni JL, Dox I, Melloni HP, Melloni BJ. *Melloni's Illustrated Review of Human Anatomy.* Philadelphia: JB Lippincott, 1988.

Northrup C. *Women's Bodies, Women's Wisdom.* New York: Bantam Books, 1998.

Paulino J, Griffith CJ. *The Headache Sourcebook.* New York: Contemporary Books/McGraw Hill, 2001.

Pharmacology for Massage Therapy and Massage Therapy and Medications.

Physicians' Desk Reference Pocket Guide to Prescription Drugs. 5th ed. New York: Pocket Books, 2002.

Persad RS. *Massage Therapy and Medications General Treatment Principles.* Toronto: Curties-Overzet, 2001.

Rattray F, Ludwig L. *Clinical Massage Therapy: Understanding, Assessing and Treating over 70 Conditions.* Toronto: Talus, 2000.

Starlanyl D, Copeland ME. *Fibromyalgia and Chronic Myofascial Pain: A Survival Manual.* 2nd ed. New York: New Harbinger Publications, 2001.

Takahashi T (editorial supervisor). *Atlas of the Human Body.* New York: HarperCollins, 1994.

Theodosakis MD, Adderly B, Fox B. *The Arthritis Cure.* New York: St. Martin's Press, 1997.

Travell JG, Simons DG. *Myofascial Pain and Dysfunction: The Trigger Point Manual.* Vol 1. Philadelphia: Lippincott Williams & Wilkins, 1983.

Travell JG, Simons DG. *Myofascial Pain and Dysfunction: The Trigger Point Manual.* Vol 2. Philadelphia: Lippincott Williams & Wilkins, 1992.

Utting, B. Lecture notes presented at: Utting School of Massage; 1994; Seattle, WA.

Versagi C. *Step-by-Step Massage Therapy Protocols for Common Conditions.* Philadelphia: Lippincott Williams & Wilkins, 2012.

Watkins J. *Structure and Function of the Musculoskeletal System.* Champaign, IL: Human Kinetics, 1999.

Werner R. *A Massage Therapist's Guide to Pathology.* Baltimore: Lippincott Williams & Wilkins, 1998.

Werner R. *A Massage Therapist's Guide to Pathology.* 3rd ed. Baltimore: Lippincott Williams & Wilkins, 2005.

Werner R. *A Massage Therapist's Guide to Pathology.* 5th ed. Baltimore: Lippincott Williams & Wilkins, 2013.

Willis MC. *Medical Terminology: The Language of Healthcare.* Baltimore: Lippincott Williams & Wilkins, 1996.

http://firstaid.webmd.com/body-temperature, accessed 2.21.12.

http://www.ahealthyme.com, accessed 3.5.06.

http://www.bartleby.com/107/pages/page502.html, accessed 3.5.06.

http://www.cancer.gov, accessed 3.5.06.

http://www.cancer.org, accessed 2.22.12.

http://www.cdc.gov, accessed 3.5.06.

http://www.cell-biology.com, accessed 3.5.06.

http://www.dermnet.org.nz/index.html, accessed 3.5.06.

http://www.e-histology.net, accessed 3.5.06.

http://www.estrellamountain.edu/faculty/farabee/biobk/biobooktoc .html, accessed 3.5.06.

http://www.factmonster.com/ce6/sci/A0843878.html, accessed 3.5.06.

http://www.infoplease.com/ce6/sci/A0818305.html, accessed 3.5.06.

http://www.intelihealth.com/IH/ihtIH, accessed 3.5.06.

http://www.mayoclinic.com/health/fibromyalgia-symptoms/AR00054, accessed 2.25.12.

http://www.mayoclinic.com/invoke.cfm?objectid~43CB5F79-2B33-4F96 -B7D06EC696826071, accessed 3.5.06.

http://www.medterms.com/script/main/art.asp?articlekey=2155, accessed 3.10.06.

http://www.nih.gov/icd/, accessed 3.5.06.

http://www.nlm.nih.gov/medlineplus/, accessed 3.5.06.

http://www.rheumatology.org/practice/clinical/patients/diseases_and _conditions/fibromyalgia.asp, accessed 2.25.12.

http://www.unomaha.edu/;swick/2740connectivetissue.html#ret, accessed 3.5.06.

http://www.webmd.com, accessed 3.5.06.

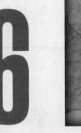

6

Communication and Documentation

Objectives

Upon completion of this chapter, the student will be able to:

- Identify the three word elements
- Translate at least five medical terms by using the 5-step guideline
- Describe at least four factors of effective communication and interviewing skills
- Define reflective listening
- List at least five specific examples of nonverbal communication

- Give at least five reasons why a massage therapist should document every massage session
- Describe the information recorded in each section of a SOAP note
- List at least 15 questions to include in a client history
- Describe the difference between short- and long-term goals
- List at least 10 abbreviations commonly used in massage treatment records

Key Terms

Activity and analysis information: The massage activity and an analysis of the treatment session documented on the SOAP note.

Confidentiality: Keeping information private unless the client expressly permits you to share it.

HIPAA: Health Insurance Portability and Accountability Act, enacted in 1996 to help employees and their families obtain and transfer health insurance coverage when their employment changes or is terminated.

Massage treatment record: The document containing input from clients, your objective assessments of the clients' condition, the massage techniques you use, results of the treatment session, and plans for future massage treatment.

Objective information: Your visual, palpation, range-of-motion, and gait assessments of the client's body and soft tissues documented on the SOAP note.

Plan information: The section of the SOAP note including plans for future treatment and self-care recommendations.

Privacy Rule (Standards for Privacy of Individually Identifiable Health Information): A modification of the original HIPAA that legally protects health-related information from being shared without clients' written permission by requiring all healthcare practitioners to keep their clients' health information private and protected.

SOAP: An acronym for Subjective, Objective, Activity and analysis, and Plan that refers to a format for documentation.

Subjective information: Verbal and written information clients share with you regarding their health documented in the SOAP note.

Treatment goal: A specific goal that is determined after therapeutic massage treatment to clarify progress toward overcoming functional limitations.

This chapter introduces key medical terminology used in the field of massage therapy as well as pertinent elements of communication and documentation. Together, they provide the foundation for communicating with clients and other healthcare professionals. With practice and commitment, your mastery of these components will enhance your professionalism and help you earn your due respect as a healthcare practitioner.

Learning this language may be challenging, but it is very possible if you commit to the learning process and are willing to practice, practice, practice. It is worth the time and effort because a working knowledge of medical terminology has many benefits for the massage therapist. It will save time in communication with clients and other healthcare professionals and in record keeping, and it can minimize confusion, help maintain a professional image, and increase your knowledge base. **Knowledge is power!**

Begin by learning the basic rules of the medical language, and then learn some individual words. Over time and with practice, you will develop the confidence to use the words comfortably when speaking about healthcare.

Most of the medical terms can be broken down into separate word elements that help simplify the meanings, and numerous medical dictionaries are available to help with spelling, pronunciation, and definitions. Having the appropriate references available and knowing how to use them is a more powerful tool than trying to memorize all the words.

Once you are familiar with the terminology, you can start to develop your communication skills. Effective communication, interviewing skills, and documentation are vital to the therapeutic process for both the massage therapist and the client. While massage therapy evolves as part of complementary medicine, documentation contributes to the professional quality of your work.

Good documentation also helps you assess the client's condition to determine the appropriateness and type of treatment, improvements, setbacks, treatment goals, and clinical reasoning. More than just a written record, documentation provides clues regarding the client's health history as well as a "road map" to effective initial and session-to-session treatment.

Medical Terminology

Communication is a key element to a successful massage therapy business. For massage therapists, communication requires a working knowledge of medical terminology because you converse with many healthcare professionals. To be respected and considered professional, you need to understand what other health professionals are saying when they refer to a treatment or a body part, and you need to be able to use the same terms. In short, you must learn to speak a common language. Since modern medical terminology has its origins in Greek and Latin words, the language is consistent across the world, which makes it one of the most practical languages to learn. Medical language continues to evolve, and terms are added that are not based on either Greek or Latin. Some of these terms are named for people who discover a body part (Broca's area of the brain) or disease (Alzheimer's disease) or who develop a procedure (Heimlich maneuver), test (Tinel's test), or device (Foley catheter).

Using these unfamiliar terms in class and practicing them at home can raise your comfort level with your new language. You can increase your learning by reinforcing it

with different combinations of processes. For instance, you can practice the language by writing terms on paper and spelling them aloud; by reading silently and saying the terms aloud; by reading the definitions, closing your eyes, and reciting the definitions; and by making up sentences that use the terms. The more ways you practice, using your eyes, ears, mouth, and hands, the more effective the learning. Eventually, you will be able to communicate with clients, keep professional records, and communicate with other healthcare professionals comfortably and easily.

The learning process does not end when you are able to use the language on a functional level. As long as you practice massage, you will need to communicate with clients and other healthcare professionals, and you will not know every medical term that exists. One of the most useful tools for learning language is a dictionary that provides English translations and definitions. Medical dictionaries, which provide definitions and pronunciations for scientific and medical terminology, are widely available and are an excellent tool to have in the office. When clients and other healthcare professionals refer to conditions, diseases, anatomical parts, or directional terms that you may not recognize or remember, you can use your medical dictionary to figure them out.

In addition to being a useful tool for you, a medical dictionary can be an educational tool for your clients. All massage therapists should understand medical language and be able to use it on a functional level, but the words and terminology each therapist uses with her clients is an individual choice. Some clients expect their therapists to use medical terminology, but others are intimidated by it. Gauge your client's comfort level and use language that keeps your client at ease but still promotes professionalism. Sometimes primary care physicians use medical terms their patients do not understand, and those patients may be uncomfortable asking the healthcare professionals for explanations. People occasionally ask their massage therapists for explanations or definitions of medical words. Pulling out a medical dictionary and finding information with your client is an opportunity to learn and teach at the same time. Demonstrating your interest in the client's concerns while admitting that you do not know everything, but are willing to learn, generates trust and respect from your client.

Word Elements

The challenging process of learning this new language can be simplified by breaking medical terms down into smaller parts. Compound words are created by combining two or more words, and the definition of the compound word generally is a combination of the meanings of the two independent words. For example, the word "headache" is a compound word made up of the words "head" and "ache," and the definition is a simple combination of those two words. Likewise, most medical terms are created by combining two or three of the following word elements: the root, the prefix, and the suffix.

Roots

The root is the core building block that provides the basic meaning for the word. Typically, it refers to an organ, anatomical structure, body region, or disease. For example:

Organs
- hepat(o) refers to the liver
- cardi(o) refers to the heart

Anatomical structures
- brachi(o) refers to the arm
- cost(o) refers to the ribs
- my(o) refers to the muscle

Body regions
- abdomin(o) refers to the abdomen
- thorac(o) refers to the chest or thorax

Diseases
- carcin(o) refers to cancer
- toxic(o) and tox(o) refer to poison

The derivation of some roots is not always so scientific. For instance, the word "muscle" comes from the Latin word meaning mouse, because the movement of a muscle under the skin resembles the scampering movement of a mouse. The coccyx is named after the cuckoo bird, because the shape of the bone resembles the cuckoo's bill.

Just as there are exceptions to every rule, there are odd situations in which context and medical dictionaries are especially helpful. For instance, some roots have two different meanings, as illustrated below:

myel(o) refers to both
- spinal cord
- bone marrow

scler(o) refers to both
- hardening
- the white of the eye

cyst(i) and cyst(o) refer to both
- filled sac
- urinary bladder

There are also some instances in which two different roots refer to the same term. Since Greek and Latin serve as the basis for medical terms, sometimes each language provides a root for the same term. For example, the Greek root "nephr(o)" and the Latin root "ren" both refer to the kidney. Table 6-1 lists commonly used roots, their meanings, and examples of their usage.

Prefixes

Prefixes are the word elements that come before the root. They change, further specify, or alter the meaning of the root by referring to numbers, amounts, directions, positions, changes, and comparisons. For example:

Numbers or amounts
- bi- two
- hyper- excessive or too much
- hypo- not enough or under
- poly- many or much
- semi- half or partial
- tri- three

Directions and positions
- ab- away from
- ad- toward
- ante- before

Table 6-1   Commonly Used Roots (more common ones in bold)

ROOT	MEANING	EXAMPLE	DEFINITION
abdomin(o)	abdomen	rectus abdominus	abdominal muscle along midline of body
adrenal(o), adren(o)	adrenal	adrenaline	chemical produced by the adrenal gland
angi(o)	vessel	angioplasty	reconstructive surgery on blood vessels
arteri(o), arter(o)	artery	arterial	pertaining to the arteries
arthr(o)	joint	arthritis	inflammation of a joint
brachi(o)	arm	brachialis	muscle of the arm
bronch(i), bronch(o)	bronchus	bronchitis	inflammation of the bronchi in the lungs
cardi(o)	heart	cardiology	study of the heart
cephal(o)	head	cephalad	toward the head
cerebr(o)	cerebrum	cerebrospinal fluid	fluid that bathes the brain and spinal cord
cervic(o)	neck	cervical vertebrae	spinal segments of the neck
chondr(o)	cartilage	chondritis	inflammation of cartilage
cost(o)	rib	intercostals	muscles between ribs
crani(o)	skull	cranial nerves	major nerves in the skull
cyt(o)	cell	cytoplasm	fluid within the cell
dent(i), dent(o)	teeth	dentist	tooth and gum specialist
dermat(o), derm(o)	skin	dermatitis	inflammation of the skin
fibr(o)	fiber, fibrous	fibrositis	inflammation of fibrous connective tissue, muscles
gastr(o)	stomach	gastritis	inflammation of the stomach
gynec(o), gyn(o)	woman	gynecology	study of the female reproductive organs
hem(o), hemat(o)	blood	hematoma	localized collection or clot of blood
hepat(o)	liver	hepatology	study of the liver
hist(o)	tissue	histology	study of cells and tissues
hydr(o)	water	hydrotherapy	treatment using water internally and/or externally
ili(o)	ilium	iliacus	muscle that attaches to the ilium
laryng(o)	larynx	laryngitis	inflammation of the larynx
my(o)	muscle	myositis	inflammation of the muscle
myel(o)	spinal cord, bone marrow	myelin	protective covering of nerves
nephr(o)	kidney	nephrology	study of the kidney
neur(i), neur(o)	nerve	neurology	study of the nervous system

continues on following page

Table 6-1 Commonly Used Roots (most common ones in bold) *continued*

ROOT	MEANING	EXAMPLE	DEFINITION
ocul(o)	eye	oculomotor nerve	nerve that controls eye movement
oss, oste(o)	bone	osteoporosis	condition where bones become porous and fragile
ot(o)	ear	otitis	inflammation in the ear
ped(i), ped(o)	child	pediatrics	branch of medicine specializing in children
pneumat(o), pneum(o)	breathing, respiration	pneumonia	inflammation in the lungs
pod(o)	foot	podiatrist	foot specialist
psych(o)	mind	psychology	study of the mind
pulm(o), pulmon(o)	lung	pulmonologist	lung specialist
rhin(o)	nose	rhinoplasty	reconstructive surgery of the nose
stern(o)	chest,	sternum	flat bone between ribs in center of chest
therm(o)	heat	thermometer	device for measuring heat
thorac(o)	chest, thorax	thoracic vertebrae	vertebral segments of the thorax
thyr(o)	thyroid	hypothyroidism	condition in which thyroid produces insufficient hormones
toxic(o), tox(o)	poison, toxin	toxicology	study of toxins, poisons
trache(o)	trachea	tracheostomy	surgical opening in trachea
troph(o)	growth	hypertrophy	excessive growth
ur(o), urin(o)	urinary tract, urination	urologist	urinary system specialist
ven(o)	vein	venule	a little vein
vertebr(o)	vertebra, spine	intervertebral disk	special tissue disks between vertebrae

- endo- inside
- inter- between
- post- after or behind
- pre- before or in front of
- syn- together
- trans- across or through

Changes
- a- not or without
- anti- against
- contra- against
- dis- separation or absence

Comparisons
- infra- below
- iso- the same or equal to
- micro- small
- ortho- straight or correct
- pseudo- false
- re- again or back

Observe how prefixes modify roots in the following examples:
- ab- + duct = abduct, which means movement away from something

Table 6-2 Commonly Used Prefixes (most common ones in bold)

PREFIX	MEANING	EXAMPLE	DEFINITION
a-, an-	without, not, absent	anaerobic	without oxygen
ab-	away from	abduct	move away from
ad-	to, toward	adduct	move toward
ante-	before	anterior	on the front side or in front of
anti-	against	antibody	protein that fights against antigens and foreign substances
auto-	self	autoimmune	immune system attacks own body tissues
bi-	two	biceps brachii	arm muscle with two origins
bio-	life	biology	study of living objects
circum-	around	circumduct	to lead around, through full range of motion
contra-	against	contraindication	situation in which treatment should be avoided
de-	down, remove, loss	degenerative	condition of breakdown
dia-	across, through	diaphragm	muscle whose origin crosses entire thorax
dis-	apart, away from	disease	condition away from health
dys-	difficult, painful	dysfunction	function that is abnormal or painful
epi-	over, upon	epidermis	top layer of skin
ex-	out of	exhale	release air out of lungs
extra-	in addition, beyond	extracellular	area beyond or outside the cell
flex-	bent	flexion	movement that reduces angle at a joint
hemi	half	hemisphere	half of a sphere
hetero	the other	heterogeneous	characteristic of having dissimilar constituents
homeo	same	homeostasis	state of keeping everything the same or balanced
hyper	above, extreme, excessive	hypertonic	excessive tone or concentration
hypo-	under, below	hypotonic	insufficient tone or concentration
infra-	below	infraspinatus	below the spine
inter-	between	intercostals	muscles between the ribs
intra-	within, inside	intracellular	area between the cells
leuk-	white	leukocyte	white blood cell
macro-	large	macrophage	large cell that destroys foreign substances
mal-	abnormal, bad	malfunction	abnormal or bad function
medi-	middle	medial	beginning or occurring in the middle
micr(o)-	small	microscope	device that allows you to see small things

continues on following page

Table 6-2 Commonly Used Prefixes (most common ones in bold) *continued*

PREFIX	MEANING	EXAMPLE	DEFINITION
mono-	one, single	monoarticular	involving one joint
poly-	many	polyarticular	involving many joints
post-	after	posterior	the back or behind
pre-, pro	before, in front of	precursor	forerunner, or event that happened before
quad-	four	quadriceps femoris	leg muscle with four origins
re-	again, back	recur	occur again
retro-	backward	retroactive	applying to events that occurred in the past
semi-	part	semipermeable	only allowing some things to permeate or move through
sub-	under, below	subcutaneous	below the skin
super-	above, in addition	superficial	on the surface or more toward the surface
supra-	above, over	suprahyoids	muscles that are above the hyoid bone
syn-	together	synergistic	working together
trans-	across	transverse process	projection of vertebrae that points outward, across the body
tri-	three	triceps brachii	arm muscle with three origins
uni-	one, single	unilateral	on one side

- ad- + duct = adduct, which means movement toward something
- bi- + cycle = bicycle, or a cycle with two wheels
- hyper- + troph(o) = hypertrophy, which means excessive growth
- hypo- + therm = hypothermia, which is a condition of below normal temperature
- inter- + cost(o) = intercostal, or between the ribs
- trans- + derm(o) = transdermal, which means through the skin

Table 6-2 lists commonly used prefixes, their definitions, and examples.

Suffixes

Suffixes are word elements tacked on to the end of a root. Because they can help determine whether the unknown term is a noun or an adjective as well as describe how the root is used, they tend to be the starting point for interpreting medical terms. Suffixes can indicate a specific condition or a descriptive condition that refers to the root.

Noun indicators

- -algia characterized by pain in
- -esthesia a sensation of
- -iatry a medical specialty of
- -ism a condition of
- -ist a specialist of
- -itis an inflammation of
- -logy the study of

Descriptive indicators

- -ac pertaining to
- -al pertaining to
- -form like or resembling

- -oid resembling
- -ous pertaining to
- -es plural for -is
- -nges plural for -nx

Table 6-3 is a list of commonly used suffixes, their definitions, and examples of terms that include them.

Combining Vowels

Pronunciation can be awkward when two word elements are combined that do not flow together well. When one element ends with a consonant and the next begins with a consonant, a combining vowel is placed between the two to make the word easier to pronounce. In many of the

Table 6-3 Commonly Used Suffixes (most common ones in bold)

SUFFIX	MEANING	EXAMPLE	DEFINITION
-al	pertaining to area	skeletal	pertaining to the skeleton
-algia	pain, painful condition of	neuralgia	painful condition of the nerves
-ar	pertaining to area	muscular	pertaining to the muscles
-ase	enzyme	lactase	breaks down lactose
-cyte	cell	leukocyte	white blood cell
-ectomy	removal of, excision	hysterectomy	surgical removal of uterus
-emia	blood condition	anemia	low numbers of red blood cells
-genic	causing, producing	allergenic	causing allergic reaction
-gram	record	electrocardiogram	recording of the electrical activity of the heart
-ic	pertaining to	optic	pertaining to the eye
-itis	inflammation of	arthritis	inflammation of the joint
-logy	study of	biology	study of living things
-oid	resembling	fibroid	resembling fibers
-oma	tumor	lipoma	fatty tumor
-osis	condition of	lordosis	condition of increased lordotic curve
-pathy	disease or suffering	sympathy	suffering together
-phobia	irrational fear of	hydrophobia	fear of water
-plasty	surgical repair of	arthroplasty	surgical repair of a joint
-plegia	paralysis	paraplegia	paralysis of two limbs
-rrhage	excessive flow	hemorrhage	excessive loss of blood
-scope	instrument for viewing	microscope	tool for viewing very small things
-stomy	opening	tracheostomy	surgical opening in trachea
-tomy	Incision	laparotomy	incision of the abdomen
-y	characterized by	bony	characterized by bones

examples above, roots are followed with an (o), which is the most common combining vowel. For example, the root "electr" means electricity, the root "cardi" means heart, and "gram" means record. Compare the pronunciation of "electrcardigram" to "electrocardiogram" to see the benefit of combining vowels.

Translating Terms

The three word elements—prefix, root, and suffix—are the building blocks for medical terminology. Once you understand how each word element works, it becomes easy to figure out what a word means. Not all medical terms have a prefix, root, and suffix; some have only two of the elements while others have two roots and a suffix.

Terms can be translated in five methodical steps. The first step in translating medical terms is breaking up the term into its word elements. The second step is defining the suffix, particularly because suffixes indicate how the term is used. Third, go to the beginning of the term and define the elements in order. String all the definitions together and check the translation against a medical dictionary. Translation of the word "fibromyalgia" can be done as follows:

1. Break up the word into its elements.
   Fibromyalgia = "fibro" "my" "algia"
2. Start with the definition of the suffix.
   "-algia" = painful condition of
3. Go to the beginning of the word and define each element.
   "fibro" = fibrous
   "my" = muscle
4. String the definitions together.
   painful condition of fibrous muscle
5. Check your definition against a medical dictionary or other source.
   "painful condition of muscles, tendons, and joints"

Another example is the translation of "hypertonic":

1. "hyper" "ton" "ic"
2. "ic" = pertaining to
3. "hyper" = excessive
   "ton" = tone
4. pertaining to + excessive + tone

5. excessive tone in the muscles or excessive salt concentration in solution

One more example is the translation of "osteoarthritis":

1. "osteo" "arthr" "itis"
2. "itis" = inflammation of
3. "osteo" = bone
   "arthr" = joint
4. inflammation of + bone + joint
5. inflammation of the joints, especially the weight-bearing joints, characterized by degenerative condition of the articular cartilage

Some of the word elements that are used more commonly in massage therapy include

- Prefixes: dys-, hyper-, hypo-, pre-, post-
- Roots: my(o), vertebr(o), cervic(o), fibr(o)
- Suffixes: -al, -algia, -itis

See Table 6-4 for some translations of terms used in the field of massage therapy.

The process of translating terms is straightforward, but you may need practice to become proficient. Medical dictionaries contain thousands of terms and by learning the meanings of some of the more commonly used prefixes, roots, and suffixes, you will not need to look up as many medical terms for their definitions.

Spelling and Pronunciation

Proper translation and communication requires proper spelling and pronunciation. Because of the Greek and Latin derivation of so many medical terms, their spelling and pronunciation may seem strange and unfamiliar, and regional accents can make familiar words sound unfamiliar. Slight differences in spelling can lead to very different meanings as well. For example, the word "ilium" is a bone of the pelvis, and the word "ileum" is a part of the digestive tract. These completely different anatomical structures have the same pronunciation, so context is important. Correct spelling must also be used in documentation to keep accurate and useful records. Again, a medical dictionary is an indispensable tool for every massage therapist. Table 6-5 provides some general tips for pronouncing medical terms.

Communication

Effective communication with clients is essential for obtaining accurate and pertinent data for the initial and subsequent massage treatment sessions. Before meeting with a client, focus your attention on the appointment and do your best to leave personal distractions out of the treatment room. Be fully aware of your clients and their

Table 6-4 Translations of Terms Used in Massage Therapy

WORD	PREFIX	ROOT	SUFFIX	DEFINITION (SPECIFIC REFERENCE TO MASSAGE)
antagonist	ant- (against)	agon (struggle)	-ist (concerned with)	one that works against (a muscle with an opposing action)
atrophy	a- (without, not)	troph (growth)	-y (condition of)	(condition of muscular deterioration or no growth)
biceps brachii	bi- (two)	ceps (head) brachi (arm)	-i (plural)	two heads (specific arm muscle with two origins)
circumduction	circum- (around)	duct (to lead)	-tion (action of)	lead all the way around (circular movement of a body part through its range of motion)
contraindication	contra- (against)	indicate (to point)	-tion (action of)	indicating the other way (a situation in which treatment is inappropriate)
extension	ex- (away from)	ten (tendon)	-sion (action of)	action of away from the tendon (movement that opens the angle at a joint and stretches the tendon)
fibromyalgia		fibro (fiber) my (muscle)	-algia (painful condition of)	pain in fibers and muscles (condition with pain in muscles, tendons and joints)
hypertonic	hyper- (excessive)	ton (tone)	-ic (pertaining to)	condition of excessive tone (muscle that is too tense)
infraspinatus	infra- (below)	spin (spine)	-atus (refers to)	refers to below the spine (specific muscle that originates below the spine of the scapula)
isometric	iso- (equal)	metr (measure)	-ic (pertaining to)	pertaining to equal measure (muscle activity in which antagonists work equally and no movement occurs)
neuralgia		neur (nerve)	-algia (painful condition of)	nerve pain (condition of pain along the nerves)
osteoarthritis		oste (bone) arthr (joint)	-itis (inflammation of)	inflammation of bone and joint (condition of inflamed and degenerative joints)
proprioception		proprius (your own) cep (take)	-tion (action of)	action of taking your own (ability to sense stimuli from your own body's position in space)
tendinitis		tendin (tendon)	-itis (inflammation of)	inflammation of tendons

needs. Engaging the client in a good conversation helps you gather the necessary information to provide safe and effective treatment. A genuine interest in the client helps the client feel heard and understood, leading to a more trusting relationship. This is important for assisting the client throughout the healing process and helps clients cultivate a broader understanding of health. Always keep clients and their needs at the center of the treatment process to establish and support a safe, trusting, effective relationship.

Table 6-5 Tips on Pronunciation

LETTERS	COMMONLY PRONOUNCED	EXAMPLE
c (before e, i, y)	S	quadriceps (KWAH-drih-seps)
c (before all other letters)	K	contraction (kon-TRAK-shun)
ch	K	cholesterol (koh-LESS-ter-ahl)
es (at the end of a word)	EEZ	meninges (meh-NIN-jeez)
eu	OO YOO	aponeurosis (AP-oh-noo-ROH-sis) eustachian tube (yoo-STAY-shun toob)
g (before e, i, y)	J	gemellus (juh-MELL-us)
g (before all other letters)	G (hard sound)	gluteus (GLOO-tee-us)
gm	M	diaphragm (DAHY-uh-fram)
gn	N	benign (bee-NAHYN)
i (at the end of a word)	AHY	nuclei (NOOK-lee-ahy)
pn	N	pneumonia (noo-MOHN-yuh)
ps	S	psoas (SOH-az)
pt	T	pterygoid (TAIR-ih-goyd)
x	Z	xyphoid (ZAHY-foyd)

Effective Communication and Interviewing Skills

There are several factors in effective communication skills and the interview process. These include establishing rapport (rah-POR), or mutual trust, through communication, making certain assumptions about the client, using reflective listening skills, asking open-ended and leading questions, and looking beyond the client's verbal report for nonverbal information.

The saying goes, "You never get a second chance to make a first impression." First impressions are lasting ones. It is important to present and maintain a professional atmosphere from the beginning of the therapist–client relationship. The first meeting with a client is critically important, as it provides the foundation for the professional relationship, so the following actions should always be incorporated:

- Formal introductions that include names, a handshake, eye contact, and a statement that clearly identifies the therapist

- Verbal communication that gives the client control over the treatment. For example, a therapist may indicate when a change to a deeper or more invasive technique will occur. You should offer a safety mechanism that allows clients to inform you if they are uncomfortable in any way, which gives them permission to request that a particular technique be altered or stopped.

- Disclosure of some of the effects of the session that could develop in the next few days, especially if the client was not familiar with the techniques used.

Establishing rapport is perhaps the single most important skill a massage therapist must have for the interviewing process. The first step to establishing rapport with a client is to offer a confident, caring handshake and a greeting using the person's first name. Know the correct pronunciation and spelling of the client's name, and nickname, if they prefer. One of the keys to establishing rapport is maintaining eye contact. Look clients in the eye while discussing the details of their condition and history to communicate your interest in their explanation. This also increases the client's feelings of validation and positive attention. Another technique for creating rapport is to establish and continue to build trust by acknowledging the client's input and maintaining confidentiality. Phrases such as "I hear you" or "I understand" show that you are paying attention to what the client said, again offering validation.

Another factor in creating and building trust and rapport in the therapist–client relationship is **confidentiality**. Any information the client provides should remain confidential, meaning that the information is to be kept private and not shared with anyone else unless the client expressly permits it. There are special situations when information in client files is shared. The client may choose to use you as part of a healthcare team, which could require you to share session information with the other healthcare practitioners. Insurance companies sometimes request session information to reimburse you or your clients. Client information may be released to an attorney or judge upon court order as part of litigation, as in auto accident cases. For you to release the client's records, the client must authorize and sign a release form (Fig. 6-1). There are a number of occupations, including licensed massage therapy, that legally require reporting abusive situations and threats of deadly harm to the appropriate authorities, such as the police or other governmental agency that protects children and families. You can inform clients of this possibility when you get informed consent for care.

Clients who sense their importance to you are more likely to trust you and, as a result, provide more pertinent information. Another way to establish rapport is to explain to clients exactly what they can expect to have happen in the therapy session. Knowing what to expect takes the mystery out of the process and makes clients more comfortable.

Certain assumptions about clients support the communication process by making sure you use a humanistic view of your clients instead of a clinical, unfeeling approach:

- Each client is unique: The extent to which you consider the individual story of each client directly affects the client's chances for improvement.

- Each client has skills: Communicating your recognition of the client's skills and using those skills as a personal strength enhances information gathering.

- Each client interacts with the environment: Recognizing that clients are significantly affected by their lives outside the massage therapy treatment area and gathering more information about their lives leads to more pertinent communication.

- Clients are like us: Considering clients as equal human beings, with similar reactions and difficulties, and maintaining equal footing with clients instead of creating a dependent relationship, facilitates the healing process.

- Clients are honest: Typically, clients give the best information they can, but it is up to you to ask the right questions to help them recall that information.

- Each client sincerely desires success: Clients do their best to achieve their treatment goals. Sometimes environmental factors prevent complete cooperation, and you must recognize these factors.

- Each client shares responsibility with you during the interview: Although you are likely more experienced with interviewing, clients also have a responsibility to help the interview be successful.

- Each client desires interaction and negotiation: Most clients attempt to understand your intent and evaluate your skills and knowledge by asking questions or negotiating instructions.

- Each client knows what the problem is: Clients are typically aware of factors contributing to their difficulties, and the therapist can learn these factors by listening carefully.

- Each client knows when success has occurred: Clients are often the best judges of whether treatment has been successful, so recognize that their concepts of success might be different from yours.

Although these assumptions are generalizations, they will help you maintain a client-centered focus and will support your work toward successfully reaching treatment goals.

Reflective Listening

Good listening skills help you to further your rapport and ensure that the information from the client is documented accurately and completely. Maintaining a client-centered focus throughout the interview process often requires the skill of reflective listening. Reflective listening is a technique with which you repeat or reiterate the client's words to convey your comprehension or to clarify a misunderstanding. For example, a client may say, "The pain in my shoulder gets worse after I sleep on my side all night." You may then respond to the client, "So when you sleep on one side through the entire night, the pain in your right shoulder has increased by the time you wake up?" This question determines if you have heard the client correctly and gives the client an opportunity to clarify a misunderstanding. Additionally, it helps you document the correct information. As you gain more practice with the interviewing process and use the fundamental skill of reflective listening, you will become a more effective interviewer.

Open-ended Questions

Using your own style with reflective listening will help you formulate questions to elicit as much information from

PATIENT'S RELEASE OF HEALTH CARE INFORMATION

Patient's Name _____

Social Security Number _____ Date of Birth _____

I hereby instruct my providers to provide full and complete information to _____ _____ and to accept this authorization form and release the protected information requested without requiring any additional authorizations. I specifically waive any "minimally necessary" limitations of HIPAA.

Health Care Provider/Facility _____
is hereby authorized to release health care information, including intake forms, chart notes, reports, correspondence, billing statements, and other written information to my attorneys, employees, and designated agents of my attorneys, to wit:

Attorney's Name _____ Phone _____
Address _____
City _____ State _____ Zip _____

This request and authorization applies to:
____ Health care information relating to the following treatment, condition, or dates of treatment: _____
____ All health care information:
____ Other: _____

How the Information will be used: Said information shall be used for any and all purposes for _____ to pursue payment of care expenses and in providing legal services to me in conjunction with my case. Following said disclosure the information may no longer be subject to HIPAA protection, as it may be subject to re-disclosure that is unprotected absent specific laws protecting specific sensitive information.

Revocation of Prior Authorization: All medical authorizations by the patient or patient's authorized representatives given before the date of this release for any reason whatsoever are hereby revoked.

Unlawful Disclosure Prohibited: State and Federal prohibits any health care provider from releasing any health care information about a patient to another person without the consent of the patient. You are requested to disclose no such information to any insurance adjuster or any other person without written authority from me which is printed on the letterhead of my attorny.

Effect of Photocopy: A photocopy of this release shall have the same force and effect as a signed original.

Authorization expires 90 days from date of signature. Thereafter, no authorization exists unless an updated release is provided by: _____

I understand that I have the right to revoke this release for any information not yet provided to _____ by providing notice of revocation in writing to the above named care provider. I also understand that I have the right to refuse to authorize disclosure at all.

_____   _____
Signature of Patient or Patient's Authorized Representative   Date

Figure 6-1. Client records release forms. **(A)** Patient's Release of Health Care Information.

Authorization to Use and Disclose Health Care Information

Name _____ ID#/DOB _____ Date _____

I: _____, authorize my manual therapist: _____,
to disclose my health care information with the following health care providers and/or insurance
companies:

Name(s): _____

Address: _____

The following information may be disclosed (check all that apply):

☐ All health care information in my medical chart.

☐ Only health care information relating to the following injury, illness, or treatment: _____

_____

☐ Only health care information for the following dates or time periods: _____

_____

☐ Including information regarding HIV, STD, mental health, drug or alcohol abuse.

I give my authorization to release health care information for the following purposes (check all
that apply):

☐ To share information with my health care team in an attempt to coordinate care

☐ To obtain payment of care expenses I have incurred for my treatments.

☐ To take part in research

☐ Other: _____

This authorization expires on:

Date: _____ (no longer than 90 days from the date signed)

Event: _____

I understand that I may refuse to sign this authorization.

I may also revoke this authorization at any time by writing a letter to my manual therapist.

I understand that once my health care information is disclosed, the recipient may redisclose the
information and it may no longer be protected HIPAA or state privacy laws.

I also understand my obtaining care can not be conditioned on my signing this release.

Signature _____ Date _____

Figure 6-1. *(continued)* **(B)** Authorization to Use and Disclose Health Information. (Reprinted with permission from Thompson DL. Hands Heal: Communication, Documentation, and Insurance Billing for Manual Therapists. 3rd ed. Baltimore: Lippincott Williams & Wilkins, 2006.)

clients as possible regarding their present condition and cumulative stressors that have affected it. The best method of gathering information uses open-ended questions. Open-ended questions are those that require a descriptive answer instead of a one-word answer. They encourage and broaden the conversation, often helping clients remember any details they might have forgotten. For example, the closed question, "Does your shoulder hurt today?" is likely to lead to a short answer such as yes or no. In contrast, the open-ended question, "What makes your shoulder pain better or worse?" may elicit a more thoughtful, thorough response that provides more information about which soft tissues might be involved. Other examples of open-ended questions include:

- How would you describe your pain or discomfort?
- How did the pain or discomfort change during the day?
- What kinds of activities made the pain or discomfort more noticeable?

Leading Questions

After exploring open-ended questions, you might use leading questions to refocus the conversation to the chief complaint. Leading questions focus the client's attention to clarify or to give more specific types of information and to recall missing or forgotten details. For example, if a client's chief complaint is right-sided neck pain, your reflective listening skills and open-ended questions might evoke a story about a typical workday and a number of events that happened at work last week that brought the client in for a massage. You can ask leading questions regarding the neck pain to help you understand which soft tissues might be involved:

- Is there any activity that you typically do with your right side, such as carry your child or talk a lot on the phone with the phone on your right side?
- Is there an activity where you turn your head mostly to one side during a typical day?
- What position do you tend to sleep in?
- Can you show me the movements that hurt the most?

These questions will help refocus the discussion to determine the plan for the upcoming massage treatment.

Nonverbal Communication

Gathering information from clients involves more than just collecting verbal data. Look beyond the client's words written on the history form and the client's answers from the interview to gather the whole picture, paying attention to nonverbal communication. These nonverbal cues help you better understand how the clients perceive and manage their conditions.

You can evaluate clients' perceptions of their conditions by observing their tone of voice, breathing patterns, and body language, including facial expression, eye contact, areas of muscular tension, and body positioning. Try to notice anything that is out of the norm. A normal tone of voice is recognized as steady instead of shaky, not too loud or soft, not too rushed or hesitant, and not excessively emotional. Body language can be especially helpful to massage therapists because people tend to accompany the verbal description of the condition of their soft tissues with clues

for massage treatment. Sometimes clients will describe pain or areas of restricted movement while they rub the affected tissues a certain way, poke at themselves, hold their hand over affected areas, or stretch restricted soft tissues. These nonverbal messages can tell you which areas to include in the session and which techniques to use. Body language is not the only thing that indicates the techniques you should use or that only certain techniques will work, nor does it necessarily indicate the specific areas that are causing the pain or restricted function, but it does suggest that these techniques will be well received by the client and that those tissues are most likely involved in the pain or restriction.

Sometimes the nonverbal communication reinforces the spoken words, but many times, the nonverbal cues contradict the client's words, and you have to recognize the discrepancy to sort through the input and determine the most effective approach to treatment. Consider a client who comes in and briefly requests a massage just to relax and denies any areas of pain or discomfort at the time. However, the client's words are quiet and shaky, there is no eye contact, and the client is slumped in the chair and breathing shallowly. While filling out the intake form, the client rubs his or her temples, squeezes the eyes shut from time to time, sits up straight a couple of times to hyperextend and laterally flex, and rubs the posterior aspect of the neck. The nonverbal body language suggests pain and some muscular tension in the head or neck. It also suggests that the client might respond well to massaging the posterior and lateral soft tissues of the neck and lateral flexion stretches to the neck.

Clients' nonverbal and emotional cues can also offer information about their stress levels and healing or recovery time. Generally, the higher the client's stress level, the more symptoms he or she may have, and the longer the recovery time will be. Conversely, lower levels of stress may be associated with fewer symptoms and shorter recovery times.

Although it is beyond the therapist's scope of practice to counsel clients, you may take note of their emotions and emotional reactions to their conditions. For example, you have a client who starts crying when describing the effect of back pain on his or her life and the feelings of worthlessness it causes. Without diagnosing any specific medical or psychological condition, you could note that the client is very distressed as a result of the back pain. This notation may offer you and other healthcare providers insight into the client's condition and response to healing.

Alert

Be extremely careful to stay within your role as a massage therapist; your scope of practice does not include diagnosing or counseling.

It is much better to offer genuine caring and concern about the client's condition than to offer inappropriate advice.

Good documentation depends on good communication as you engage clients in effective interviews. Establishing rapport through communication, making certain assumptions about the client, using reflective listening skills, asking open-ended and leading questions, and paying attention to nonverbal messages all help you gather accurate, complete information for documentation.

Documentation

Within the healthcare community, documentation is used to create and maintain a patient's record and to develop initial treatment plans as well as session-to-session treatment plans. Documentation is a guideline for safe and effective treatment and proof of the client's progress, and it is the basis for communication between healthcare professionals regarding a client's health. As massage continues to develop as a healthcare profession and governmental licensure becomes prevalent, the need to learn documentation becomes more critical because licensed healthcare practitioners are legally required to document patient progress. Many insurance companies require professional documentation for reimbursement. There are therapists who do not keep accurate records of client progress because they consider it unnecessary at the time, think it takes too much time, or do not want to bother clients with paperwork and interviews. Realistically, most clients are not interested in filling out forms or sitting through an interview. Most of them just want to get on the massage table, receive treatment, and go home.

Reasons for Documentation

Despite the impatience of clients who "just want to get a massage," maintaining a client-centered and successful practice requires documentation of both wellness and therapeutic massage for many reasons:

- You must understand the clients' health history to ensure that there are no contraindications for massage.
- You can treat repeat clients more efficiently when you know which techniques were effective.
- You can encourage clients' participation by inquiring about their self-care activities.
- You have written proof to illustrate progress toward the clients' goals.
- You promote professional massage therapy as a legitimate, aboveboard healthcare practice.

- You convey and breed trust by conducting a professional interview that ensures that your treatment will be purely professional.
- You convey the importance of health history and progress by writing it down instead of trying to remember it.
- You can show clients that their goals were reached with money well spent.
- You have written records to share with insurance companies, both to get reimbursed and for accident and injury settlements.
- You have written records to share with the clients' other healthcare practitioners to ensure that treatments are cooperative rather than contradictory.
- You have written records to share with healthcare practitioners who refer clients to you, thus closing the communication loop and marketing and presenting yourself as a professional.
- You have written records to protect you in the rare case of a malpractice suit.

As you can see, keeping written records in an organized file system is a worthwhile investment for the safety of your clients, the education of your clients, the financial success of your practice, and the professional image of your practice. Client files must represent accurate information that is pertinent to treatment. The file should include client contact information, the client's signed informed consent for care (discussed in the Ethics and Professionalism chapter), and basic treatment information, whether in a SOAP note or in another format. It should include any referrals made and any self-care recommended.

Alert

The file should not include your subjective or judgmental statements, suspected diagnoses, or written observations regarding behavioral inconsistencies.

The files can be used to keep track of the techniques you use, techniques clients like or do not like, techniques that work especially well for a particular client, and the condition of soft tissues from session to session. Documentation is not only a tool for you; it is also an important method of communication with other massage therapists or healthcare practitioners. You may work in a situation, perhaps a spa or massage clinic, where other therapists may see the same clients. Good documentation will help the treating therapist gain an understanding of the client's history and progress and learn what techniques work well with a particular client. Additionally, the uniqueness of individuals makes it impossible for any one treatment to work for every person, so clients may choose to use one or several healthcare practitioners as a collective team. The team approach can be especially beneficial, as long as the participants share pertinent and valid information. You need to keep records that a primary care physician or other healthcare practitioner can understand and, with the client's signed release of records form, share any records with referring practitioners as a professional courtesy.

The Health Insurance Portability and Accountability Act of 1996 (HIPAA)

In 1996, the Health Insurance Portability and Accountability Act, better known as HIPAA, was enacted to help employees and their families obtain and transfer health insurance coverage when their employment changes or is terminated. The law was later modified to include Standards for Privacy of Individually Identifiable Health Information, more commonly called the Privacy Rule. The modified law not only gives people better access to health insurance coverage, it also gives them ownership of their health information and legally protects that information from being shared without their written permission. Unfortunately, there is a lot of confusion regarding HIPAA and the Privacy Rule.

The Department of Health and Human Services (HHS) has a web site devoted to HIPAA, http://www.hhs.gov/ocr/privacy/hipaa/understanding/index.html, that attempts to simplify and explain the law. Included is a series of questions designed to help people determine whether or not they must follow the law, but the terminology throughout the questions is confusing and wordy, and even though the web site defines some of the terms, the definitions can be unclear. Essentially, you are asked whether your business provides any kind of healthcare. If so, you are asked whether anything your business does is considered a "Covered Transaction" as defined in the law. Covered Transactions include using any electronic means to transmit a person's health insurance information such as claims, enrollment, eligibility, explanation of benefits, premium payments, claim status, referral certification or authorization, and coordination of plan benefits. If your business performs any Covered Transactions electronically (computer, electronic media storage, email, internet, personal data assistants, etc.), then your business is considered a Covered Entity, meaning that it must comply with HIPAA and follow all of the rules. If not, which is often the answer for massage therapists, the questionnaire suggests that your business is not a Covered Entity and is not required to follow HIPAA law. However, there is a "chain of trust" that requires any business associate of a Covered Entity to be HIPAA compliant. Business associates include persons, companies, or entities hired by the practitioner to perform duties that access, use, or disclose a client's protected health information (PHI). In other words, if your practice is not a Covered Entity but you accept referrals from a doctor or clinic, or you share a client's progress with his physician, you must comply with HIPAA regulations. The Covered Entity should ask you to sign a Business Associate form as part of HIPAA compliance.

Besides the chain of trust, the regulations of the HIPAA Privacy Rule require all healthcare practitioners to keep their clients' health information private and protected. This means that all massage therapists must protect their client records according to HIPAA regulations. Marilyn Allen, a well-known expert in acupuncture and medical malpractice, states that it is mandatory that every client's PHI be kept private, and that you are considered a Covered Entity if you gather information directly from clients, through written or oral communications, or transmit records electronically or by any other means (including paper and fax).

HIPAA Compliance

To establish and maintain HIPAA compliance, you will need a way to keep client information protected and private, and there are specific forms and medical codes you will need to use. All Covered Entities will use the same medical codes, as found in the *Current Procedural Terminology* codebook, the *International Classification of Diseases*, Ninth Revision diagnosis codebook, and the federal medical devices codebook. In addition to textbooks for self-teaching, there are a number of courses that train people for HIPAA compliance. Following is a list of some of the steps you will need to take to be compliant:

- Designate someone from within or outside the business as the Privacy Officer (the person responsible for your policies and procedures for handling PHI).

- Establish policies and procedures for keeping PHI private, and ensure that all employees understand and follow these rules.

- Develop a manual for HIPAA policies and procedures, including how you will keep or destroy client records and email communications.

- Use computer firewalls and security software to prevent PHI from being stolen or destroyed.

- Implement the use of passwords and user identifications for anyone who has access to electronic forms of PHI.

- Obtain written authorization from the client before emailing any PHI, and make sure the information is encrypted.

- Include a confidentiality notice on all email, fax, and paper transmissions of PHI.

- Provide each client with a Notification of Privacy Policies (NOPP) form as well as a form with their signature indicating that they have received the NOPP.

6 Communication and Documentation

Anything that has health information related to a particular client must be protected from unauthorized access. For example, it is unacceptable to set a client's file on your desk or anywhere someone could pick it up and look at it. Likewise, it is not compliant to have client information on a computer that is accessible to passersby or other unauthorized personnel. Another example of noncompliance is a sign-in sheet that lists more than just the client's name, such as their health insurance company or the primary reason for their massage appointment.

There are several forms you will need for HIPAA compliance. The first is called the Notification of Privacy Policies. It informs clients of the policies and procedures you follow to keep their PHI private. You can also include the clients' rights on the NOPP:

- Clients are entitled to see and receive copies of their records.
- Clients are entitled to suggest or request amendments to the health information in their files, but the therapist has the right to not include those amendments in the file, and clients have the right to disagree with the therapist's refusal.
- Clients are entitled to have a copy of the therapist's Notice of Privacy Policies.
- Clients are entitled to object to the privacy policies, and the therapist then has the right to refuse treatment to those clients.

Once clients have seen your NOPP, they must sign a separate form indicating their understanding of those policies. Any activity that exposes a client's PHI or changes information in their file requires consent and authorization forms and signatures, and the paper trail of these forms must be protected and kept private.

Client confidentiality is essential for you as a massage therapist. It is the ethical way to practice, and the government has only just begun regulating the privacy of health information. The fine for noncompliance ranges from $100 to $50,000, so check the HHS web site (www.hhs.gov) or search online for "HIPAA compliance" to familiarize yourself with and follow the law.

Documentation Forms

There are different forms and formats you can use to document client assessment and massage treatment. You can choose or create the appropriate forms based on the information you will document. Essentially, you need to include contact information for your clients, health history information, informed consent for care, subjective ideas from your clients about how they feel and what they want to accomplish, your objective evaluations of clients' bodies and the condition of their soft tissues, massage activity and analysis of treatments, and future massage treatment plans.

The contact information, health history, and informed consent for care can be consolidated onto one form. Sometimes called intake forms, these are filled out by clients at their first appointment, and the forms are kept in your client files. (Figure 6-6 shows an example of an intake form.)

The massage treatment record contains the rest of the information you need to document: input from the client, your objective assessments, the massage techniques you use, results of the treatment session, and plans for future massage treatment. All of the information can be recorded on a printed form or just written down on a blank document, as long as the appropriate information is included.

SOAP

A common format for documenting massage sessions is SOAP, an acronym for Subjective, Objective, Activity and analysis, and Plan information. Figure 6-2 is an example of a printed SOAP chart, also called a SOAP note, and indicates the pertinent information to document in each section.

Subjective Information

Generally, subjective information includes any written or verbal information the client shares with you. In addition to the health history information that clients share on the intake form, they may tell you what hurts, what they want to accomplish

from the session, the physiological or psychosocial factors that are affecting their health, and activities they think are affected by muscular tension or pain. Use effective communication skills to obtain as much pertinent information as you can from the client to determine any potential contraindications and to create the best treatment plan. This chapter focuses on communication skills and the "S" portion of the SOAP note.

Client History

To know where to begin treatment, you need to know where clients have been—know their history. The history is the first step in evaluating the client's condition, and this

SOAP NOTE

Name: _____ **Date:** _____

Current illness, injury, medication:

_____

_____

Primary reason for visit:

_____

SUBJECTIVE

The clients' chief complaint or concern (the reason they came for massage)
- what clients say about their condition
- their perception of the condition since the last massage treatment

Information from the health history that is pertinent to the chief complaint

OBJECTIVE (Obvious differences you notice before, during, and after the massage)

Postural assessments
- levelness and evenness of bilateral landmarks, rotational deviations, landmarks that are anterior or posterior to their normal position, feet

Gait assessments
- quantity, quality, fluidity of steps and arm swing (bilateral similarities, evenness, smoothness), upright alignment (head over spine, shoulders not hunched, etc.), feet (medial or lateral deviation), knee flexion (slight flexion for shock absorption resembles a bounce in the step)

Range of motion assessments
- active range of motion, passive range of motion

Your visual observations of the clients' bodies and their soft tissues
- color, fullness, bilateral symmetry

Your palpation observations of the clients' bodies and their soft tissues
- temperature abnormalities, differences in texture and movement of skin and soft tissues, areas of abnormal fullness or swelling, body rhythms

ACTIVITY AND ANALYSIS

Massage activity
- specify where and which techniques you applied

Massage session analysis
- results of the current massage session
- prioritized functional limitations
- long and short term goals

PLAN

Plan for future massage treatment
- techniques to use or avoid, duration and frequency of future sessions
- self-care recommendations
- referrals to other healthcare practitioners
- reminders for follow-up on areas treated

Therapist's Signature: _____ **Date:** _____

Figure 6-2. Pertinent information for SOAP notes.

information is documented as subjective data on the SOAP note. Information from the client history form provides many clues about the condition of a client's structures and soft tissues even before your formal assessment. The history form should include the following client data: personal identification and contact information; current health information, health concerns, and goals for health; goals for treatment; history of injuries, illnesses, and surgeries; and consent to exchange health information with other healthcare providers as well as consent for care. Finally, clients should sign and date the form as acknowledgment and proof that they had the opportunity to discuss anything on the form with you and gave their consent for massage treatment. (See Figs. 6-6 and 6-9 for examples of health history forms.)

Some intake forms include body diagrams, which can be a helpful tool for clients because verbalizing their symptoms and physical sensations of discomfort may be difficult. Additionally, when the client is given the opportunity to draw on the body diagram before the interview, it can simplify and expedite the interview process. Figure 6-3 is a sample health report form indicating a client's current symptoms. **Know that clients almost always have more information than they initially write down.** More often than not, people forget about accidents and injuries. The muscular and nervous systems, however, do not forget. In fact, soft tissue condition and postural compensations directly reflect their cumulative stresses. Any one accident, injury, condition, hobby, or activity may not seem stressful for the body, but cumulatively or unresolved, individual stressors will manifest in the body as postural compensation patterns and physical symptoms in soft tissues.

Interview

After the client has filled out the history form and indicated symptoms on the body diagram, you begin sorting through the information. Leading questions help clarify the client's input, allowing you to identify contraindications, set appropriate session goals, and develop an effective treatment plan. Daily activities, hobbies, and environmental factors such as climbing stairs or long commutes to and from work are often the culprit behind muscular tension and pain. Some categories that are commonly covered when interviewing massage clients[1]:

- General: allergies, fatigue, fever, function, illness, pain, stress
- Circulatory: cold extremities, cramps, edema, inflammation, swollen lymph nodes, varicose veins
- Musculoskeletal: aches, joint pain, muscle pain, stiffness, swelling, tension, weakness

- Neurological: numbness, radiating pain, tingling, localized weakness
- Psychosocial: lifestyle, important experiences, personal life, social life, work situation

The history is your first and perhaps most important assessment tool to understand the condition of the client and whether massage is the safest and most effective treatment.

Functional Stress Assessment

Stress can be anything that takes a person out of homeostasis or balance or it can be defined as a state of bodily or mental tension resulting from factors that hinder the body from maintaining homeostasis. Stress is not necessarily a bad thing and, in fact, small doses of stress can encourage the body to become stronger. Antigens that are incompatible with our own tissues are a form of stress because they jeopardize homeostasis, but the only way our bodies can develop the appropriate antibodies is by being exposed to those antigens. The resulting antibodies effectively strengthen the immune system. Bones remodel and become stronger in response to mechanical forces, or forms of stress that push, pull, twist, or compress them.

Stress may cause problems when it is prolonged or when many individual stress factors accumulate and the body is challenged to maintain homeostasis. For example, people who work long hours and have to stay intense and alert for weeks on end overwork their sympathetic nervous systems. Without enough rest, the activities of the sympathetic and parasympathetic nervous systems become imbalanced, creating internal stress that threatens the ability to maintain homeostasis. Mechanical forms of stress can be caused by overusing one set of muscles on one side of the body without using the antagonists or the same set of muscles on the other side of the body as much. To maintain balance and homeostasis, the body adopts an abnormal posture that compensates for the imbalance. Another form of mechanical stress is pain, which may force the body to accommodate for the pain with an abnormal posture and compensation patterns.

Massage therapists consider the effects of stress from a functional perspective, evaluating the extent to which a client is out of balance and how the imbalance affects the client's soft tissue and postural compensation patterns as well as everyday activities. When assessing a client, you must consider specific sources of stress, such as dysfunctions or pathology, previous accidents or surgeries, activities, and nutritional habits and the overall effect of the accumulated stress factors. Several types of stress may affect the client in many areas of life, and you must recognize how each source of stress affects soft tissues and postural compensation patterns so you can develop the most

Manual Therapist _Sophie Ellis_

HEALTH REPORT

Patient Name _CRAIG SHERMAN_ Date _AUG. 5, 2003_

Date of Injury _N/A_ ID#/DOB _APRIL 20, 1974_

A. Draw today's symptoms on the figures.

1. Identify CURRENT symptomatic areas in your body by marking letters on the figures below. Use the letters provided in the key to identify the symptoms you are feeling today.
2. Circle the area around each letter, representing the size and shape of each symptom location.

Key
P = pain or tenderness
S = joint or muscle stiffness
N = numbness or tingling

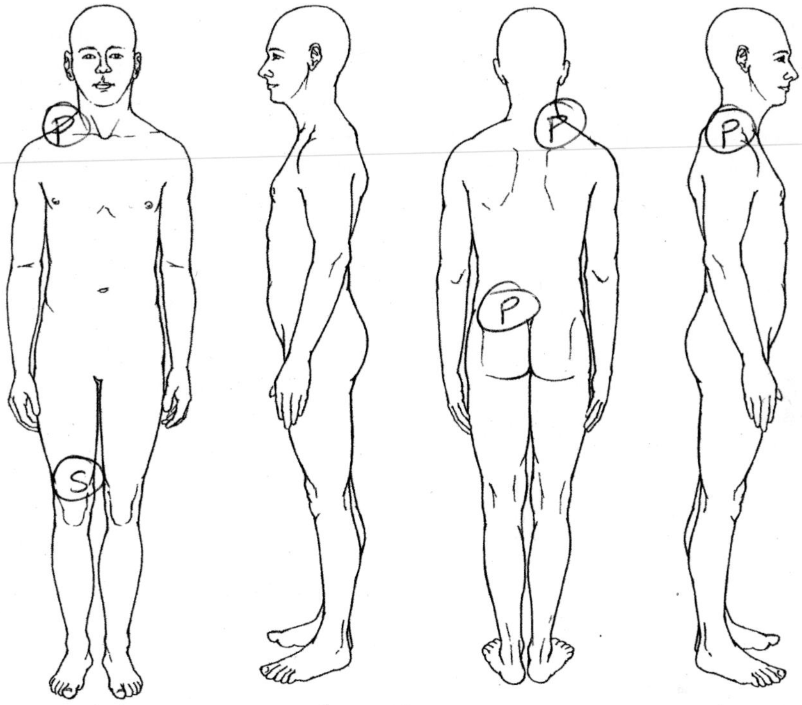

B. Identify the intensity of your symptoms.

1. Pain Scale: Mark a line on the scale to show the amount of pain you are experiencing today.

No Pain ├────────────X────────────┤ Unbearable Pain

2. Activities Scale: Mark a line on the scale to show the limitations you are experiencing today in your daily activities.

Can Do Anything I Want ├──X────────────────────┤ Cannot Do Anything

C. Comments

STIFF KNEE FROM BASKETBALL

Signature _(signature)_ Date _8-5-03_

Figure 6-3 Health report, filled out. (Reprinted with permission from Thompson DL. Hands Heal: Communication, Documentation, and Insurance Billing for Manual Therapists. 3rd ed. Baltimore: Lippincott Williams & Wilkins, 2006.)

effective treatment plan for each client. You should evaluate, using leading questions, if necessary, the following stress factors:

Health Conditions

- What current soft tissue or pathological conditions is the client experiencing?
- Are the client's conditions acute or chronic? (This provides information about the condition of soft tissues.)
- Are the conditions genetic?
- Has the client seen any other healthcare practitioner or had other forms of treatment for the condition? If so, what did the other healthcare practitioner conclude? What kind of treatment is currently being given?

Accidents and Surgeries

- How many and what kinds of accidents or surgeries has the client had?
- What kind of treatment, if any, has the client had for the accidents?
- What are the residual soft tissue injuries or compensations?
- How many and what kinds of surgeries has the client had? Does the client have residual scarring in the area?

Age Considerations

- Tissue changes at different ages
- The effects of gravity over time on postural compensation patterns

Lifestyle

- Are there any activities the client does daily that use repetitive movements or positions that are held for extended periods of time? What postures or positions is the client in and for how many hours a day?
- What exercise activities does the client participate in? What muscles are used most in those particular activities?

Postural Factors

- Are there any daily postures or positions that the client holds for extended periods of time?
- How many hours does the client work per day?
- What position does the client sleep in?
- How many hours does the client sleep per night?

Nutrition and Medication

- What are the client's nutritional habits?
- How much water does the client drink per day?
- How much caffeine does the client consume per day?
- What vitamins or nutritional supplements does the client take?

- Does the client take any medication, prescription or over-the-counter? If so, what does the client take it for?

Emotional and Psychological Factors

- As stated above, treating emotional and psychological factors is *not* within the massage therapist's scope of practice, but any increase in stress level because of these factors can weaken the body's ability to maintain homeostasis or balance. In turn, this can affect the client's soft tissues or postural compensation patterns. Although specific psychological conditions should not be documented, you can make notes regarding general emotions to consider when creating a treatment plan.

Generally, the higher the client's stress level, the longer it will take to return to balance or homeostasis.

Cumulative Effects of Stress

After discussing the client's history, you can educate the client about how stress has accumulated and describe your plan for the current and future massage sessions. The client may be seeking relief from current pain or discomfort, but an effective therapist will also consider past and potential stressors. All past, present, and potential or perceived future stressors can affect the client's condition. Explain to the client that if it took years to develop a muscular or soft tissue condition, it could take numerous sessions to reduce the severity of the condition. Again, the number and accumulation of stressors influence the length of time it will take soft tissues and postural compensation patterns to return to balance or homeostasis. Although there are general principles regarding soft tissue rehabilitation and recovery time, each client is affected by a unique set of accumulated stressors. Some clients may think that one massage will miraculously cure them of their aches and pains. Unless they understand how the cumulative effects of stress relate to the development of a chronic condition, clients may be quickly discouraged or decide that massage is not helpful after only one session. (See Box 6-1, Procedure: Client Interview.)

Objective Information

Objective information includes your assessments of a client's body and the condition of the soft tissues. Any observations and evaluations you make before, during, or after the actual massage treatment are documented in this section of the SOAP note. Visual observations to record might include areas of swelling or inflammation, unevenness of bilateral bony landmarks or muscles, postural abnormalities, compensation patterns, gait (walking) assessments, and localized areas of abnormal skin coloration, especially

BOX 6.1 PROCEDURE Client Interview

1. Greet first-time clients with good eye contact and a friendly, confident handshake.

2. Explain your policies and intake form(s) and offer reasons for documentation.

3. Ask clients to fill out forms. Meanwhile, start filling out their SOAP note.

4. Interview clients:
   a. Clarify their purpose for coming to you for a massage.
      i. Is there any area in particular they want you to address or avoid?
      ii. Are there any techniques they prefer or dislike?
   b. Clarify their chief complaint, if there is one. This helps you better understand the client's current condition to know if any progress was made when you perform the posttreatment assessment.
      i. Is there anything that makes the pain worse or better?
      ii. Do they notice the discomfort all of the time, only during certain activities, or only after certain activities?
      iii. How long have they had this condition?
      iv. Ask them to try to rate the discomfort, using a scale of 1 to 10 or on a scale of mild to severe.
      v. Ask them to try to describe the discomfort (sharp, achy, numb, tingling, heavy, throbbing, etc.).
   c. Question any conditions on the history form that might present contraindications—injuries, illness, surgeries, bruises, circulatory problems.
   d. Inquire about daily activities, hobbies, and environmental factors, looking for repetitive movements or sustained positions to try to identify the soft tissues that might be involved.
      i. Do they drive/sit/stand/type/carry an infant a lot during a typical workday?
      ii. Do they garden/knit/ride horses/drive a race car most of the weekend?
      iii. Do they hold an instrument/walk a lot of stairs/breathe smoke-filled air/shift a manual transmission/look up at a screen high on the wall repeatedly?
   e. Discuss the general, circulatory, musculoskeletal, neurological, and psychosocial aspects of their health to find out if there is anything that might influence the treatment you give or the results of the treatment.

5. Evaluate their functional stress:
   a. Health conditions
   b. Accidents and surgeries
   c. Nutrition and medication
   d. Age, lifestyle, postural factors, emotional and psychological factors

6. Explain that the uniqueness of individuals, especially their stress factors, can affect the length of time it takes to restore function or create a noticeable change.

redness. Palpation observations are noticed when you touch the client's body and feel the soft tissues. Some pertinent palpation observations to record include hypertonic muscles, atrophied muscles, and abnormal skin temperatures, either localized or over the entire body.

You may also evaluate the client's range of motion (ROM) at one or more joints, especially if he or she complains of restricted movement, normal activities that cannot be performed, or "tightness." A goniometer (GOH-nee-AH-meh-ter) is a specific device that measures the ROM in degrees. With specific training, some massage therapists use this device; however, most massage therapists evaluate ROM as a relative difference. Usually, clients explain that they have difficulty moving a specific joint or difficulty performing an activity that they normally do without any trouble. You can easily compare the ROM of the affected joint to the ROM of the same joint on the opposite side of the body. Likewise, you can consider the ROM of the joints involved in the activities that they cannot perform or have difficulty performing and compare the client's normal ROM to the now limited function and its associated limited ROM. With additional training, you can use functional assessment tests such as manual resisted (manual muscle) and special orthopedic tests to help determine any potential contraindications or the need for referral to another healthcare practitioner. The information you need to document in the "O" section of the SOAP note is covered in Chapter 7.

Activity and Analysis Information

Activity and analysis information covers the massage activity and an analysis of the session. The "A" portion of the SOAP note includes information about which techniques were used, where they were applied, and what the results were. You can also include effective or ineffective techniques, techniques the client preferred or disliked, and any changes you might have made during the session. Massage strokes, the flow of the massage, therapeutic techniques, complementary therapies, and special techniques are covered later in Chapters 9 through 12.

The analysis of the session requires that you perform a posttreatment assessment to determine if there are any changes following the massage, including increased or reduced pain levels, ROMs, stress levels, muscular tension, and progress toward the client's goals. These assessment skills are detailed in Chapter 7.

The next two steps of the analysis of the session, prioritizing functional limitations and setting treatment goals, apply to both therapeutic and wellness massage sessions. Try to avoid categorizing clients as either wellness massage clients or therapeutic massage clients, because in actuality, there is overlap. Even though wellness massage does not address any specific soft tissue conditions or limitations, you should document the functional limitations and treatment goals. People who go to spas for wellness massage on a regular basis may occasionally have soft tissue injuries. When that happens, a massage therapist can perform a therapeutic massage and establish the necessary treatment goals on the basis of the prioritized functional limitations.

Prioritizing Functional Limitations

After you have performed the posttreatment assessment, you can review all of the subjective, objective, and activity and analysis information to help clients prioritize their functional limitations, which are normal daily activities limited by muscular or connective tissue conditions. Using the information gathered from the intake forms, interview, and general assessments, you can help clients prioritize their functional limitations, deciding which activity is most

important to restore. Consider a client who has trouble flexing his left hip. Functional limitations may include a struggle to get in and out of his car without severe pain, an inability to go running, and difficulty getting in and out of his bed. His main concern might be getting in and out of the car because his job, which requires a lot of driving, is significantly affected. The secondary concerns might be running and climbing in and out of bed. You may have some information about the client's past and present involvement with these limited activities: how much the client ran before the limitation or how the lack of running has affected him. All of this information will help you devise the treatment goals and treatment plan.

Setting Treatment Goals

When clients come to you for massage treatment, they typically want to relax, reduce pain, reduce stress, reduce muscular tension, and/or increase movement. These pretreatment requests, sometimes considered goals, are subjective input that can be documented in the "S" portion of the SOAP note. After the massage and posttreatment assessment, however, you and your client will integrate the client's goals with the analysis of the session to determine short- and long-term treatment goals. These treatment goals are functional goals that clarify a client's progress toward overcoming functional limitations. Although not necessary, client participation in goal setting is helpful because it gets them involved in their healing and treatment process. When establishing goals, the following components must be included:

- Identify a specific activity.
- Include results that can be easily recognized or are quantifiable.
- Include measurable tasks that can be accomplished by the client.
- Include a functional limitation that is pertinent to the client's lifestyle.
- Set a limited amount of time in which to accomplish the goal.

The most important quality of these goals is that you and your clients can recognize when the goals are met and the outcome has been achieved. Specifying measurable quantities and identifiable qualities makes it easy for clients to see that the goal has been accomplished. Make sure the goals are reasonable and attainable. Otherwise, clients might feel too discouraged to participate in their healthcare or could be disappointed when the goals are not quickly reached. If the client is not convinced that a goal will lead to lifestyle improvements, and there is no distinguishable way to know if the goal is achievable or when it has been achieved, then that goal is useless for the therapeutic process. Creating effective and useful goals takes some practice but is important for the therapeutic process.

When clients have a solid goal before them that is attainable and easily recognized, they are usually more motivated to participate in their healthcare.

Long- and Short-term Goals

Long-term goals (LTGs) are set up for clients to achieve within 1 to 2 months and are based on their primary areas of concern. This time frame varies with functional stress, chronic conditions that require time to heal, and a client's desire to return to the most functional state of health over time. With time frames longer than 2 months, clients can easily lose sight of the goal and may discontinue treatment. An LTG for the above client with hip problems might be being able to run 3 miles, three times a week without pain after 2 months of treatment.

To keep clients from becoming discouraged with slow progress or from doubting progress altogether, you assign short-term goals (STGs). STGs are those that can be accomplished in 1 to 2 weeks. They are a good source of motivation for clients to continue treatment and continue working toward overcoming functional limitations. They focus on the client's primary area of concern, overcoming functional limitations that are top priority, or getting clients out of an acute phase of an injury. Each STG should support the LTG, and they are typically designed to be progressive so the client is aware of the progress. For instance, consider a dog groomer who experiences shoulder pain when lifting dogs onto the grooming table. You and the client can decide on the LTG of being able to lift a 20-pound dog onto the grooming table, four times a day, 5 days a week without pain. A series of STGs to support this LTG might be:

1. Within 10 days, be able to lift a dog of less than 5 pounds onto the grooming table, twice a day, 3 days a week without pain.

2. Within 10 days, be able to lift a dog of between 5 and 10 pounds onto the grooming table, twice a day, 5 days a week without pain.

3. Within 10 days, be able to lift a 10-pound dog onto the grooming table, four times a day, 5 days a week without pain.

Following are some effective STGs to support LTGs:

- STG: Climb in and out of a car three times a day with mild pain within 2 weeks
  - LTG: Run 3 miles, three times a week without pain after 2 months
- STG: Drive the car for 10 minutes, 3 days in a row, without pain within 1 week
  - LTG: Drive the car for the 1-hour commute to work, 5 days a week without pain within 2 months
- STG: Sleep for 3 hours in a row, without back pain upon waking, 3 days a week within 2 weeks
  - LTG: Sleep for 6 hours in a row and wake up without back pain, 3 days a week within 2 months

- STG: Talk on the phone for 15 minutes without getting a headache, 3 days in a row, within 12 days
  - LTG: Talk on the phone for 30 minutes, five times a day, 5 days a week without getting a headache, within 6 weeks
- STG: Carry the baby for 10 minutes at a time, once a day without neck and shoulder pain, 3 days in a row, within 1 week
  - LTG: Carry the baby for 15 minutes at a time, five times a day without neck and shoulder pain, 7 days a week within 2 months

Recall the effects of cumulative stress. Healing time and the length of time improvements will last depend on the accumulated stress and stress factors, the amount of self-care a client performs, and the client's physical activity. You must explain to clients that accomplishing their treatment goals depends on a number of factors: the uniqueness of the individual plays a large part in restoring normal function, and although the treatment goals are reasonable and attainable, client participation with self-care activities will be helpful.

Examples of the activity and analysis of massage sessions are shown in Box 6-2.

Plan Information

The **plan information** of the SOAP note includes a plan for future treatment and recommendations for self-care. This future treatment refers to the frequency of future treatments, duration of those treatments, techniques to try, and techniques to avoid. If you refer clients to any other healthcare practitioners, you can document it in this section.

The plan section identifies the specific self-care activities that you assign and how often clients are supposed to do the activities. You can check the SOAP note from the client's previous session to know what kind of self-care the client might have used between sessions and ask whether it was used. Many clients are only interested in receiving massage to feel better and are not interested in participating in their own healthcare, so try to not get frustrated with clients who do not use the self-care activities you recommend. You can gently remind clients that self-care activities will help reduce the time it takes to accomplish goals and will increase the length of time the benefits of the massage last. One form of self-care is to redirect clients' focus from illness and pain to health and absence of pain. When clients start paying attention to how much better they feel, they better appreciate the benefits of massage and may be more likely to participate in their own healthcare. Treatment goals that focus on the absence of pain or discomfort support this redirected pattern of thinking. The treatment plan is further discussed in Chapter 8.

BOX 6-2
Examples of Activity and Analysis

ANDY

Andy begins the session by wanting to minimize his right-sided neck tension and pain. He has difficulty looking over his shoulder to check his blind spot when he drives, and he states that he drives in city traffic all day long for his job. Aspirin seems to reduce the pain temporarily, and as the day wears on, he can move his neck more. You observe limited range of motion (ROM) of the neck upon rotation and lateral flexion, especially to the left.

During the session, you notice that the muscles for neck rotation and lateral flexion are hypertonic, and you find some trigger points that radiate pain in his levator scapula muscles. You apply some light friction and trigger point release along with general massage techniques.

The posttreatment assessment shows several improvements. Andy reports reduced pain and expresses relief and gratitude. With palpation and retesting, you notice that the tension in the neck has decreased and the ROM has increased when tested for lateral flexion. Andy says that his only concern is to be able to check his blind spot without wincing in pain, which becomes his top priority functional limitation. Together, you determine his long-term goal to be to be able to check his blind spot throughout the entire day, 5 days a week without pain. Some short-term goals you set from session to session might be to

1. Check his blind spot for the first hour of driving without pain at least 3 days a week, within the next week.
2. Check his blind spot all morning without pain at least 3 days a week, within 10 days.
3. Check his blind spot all day without pain at least 3 days a week, within 10 days.

SARA

Sara comes to you for massage. She says she is having trouble lifting her baby in and out of the crib, car, swing, and high chair. She complains that her neck and shoulders hurt all the time, but these particular movements create so much pain in her shoulders that she is afraid she will drop the baby. She says she suffers the same pain when doing laundry and trying to wash her hair. Before the massage, your general assessments reveal bilateral limited shoulder flexion and bilateral shoulder abduction, although worse on the right side.

During the massage, you detect hypertonic areas anterior to her glenohumeral joints, hypertonic upper trapezius muscles, and hypertonic levator scapula muscles. Adding therapeutic techniques to your typical relaxation massage flow, you feel the hypertonic tissues soften with massage.

Following the massage, Sara admits that the pain that she felt all the time is gone. You reevaluate the affected ROMs and find that she can flex and abduct both shoulders much farther than before treatment and barely notices the pain at the end of the ROM. Verbally summarizing the subjective, objective, activity and analysis information, you can then review Sara's functional limitations: lifting the baby in and out of different things, doing laundry, and washing her hair. She states that it is most important that she be able to lift the baby in and out of the crib confidently because people are usually around to help her with the other things, such as getting the baby out of the car and doing the laundry.

Together, you determine her long-term goal to be to lift the baby in and out of the crib three times a day for a week without pain. Over a series of sessions, you establish the following short-term goals:

1. Within a week, be able to place four dishes on the top shelf of the kitchen cabinet daily, one at a time, without pain
2. Within a week, be able to place eight dishes on the top shelf of the kitchen cabinet daily, two at a time, without pain
3. Within 2 weeks, be able to lift the baby out of the high chair twice a day, every day, without pain
4. Within 2 weeks, be able to lift the baby out of the crib once a day, every day, without pain

Putting the SOAP Together

The massage treatment record you use does not have to be the SOAP format included in this text; however, it is commonly used in many healthcare fields, and it can be helpful for sharing information with other healthcare practitioners. There are several guidelines for documenting in your practice to ensure validity and dependability of the records:

- Information should be pertinent to the client's chief complaint/s or massage treatment.

- Information should be clear but brief.

- Abbreviations used should be generally accepted industry standards.

- Writing should be in pen, neat, and legible.

- Only correct a mistake by drawing a single line through it and writing your initials and date near or over the line. Never use an eraser or correction fluid.

- Records should be kept in a safe place and away from public access.

When you first start writing SOAP notes, you may find it challenging to write all the necessary information in a limited space and within the limited time for every massage session. There are times when you might have 15 minutes between clients to clean the table, wash your hands, put new sheets on the table for the next client, and document the session you just finished. Although it is tempting to skip the documentation for some sessions, it is important to your clients, your financial success, and the profession that each session is recorded. Brief statements, body diagrams, abbreviations, and symbols can speed up the documentation process and make SOAP notes easier to interpret. SOAP notes can be preprinted forms or blank documents that you fill out.

Some preprinted massage treatment records include a body diagram to indicate where on the body the client feels symptoms. (See Fig. 6-4 for an example SOAP note for a client from Box 6-2.) Symbols are often used on these diagrams, and a key to the symbols is typically at the bottom of the page.

These diagrams and symbols can be useful for visually tracking changes on the body, and they eliminate the need to use words to describe an area on the body or a change that occurred.

Many abbreviations and symbols are used for efficient and effective documentation. (Table 6-6 lists abbreviations

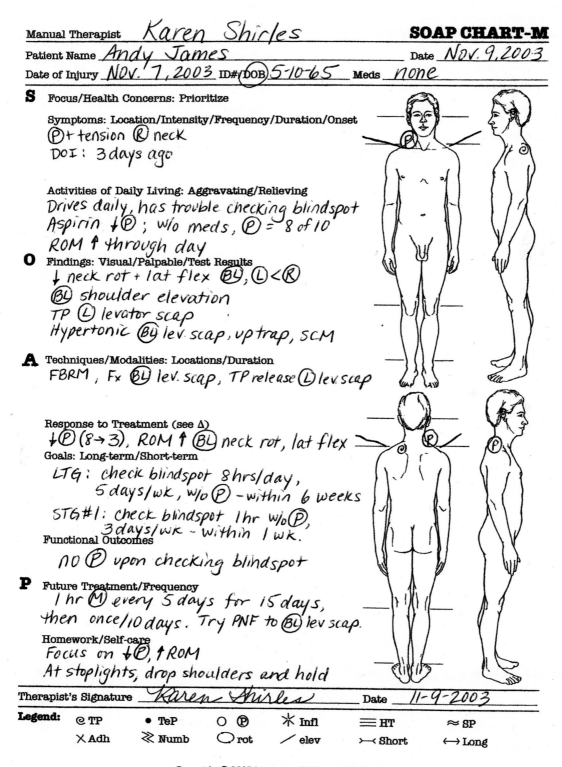

Manual Therapist **Karen Shirles**

SOAP CHART-M

Patient Name **Andy James** Date **Nov. 9, 2003**

Date of Injury **Nov. 7, 2003** ID#/DOB **5-10-65** Meds **none**

S Focus/Health Concerns: Prioritize

Symptoms: Location/Intensity/Frequency/Duration/Onset
Ⓟ + tension Ⓡ neck
DOI: 3 days ago

Activities of Daily Living: Aggravating/Relieving
Drives daily, has trouble checking blindspot
Aspirin ↓Ⓟ ; w/o meds, Ⓟ = 8 of 10
ROM ↑ through day

O Findings: Visual/Palpable/Test Results
↓ neck rot + lat flex ⒷⓁ, Ⓛ<Ⓡ
ⒷⓁ shoulder elevation
TP Ⓛ levator scap
Hypertonic ⒷⓁ lev. scap, up trap, SCM

A Techniques/Modalities: Locations/Duration
FBRM , Fx ⒷⓁ lev. scap, TP release Ⓛ lev scap

Response to Treatment (see Δ)
↓Ⓟ (8→3), ROM ↑ ⒷⓁ neck rot, lat flex
Goals: Long-term/Short-term
LTG: check blindspot 8 hrs/day,
    5 days/wk, w/o Ⓟ - within 6 weeks
STG#1: check blindspot 1 hr w/o Ⓟ,
    3 days/wk - within 1 wk.
Functional Outcomes
    no Ⓟ upon checking blindspot

P Future Treatment/Frequency
    1 hr Ⓜ every 5 days for 15 days,
    then once/10 days. Try PNF to ⒷⓁ lev scap.
Homework/Self-care
Focus on ↓Ⓟ, ↑ROM
At stoplights, drop shoulders and hold

Therapist's Signature **Karen Shirles** Date **11-9-2003**

Legend: ℮ TP ● TeP ○ Ⓟ ✳ Infl ≡ HT ≈ SP
X Adh ≋ Numb ◯ rot ╱ elev ⊁ Short ⟷ Long

Figure 6-4. SOAP with body diagram filled out for sample client in Box 6-2. (Reprinted with permission from Thompson DL. Hands Heal: Communication, Documentation, and Insurance Billing for Manual Therapists. 3rd ed. Baltimore: Lippincott Williams & Wilkins, 2006.)

Table 6-6 Abbreviations and Symbols for Massage Therapy (common ones in bold)

TERM	SYMBOL	TERM	SYMBOL
Massage Terms, Modalities, Findings		tension	**tens**
client	**Cl**	**treatment**	**Tx**
connective tissue	**CT**	*Symbols*	
contraindication	**CI**	**adhesion**	**X**
craniosacral therapy	**CST**	**after**	**p, post**
cross-fiber friction	**XFF**	**and**	**&, +**
deep tissue	**DT**	**approximate**	**≈, ~**
direct manipulation	**DM**	**at**	**@**
direct pressure	DP	**before**	**ā, pre**
effleurage	**eff**	**change**	**Δ**
energy work	**EW**	**down, decrease**	**↓**
friction	**Fx**	**elevation**	**/**
ice, compression, elevation, support	ICES	**equals**	**=**
manual lymphatic drainage	**MLD**	female	♀
massage	**Ⓜ**	greater than	>
massage therapist	**MT**	hypertonic, tension	≡
muscle energy technique	**MET**	**leading to, resulting**	**→**
myofascial release	**MFR**	less than	<
neuromuscular therapy	**NMT**	longer than normal	↔
not applicable	N/A	male	♂
palpation	**palp**	numbness, tingling	⋛
pétrissage	**pet**	**pain**	**P, Ⓟ**
physical therapy	PT	rotation	↺, ↻, ↻
positional release	**PR**	shorter than normal	⋈
proprioceptive neuromuscular facilitation	**PNF**	spasm	≈
reciprocal inhibition	**RI**	swelling, inflammation	✳
reflexology	reflex	tender point	•
somatoemotional release	SER	trigger point	℮
tense and relax	**T&R**	**times, repetitions**	**X**

continues on following page

Table 6-6 Abbreviations and Symbols for Massage Therapy (common ones in bold) *continued*

TERM	SYMBOL	TERM	SYMBOL
up, increase	↑	quadriceps femoris	quads
with	w/, c̄	rhomboid muscles	rhomb
without	w/o	scalene muscles	scal
Anatomy		sternocleidomastoid	SCM
abdominals	abs	sacroiliac	SI
anterior superior iliac spine	**ASIS**	soft tissue	ST
biceps brachii	bi	**thoracic, thoracic vertebrae**	**T, T1–T12**
cervical, cervical vertebrae	**C, C1–C7**	**tensor fascia latae**	**TFL**
connective tissue	**CT**	**temporomandibular joint**	**TMJ**
cranium	Cr	**trapezius muscles**	**traps**
deltoid	**delt**	triceps brachii	tri
diaphragm	dia	*Medical Record Terminology, Measurements*	
energy	E	as needed	prn
erector spinae	ES	beats per minute	bpm
gastrocnemius	**gastroc**	**complains of**	**c/o**
gluteal muscles	**gluts, glutes**	continue same	CSTx
		could not test	CNT
hamstrings	**hams**	**date of injury**	**DOI**
head and neck	H&N	did not test	DNT
iliotibial band	**ITB, IT band**	**full body**	**FB**
latissimus dorsi	**lats**	**full-body relaxation massage**	**FBRM**
levator scapulae	**lev scap**	**history**	**Hx**
low back	**LB**	**long-term goal**	**LTG**
lumbar, lumbar vertebrae	**L, L1–L5**	**medications**	**meds**
muscles	**mm**	next visit	nv
occiput	occ	**prescriptions**	**Rx**
pectoralis muscles	**pecs**	**recommendation**	**rec**
posterior superior iliac spine	**PSIS**	same as	S/A
quadratus lumborum	**QL**	same treatment	SATx
		treatment	**Tx**

continues on following page

Table 6-6 Abbreviations and Symbols for Massage Therapy (common ones in bold) *continued*

TERM	SYMBOL	TERM	SYMBOL
Symptoms, Maladies		posterior	**post**
adhesion	**adh**	prone	pr
backache	BA	**proximal**	**prox**
chronic fatigue syndrome	CFS	**right**	**Ⓡ**
diagnosis	Dx	**severe**	**sev**
edema	ed	side-lying	SL
fibromyalgia syndrome	FM, FMS	superior, supine	sup
fibrous tissue	FT	within normal limits	WNL
headache	**HA**	*Actions*	
pain	**P, Ⓟ**	**abduction**	**abd**
sleep disturbance	SD	**adduction**	**add**
symptoms	Sx	**circumduction**	**circ**
tender point	**TeP**	depression	dep
tension	**tens**	dorsiflexion	DF
trigger point	**TP, TrP**	elevation	ele
Directional, Descriptive Terms		eversion	ever
anterior	**ant**	**extension**	**ext**
bilateral, both	**Ⓑ⃝L, Ⓑ**	**flexion**	**flex**
constant	const	inversion	inv
excessive	xs	**lateral flexion**	**lat flex**
external	**ext**	**opposition**	**opp**
internal	**int**	plantarflexion	PF
lateral	lat	pronation	pro

left	**Ⓛ**	range of motion
		    active range of motion
		    active assisted range of motion
		    passive range of motion
		    resisted range of motion
			ROM
			AROM
			AAROM
			PROM
			RROM

light, low, mild	L		
medial	**med**	**rotation**	**rot**
moderate	**mod**	side-bending	SB
normal	N	supination	sup

and symbols for massage treatment records, identifying the more common ones.) Some of the more helpful symbols you may use include delta (Δ), the standard symbol for change, or an arrow ($\rightarrow$) to indicate posttreatment assessment findings. The changes you indicate will typically be positive changes due to treatment, but if symptoms worsen, you can still use these symbols. For instance:

- Full-body relaxation massage resulted in reduced pain and increased left lateral flexion of the neck:
    - FBRM $\rightarrow$ $\downarrow$P + $\uparrow$(L)lat flex neck
- The client complains of moderate pain in the right shoulder:
    - Cl c/o mod P (R)shoulder
- The left anterior superior iliac spine was higher than the right before the massage, but they were even after the massage:
    - (L)ASIS $\uparrow$ Δ (L)ASIS = (R)ASIS

Typically, not much time is available to fill out a SOAP note, so you may be inclined to wait until the end of the day to document all the SOAP notes. The longer you wait to fill out the SOAP, however, the less accurate your documentation will be, especially if you have to fill out numerous SOAP notes at one time. After several different clients have come and gone, it is often difficult to remember details specific to each client. Information is more accurate when you document immediately after the session. Because these documents are used as the basis for future treatments and may also be used by other healthcare professionals as well as attorneys and insurance companies, your accuracy is critical. Using appropriate abbreviations can speed up the process of documentation, allowing you to fill out the SOAP note immediately after each massage session.

SOAP Note Variations

All of the previous examples of SOAP notes are full-page forms that provide space for recording the pertinent details for therapeutic massage sessions. There are a number of variations available. A shortened form can be used when a client is treated for general concerns or given a wellness massage. One of the shortened forms is called the Wellness Chart (Fig. 6-5). Tx refers to treatment, in which you document general information on treatment and results. C refers to comments, including brief recommendations for another treatment and self-care. The form shown here includes a body diagram for you to note specific data.

Case Studies

Introducing . . . The Case Studies

Three different case studies are presented throughout this text. The participants are introduced with brief biographies followed by the documentation forms used to record their information: health history and SOAP notes. The SOAP note will be highlighted differently in each chapter that includes the Case Studies, showcasing the information that is most appropriate for those chapters. Here, we introduce Rob Blackwell, Timothy Roberts, and Kirsten Van Marter.

Progressive Case Study 1:
Rob Blackwell

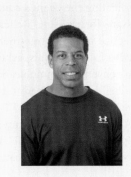

Rob Blackwell is a 42-year-old man who is trying massage for the first time and hopes to restore his sleep and reduce pain in his neck, shoulder, back, and knees so he can lift weights and golf as he used to. Rob says his shoulder pain interferes with his activities the most. He complains that his sleep is affected by his pain, and his health history reveals osteoarthritis and tendinitis in his knees, multiple sprains in his ankles, sinus trouble, and multiple head injuries. Your interview determines that the osteoarthritis diagnosis was made more than 10 years ago. On a pain scale of 1 to 10, with 10 being the worst pain, Rob says all of his areas of concern are about 4. He soaks in the hot tub, which helps the pain, and he occasionally takes ibuprofen, which could affect his pain perception during massage. All of the information Rob tells you is subjective information, and you record anything that is pertinent to his chief complaints (Figs. 6-6 and 6-7).

The massage for Rob is designed to reduce pain and tension and find fascial adhesions, but you focus on the condition of the soft tissues in his shoulders. You use your standard massage flow, with the addition of some therapeutic techniques. After the massage, you perform the posttreatment assessment, prioritize Rob's functional limitations, and determine short- and long-term treatment goals. You make treatment plan recommendations regarding future treatment, self-care, and referrals to other healthcare practitioners.

Progressive Case Study 2:
Timothy Roberts

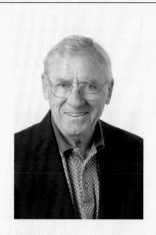

Timothy Roberts is an elderly gentleman who is primarily interested in relaxation. A person his age is considered part of the senior (geriatric) population, but treatment should be based on the condition of the soft tissues and general state of health. He indicates no specific areas of concern or chief complaints, but you notice that he takes blood pressure medication and has a history of skin cancer (Fig. 6-8).

The main focus of Timothy's massage will be relaxation and circulatory enhancement. During the massage, you find fascial restrictions and reduced passive ROM in his left ankle. Following the massage, you briefly discuss plans for future massage treatment and self-care activities.

Progressive Case Study 3:
Kirsten Van Marter

Kirsten Van Marter is a 38-year-old woman in her third trimester of pregnancy. She has received monthly massage treatments in the past but is a

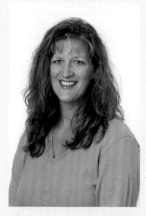

first-time client for you. Her primary complaint is mild but constant back pain. Her secondary concern is mild pain in her hips, pelvis, neck, and shoulders. She is looking for pain relief in her areas of concern as well as restored sleep, restored normal fitness level, and she wants to be able to pick up her child without pain. She says that she worries that she will drop her daughter because of the pain. She is physically active and in good health, except for anemia and gestational diabetes during this pregnancy. You record any information Kirsten shares with you that is pertinent to her areas of concern as subjective information (Figs. 6-9 and 6-10).

There are a number of techniques and areas to avoid for prenatal massage and special considerations to make. You keep Kirsten in the side-lying position for most of the massage and provide a relaxation massage with some therapeutic techniques. After the massage, you perform a posttreatment assessment, prioritize her functional limitations, and determine short- and long-term treatment goals. You make specific recommendations for future treatment and self-care.

CHAPTER SUMMARY

The language of massage therapy contains many medical and scientific terms. To learn this language, you need commitment and lots of practice. Use your eyes, ear, mouth, and body in the process to reinforce and facilitate learning, but make sure you are learning correctly. In all modes of communication, whether oral or written, with the client or another healthcare professional, you must use correct spelling, pronunciation, and context. Knowing how to break down a word to determine its meaning will help you understand the universal language of healthcare and may make it easier to learn the basics of anatomy, physiology, pathology, and pharmacology.

Based on the events in the history of massage and the concepts of ethics and professionalism, you can see why effective communication and documentation are important. Without effective communication, you cannot gather appropriate and important information or accurately document activity that occurred. Inaccurate records provide an undependable history, they can lead to misunderstanding,

and they can compromise your integrity and professionalism. Ethics and professionalism are cornerstones for a successful practice. Your understanding of medical terminology, anatomy, and physiology help you read and write useful massage treatment records that contain helpful information for you and the other members of your clients' healthcare team.

Gathering information through effective communication with clients is vital to good documentation. Establishing rapport and mutual trust and validating the client's condition and perceptions are necessary for creating a client-centered focus for safe and effective massage treatment. Effective communication, reflective listening skills, asking useful questions, and considering nonverbal communication all help make the interview more effective and lead to the most thorough picture of a client's current condition. This information is recorded on a SOAP chart or other documentation format. Documentation is essential for the safe and effective treatment of clients as well as for communication with other healthcare providers.

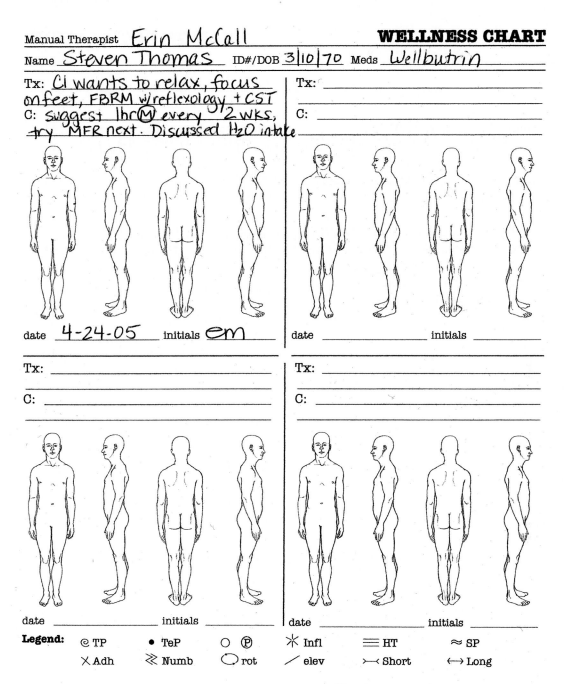

Manual Therapist **Erin McCall**   **WELLNESS CHART**

Name **Steven Thomas**   ID#/DOB **3/10/70**   Meds **Wellbutrin**

Tx: **Cl wants to relax, focus on feet, FBRM w/reflexology + CST**

C: **suggest 1hr M every 2 wks, try MFR next. Discussed H₂O intake**

Tx: _____

C: _____

date **4-24-05**   initials **em**

date _____   initials _____

Tx: _____

C: _____

Tx: _____

C: _____

date _____   initials _____

date _____   initials _____

Legend:

℮ TP	• TeP	○ ℗	✳ Infl	≡ HT	≈ SP
✕ Adh	≫ Numb	↻ rot	⁄ elev	⊁ Short	↔ Long

Figure 6-5. Wellness chart. (Reprinted with permission from Thompson DL. Hands Heal: Communication, Documentation, and Insurance Billing for Manual Therapists. 3rd ed. Baltimore: Lippincott Williams & Wilkins, 2006.)

Manual Therapist   **HEALTH INFORMATION**

Patient Name _ROB BLACKWELL_____   Date _4-2-02___

Date of Injury _____—_____ ID#/DOB __—____

A. Patient Information

Address _120 MAIN ST._____

City _INDY____ State_IN_ Zip_46220_

Phone: Home _555-2345_____

   Work ___—___ Cell_555-3333___

Employer _(self)_____

Work Address _____

Occupation _PERSONAL TRAINER_

Emergency Contact_STEPHANIE (WIFE)_

Phone: Home _(SAME)_____

   Work_555-1880_Cell_555-6960___

Primary Health Care Provider

Name ____NONE_____

Address _____

City/State/Zip_____

Phone: _____ Fax _____

I give my massage therapist permission to
consult with my health care providers
regarding my health and treatment.

Comments _____

Initials _____ Date _____

B. Current Health Information

List Health Concerns Check all that apply

Primary _NECK/SHOULDER_____

☒ mild ☐ moderate ☐ disabling

☒ constant ☐ intermittant

☒ symptoms ↑ w/activity   ☐ ↓ w/activity

☐ getting worse ☐ getting better ☒ no change

treatment received _NONE_____

Secondary _BACK_____

☒ mild ☐ moderate ☐ disabling

☒ constant ☐ intermittant

☒ symptoms ↑ w/activity   ☐ ↓ w/activity

☐ getting worse ☐ getting better ☒ no change

treatment received _NONE_____

Additional _KNEE_____

☐ mild ☒ moderate ☐ disabling

☐ constant ☒ intermittant

☐ symptoms ↑ w/activity   ☒ ↓ w/activity

☐ getting worse ☐ getting better ☒ no change

treatment received _NONE_____

List Daily Activities Limited by Condition

Work _PHYSICAL TRAINING_
8+ HRS/DAY

Home/Family _____

~~Sleep~~/Self-care _____

Social/Recreational _WORKOUT, WEIGHTS,_
BICYCLE, BASKETBALL 3X/MO,
GOLF

List Self-Care Routines

How do you reduce stress? _EXERCISE_

Pain? _IBUPROFEN, HOT TUB_

List current medications (include pain relievers
and herbal remedies) _____

_____

_____

_____

Have you ever received massage therapy
before? _NO_ Frequency? _____

What are your goals for receiving massage
therapy? _RESTORE SLEEP, REDUCE_
PAIN, RETURN TO PRIOR LEVEL
WEIGHTLIFTING, GOLF AGAIN

C. Health History

List and Explain. Include dates and treatment
received.

Surgeries _APPENDIX 9/78_

_____

_____

Injuries _____

_____

_____

Major Illnesses _N/A_

_____

_____

Copyright © 2005 Lippincott Williams & Wilkins

Figure 6-6. Health Information Form for Rob Blackwell. (Reprinted with permission from Thompson DL. Hands Heal: Communication, Documentation, and Insurance Billing for Manual Therapists. 3rd ed. Baltimore: Lippincott Williams & Wilkins, 2006.)

HEALTH INFORMATION page 2

Check All Current and Previous Conditions Please Explain

General

current	past		comments
☐	☐	headaches	
☒	☐	pain	
☒	☐	sleep disturbances	
☒	☐	fatigue	
☐	☐	infections	
☐	☐	fever	
☐	☒	sinus	
☐	☐	other	

Skin Conditions

current	past		comments
☐	☐	rashes	
☐	☒	athlete's foot, warts	
☐	☐	other	

Muscles and Joints

current	past		comments
☐	☐	rheumatoid arthritis	
☒	☐	osteoarthritis *KNEES*	
☐	☐	osteoporosis	
☐	☐	scoliosis	
☐	☐	broken bones	
☐	☐	spinal problems	
☐	☐	disk problems	
☐	☐	lupus	
☐	☐	TMJ, jaw pain	
☐	☐	spasms, cramps	
☐	☒	sprains, strains	
☐	☒	tendonitis, bursitis *KNEES*	
☒	☐	stiff or painful joints	
☐	☐	weak or sore muscles	
☒	☐	ⓝⓔⓒⓚ ⓢⓗⓞⓤⓛⓓⓔⓡ, arm pain	
☐	☐	low back, hip, leg pain	
☐	☐	other	

Nervous System

current	past		comments
☐	☒	head injuries, concussions *1980, 81, 82*	
☐	☐	dizziness, ringing in ears	
☐	☐	loss of memory, confusion	
☒	☐	numbness, tingling	
☐	☐	sciatica, shooting pain	
☐	☐	chronic pain	
☐	☐	depression	
☐	☐	other	

Respiratory, Cardiovascular

current	past		comments
☐	☐	heart disease	
☐	☐	blood clots	
☐	☐	stroke	
☐	☐	lymphadema	
☐	☐	high, low blood pressure	
☐	☐	irregular heart beat	
☐	☐	poor circulation	
☐	☐	swollen ankles	
☐	☐	varicose veins	
☐	☐	chest pain, shortness of breath	
☐	☐	asthma	

Allergies

current	past		comments
☐	☐	scents, oils, lotions	
☐	☐	detergents	
☐	☐	other	

Digestive/Elimination System

current	past		comments
☐	☐	bowel problems	
☐	☐	gas, bloating	
☐	☐	bladder/kidney/prostrate	
☐	☐	abdominal pain	
☐	☐	other	

Endocrine System

current	past		comments
☐	☐	thyroid	
☐	☐	diabetes	

Reproductive System

current	past		comments
☐	☐	pregnancy	
☐	☐	painful, emotional menses	
☐	☐	fibrotic cysts	

Cancer/Tumors

current	past		comments
☐	☐	benign	
☐	☐	malignant	

Habits

current	past		comments
☐	☐	tobacco	
☐	☐	alcohol	
☐	☐	drugs	
☐	☐	coffee, soda	

Contract for Care

I promise to participate fully as a member of my health care team. I will make sound choices regarding my treatment plan based on the information provided by my manual therapist and other members of my health care team, and my experience of those suggestions. I agree to participate in the self care program we select. I promise to inform my practitioner any time I feel my well-being is threatened or compromised. I expect my manual therapist to provide safe and effective treatment.

Consent for Care

It is my choice to receive manual therapy, and I give my consent to receive treatment. I have reported all health conditions that I am aware of and will inform my practitioner of any changes in my health.

Signature _Robert Backwell_ Date _4-2-02_

Figure 6-6. (*continued*)

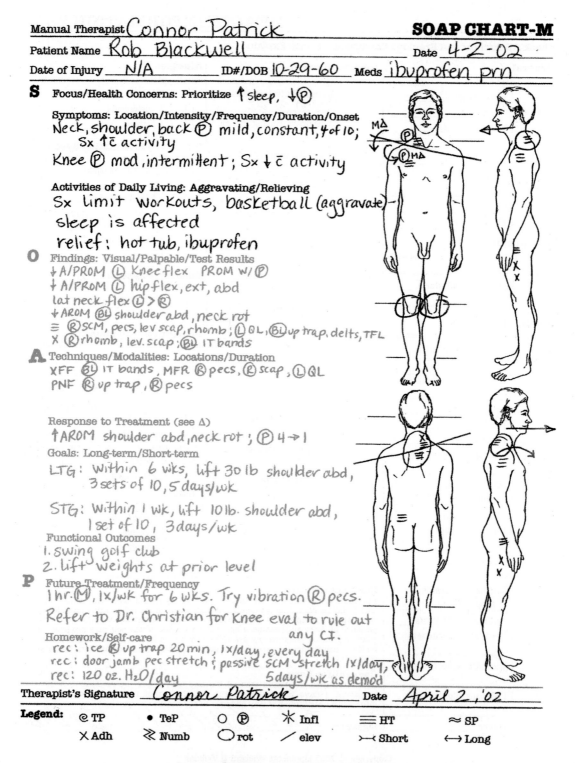

Manual Therapist **Connor Patrick**   **SOAP CHART-M**

Patient Name **Rob Blackwell**   Date **4-2-02**

Date of Injury **N/A**   ID#/DOB **10-29-60**   Meds **ibuprofen prn**

S Focus/Health Concerns: Prioritize ↑sleep, ↓Ⓟ

Symptoms: Location/Intensity/Frequency/Duration/Onset
Neck, shoulder, back Ⓟ mild, constant, 4 of 10;
   Sx ↑c̄ activity
Knee Ⓟ mod, intermittent; Sx ↓c̄ activity

Activities of Daily Living: Aggravating/Relieving
Sx limit workouts, basketball (aggravate)
sleep is affected
relief: hot tub, ibuprofen

O Findings: Visual/Palpable/Test Results
↓A/PROM Ⓛ knee flex PROM w/Ⓟ
↓A/PROM Ⓛ hip flex, ext, abd
lat neck flex Ⓛ > Ⓡ
↓AROM Ⓑ shoulder abd, neck rot
≡ Ⓡ SCM, pecs, lev scap, rhomb; Ⓛ QL, Ⓑ up trap, delts, TFL
✗ Ⓡ rhomb, lev. scap; Ⓑ IT bands

A Techniques/Modalities: Locations/Duration
XFF Ⓑ IT bands, MFR Ⓡ pecs, Ⓡ scap, Ⓛ QL
PNF Ⓡ up trap, Ⓡ pecs

Response to Treatment (see Δ)
↑AROM shoulder abd, neck rot ; Ⓟ 4→1
Goals: Long-term/Short-term
LTG: Within 6 wks, lift 30 lb shoulder abd,
        3 sets of 10, 5 days/wk

STG: Within 1 wk, lift 10 lb. shoulder abd,
        1 set of 10, 3 days/wk
Functional Outcomes
1. swing golf club
2. lift weights at prior level

P Future Treatment/Frequency
1 hr. Ⓜ, 1x/wk for 6 wks. Try vibration Ⓡ pecs.
Refer to Dr. Christian for knee eval to rule out
                                any CI.
Homework/Self-care
   rec: ice Ⓡ up trap 20 min, 1x/day, every day
   rec: door jamb pec stretch ; passive SCM stretch 1x/day,
   rec: 120 oz. H₂O/day   5 days/wk as demo'd

Therapist's Signature **Connor Patrick**   Date **April 2, '02**

Legend: ℮ TP   • TeP   O Ⓟ   ✳ Infl   ≡ HT   ≈ SP
            ✗ Adh   ≋ Numb   ◯ rot   ╱ elev   >—< Short   ↔ Long

Copyright © 2005 Lippincott Williams & Wilkins

Figure 6-7. SOAP Chart for Rob Blackwell, subjective information highlighted. (Reprinted with permission from Thompson DL. Hands Heal: Communication, Documentation, and Insurance Billing for Manual Therapists. 3rd ed. Baltimore: Lippincott Williams & Wilkins, 2006.)

Manual Therapist *Max Harr*

WELLNESS CHART-M

Name *Timothy Roberts*   ID#/DOB *9-10-30*   Date *12-18-03*

Phone *555-4220*   Address *7000 Osprey Ln.*

1. What are your goals for health, and how may I assist you in achieving your goals? _____
   relaxation

2. List typical daily activities—work, exercise, home.   *golf, house projects*

3. Are you currently experiencing any of the following? If yes, please explain.

   pain, tenderness   ☑ No ☐ Yes: _____   stiffness ☑ No ☐ Yes: _____
   numbness or tingling ☑ No ☐ Yes: _____   swelling ☑ No ☐ Yes: _____
   allergies   ☑ No ☐ Yes: _____

4. List all illnesses, injuries, and health concerns you have now or have had in the past 3 years.
   (Examples: arthritis, diabetes, car crash) *moderate blood pressure,*
   skin cancers, broken left ankle

5. List medications and pain relievers taken this week. *blood pressure meds*

6. I have provided all my known medical information. I acknowledge that massage therapy is
   not a substitute for medical diagnosis and treatment. I give my consent to receive treatment.

   Signature *Timothy Roberts*   Date *12-18-03*

   Tx: *FBRM c̄ circulatory enhancement focus;*
   during (M) noticed ↓ROM + X (L) ankle (dorsiflex, evert)
   C: *cl has no specific complaints today*
   next session try XFF (L) ankle

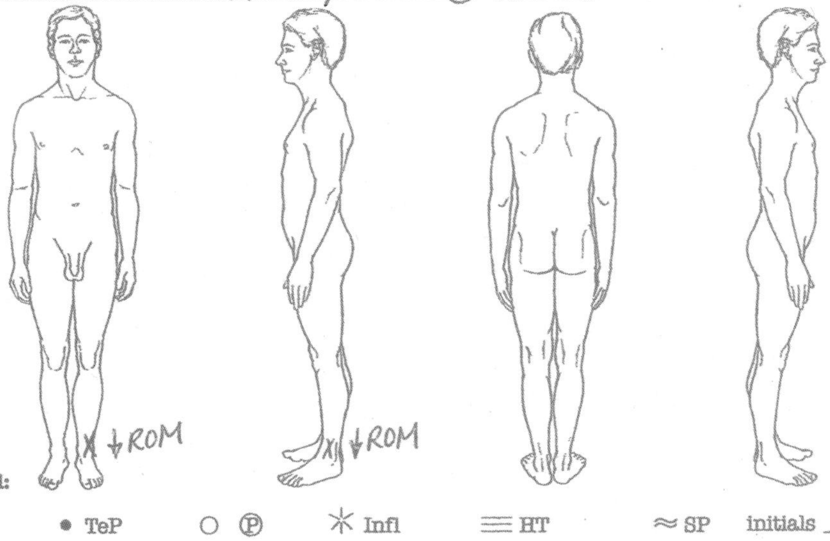

X ↓ROM   *X ↓ROM*

Legend:

ⓔ TP   • TeP   ○ ⓟ   ✳ Infl   ≡ HT   ≈ SP   initials *MH*

✗ Adh   ≋ Numb   ⊘ rot   ╱ elev   >—< Short   ←→ Long

Figure 6-8. Wellness chart for Timothy Roberts, subjective information highlighted. (Modified with permission from Thompson DL. Hands Heal: Communication, Documentation, and Insurance Billing for Manual Therapists. 3rd ed. Baltimore: Lippincott Williams & Wilkins, 2006.)

Manual Therapist _Parker Bellman_   **HEALTH INFORMATION**

Patient Name _Kirsten Van Marter_   Date _4-9-02_

Date of Injury _N/A_   ID#/(DOB) _6-17-63_

A. Patient Information

Address _130 Main St._

City _Indianapolis_ State _IN_ Zip _46260_

Phone: Home _555-3456_

   Work _555-4455_ Cell _555-5961_

Employer _ABC Hospital_

Work Address _N. Senate Ave._

Occupation _Health Program Coordinator_

Emergency Contact _Tony (husband)_

Phone: Home _(same)_

   Work _555-6789_ Cell _555-5962_

Primary Health Care Provider

Name _Dr. Daniels_

Address _5995 N. America_

City/State/Zip _Indpls, IN 46254_

Phone _555-6135_ Fax _—_

I give my massage therapist permission to consult with my health care providers regarding my health and treatment.

Comments

Initials _KVM_   Date _4-9-02_

B. Current Health Information

List Health Concerns Check all that apply

Primary _Back pain_

[X] mild [ ] moderate [ ] disabling

[ ] constant [X] intermittant

[X] symptoms ↑ w/activity   [ ] ↓ w/activity

[ ] getting worse [ ] getting better [X] no change

treatment received _massage_

Secondary _hip pain_

[X] mild [ ] moderate [ ] disabling

[ ] constant [X] intermittant

[X] symptoms ↑ w/activity   [ ] ↓ w/activity

[ ] getting worse [ ] getting better [X] no change

treatment received _massage_

Additional _neck/shoulder_

[X] mild [ ] moderate [ ] disabling

[ ] constant [X] intermittant

[X] symptoms ↑ w/activity   [ ] ↓ w/activity

[ ] getting worse [ ] getting better [X] no change

treatment received _massage_

List Daily Activities Limited by Condition

Work _computer entry, fitness instructor 3x/wk._

Home/Family _housework, care for 2½ yr. old_

Sleep/Self-care _sleep difficulties_

Social/Recreational _walk 1-2x/wk strength train 1x/wk_

List Self-Care Routines

How do you reduce stress? _exercise, massage_

Pain? _stretching, pain meds_

List current medications (include pain relievers and herbal remedies) _prenatal vits, iron supplement_

Have you ever received massage therapy before? _yes_ Frequency? _1x/mo_

What are your goals for receiving massage therapy? _reduce back & hip pain, neck/shoulder pain, restore sleep, restore fitness, lift daughter_

C. Health History

List and Explain. Include dates and treatment received.

Surgeries _1979- right knee - cartilage removed 1999- c-section_

Injuries _—_

Major Illnesses _Hepatitis A (8/2000)_

Figure 6-9. Health Information Form for Kirsten Van Marter. (Modified with permission from Thompson DL. Hands Heal: Communication, Documentation, and Insurance Billing for Manual Therapists. 3rd ed. Baltimore: Lippincott Williams & Wilkins, 2006.)

HEALTH INFORMATION page 2

Check All Current and Previous Conditions Please Explain

General

current	past		comments
☒	☐	headaches	*pregnancy*
☒	☐	pain	"
☒	☐	sleep disturbances	"
☒	☐	fatigue	"
☐	☒	infections	
☐	☒	fever	
☐	☒	sinus	
☐	☐	other	

Skin Conditions

current	past		comments
☐	☐	rashes	
☐	☒	athlete's foot (warts)	
☐	☐	other	

Muscles and Joints

current	past		comments
☐	☐	rheumatoid arthritis	
☐	☐	osteoarthritis	
☐	☐	osteoporosis	
☐	☐	scoliosis	
☐	☐	broken bones	
☐	☐	spinal problems	
☐	☐	disk problems	
☐	☐	lupus	
☐	☐	TMJ, jaw pain	
☐	☐	spasms, cramps	
☒	☐	sprains, strains	*left ankle*
☐	☐	tendonitis, bursitis	
☐	☐	stiff or painful joints	
☐	☐	weak or sore muscles	
☒	☐	neck, shoulder, arm pain	
☒	☐	low back, hip, leg pain	
☐	☐	other	

Nervous System

current	past		comments
☐	☒	head injuries, concussions	*7 yrs old*
☐	☐	dizziness, ringing in ears	
☐	☐	loss of memory, confusion	
☐	☐	numbness, tingling	
☐	☐	sciatica, shooting pain	
☐	☐	chronic pain	
☐	☐	depression	
☒	☐	other	*anemia-due to pregnancy*

Respiratory, Cardiovascular

current	past		comments
☐	☐	heart disease	
☐	☐	blood clots	
☐	☐	stroke	
☐	☐	lymphadema	
☐	☐	high, low blood pressure	
☐	☐	irregular heart beat	
☐	☐	poor circulation	
☐	☐	swollen ankles	
☐	☐	varicose veins	
☐	☐	chest pain, shortness of breath	
☐	☐	asthma	

Allergies

current	past		comments
☐	☐	scents, oils, lotions	
☐	☐	detergents	
☒	☐	other	*sulfa drugs*

Digestive/Elimination System

current	past		comments
☐	☐	bowel problems	
☐	☐	gas, bloating	
☐	☐	bladder/kidney/prostrate	
☐	☐	abdominal pain	
☐	☐	other	

Endocrine System

current	past		comments
☐	☐	thyroid	
☐	☒	diabetes	*gestational*

Reproductive System

current	past		comments
☐	☐	pregnancy	
☐	☐	painful, emotional menses	
☐	☐	fibrotic cysts	

Cancer/Tumors

current	past		comments
☐	☐	benign	
☐	☐	malignant	

Habits

current	past		comments
☐	☐	tobacco	
☐	☐	alcohol	
☐	☐	drugs	
☒	☐	coffee, soda	*tea*

Contract for Care

I promise to participate fully as a member of my health care team. I will make sound choices regarding my treatment plan based on the information provided by my manual therapist and other members of my health care team, and my experience of those suggestions. I agree to participate in the self care program we select. I promise to inform my practitioner any time I feel my well-being is threatened or compromised. I expect my manual therapist to provide safe and effective treatment.

Consent for Care

It is my choice to receive manual therapy, and I give my consent to receive treatment. I have reported all health conditions that I am aware of and will inform my practitioner of any changes in my health.

Signature *Kirsten Van Marter* Date *4-9-02*

Figure 6-9. (*continued*)

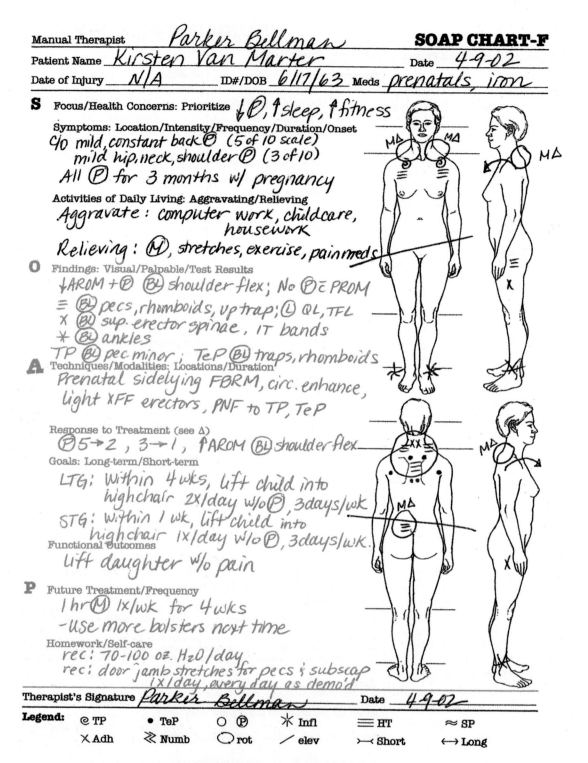

Manual Therapist __Parker Bellman__   **SOAP CHART-F**

Patient Name __Kirsten Van Marter__   Date __4-9-02__

Date of Injury __N/A__   ID#/DOB __6/17/63__   Meds __prenatals, iron__

S Focus/Health Concerns: Prioritize ↓℗, ↑sleep, ↑fitness

Symptoms: Location/Intensity/Frequency/Duration/Onset

c/o mild, constant back ℗ (5 of 10 scale)
mild hip, neck, shoulder ℗ (3 of 10)
All ℗ for 3 months w/ pregnancy

Activities of Daily Living: Aggravating/Relieving

Aggravate: computer work, childcare,
                    housework
Relieving: Ⓜ, stretches, exercise, pain meds

O Findings: Visual/Palpable/Test Results

↓AROM +℗ Ⓑ shoulder flex; No ℗ c̄ PROM
≡ Ⓑ pecs, rhomboids, up trap; Ⓛ QL, TFL
✗ Ⓑ sup. erector spinae, IT bands
✳ Ⓑ ankles
TP Ⓑ pec minor; TeP Ⓑ traps, rhomboids

A Techniques/Modalities: Locations/Duration

Prenatal sidelying FBRM, circ. enhance,
light XFF erectors, PNF to TP, TeP

Response to Treatment (see Δ)

℗ 5→2 , 3→1 , ↑AROM Ⓑ shoulder flex

Goals: Long-term/Short-term

LTG: Within 4 wks, lift child into
         highchair 2x/day w/o ℗, 3days/wk
STG: Within 1 wk, lift child into
         highchair 1x/day w/o ℗, 3days/wk

Functional Outcomes

lift daughter w/o pain

P Future Treatment/Frequency

1 hr Ⓜ 1x/wk for 4 wks
- use more bolsters next time

Homework/Self-care

rec: 70-100 oz. H₂O/day
rec: door jamb stretches for pecs & subscap
         1x/day, every day as demo'd

Therapist's Signature __Parker Bellman__   Date __4-9-02__

Legend: ⓒ TP   • TeP   ○ ℗   ✳ Infl   ≡ HT   ≈ SP
              ✗ Adh   ≋ Numb   ◯ rot   ∕ elev   ⊢ Short   ↔ Long

Copyright © 2005 Lippincott Williams & Wilkins

Figure 6-10. SOAP chart for Kirsten Van Marter, subjective information highlighted. (Reprinted with permission from Thompson DL. Hands Heal: Communication, Documentation, and Insurance Billing for Manual Therapists. 3rd ed. Baltimore: Lippincott Williams & Wilkins, 2006.)

CHAPTER EXERCISES

1. Name the three word elements and explain how they are used in a medical term.

2. Define each of the following prefixes:

   - ab-
   - ad-
   - bi-
   - circum-
   - contra-
   - dys-
   - hyper-
   - hypo-
   - infra-
   - inter-
   - poly-
   - post-
   - pre-
   - supra-

3. Define the following roots:

   - arthr(o)-
   - brachi(o)-
   - cervic(o)-
   - cost(o)-
   - crani(o)-
   - dermat(o)-
   - fibr(o)-
   - my(o)-
   - neur(o)-
   - oste(o)-
   - stern(o)-
   - thorac(o)-
   - vertebr(o)-

4. Define the following suffixes:

   - -algia
   - -asis
   - -iasis
   - -ism
   - -itis
   - -oma
   - -osis
   - -pathy
   - -stasis
   - -al
   - -ar

5. Break down the following words into separate elements and define:

   - osteoarthritis
   - fibromyalgia
   - neuropathy
   - tendinitis
   - intervertebral
   - unilateral
   - hypertonic
   - contralateral
   - atrophy

6. Using the procedure outlined in this chapter, perform at least five different client intake interviews with friends or family members.

7. Using the procedure outlined in this chapter, take at least five different client histories from friends or family members.

8. Identify the stress factors for yourself and five other people.

9. Identify the appropriate section of the SOAP note (Subjective, Objective, Activity and analysis, Plan) for documenting the following information:

   - Within the next week, the client should be able to lift 10 pounds at a time, three times a day, for 5 days with no shoulder pain.

   - Applied a full-body relaxation massage using therapeutic techniques on the left quadriceps femoris muscles.

   - Client complains of low back pain.

   - Client was referred to Dr. Bob Smith for skin abnormality.

   - Upon posttreatment assessment, the client's lateral neck flexion and neck rotation to the right increased.

   - Next session, try to address the right biceps femoris muscle with therapeutic techniques.

   - The client's skin was red and hot around the left scapula.

   - The client barely swings her left arm when walking.

- After the massage, the client says he has to be able to lift 50 pounds at a time, repeatedly throughout the day, for his job.
- The client responded well to vibration over the levator scapula muscles.

10. List the signs and symptoms of the following categories that you should ask about during a client interview: General, Circulatory, Musculoskeletal, Neurological, Psychosocial.

11. Identify at least five of the steps required for HIPAA compliance.

12. Identify four of the client's rights that can be included on your Notification of Privacy Policies (NOPP) form.

13. Identify the five components of an effective goal.

14. Use abbreviations and symbols from Table 6-6 to shorten the following sentences:

- The client complains of pain in the right levator scapula muscle.
- Lateral flexion of the neck increased with massage.
- I applied a full-body relaxation massage with a lot of effleurage bilaterally over the quadratus lumborum muscles.
- The client has decreased ROM at the left ankle, and no dorsiflexion is possible.
- The client came in with a headache and a fever, which is a contraindication, so I explained that he could return for a safe massage treatment when his fever has subsided.

15. Design your own client intake form by following the steps below:

- What client contact information do you want to record?
- Do you want clients' insurance information?
- What questions do you want to include regarding the current condition of the clients' soft tissues?
- What health history information do you want to know about?
- Do you want to know about daily activities?
- Do you want to include a body diagram for the client to use?
- Do you want to include the informed consent for care on your intake form?

REFERENCES

1. Thompson DL. *Hands Heal: Communication, Documentation, and Insurance Billing for Manual Therapists*. 3rd ed. Baltimore: Lippincott Williams & Wilkins, 2006.

SUGGESTED READING

Austrin MG, Austrin HR. *Learning Medical Terminology: A Worktext*. 7th ed. St. Louis, MO: Mosby Year Book, 1991.

Chabner DE. *Medical Terminology: A Short Course*. Philadelphia: WB Saunders, 1999.

Cohen BJ. *Medical Terminology: An Illustrated Guide*. 3rd ed. Philadelphia: Lippincott-Raven, 1998.

Fisher JP. *Basic Medical Terminology*. 5th ed. Westerville, OH: Glencoe-McGraw Hill, 1999.

Ford RD, ed. *Health Assessment Handbook*. Springhouse, PA: Springhouse Corporation, 1985.

Loeb S (executive editorial director). *Mastering Documentation*. Springhouse, PA: Springhouse Corporation, 1995.

McCann JAS. *Medical Terminology Made Incredibly Easy*. Springhouse, PA: Springhouse Corporation, 2001.

Moisio MA, Moisio EW. *Medical Terminology A Student-Centered Approach*. Albany, NY: Delmar Thomson Learning, 2002.

Newell R. *Interviewing Skills for Nurses and Other Health Care Professionals: A Structured Approach*. New York: Routledge, 1994.

Random House Webster's College Dictionary. New York: Random House, 1997.

Salvo S. *Massage Therapy, Principles and Practice*. 2nd ed. St. Louis, MO: WB Saunders, 2003.

Sheaffer BP (project coord). *Mary's Story: A Curriculum for Teaching Medical Terminology*, Institute for the Study of Adult Literacy. University Park, PA: Penn State University, 1991–1992.

Stedman's Concise Medical Dictionary for the Health Professions. 4th ed. Baltimore: Lippincott Williams & Wilkins, 2001.

Rattray F, Ludwig L. *Clinical Massage Therapy: Understanding, Assessing and Treating over 70 Conditions*. Toronto: Talus Incorporated, 2000.

Thompson DL. *Hands Heal: Documentation for Massage Therapy, A Guide to SOAP Charting*. Seattle, WA: Diana L. Thompson, 1993.

Thompson DL. *Hands Heal: Communication, Documentation, and Insurance Billing for Manual Therapists*. 2nd ed. Baltimore: Lippincott Williams & Wilkins, 2002.

Thompson DL. *Hands Heal: Communication, Documentation, and Insurance Billing for Manual Therapists*. 3rd ed. Baltimore: Lippincott Williams & Wilkins, 2006.

Thompson DL. *Hands Heal Essentials: Documentation for Massage Therapists*. Baltimore: Lippincott Williams & Wilkins, 2006.

Werner R. *A Massage Therapist's Guide to Pathology*. Philadelphia: Lippincott Williams & Wilkins, 1998.

Willis MC. *Medical Terminology The Language of Healthcare*. Philadelphia: Lippincott Williams & Wilkins, 1996.

http://www.acupuncturetoday.com, accessed 6.12.05.

http://www.cms.hhs.gov/hipaa/, accessed 2.23.05.

http://www.ctconline.net/hipaa_sense.htm, accessed 6.12.05.

http://www.hhs.gov/ocr/hipaa/consumer_summary.pdf, accessed 2.23.05.

http://www.hhs.gov/ocr/hipaa/finalreg.html, accessed 4.4.05.

http://www.hhs.gov/ocr/hipaa/privruletxt.txt, accessed 2.23.05.

http://www.hhs.gov/ocr/privacy/hipaa/understanding/summary/index.html, accessed 12.28.11.

http://www.hipaacomplianceguide.com, accessed 6.12.05.

http://www.massagetoday.com/archives/2003/01/05.html, accessed 6.05.05.

http://www.ncvhs.hhs.gov/020911p2.htm, accessed 6.05.05.

http://www.sohnen-moe.com/articles/abmp-1-2003.php, accessed 6.12.05.

Assessment

Objectives

Upon completion of this chapter, the student will be able to:

- List the five kinds of observations included in general assessments
- Describe why massage therapists should understand fascial adhesions
- Define compensation pattern
- Identify at least three characteristics to evaluate during postural assessment

- Name the six aspects of gait assessment
- Name the two different kinds of range-of-motion evaluations
- Define end feel
- Name the three characteristics to assess with palpation
- Describe the purpose of functional assessments

Key Terms

Active range of motion (AROM): Joint movement that requires clients to actively use their own energy to demonstrate how much of the full range can be completed comfortably and without restriction.

Assessment: The process of evaluating a client's condition.

Compensation pattern: A postural offset that is the body's attempt to correct an imbalance or protect a primary dysfunction or injury.

Direction of ease: The direction in which tissues move with least resistance.

End feel: A unique feel when a joint reaches the end of its passive range of motion (PROM) determined by specific structures that stop the movement.

Fascial adhesion (fascial restriction): An area where the fascia has adhered to nearby tissues or has been crumpled or kinked.

Gait: A walking pattern.

Palpation: The skillful art of client evaluation that uses touch to locate and assess the quality of different structures.

Passive range of motion (PROM): Joint movement that requires the therapist to move the relaxed client through a range of motion to determine how much of the full range can be completed comfortably and without restriction.

Range of motion (ROM): The end-to-end distance of a specific joint movement that is structurally possible.

Well-trained massage therapists are soft tissue experts with a solid understanding of muscular system anatomy and physiology. **Assessment** is the process of evaluating a client's condition to determine which muscles and soft tissues of the client's body to work on and which massage techniques to use. Good assessment skills go hand in hand with skilled and effective treatments. They help you evaluate the condition of the client's soft tissues to:

- Determine which techniques to use to reach the client's treatment goals

- Identify compensation patterns

- Determine whether massage therapy is indicated or the client needs to be referred to a healthcare professional for further evaluation

The physical condition of clients, in addition to their treatment goals, will guide your approach to treatment. Using techniques that are too aggressive or too subtle can be inappropriate or ineffective, as can massage sessions that are too short or too long and techniques that are too slow or too fast.

Although assessment skills help you determine the condition of the client's tissues for massage and discover contraindications, you do not use them to diagnose any specific medical conditions or prescribe treatments. **Medical diagnosis and prescription are out of the massage therapy scope of practice and should not be performed by massage therapists under any circumstance.**

Many assessment tools can be used to evaluate the condition of soft tissues. The massage therapist's first assessment tool is the client's health history. The initial interview process gives you a general idea of the condition of the soft tissues and the past and present stress factors that influence the healing process. Clients often come to you with specific areas of concern and functional limitations that serve as a starting point for your assessment. Some common areas of concern are neck tension, low back pain, and shoulder stiffness. The accompanying functional limitations can include the inability to turn the neck to check blind spots while driving, the inability to sit for long periods of time, and difficulty brushing and washing hair.

Along with the health history that provides information about the client's condition, there are general assessments and functional assessments (FAs). General assessments include postural, gait, range-of-motion (ROM), visual, and palpation (tactile) observations. More advanced, FAs can help you determine whether a specific pain or injury condition warrants massage or whether massage may be contraindicated. FAs include manual muscle testing, manual resistive testing, and orthopedic tests. They require additional training because to elicit accurate and useful information, you need careful technique and supervised practice. Referring clients for further evaluation to rule out contraindications conveys the message that you know your limits and that the client's health and well-being is at the center of care. **Understand that massage is not necessarily the appropriate treatment for all soft tissue conditions.** Often, though, when medical conditions that present contraindications have been ruled out, massage is one of the best treatments for soft tissue conditions.

General Assessments

The general assessments you perform prior to all wellness and therapeutic massage sessions include postural, gait, ROM, visual, and palpation (tactile) observations. For clients seeking nonspecific relaxation massage for wellness, the general assessment process does not need to be extensive or time consuming, but it still needs to be done. Without an initial assessment, it is more difficult for you and your client to recognize the results of the massage treatment, and it is also more difficult to write an effective treatment plan. The assessments pertinent to the areas of concern are documented on your massage treatment records. When clients have concerns about health conditions beyond the massage scope of practice (soft connective tissues), you should refer them to the appropriate healthcare professionals who can perform the necessary examinations to determine whether there are any contraindications for massage.

Wellness versus Therapeutic Massage Assessments

The general assessment process for wellness and relaxation massage is usually completed in less than 2 to 3 minutes. You can use the following guidelines for a short but complete assessment:

1. Ask a series of two or three questions to elicit the client's goal(s) for the treatment session.

2. Ask a couple of questions to determine if there are any functional limitations, areas to concentrate on, or areas to avoid.

3. Look for obvious visible differences in the evenness or levelness of the body, especially in the client's area of concern or area of functional limitation.

4. Before or during the massage, evaluate one or two movements that relate to the functional limitation or area of previous injury.

5. During the massage session, pay attention to the general texture and movement of soft tissues.

Many clients who initially come to you for relaxation massage on a regular basis can benefit from therapeutic massage if their pain pattern becomes worse or if they sustain an injury. When these clients look for more than a relaxation massage, your general assessments can last 5 minutes or longer because you need more information to determine safe and effective treatment. The assessment process for therapeutic massage can include the following:

1. Determine the client's goal(s) for the session.

2. Ask a series of leading questions to understand the condition of the client's soft tissues.

3. Ask a series of leading questions to determine the client's functional limitations and how they affect the client's lifestyle.

4. Before the massage, perform the general assessments shown in Procedure Box 7-1 to evaluate posture, gait, and ROMs.

5. Evaluate each movement of the joint(s) involved in the functional limitations.

6. During the massage session, pay attention to the textures and movement of soft tissues throughout the body.

The general assessments give you a better idea of whether or not a client presents any contraindications for massage, which soft tissues you should address, and how you should address them.

There are also occasions when therapeutic massage clients reach a point at which relaxation massage is indicated and a brief assessment is sufficient. Either way, you need to have a thorough understanding of the assessment process to determine how much assessment is necessary to ensure the most appropriate massage treatment.

Fascia

When assessing the soft tissue, keep in mind the widespread nature of fascia. As described in the body systems chapter, fascia is very pervasive, wrapping around and running between all the organs, muscles, and layers of tissue. Its tough, pliable, plastic structure provides support and

protection and forms a sort of spider web throughout the body. The protein fibers in fascia can get crumpled, kinked, or stuck together, making it difficult for muscle fibers to slide back and forth for smooth contraction and movement. These fascial adhesions, also called fascial restrictions, are disruptions in the smooth fascia that can result from:

- Insufficient hydration
- Injury
- Accumulated scar tissue
- Tissue dehydration
- Repetitive motions
- Sustained positions
- Postural deviations

In addition to the local restrictions and tightness, fascial adhesions have far-reaching effects on other soft tissues because of the intertwined, three-dimensionality of fascia.

For massage, fascial adhesions are particularly important to understand because fascia's involvement with muscle tissues can cause the location of your clients' pain to differ from where the pain originates. Fascia is much like a sheet of plastic wrap. When a sheet of plastic wrap is pulled on at one corner, the tension creates deformities that extend across the plastic in lines. When a section in the middle of a sheet of plastic is crumpled, it creates several lines of tension that radiate out from the crumpled area. If there is a local restriction in the muscle and soft tissues, there will be similar lines of tension called fascial lines that extend out to other areas of the body. Figure 7-1 illustrates lines of tension that reach out from a restriction to other areas, similar to the way a fascial adhesion can pull on structures far away. Restricted movement, compensation patterns, reduced circulation, muscular tension, and pain in seemingly unrelated areas can all result from fascial tension. Generally, the longer the restriction exists, the more the fascia will be deformed and the longer it will take for the client's tissues to return to normal. For example, right shoulder pain can be caused not only by structures in and immediately around the glenohumeral joint but also by fascial tension that originates in the abdomen or near the spine. The length of time the pain and restriction have existed, in addition to stress factors and client participation, will determine the best treatment techniques and the amount of time it could take to "unwind" the restriction.

Compensation Patterns

The body's objective is to have all the muscles in balance to remain upright, in ideal posture and moving efficiently. When the body deviates from this balanced state, muscles become shortened or overstretched to compensate for the imbalance.

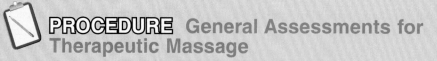

BOX 7-1 **PROCEDURE** General Assessments for Therapeutic Massage

Standing Postural Assessment

(You can use the body diagram on the general assessment form)

1. With the client fully clothed, shoes off, ask the client to stand comfortably with heels about 3 inches apart, arms hanging in a relaxed position.

    You can use a door frame as a vertical reference line by asking the client to stand in front of it so that the vertical part of the frame can be seen centered between the client's feet.

2. View the client's anterior aspect to look for obvious differences in the height of bilateral surface or bony landmarks or obvious deviations off the midsagittal plane (off to one side).
    a. Head (nose, chin, ears)
    b. Shoulders (acromion process)
    c. Sternum
    d. Navel
    e. Pelvis (ASIS and iliac crest)
    f. Hands (fingertips, wrists)
    g. Knees (patella)
    h. Feet—flat, normal, or high arches, lateral deviation (toes point out) or medial deviation (toes point in), how client wears out soles of shoes

3. Ask the client to turn around and face the door frame in the same relaxed position.

4. View the client's posterior aspect to look for obvious differences in height of bilateral surface or bony structures, or obvious deviations off the midsagittal plane.
    a. Head (ears)
    b. Shoulders (acromion process)
    c. Spine
    d. Pelvis (iliac crest or PSIS)
    e. Hands (fingertips, wrists)

5. Ask the client to turn so the door frame is behind the ankle and stand in the same relaxed position.

6. View the client's lateral aspect to look for obvious deviations toward the anterior or posterior.
    a. Head (ear just anterior to midsagittal line)
    b. Shoulders (center of glenohumeral joint on midsagittal line)
    c. Hands (palms directed medially)
    d. Pelvis (greater trochanters on midsagittal line)
    e. Knees (center of joint on midsagittal line)

7. Ask the client to turn and face the other direction, in the same relaxed position, with the door frame behind the ankle.

8. View the second side to confirm the anterior or posterior deviations observed on the first side or to show differences from right to left, suggesting rotation.
    a. Head (left ear is anterior to the right ear, or vice versa)
    b. Shoulder girdle (left acromion process is anterior to right, or vice versa)
    c. Pelvis (right ASIS is anterior to the left, or vice versa)

9. Document any obvious differences or deviations on the general assessment form and in the objective portion of the SOAP chart.

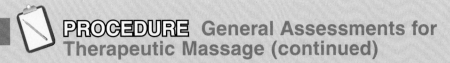

BOX 7-1 PROCEDURE General Assessments for Therapeutic Massage (continued)

Gait Assessment

1. Ask the client to walk across the floor.

2. Observe how the client walks, paying attention to the quantity, quality, and fluidity of steps (bilateral symmetry, evenness of steps, smoothness).

3. Observe the alignment of the head over the spine and the position of the shoulders.

4. Observe the arm swing for bilateral symmetry and smooth movement.

5. Observe the medial or lateral deviation of the feet (indicating rotation of the hip).

6. Observe the knee flexion upon a step and the bounce in the step or lack thereof.

7. Document any deviation from the normal gait pattern on the general assessment form and in the SOAP note's Objective section.

Active Range-of-Motion Assessment

1. Determine the possible movements of the joint.

2. Starting and ending in the anatomical position, demonstrate the ROM to clients, moving slowly and steadily, keeping the body very still to isolate the joint movement.

3. Explain that there are no successful results or failures possible because it is not a test. Ask clients to tell you if there is any sensation of discomfort or pain.

4. Ask clients to demonstrate the ROM slowly and steadily, starting with the joint on the side that is unaffected or least affected, and ending when there is any sensation of restriction, tightness, or discomfort.

5. Evaluate clients' movement.
   a. Glitches or hesitations
   b. Facial expressions
   c. Changes in breathing patterns
   d. Variations in speed or fluidity
   e. Recruitment of other muscles to complete the range
   f. Completeness or limitations to the ROM

6. Ask clients to repeat the ROM using the affected joint, with a slow, steady movement while holding the body still.

7. Evaluate clients' movement of the affected side as in step 5.

8. Document any findings from your evaluations of AROM on the general assessment form and in the SOAP note's Objective section.

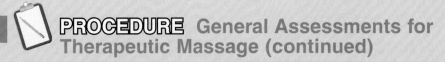

Passive Range-of-Motion Assessment

1. Identify the movements possible at the particular joint and the muscles and passive structures involved with the joint movement.

2. Explain that clients relax their bodies while you slowly and gently move them through an ROM and to let you do the work. Reassure clients with your confidence and sufficient stabilization, holding them securely and using a gentle but knowledgeable tone of voice.

3. Explain that there are no successful results or failures possible because it is not a test. Ask clients to tell you if there is any sensation of discomfort or pain.

4. Ask clients to sit or lie comfortably while you start with the joint on the uninvolved or less involved side.

5. Holding the client's body securely, slowly, steadily, and gently move through the ROM of the joint.

6. Evaluate the movement.
   a. Glitches or hesitations
   b. Resistance
   c. Changes in breathing patterns
   d. Variations in fluidity of movement

7. Move to the affected side, telling the client to remain relaxed while you repeat the process on the other side.

8. Holding the client's body securely, slowly, steadily, and gently move the affected joint through the ROM.

9. Evaluate the movement for the same factors as in step 6.

10. Document any findings from your evaluations of PROM on the general assessment form and in the SOAP note's Objective section.

Appearance of Tissues

1. Before and during the massage, visually evaluate clients.
   a. Differences in color (areas of redness or paleness)
   b. Differences in fullness or thickness of soft tissues
   c. Bilateral symmetry of soft tissues
   d. Marks, bruises, moles, wounds, scars

2. Document any visual findings on the general assessment form and Objective portion of the SOAP note.

Palpation Assessments

1. During the massage, take note of what you feel.
   a. Differences in temperatures (cold areas or hot areas)
   b. Textural differences in skin and soft tissues
   c. Movement of skin and soft tissues
   d. Areas of fullness or swelling
   e. Body rhythms

2. Document any palpation findings on the general assessment form and the Objective portion of the SOAP note.

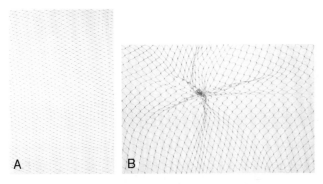

Figure 7-1. Fascia photo showing fascial lines. **(A)** Representation of unrestricted fascia. **(B)** Representation of fascial restriction; notice the fascial lines created by the fascial restriction.

Compensation patterns are postural offsets that attempt to protect a primary dysfunction or injury or correct an imbalance. Some examples of injury compensation patterns are a limp for a sore ankle, the excessive use of one arm because the other is in a cast, and turning the entire thorax to look over your shoulder because neck rotation is limited and painful.

Sustained postures and repetitive motions can also cause compensation patterns. When muscles continually hold the body in place or are continually used to perform the same movement, they are actively contracted on a regular basis without being lengthened regularly by their antagonists. As a result, the muscles that repeatedly contract or hold contractions for extended periods of time adopt a shorter resting length (they are posturally shortened), and their antagonists develop longer resting lengths (they are overstretched). The body must make up for the imbalance between the antagonistic muscles by adjusting the posture in other areas with functional compensation patterns. Sitting at a computer all day using a mouse requires your body to hold a single position for an extended period of time. Cashiers repetitively turn to their left and sweep products from right to left. Musicians are especially prone to functional compensation patterns because they have to hold their bodies in asymmetric positions for extended periods while they perform repetitive motions with their hands and fingers. All of these activities result in functional compensation patterns that show up as postural asymmetries or deviations. See Procedure Box 7-2 for the steps to determine compensation patterns.

Compensation patterns begin when the imbalance or injury occurs. Ideally, as balance is restored and the injury heals, the compensation patterns work themselves out. Unfortunately, a lot of compensation patterns do not go away completely and can develop areas of chronic hypertonic muscles and restricted fascia. A sprained ankle ligament that occurred a week ago will have an associated compensation pattern that could dissipate over several months, as long as the ligament healed well and the ROM was restored safely and completely. On the other hand, a 40-year-old man who has had flat feet all his life and has never been medically treated for them will have developed and reinforced a compensation pattern over several decades. Restoring the shortened and overstretched muscles to their normal resting lengths and breaking up the fascial adhesions that have settled into the tissues could take years, especially if the man continued to go without medical corrective treatment and continued to reinforce the source of the imbalance.

The body's compensation is registered not only in the muscles but also in the nervous system via nerve tracks, which are discussed in the nervous system section of the Body Systems chapter. The longer a compensation pattern has existed, the more the compensated body positions and the functionally shortened and overstretched muscles are locked into these figurative grooves in the nervous system. Imagine drawing a circle in the sand with a stick. The more circles you draw, the deeper the groove becomes. Over time, compensations are reinforced and become more difficult to change.

Implications for Massage

Once you discover compensation patterns in your postural assessment, you can determine which muscles are functionally shortened or overstretched. Postural deviations, imbalances, or restrictions in movement can be documented with symbols and abbreviations on body diagrams or in the text of your massage treatment records.

Your findings can determine the type of techniques to use and the length of time it may take to restore the most functional balance for the client. Several factors affect massage treatment and the time it will take for healing and restoration of balance and functional movement to occur:

- Lifestyle
- General health
- Length of time the client has been compensating
- Number of planes involved in the compensation
- The client's continuation to repeat any activity that reinforces the imbalance or compensation pattern
- Reinjuring the affected muscles

Assessment Documentation

Your initial observations of postural symmetry, gait, ROM, soft tissue appearance, and soft tissue textures can be recorded as objective information in the SOAP note or on specific forms that only include general assessment data. Figure 7-2 shows an example of a general assessment form. If you use a general assessment form for the client's initial visit, you can record general assessments made in subsequent massage sessions in the Objective portion of the SOAP chart. See Chapter 6, Communication and Documentation, for more in-depth coverage of documentation.

BOX 7-2   **PROCEDURE** Compensation Patterns

1. Identify the client's primary area(s) of complaint.

2. Identify the client's postural deviations as noted on the general assessment form and/or the objective portion of the SOAP chart.

3. Consider relationships between the postural deviations, the area(s) of concern, and pain patterns.

4. Determine the original imbalance or primary dysfunction or injury that caused the postural offsets:
   a. Ask if there is an area that has been painful longer than the others.
   b. Ask if there was an event (such as an injury, trauma, fall, twisted joint, prolonged period in one position, extended period of repetitive motion) that started the pain pattern.

5. Identify the joint(s) involved in the original imbalance or primary dysfunction.

6. Evaluate AROM and PROM of the movements of those joints, looking for restrictions or limitations, and for pain upon PROM, suggesting problems with the passive structures that require a medical referral.

7. Evaluate AROM and PROM of the movements of nearby joints, looking for restrictions that may have resulted from the original imbalance.
   For example, an injury to the right foot could be compensated by a limp to relieve pressure on the right foot. The limp could require extra work from the hamstring muscles to flex the knee, the rectus femoris muscle to flex the right hip, the right quadratus lumborum to elevate the right side of the pelvis, and the left levator scapula and upper trapezius to elevate the left shoulder. The muscles that are overworked will likely be posturally shortened and will restrict ROM of the joints they move.

8. Document compensation patterns in the Objective section of the SOAP chart.

9. Document any medical referrals in the Plan section of the SOAP chart.

Postural Assessment

Posture is the position of the upright, relaxed body. Although many people pay little attention to posture, it can significantly affect a person's health and well-being. The efficiency of the entire organism, or person, depends on cooperation of all the separate anatomical structures working efficiently, with little friction and minimal energy. Any interference can create muscular and soft tissue strain, extra energy requirements, and reduced efficiency in movement. These interferences can result in stress, exhaustion, and health problems that affect the circulatory and digestive systems, spleen, liver, and kidneys. Correct posture provides the best conditions for the bones, joints, muscles, and organs. Incorrect posture can lead to discomfort, pain, organ dysfunction, and disability.

You can evaluate posture to see how "straight" clients stand by looking at how surface landmarks and bony landmarks are positioned, relative to vertical and horizontal reference lines. Your vertical reference can be a plumb line, a line that hangs perfectly vertically as the result of gravity. It can be fashioned with a small weight at the end of a string that hangs from a level higher than the client's head. The client's stance is positioned such that the line falls exactly between the feet. (Fig. 7-3 shows a plumb line relative to a client's posture.) As simple as it is to hang a plumb line, most

General Assessment Form

Client Name: _____

Standing Postural Assessment (Evaluate level and position of the following)

    Cranium (ears)

    Shoulder girdle (acromion process)

    Pelvic girdle (ASIS, iliac crest, PSIS)

    Hands and fingers

    Knees (patella)

    Feet :   flat, normal, high arch
              lateral or medial deviation
              wear pattern on soles of shoes
              supination/pronation

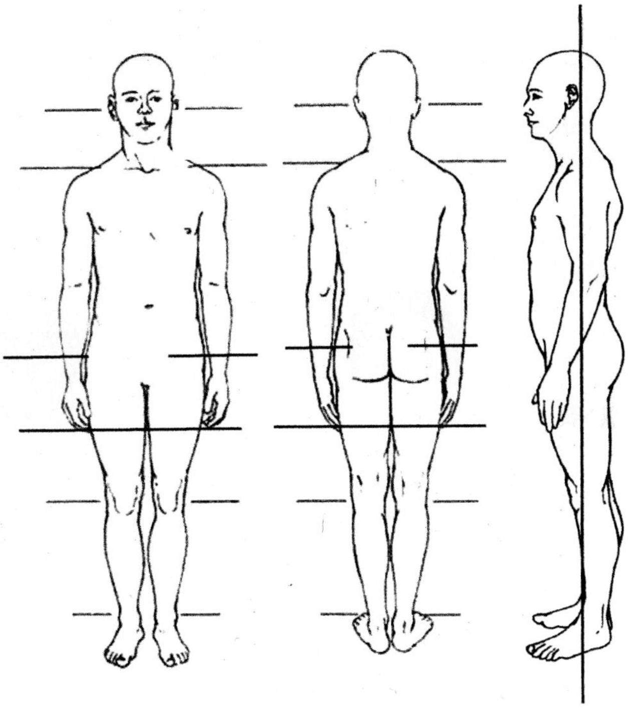

Gait Analysis (quantity, quality, fluidity, alignment, arm swing, foot deviation, knee flexion):

Range of Motion Evaluation:
    Joint: _____ Movement: _____ Normal or reduced
    Pain or discomfort with AROM? ___ PROM? ____

    Joint: _____ Movement: _____ Normal or reduced
    Pain or discomfort with AROM? ___ PROM? ____

    Joint: _____ Movement: _____ Normal or reduced
    Pain or discomfort with AROM? ___ PROM? ____

    Joint: _____ Movement: _____ Normal or reduced
    Pain or discomfort with AROM? ___ PROM? ____

Appearance of Tissues (color, fullness, bilateral symmetry):

Palpation Findings (temperature, texture, movement, fullness, rhythms):

Therapist's signature: _____ Date: _____

Figure 7-2. Blank general assessment form. (Modified with permission from Thompson DL. Hands Heal: Communication, Documentation, and Insurance Billing for Manual Therapists. 2nd ed. Baltimore: Lippincott Williams & Wilkins, 2002.)

massage therapists do not have one in their office. Instead, you can use a door frame, which is readily available in every massage treatment room, as a vertical reference. Some door frames are not perfectly vertical, but they still give you a reference line to work with.

Ideal Posture

Ideal posture minimizes stress and strain while maximizing efficiency. To evaluate posture for massage, you will look at the anterior, posterior, and lateral aspects of your client and check the alignment and position of surface landmarks.

Figure 7-3 illustrates anterior, posterior, and lateral views of ideal posture.

Looking at the anterior aspect of ideal posture, there are a number of surface and bony landmarks that fall on the midsagittal line, which runs vertically down the center of the body: nose, chin, sternum, spine, and navel.

Looking at the anterior or posterior view of ideal posture, there are a number of bilateral landmarks that are both at the same horizontal level: ears, shoulders (acromion process), pelvis (anterior superior iliac spine [ASIS], posterior superior iliac spine [PSIS], and iliac crest), hands (fingertips), and knees (patella).

When you evaluate the lateral aspect of your clients, your reference is a vertical line that runs just anterior to the

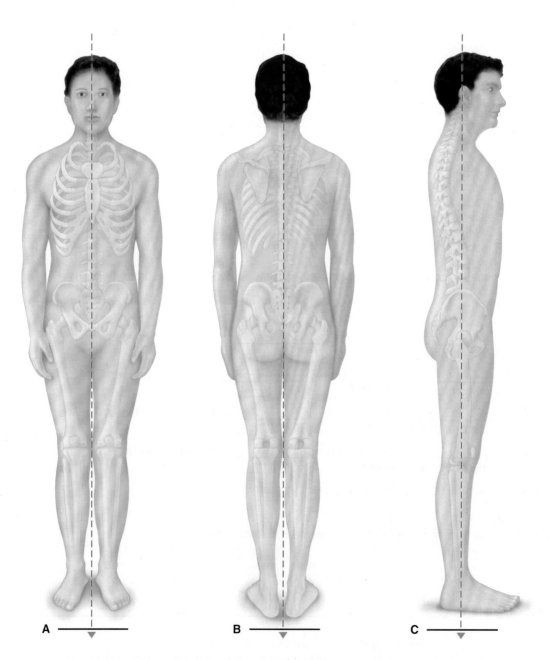

Figure 7-3. Ideal posture. **(A)** Anterior view. **(B)** Posterior view. **(C)** Lateral view.

lateral malleolus (ankle). In ideal posture, the vertical line will run through the center of the ear, through the center of the glenohumeral joint, through the bodies of the lumbar vertebrae, through the center of the greater trochanter of the femur, and through the center of the knee joint.

Anterior Postural Assessment

To view the client's anterior postural alignment, ask clients to stand comfortably, shoes off, arms hanging at the sides, and heels about 3 inches apart. Make sure that your vertical reference line falls midway between the heels and that the client's body does not touch the line. Using the position of bony landmarks in ideal posture as a comparison, evaluate the position of the client's:

- Ears (both ears at the same level)
- Nose (on the midsagittal line)
- Chin (on the midsagittal line)
- Shoulders (both clavicles at the same level and the same distance from the midsagittal line)
- Sternum (on the midsagittal line)
- Navel (on the midsagittal line)
- Pelvis (ASIS and iliac crests at the same level)
- Hands (fingertips at the same level, same amount of space between the body and each hand)
- Knees (patellae at the same level)
- Feet (even arches) (see Fig. 7.3A)

If bilateral landmarks are higher on one side than on the other, the landmarks are said to be located off the transverse plane (Chapter 4 describes planes of division). For example, a right shoulder that is noticeably higher than the left shoulder exhibits a deviation off the transverse plane. Another way to recognize bilateral landmarks at different levels is to use the term elevation. Using the previous example, the right shoulder is elevated. This can be documented on the SOAP note or general assessment form with a diagonal line on the body diagram at the shoulders that is higher on the right. (Figs. 7-10, 7-11, 7-13, and 7-14 show how to document elevation.)

If left and right landmarks are at the same horizontal level but farther to the left or the right, they are said to deviate off the sagittal plane. Some examples of deviations off the sagittal plane include a body part that is abducted or adducted more on one side than the other or a body that leans to one side. These can be recorded on the body diagram with an arrow at the location of the deviation, pointing in the direction of the deviation.

When evaluating the anterior view of your client's standing posture, consider symmetry. Determine whether the client's landmarks are in similar positions on both sides, as described earlier, but also look for side-to-side differences in fullness, space, and body surface curves. There are sometimes differences in the fullness of tissues from side to side. For instance, one arm might be noticeably larger than the other. The space between the arms and body should also be about equal, but occasionally one arm will hang much closer to the body than the other. You might notice symmetrical differences in the curves, such as the curve at the waist, or the creases of the body such as at the axilla (armpit). (Fig. 7-6, illustrating scoliosis, shows a difference in symmetry.) These observations can be noted on the general assessment form and the Objective portion of the SOAP note.

Posterior Postural Assessment

To evaluate the client's postural alignment in the posterior view, clients should stand in the same, relaxed position and not touch the vertical reference line, but instead of facing you, their back is to you. Using the ideal posture in Figure 7-3B for comparison, evaluate the position of the client's:

- Cranium (ears at the same level)
- Shoulders (scapular spines at the same level and angles)
- Spine (along the midsagittal line)
- Pelvis (PSIS and iliac crest at the same level)
- Hands (fingertips at the same level, same amount of space between the body and each hand)
- Scapula (space to spine, angles)

Check for bilateral symmetries when evaluating the posterior view of your client's standing posture, just as you did with the anterior view: positions of landmarks, fullness, space, and body curves. The differences can be recorded on the general assessment form and the Objective portion of the SOAP note.

Lateral Postural Assessment

When you evaluate the side view, the client's feet maintain the same kind of positioning, but the vertical reference line should run just anterior to the lateral malleolus. You can use Figure 7-3C, lateral view of ideal posture, as a comparative standard when evaluating your clients for:

- Cranium (line through the ear)
- Shoulder (center of the glenohumeral joint should be on the line)

- Hands (palms should be directed medially)
- Pelvis (greater trochanter should be on the line)
- Knee (center of the knee joint should be on the line)

If a landmark is found more toward the anterior or posterior of the client's body, the deviation is off the frontal plane. A client whose head and shoulders are anterior appears to stand slightly bent forward in what is sometimes called a forward posture. The deviation can be documented on a body diagram with an arrow located at the area that is noticeably deviated, with the arrow pointing in the direction of the deviation. (Figs. 7-10 and 7-11 show how to document deviation off the frontal plane.) Clients who wear shoes with a heel are shifted forward, off the frontal plane, and their bodies have to compensate by pulling the head and shoulders posteriorly. In fact, the higher the heel, the farther forward the shift, and the more the body has to compensate.

Postural Deviations

Sometimes posture contributes to, or is the source of, soft tissue dysfunction. Seemingly minor postural deviations can cause major problems in some clients, yet significant postural deviations may not be accompanied by any symptoms. Generally, however, incorrect posture is learned and reinforced from soft tissue imbalances that occur over time and lead to discomfort, pain, and compensation patterns. A deviated angle of the sacrum can distort the symmetry and balance of the body, causing rounded shoulders, spinal curve deviations, and abdominal deformations, which can affect internal organs. In animals that walk on four legs, the ventral wall of the abdomen supports the organs. In people, however, organs rest on each other and are suspended by ligaments and the mesentery. Abnormal positioning of the organs can interfere with the circulatory and digestive systems. Because all body systems are functionally interrelated, even the spleen, liver, and kidneys can be affected. Massage therapists may relax the soft tissue surrounding the postural deviation, and although that may not cure symptoms, it allows the body to use its energetic resources where they are best needed, rather than to fight against posture-created strain.

Abnormal Spinal Curvature

There are a number of postural deviations your clients may have, often accompanied by excessive spinal curvature:

- Sway-back posture—easiest to see from the lateral view: excessive kyphosis, head is anterior, shoulder is slightly anterior, palms of hands are directed posteriorly, pelvis is anterior, knees are often hyperextended (Fig. 7-4).

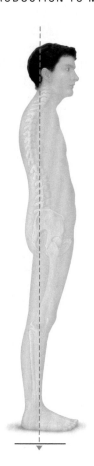

Figure 7-4. Sway-back posture.

- Flat-back posture—easiest to see from the lateral view: reduced lordotic curve, head is anterior, pelvis is anterior, knees are posterior and often hyperextended (Fig. 7-5).
- Scoliosis (lateral curvature of spine)—easiest to see from the posterior view: ears may not be at the same level, shoulders may not be at the same level, spine is not directly along midsagittal line, iliac crests are not at the same level, PSIS are not at the same level, space between hands and body differs from side to side (Fig. 7-6).
- Kyphosis–lordosis (excessive lordosis and kyphosis)—easiest to see from the lateral view: head anterior, shoulder posterior, pelvis anterior, knees posterior and slightly hyperextended (Fig. 7-7). In this case, the musculature will compensate for the abnormal curvature with shortened neck extensors and hip flexors as well as elongated, weakened neck flexors, upper sections of the erector spinae group, and external obliques.

Many clients have a forward posture, with the head anterior to the spine. Their scalenes, sternocleidomastoid, and other neck flexor muscles might be hypertonic, or excessively tight. As a result, the antagonistic neck extensor muscles are overstretched, creating tension on the musculotendinous

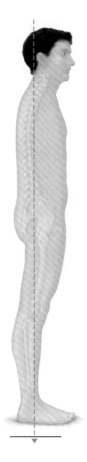

Figure 7-5. Flat-back posture.

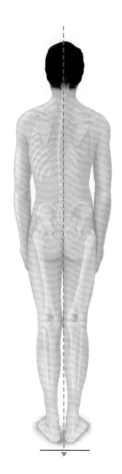

Figure 7-6. Scoliosis.

juncture or the tenoperiosteal juncture. This tension often causes pain because the overstretched muscles are continually attempting to bring the head back into balance, over the spine. Clients commonly feel pain in their upper back because of overstretched neck extensors resulting from chronically tight neck flexor muscles associated with their forward posture.

The massage therapy scope of practice includes manipulation of soft tissue but not bony structures. In other words, we do not attempt to realign the skeleton. Sometimes, in our attempt to normalize the soft tissues of the body to restore function, the client's posture and skeletal alignment improve.

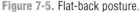

Alert

Do not make it your intent to manipulate skeletal structures.

Chiropractors and osteopathic physicians perform spinal manipulations (adjustments) to realign the spine and bony structures of the body. Their work is very complementary to massage because the skeletal structures and soft tissue structures are so interactive in maintaining posture and creating movement.

Rotation

Rotation, or torque, occurs around the vertical or longitudinal axis. This is an imaginary axis that runs straight up and down through the center of the body or through the center of a long bone. For example, if a client is standing up, facing forward with feet parallel, and the shoulders appear to be turning to face another direction, the client is exhibiting rotation of the thorax. The left and right acromion processes are both on the same horizontal level, but one is anterior to the frontal plane and one is posterior. In another example, a person standing in the anatomical position has a patella that is directed more laterally than anteriorly, possibly indicating a laterally rotated femur. Rotation is a significant factor in soft tissue compensation, although it is unfortunately often ignored. Document your initial observations on the general assessment form as well as in the Objective section of the SOAP chart.

A complex movement at the glenohumeral joint that rolls the structures of the shoulder joint forward and down is sometimes called shoulder rotation, but it is not a true rotation. A more appropriate description is an anterior roll, which is recorded as "shoulders rolled forward." You can document a shoulder roll by drawing a curved line in the direction of the roll on the body diagram. (Figs. 7-10, 7-11, 7-13, and 7-14 show documentation for rolled shoulders.)

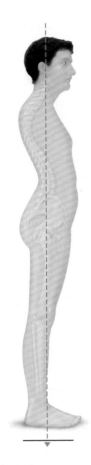

Figure 7-7. Kyphosis–lordosis.

Feet

As the foundation for our balance, the feet are important to healthy posture. If you have ever stepped on something sharp or injured a toe, you know how your body compensates to keep you from putting any pressure on the injury. **Imbalances of the feet can result in the development of multiple compensation patterns because our structure balances on top of our feet.** When the compensation patterns are not relieved (rebalanced) within a month or two, muscles develop shorter resting lengths and fascial restrictions are established.

Postural assessment is performed with shoes off, giving you an opportunity to take a look at your clients' feet. You can check the height of their arches, see if the feet are deviated medially (toes point in, or commonly, duck footed) or laterally (toes point out, or commonly, pigeon toed), and observe the wear pattern on the soles of their shoes. The arch affects how people stand on their feet, as does the wear pattern on the soles of the shoes, and the deviation can indicate rotation of the femur.

Arches and wear patterns can provide information about stance. Pronation causes wear on the medial edge of the sole, and supination wears the lateral edge of the sole. If the client's feet pronate, the peroneus muscles will develop a shorter resting length, and the antagonistic muscles will be overstretched. As a result of this imbalance starting at the feet, compensation patterns can develop all the way up the body as we try to maintain balance. If you judge that supination or pronation may be causing compensation patterns throughout the body, you may refer the client to a podiatrist (poh-DAHY-ah-trist), chiropractor, or other healthcare professional. There are some medical devices and treatments that can rectify pronation and supination. Massage therapy can provide temporary relief for these compensation patterns, but unless the client can walk and stand in a new, balanced state, the compensation patterns will be perpetuated. Wearing old, worn-out shoes is one of the worst things a client suffering from foot imbalances can do, because those shoes reinforce the imbalance and can even make the situation worse. Proper stance and muscle balance, on the other hand, facilitate good health. This information can be used to educate clients and is a source of good self-care. Once you make observations of the feet, record your findings on the general assessment form and in the Objective portion of the SOAP note. For example, supination of both feet can be recorded as (BL) foot sup.

Gait Assessment

Observing the body in motion is another assessment tool you can use. Evaluating gait, or the walking pattern, is a process of observing how the client walks. Pay attention to the following aspects:

- Quantity, quality, fluidity, and evenness of steps
- Alignment of the head over the spine
- Position of the shoulders

- Shoulders and shoulder girdle movement is even and fluid
- Arm swing is equal from side to side
- Medial or lateral deviation of the feet
- Extent of knee flexion upon a step and the amount of bounce in the step
- Hip movement is even and fluid

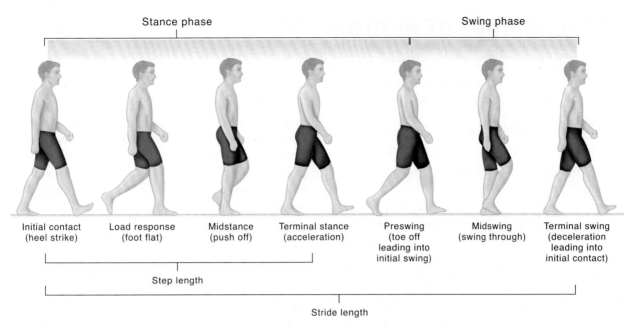

Figure 7-8. Gait pattern.

The proper, normal gait pattern is shown in Figure 7-8. Some clients will swing one arm less than the other, some will walk with their head anterior to the spine, and others will use their toes to absorb the shock of a step instead of their knees. Document any deviations from the normal gait pattern on the general assessment form and in the SOAP note's Objective section.

Range of Motion Assessment

Evaluating ROM is another way of assessing the body in motion. When your clients tell you what their primary area of concern is, you use that information to determine which joint movements are affected, how they are affected, and which soft tissues might be involved. The first joint you check is the one closest to the client's area of concern. Assess each movement of that joint for limitations and the quality of movement and use the information for your analysis of the massage session.

Each joint can move in specific directions to varying extents. The range of motion (ROM) is the end-to-end distance of a specific joint movement that is structurally possible. It can be quantitatively measured in degrees by a device called a goniometer (GOH-nee-AH-meh-ter), but massage therapists generally evaluate the quality and restriction of a client's joint movement instead of measuring the actual quantity of movement.

There are two kinds of ROM: active and passive. Active range of motion (AROM) is joint movement that requires clients to actively use their own energy to demonstrate how much of the full range can be completed comfortably and without restriction. It provides information regarding condition of the active structures of movement, such as the muscles and tendons. Passive range of motion (PROM) is joint movement that requires the therapist to move the relaxed client through a ROM to determine how much of the full range can be completed comfortably and without restriction. PROM evaluations can help determine the likelihood that there is a dysfunction in anatomical structures that are passively involved in movement, such as ligaments and joints. **AROM assesses active structures and PROM assesses passive structures.**

Massage therapists work with muscles and soft tissues, not bones and structures of the joints. Pain and discomfort caused by PROM can suggest problems with the ligaments and joint structures, which are outside the massage scope of practice. If you suspect that a client's area of concern could be a contraindication for massage, you can use ROM evaluations to help you make the determination and refer to the appropriate healthcare professional. Medical, osteopathic, and chiropractic doctors can diagnose medical conditions and prescribe treatment for injuries to bones and joint structures.

Active Range of Motion

AROM assesses the muscles and tendons actively involved in the joint movement. The following factors are critical to evaluating AROM and gathering useful information:

- Movement should be slow.
- Movement should be performed at a steady speed.
- Movement must be isolated, and the rest of the body must be still.
- Movement should continue through the normal range until the client feels restriction, tightness, or discomfort.

When the movement is not slow and steady, you will not easily notice hesitations, glitches, facial expressions, changes in breathing patterns, variations in speed or fluidity, recruitment of other muscles to complete the range, or limitations to the ROM. Isolating the movement is a finer point of the evaluation. Clients often recruit other muscles to perform AROM, partly because of their natural compensation patterns and sometimes because of a desire to successfully "pass the test." For example, neck rotation is easily and commonly altered with lateral flexion of the neck, and shoulder flexion is often accompanied by shoulder elevation. Keeping the body still, except for the movement of the joint being evaluated, helps reveal any recruitment of other muscles to accomplish the whole range of joint movement (Fig. 7-9A).

To evaluate AROM, there are a series of steps to follow (see Procedure Box 7-1). You should always demonstrate the movement before asking your client to perform the movement. During your demonstration you can point out the slow, steady speed and the stillness of your body that helps isolate the joint movement. Let clients know that if there is any restriction, pain, or discomfort, they should tell you. Clients then slowly move one joint through the specified range and back to anatomical position, minimizing any other body movement during the evaluation, while you look for compensation and recruitment activities. Then they demonstrate AROM for the joint on other side and you compare the quality and quantity of the two sides.

When AROM is evaluated to rule out the possibility of a condition that would contraindicate massage, the uninvolved or unaffected side should be observed first to determine the client's normal ROM. Explain this concept to clients, emphasizing that you are only comparing their left and right sides. Sometimes this helps clients

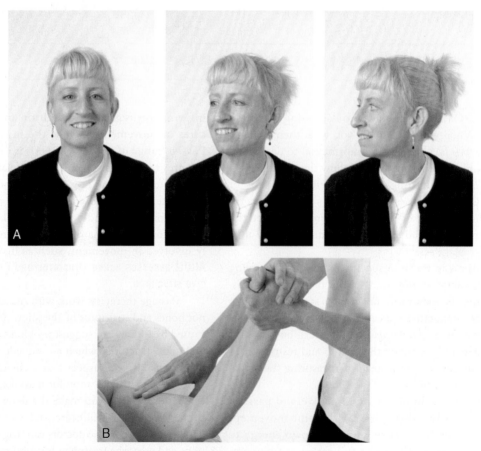

Figure 7-9. (A) Active range of motion. **(B)** Passive range of motion.

realize that AROM is not a test or a competition. After the evaluation has been made on the unaffected side, you can evaluate the involved side, looking for any limitations, hesitation, fluidity, compensation, recruitment, and facial expressions.

Always ask clients to let you know if there is any restriction, discomfort, or pain during AROM. Clients perceive pain at different levels or may have a diminished awareness of pain. They may not use the word "pain" or "weakness" to describe a restriction of movement, instead thinking of it as "pressure," "tension," or a feeling of being "stuck." Be sensitive to this terminology and watch for any abnormal movement, unusual facial expressions, or movement-created sensations. Any findings can be recorded as a positive test result on the general assessment form or in the Objective section of the SOAP note. For a client who complains of pain in the right shoulder when demonstrating AROM, you can record: Cl c/o (P) in ® shoulder w/ AROM.

Passive Range of Motion

PROM evaluates passive tissues including ligaments, joints, and joint capsules. Using PROM can give you a better idea of whether the client's area of concern can benefit from massage or whether the client should be referred out for further evaluation. Clients relax during PROM while you do the work. You hold and support their body parts, slowly and gently moving their body through the individual joint ROMs. If they feel that you might drop their arm or leg, they will "help" you by holding up their own body part to prevent it from being dropped. When clients "help" you hold their body, they introduce muscular tension that interferes with the PROM evaluation. By holding clients securely and using a gentle and knowledgeable tone of voice, clients are more likely to relax their body (Fig. 7-9B illustrates the gentle but secure way to hold a client during PROM). PROM requires a certain amount of trust from your client and must be performed carefully to avoid injuring your clients.

Before you evaluate PROM, clients should demonstrate AROM for the same joint movement because it gives you a good idea of the limits of the range. With AROM, the actively contracted muscles can impede movement, but with PROM, those muscles are relaxed and can be compressed to allow a greater ROM.

Evaluating PROM follows a series of steps similar to the AROM procedure (see general assessment Procedure Box 7-1). Starting with the client's area of concern, you determine the joint that may be affected, determine the movements of that joint, and observe the client's AROM of the

joint to get a general idea of the limits to the ROM. Explain the PROM process to your clients, demonstrating passive elbow flexion on your own arm if they need clarification. Express the importance of being relaxed, encourage clients to tell you if there is any pain or discomfort, and provide sufficient stabilization.

Gently and slowly guide the client's joint through its range, watching and feeling for glitches or hesitations in movement, resistance, changes in breathing patterns, and variations in fluidity of movement. Test the uninvolved side first to determine the client's normal PROM for the joint and then test the affected side. Record any differences you notice from side to side and note any pain or discomfort as a positive test result on the general assessment form and in the Objective portion of the SOAP chart.

> **Alert**
>
> *If passive ROM elicits pain or discomfort, the client may have a condition outside the scope of massage therapy.*

Massage therapists do not treat joint or joint capsule injury, and clients with those conditions should be referred to the appropriate healthcare professional. If PROM results are negative, meaning that there is no pain or discomfort with passive movement, massage therapy is indicated.

End Feels

When moving any joint through an ROM, you need to know when to stop pushing or pulling. It is possible to injure a client with PROM if the joint is moved past its safe stopping point. It requires practice to be able to feel the limitation of a joint's ROM. An **end feel** is a sensation of hesitation, tightness, or resistance as a joint reaches the end of its PROM and the client's body resists further movement. Specific structures that stop the ROM have a unique end feel. Normal end feels are created by normal anatomical structures that stop the movements and determine the full ROM. Normal end feels are classified as hard, soft, or firm. Abnormal end feels are the result of abnormal anatomical conditions or some kind of problem in or around the joint. Abnormal end feels are classified as hard, soft, firm, springy block, empty, or spasm. More important than learning the difference between the abnormal end feels, which takes a lot of practice, is being able to recognize an end feel as normal or abnormal. Table 7-1 describes the normal and abnormal end feels and gives examples of each. You should learn the normal end feels and get comfortable with determining a firm end feel. The firm end feel is caused by muscular or fascial tension, which is within the scope of practice for massage therapy. When PROM is limited by a firm end feel,

Table 7-1 End Feels

Normal (Physiological) End Feels

End Feel	Description	Example
Hard (Bony)	When movement comes to an abrupt, hard stop and bone contacts bone	Passive elbow extension: the olecranon process contacts the olecranon fossa
Soft (Soft apposition)	When two exterior body surfaces come together and a soft compression of tissue is felt	Passive knee flexion: the posterior aspects of the calf and thigh come together
Firm (Soft tissue stretch)	When muscles are stretched and elicit a firm or springy sensation that has some give	Passive ankle dorsiflexion with the knee in extension: tension from the gastrocnemius muscle
(Capsular stretch)	When joint capsule or ligaments are stretched and provide a hard arrest with some give	Passive external rotation of humerus

Abnormal (Pathological) End Feels

End Feel	Description	Example
Hard	When bone contacts bone or there is a grating sensation like rough articular surfaces moving past each other, there will be an abrupt, hard stop to movement	A joint with loose components, degenerative joint disease or bone fracture
Soft	When movement is stopped with a squishy or yielding sensation	Presence of synovitis or soft tissue edema
Firm	When there is a springy sensation or hard stop with a little give	Muscular, capsular, or ligamentous shortening
Springy block	When the client jumps or withdraws with discomfort (a rebound) to the end feel	Torn meniscus of the knee
Empty	When the therapist cannot reach the end feel because the client experiences considerable pain and requests to stop ROM	Acute bursitis, joint inflammation, or a fracture
Spasm	When PROM comes to a hard, sudden stop the client often suffers pain	Acute or subacute arthritis or a fracture

massage is indicated to relieve the muscular tension and soft tissue restrictions. You must learn and practice these end feels with a qualified instructor to avoid injuring a client.

When a joint is put through PROM, the position at the end of the range passively contracts the muscle that is responsible for that movement. In other words, a muscle in passive contraction is in a shortened position but is not actively contracting. Passive contraction brings the muscle's origin and insertion closer together and puts the muscle in a relaxed, soft position that is especially helpful for massaging deep tissues.

Direction of Ease

There are a lot of clients who want to "help," but encouraging these clients to relax by saying, "Just relax," is not always effective. The **direction of ease** concept can be a good tool in these situations. This concept uses the direction in which the tissues move with least resistance. Let clients position themselves the way they want to (in the direction that "eases" their pain or discomfort); you can even encourage them to display that position and then slowly but gently move them into the position you prefer or ask them to actively move themselves into that position. Clients who continue to tense their muscles despite your requests and suggestions to relax during PROM may respond to the direction of ease concept. You can firmly hold their body in a fixed position and ask them to gently push or pull against your resistance, giving them the opportunity to activate their muscles, which is what their body wants to do. After 5 seconds or so, you can ask them to relax slowly and gently, which again gives them control over their body. The muscles will likely be more relaxed than before they pushed against you, and you can attempt the PROM evaluation again.

Appearance of Tissues

Once clients are on your massage table, visual assessments provide information regarding the condition of their soft tissues. Look for variations of skin coloration, differences in bilateral symmetry of tissues, and any kind of marks or wounds on the skin.

Areas of redness often indicate a localized area of increased circulation. Areas that appear paler than the rest of the skin can result from ischemia, which is a localized area of reduced blood supply. Either condition indicates some kind of dysfunction that may affect the condition of the client's soft tissues.

Sometimes you notice differences in the fullness or thickness of soft tissues or bilateral asymmetry of soft tissues. If your client's left gastrocnemius is smaller than the right one, they likely have some compensation patterns to maintain balance. Differences in the size and fullness of soft tissues can be caused by hypertonicity, a difference in muscle mass, or edema (swelling caused by accumulated interstitial tissue fluids that are not drained by the lymph system). Checking the fullness of muscles and comparing the left to right can point out hypertonic muscles or compensation patterns, which gives you more information on where you might focus your massage techniques.

Visual assessments should also include open wounds, rashes, bruises, moles, varicose veins, and scars. You may notice changes on a client's skin before he or she does. Remember that any open skin wounds, bruises, or varicose veins are local contraindications for massage. Visible scars are important because the skin and underlying tissues are usually pulled toward the scar in the healing process and they can even lead to compensation patterns. All of these visual findings are recorded on the general assessment form and the Objective portion of the SOAP note. For a client with a bruise on the right gastrocnemius, you could record "bruised ℝ gastroc."

Palpation Assessment

Palpation is the skillful art of touching and exploring the body, locating different structures, and assessing the quality of structural characteristics. It requires a thorough knowledge of the functional anatomy of the body and continually improves with practical experience. With practice, you will learn to use all of your senses with increased awareness and become more sensitive to what is underneath your hands. Good palpation skills are critical for massage therapy. Massage therapists with good palpation skills become soft tissue experts. Working with relaxed hands will help you gain even the subtlest sensory information about the client's soft tissues. **There are more nerve endings in the skin than any other body part—600,000 overall in an adult; 50,000 per square inch in the fingertips.** A single touch receptor in a fingertip can detect pressure of less than 1/1,400 of an ounce, or the weight of an average housefly.

The saying "Less is more" can be applied to palpation and treatment of soft tissues. People tolerate being poked, prodded, and invaded, but nobody is particularly comfortable with such intrusions. Moving too fast and too deep can activate the body's protective response to push the intrusion back out by contracting muscles. You can test this phenomenon by slowly poking yourself in a relaxed muscle such as the masseter, which is located in the lower cheek. Notice how your finger sinks into the relaxed muscle tissue. Now, actively contract the muscle by clenching your teeth and feel the contraction of the muscle push your finger out. This protective mechanism is activated subconsciously by the sympathetic nervous system in situations of potential and perceived danger. When you quickly jab a finger into someone's arm, they can respond with surprise, pain, discomfort, and recoil. If you very slowly push your finger into their relaxed arm, your finger can penetrate deeper and you might be able to feel the muscle relax and soften. This approach is less intrusive and less painful for clients and gives you a better feel for the condition of the soft tissues.

Your palpation assessment evaluates and notices different temperatures, textures, and movements of soft tissues:

- Temperature—localized areas of heat or cold, or a noticeably elevated body temperature
- Textures—hypertonic muscles, scar tissue, restricted fascia, trigger points, and tissue edema (swelling)
- Movements—fascial adhesions or restrictions, which can be localized or cover large areas of the body, sometimes feel stuck, sticky, or resist movement; hypertonic muscles limit ROM
- Rhythms—breathing, pulse, craniosacral

Assessment of Skin Temperature

Skin temperature can be an indicator of circulation. Excessive heat can be caused by a fever or by the increased circulation of an inflammatory process that is the body's response to an injury. Fever is a systemic contraindication for massage, meaning you should not massage clients who have a fever. If the inflammatory process is causing the elevated temperature, you need to know how long the pain and discomfort have been present. An acute injury that has existed less than 72 hours is a local contraindication for massage, but general massage will help the rest of the body relax and may decrease the likelihood of the formation of compensation patterns.

Cold skin temperatures can indicate decreased circulation. Ischemia is a condition of reduced blood supply that is sometimes caused by fascial adhesions and hypertonic muscles. These conditions restrict circulation and prevent adequate blood supply. Massage is especially beneficial for ischemia caused by restricted soft tissues because it can relax and create more space in them or normalize them and restore their blood supply.

Textures and Movement of Soft Tissues

As you gain experience with palpation and massage, you will easily notice the different textures associated with soft tissues. Scar tissue and restricted fascia can feel as if the tissues are bound down and stuck together, and sometimes they

have a grainy texture. Hypertonic muscles feel tight and resistant when they are in a relaxed position or are passively contracted. Trigger points feel like little knots within a muscle, and they elicit pain or discomfort upon palpation, which radiates to another part of the body. Without the radiating pain, these localized areas of hypertonic muscle tissue are considered tender points. Tissue edema (swelling) can feel spongy or full and squishy.

Texture and Movement of Muscles

Normal, healthy muscles feel warm and pliable; they open up to receive additional pressure, they slip smoothly past neighboring tissues, and they are not painful. When muscles lack nutrition, are injured, or are chronically contracted or overstretched, they will not feel like healthy muscle tissue. Tissues suffering from poor nutrition feel deteriorated and nonsubstantial, as if they are falling away or dissolving under the palpation pressure. Tissue that seems to dissolve under pressure feels different from tissue that opens up to receive additional pressure. The difference is subtle at first, but with experience, you can easily differentiate between the two.

Injured muscle tissue that develops fascial adhesions and scars has a ropelike feel that may elicit pain or discomfort with applied pressure and force. When your massage stroke travels across fascial restrictions, your hand or forearm may slow down or bounce over the tissue with a skidding or jumpy movement.

Muscles used for repetitive motions and muscles that are posturally shortened can become hypertonic, or excessively tight. Hypertonic muscles can create trigger points, areas of pain and hypersensitivity, and fascial adhesions. They feel tight upon palpation, even in a passive contraction, and can feel resistant, tough, inelastic, and sticky.

Rhythms

There are different body rhythms you can learn to distinguish and evaluate. These rhythms can provide you with more information about your client's overall condition. Once you recognize the normal range of the different rhythms, you can recognize aberrations. The repeated inhalation and exhalation of breathing produces a rhythm that you can feel. The regular contractions of the heart ventricles that create the cardiac pulse can be detected along the arteries. The craniosacral rhythm is a subtle ebb and flow of cerebrospinal fluid (CSF) that, with practice, can be felt in different parts of the body, but most easily on the cranium.

Breathing Rhythm

By placing your hands lightly on the back of a prone client or on the shoulders of a supine or seated client, relaxing your hands and using a light touch, you should be able to detect the breathing rhythm. The movement of the rib cage may feel easy and fluid, freely movable, restricted, hesitant, or difficult. The more freely the rib cage moves, the more deeply and effectively the client can breathe. Slow, deep breathing usually indicates relaxation and parasympathetic nervous system activity. Shallow, fast breathing generally indicates stress or sympathetic nervous system activity, and it usually involves upper chest breathing. You may notice the shoulders moving up and down, indicative of shallow breathers who use their scalenes, the accessory muscles that raise the rib cage, instead of the diaphragm muscle to pull air into the lungs. Upper chest breathing overworks the scalene and anterior neck muscles and can lead to neck and shoulder tension and headaches. The muscular involvement in breathing is a good topic for client education and self-care because getting oxygen into the body not only helps the soft tissue but also the overall health and well-being. (Remember that without oxygen, cells will eventually die.) A number of resources are available to explain breathing techniques, which you may suggest to clients.

Cardiac Pulse Rhythm

Your palpation observations can include assessment of the client's heartbeat or cardiac pulse. The pulse is the rhythmic throbbing felt along the arteries, and it indicates the rate at which the heart is pumping oxygenated blood through the arterial system. More common places to detect and evaluate the pulse are the radial artery (at the distal end of the anterior radius), carotid artery (anterolateral aspect of the neck), and temporal artery (anterior aspect of the temporal bone). Use your middle and index fingers to firmly compress the artery and then relieve the pressure gradually to feel the pulse. The average pulse rate is about 75 beats per minute, but for massage, you will be checking more for differences in the strength of the

pulse from side to side. Hypertonic muscles and fascial adhesions can restrict the blood vessels and thus reduce the blood flow to an area. For example, if you detect a stronger radial pulse on the right than on the left, you could use ROM evaluations to see if some soft tissue restrictions near the shoulder might be constricting blood flow through the brachial artery.

Craniosacral Rhythm

You may notice the extraordinarily subtle craniosacral (KRAY-nee-oh-SAY-krahl) rhythm, which is an ebb and flow of CSF, while you perform massage. The CSF surrounds the brain and spinal cord, acting as a source of protection and nourishment. It is produced in the brain, is contained within the dural tube as it bathes the spinal cord, and is reabsorbed in the brain. The CSF is released and reabsorbed in a slow rhythm, and the flow creates a wavelike pulsation that is almost imperceptible, but the rhythm can be palpated on the body.

The rhythm may be easiest to detect at the cranium by positioning your relaxed fingertips so that they touch different bones of the cranium. For example, you could touch the occipital, parietal, and temporal bones. With a very light touch, you might feel those bones move outward very slightly (1 to 2 mm) over a period of about 4 seconds, which feels like the entire cranium is expanding ever so slightly, and then a short pause that is followed by all the bones moving inward a similar distance and at a similar rate. Feeling the craniosacral rhythm depends on a delicate, refined technique that can be learned with advanced training in the field of craniosacral therapy. This rhythm can be evaluated for quality, quantity, and fluidity. The parasympathetic nervous system arises from the cranial and sacral sections of the spinal cord and is sometimes referred to as the craniosacral system. Restricted CSF flow, which can be caused by soft tissue restrictions, may hinder the parasympathetic nervous system response. Massage can relieve soft tissue restrictions and restore the parasympathetic response, which involves the activities of resting and digesting, relaxing, and restoring energy. Without these activities, a body cannot resolve stress effectively.

Functional Assessments

For the entry-level student, using massage techniques to reduce pain and tension and restore muscle balance can help minimize or eliminate functional limitations over time. The general assessments you use before the initial and subsequent massage sessions help you determine the soft tissues that might be involved with your clients' areas of concern, the techniques you should use or avoid, and a treatment plan that is focused on achieving treatment goals. FA tests

specifically evaluate the client's area of concern to discover the likelihood of specific dysfunctions and conditions that require medical diagnosis. These tests, which include manual muscle tests, manual resistive tests, and special orthopedic tests, are more definitive than general assessments. Some resources refer to active and passive ROM evaluations as FA.

Manual muscle tests require clients to perform isometric muscle contractions against your counterforce. The test results help you determine whether muscles are functioning abnormally because they are shortened, overstretched, or weak. Manual resistive tests are similar, involving active isometric muscle contractions, but they help you determine whether there may be problems with a muscle or a tendon, a breakdown in the neuromuscular communication, or a more severe neurological condition. There are orthopedic tests that are designed to discover the likelihood of specific medical conditions related to fascia, ligaments, nerves, and joints. For instance, there are orthopedic tests that examine symptoms of carpal tunnel syndrome, tendinitis, ankle sprain, and sciatica to indicate whether or not these conditions are likely.

The concepts of these FAs are introduced so you know that they are available as assessment tools. Once you have an established practice and find that many of your clients come to you with health conditions that may need further evaluation, or if you want to work specifically with clients who have injuries, you might want to take additional training on FA techniques so you can deliver safe and effective massage treatments and continue to keep the clients' health and well-being at the center of your care. Performing good FA tests requires good technique and supervised practice to elicit valid test results that can be incorporated into your treatment plan.

Posttreatment Assessment

Following the massage treatment, you need to analyze progress with posttreatment assessments or reassessment observations. These assessments are the same ones you used before the treatment, but they help you analyze the massage. For a client who begins the session complaining of a tight left shoulder, your initial assessment may discover bilateral hypertonicity in the upper trapezius and levator scapula muscles, left shoulder elevation, and reduced AROM and PROM upon left shoulder flexion and abduction. Posttreatment assessment would reevaluate your original findings to look for any changes in the hypertonic muscles, shoulder elevation, or ROMs. Tightness can be assessed during the massage after

you apply techniques to this area. Assess the shoulder elevation and ROMs after the client is off the table and dressed. Document these changes in the Activity and Analysis portion of the SOAP note. For this sample client, you could record:

- A moderate change that reduced hypertonicity in the bilateral upper trapezius and levator scapula muscles: mod. $\Delta\downarrow\equiv$ (BL) up trap + lev scap
- After a full-body relaxation massage, the left shoulder elevation was reduced: FBRM $\rightarrow$ $\downarrow$(L) shoulder elev.

(See SOAP notes with posttreatment assessment findings documented in Figs. 7-11 and 7-14.)

Case Studies

This section highlights the documentation of objective information.

Progressive Case Study 1:
Rob Blackwell

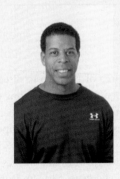

Rob Blackwell's health history form and intake interview provide the starting point for your assessment process. His goals are to restore sleep, reduce pain, and restore his previous abilities to lift weights and play golf. Your questions determine that he especially likes golf and is frustrated because his shoulder pain has significantly affected his game.

The anterior postural assessment shows some extra wrinkles in his shirt at the right axilla and elevation of the right shoulder. From the posterior aspect, you confirm right shoulder elevation. The lateral view of Rob's posture indicates that his right shoulder is rolled forward and his head is forward.

His gait pattern is smooth and symmetrical with no noticeable abnormalities.

To sort through the different areas of pain, you determine Rob's compensation patterns (see Procedure Box 7-3). Both active and passive ROM for flexion of the left knee are reduced and painful. You find reduced active and passive ROM upon left hip flexion, extension, and abduction. AROM shows lateral flexion of the spine is greater to the left than to the right. AROM is reduced for bilateral shoulder abduction and neck rotation to the left and right.

During the massage, you do not notice any visual differences. You feel a number of hypertonic muscles on the right: sternocleidomastoid, pectoralis major, levator scapula, and rhomboids. The upper trapezius, deltoids, and tensor fascia lata muscles are hypertonic bilaterally. Quadratus lumborum is hypertonic on the left. You feel fascial adhesions around the right levator scapula, right rhomboids, and bilateral iliotibial bands. All of these general assessments are recorded in the Objective section of the SOAP note. You also use a general assessment form, as shown in Figure 7-10.

You perform the appropriate massage, analyze the results, prioritize functional limitations, and determine treatment goals. You determine a treatment plan, including recommendations for future treatment and self-care activities to help him maintain the progress made during the first massage (Fig. 7-11).

Progressive Case Study 2:
Timothy Roberts

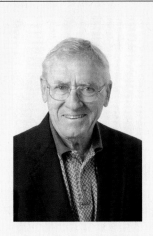

Timothy has made a first-time appointment for relaxation massage. To assess the general condition of his health and soft tissues, you look over the HxTxC form he filled out, looking for any specific complaints to confirm that he does not want therapeutic treatment. He states impatiently that he just wants a massage and asks if all the paperwork is really necessary. To strike a balance between gaining his trust and remaining professional, your assessments are brief. You quickly ask if there are any specific areas he wants you to work on, or if there are any areas he wants you to avoid. He says no and starts taking off his shoes. As he is sitting in front of you and begins to stand up, you look for any obvious postural deviations. While he is getting onto the table, you use your office references to determine that the combination of relaxation massage and blood pressure medication could lower blood pressure further. You know to be especially careful when he gets off the table.

During the massage, you notice some fascial adhesions around his left ankle and that PROM is limited for that ankle. Like many seniors, Timothy may have hypertonic areas where ROM is reduced without associated pain.

Following the massage, you make recommendations for future treatment and self-care. Your assessments and recommendations are recorded on the HxTxC form (Fig. 7-12).

Progressive Case Study 3:
Kirsten Van Marter

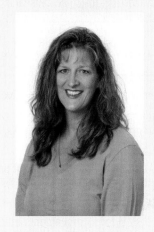

Kirsten's information from the history and intake interview provides the basis for your assessment process. She wants to reduce her back, hip, neck, and shoulder pain; restore sleep; restore her previous fitness level; and lift her child. She has been receiving massage regularly for years, and she knows that massage cannot deliver all of these benefits at once. She says that she is especially concerned that she cannot lift her child without pain and is afraid it will only get worse as the pregnancy progresses.

Postural assessments show that both shoulders are rolled forward and her left hip is elevated. When you evaluate her gait, you notice that she is starting to compensate for the growing fetus by widening her stance and pulling her shoulders back. AROM is limited with pain upon bilateral shoulder flexion, but PROM is not painful.

During the massage, you notice hypertonicity in a number of areas: bilateral pectoralis major and minor, rhomboids, and upper trapezius muscles and left quadratus lumborum and left tensor fascia latae muscles. You feel adhesions in the superior erector spinae muscles and bilateral iliotibial bands. She has trigger points in her bilateral pectoralis minor muscles and many tender points in her trapezius and rhomboid muscles. You do not notice any visual differences in tissue color, but you do notice some swelling around her ankles. All of your observations are recorded as objective information on the SOAP note or on a general assessment form (Fig. 7-13).

Following the massage, you and she prioritize her functional limitations, determine treatment goals, and come up with a treatment plan that is feasible for her (Fig. 7-14).

BOX 7-3 **PROCEDURE** Rob Blackwell's Compensation Patterns

1. Primary areas of concern are neck, back, and knees.

2. Rob's right shoulder is elevated and rotated (rolled) forward.

3. The right shoulder elevation and roll could cause the neck and back pain, but the knees do not fit into the local pain pattern.

4. Rob indicates that his bilateral knee pain has been with him the longest, for about 10 years. He was diagnosed with osteoarthritis in both knees over 10 years ago but remembers badly twisting his left knee playing basketball before then.

5. Assume that the knee is the joint originally involved in the imbalance.

6. Evaluate AROM and PROM for flexion and extension of the left knee.
   a. You find reduced AROM with discomfort.
   b. PROM is reduced and painful, indicating that passive structures are involved in addition to active structures. Treating passive structures is outside our scope of practice.

7. Evaluate AROM and PROM for all movements of the left and right hips, spine, and shoulders.
   a. You find reduced AROM and PROM of left hip flexion, extension, and abduction.
   b. You find greater AROM for lateral flexion of the spine to the left than to the right.
   c. AROM for neck rotation is reduced to both sides.
   d. You find reduced AROM upon bilateral shoulder abduction.
      His right shoulder elevation and roll could be compensation for the original left knee injury.

8. Document your general assessment findings, including the compensation pattern, in the Objective portion of the SOAP note, and/or on the general assessment form.
   a. Ⓡ shoulder elev + roll, ↓ ROM + Ⓟ w/ Ⓛ knee flex text, ↓ ROM Ⓛ hip flex text + abduct, AROM lat flex spine Ⓛ > Ⓡ, ↓ AROM ⒷⓁ neck rot + shoulder abduct
   b. Ⓡ shoulder compensation for Ⓛ knee?

9. Because there was pain upon PROM of left knee, refer Rob to a medical doctor for a more current diagnosis to make sure massage is not contraindicated. Document your referral in the Plan section of the SOAP note.

CHAPTER SUMMARY

Relaxation massage often provides temporary relief from pain and tension, but determining the underlying cause of the problem and using therapeutic techniques when they are indicated is more beneficial and offers longer lasting results. Clients should be evaluated for their chief complaints to determine the condition of their soft tissues as well as their overall health. A new mother complaining of tight shoulders, for example, probably suffers fatigue, guilt, lack of rest, and insufficient aerobic exercise. These other factors can affect her overall health as much or more than the hypertonic shoulders and associated fascial restrictions.

Although we cannot avoid stress completely, we can learn to cope with it. Holding onto tension and stress requires a lot of energy, which then depletes the body's resources for functioning properly. Compensation patterns require a part of the body to work excessively to compensate for a dysfunction or imbalance in another part of the body, and they can increase the potential for injury. By relieving compensation patterns, we can facilitate the client's ability to relax and experience more energy and vitality. Compensation patterns should always be suspected and, when they exist, treated to restore optimal function and movement. **As a guideline, treat where it hurts, where it is compensated, and at the ends of the fascial restriction.**

General Assessment Form

Client Name: _Rob Blackwell_

Standing Postural Assessment (Evaluate level and position of the following)

Cranium (ears) forward

Shoulder girdle (acromion process)
Ⓡ elevated, rolled forward

Space between body ; arm Ⓛ > Ⓡ

Pelvic girdle (ASIS, iliac crest, PSIS)

Hands and fingers
Ⓡ higher than Ⓛ
Ⓡ palm directed posteriorly
Knees (patella)

Feet : flat, ⟨normal⟩, high arch
⟨lateral⟩ or medial deviation
wear pattern on soles of shoes -even

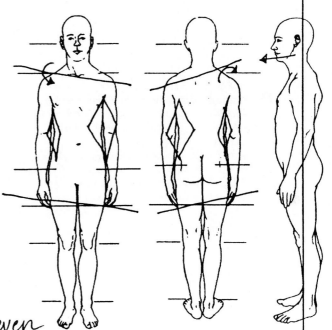

Gait Analysis (quantity, quality, fluidity, alignment, arm swing, foot deviation, knee flexion):
smooth, symmetrical

Range of Motion Evaluation:
Joint: Ⓛ Knee___ Movement: flexion + exten. Normal or ⟨reduced⟩
Pain or discomfort with AROM? ✓ PROM? ✓
Joint: ⟨BL⟩ shoulder Movement: abduction Normal or ⟨reduced⟩
Pain or discomfort with AROM? ___ PROM? ___
Joint: neck___ Movement: rotation___ Normal or ⟨reduced⟩ both sides
Pain or discomfort with AROM? ___ PROM? ___
Joint: spine___ Movement: lat flex Normal or reduced ⟨Ⓛ⟩ > Ⓡ
Pain or discomfort with AROM? ___ PROM? ___

Appearance of Tissues (color, fullness, bilateral symmetry):
∅

Palpation Findings (temperature, texture, movement, fullness, rhythms):
Hypertonic - Ⓡ SCM/pecs/lev.scap/rhomb, Ⓛ QL, ⟨BL⟩ up trap/delt/TFL
Adhesions - Ⓡ rhomb, ⟨BL⟩ IT band, Ⓡ lev scap

Therapist's signature: _Anne Therapist_ Date: 4-2-02

Figure 7-10. General assessment form for Rob.

Manual Therapist *Connor Patrick*

SOAP CHART-M

Patient Name *Rob Blackwell*   Date *4-2-02*

Date of Injury *N/A*   ID#/DOB *10-29-60*   Meds *ibuprofen prn*

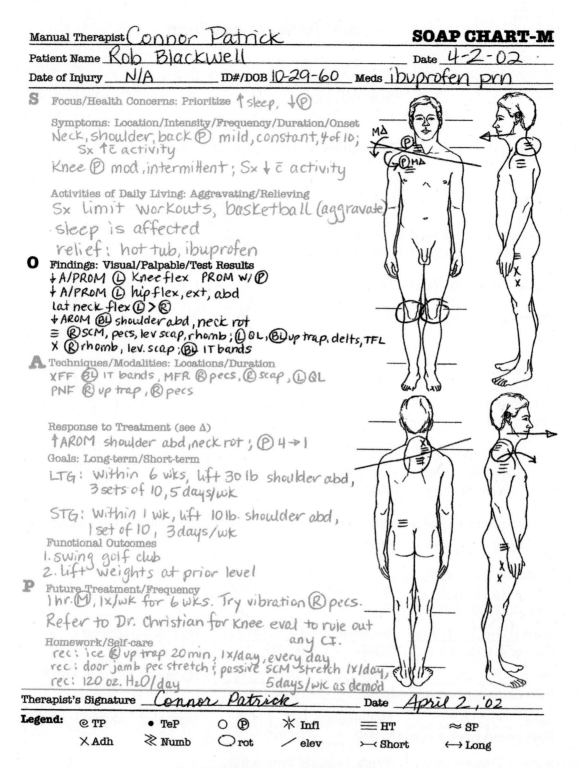

S Focus/Health Concerns: Prioritize ↑sleep, ↓℗

Symptoms: Location/Intensity/Frequency/Duration/Onset
Neck, shoulder, back ℗ mild, constant, 4 of 10;
   Sx ↑c̄ activity
Knee ℗ mod, intermittent; Sx ↓ c̄ activity

Activities of Daily Living: Aggravating/Relieving
Sx limit workouts, basketball (aggravate)
sleep is affected
relief: hot tub, ibuprofen

O Findings: Visual/Palpable/Test Results
↓A/PROM Ⓛ knee flex PROM w/ ℗
↓A/PROM Ⓛ hip flex, ext, abd
lat neck flex Ⓛ > Ⓡ
↓AROM Ⓑ shoulder abd, neck rot
≡ ⓇSCM, pecs, lev scap, rhomb; ⓁQL, Ⓑup trap, delts, TFL
✕ Ⓡrhomb, lev. scap; Ⓑ IT bands

A Techniques/Modalities: Locations/Duration
XFF Ⓑ IT bands, MFR Ⓡpecs, Ⓡscap, ⓁQL
PNF Ⓡup trap, Ⓡpecs

Response to Treatment (see Δ)
↑AROM shoulder abd, neck rot; ℗ 4→1
Goals: Long-term/Short-term
LTG: within 6 wks, lift 30 lb shoulder abd,
   3 sets of 10, 5 days/wk

STG: within 1 wk, lift 10 lb. shoulder abd,
   1 set of 10, 3 days/wk
Functional Outcomes
1. swing golf club
2. lift weights at prior level

P Future Treatment/Frequency
1 hr. Ⓜ, 1x/wk for 6 wks. Try vibration Ⓡpecs.
Refer to Dr. Christian for knee eval to rule out
                 any CI.
Homework/Self-care
rec: ice Ⓡ up trap 20 min, 1x/day, every day
rec: door jamb pec stretch ¢ passive SCM stretch 1x/day,
rec: 120 oz. H₂O/day   5 days/wk as demo'd

Therapist's Signature *Connor Patrick*   Date *April 2, '02*

Legend: ℮ TP   • TeP   ○ ℗   ✳ Infl   ≡ HT   ≈ SP
         ✕ Adh   ≋ Numb   ⟲ rot   / elev   ⤜ Short   ↔ Long

Figure 7-11. SOAP note for Rob, highlighting Objective information. (Modified with permission from Thompson DL. Hands Heal: Communication, Documentation, and Insurance Billing for Manual Therapists. 2nd ed. Baltimore: Lippincott Williams & Wilkins, 2002.)

Manual Therapist _Max Harr_   **WELLNESS CHART-M**

Name _Timothy Roberts_   ID#/DOB _9-10-30_   Date _12-18-03_

Phone _555-4220_   Address _7000 Osprey Ln._

1. What are your goals for health, and how may I assist you in achieving your goals? _____
   relaxation

2. List typical daily activities—work, exercise, home. _golf, house projects_

3. Are you currently experiencing any of the following? If yes, please explain.

   pain, tenderness   ☑ No   ☐ Yes: _____   stiffness   ☑ No   ☐ Yes: _____
   numbness or tingling   ☑ No   ☐ Yes: _____   swelling   ☑ No   ☐ Yes: _____
   allergies   ☑ No   ☐ Yes: _____

4. List all illnesses, injuries, and health concerns you have now or have had in the past 3 years.
   (Examples: arthritis, diabetes, car crash) _moderate blood pressure,_
   skin cancers, broken left ankle

5. List medications and pain relievers taken this week. _blood pressure meds_

6. I have provided all my known medical information. I acknowledge that massage therapy is
   not a substitute for medical diagnosis and treatment. I give my consent to receive treatment.

   Signature _Timothy Roberts_   Date _12-18-03_

   Tx: _FBRM c̄ circulatory enhancement focus;_
   during (M) noticed ↓ROM + X (L) ankle (dorsiflex, evert)
   C: _Cl has no specific complaints today_
   next session try XFF (L) ankle. rec 8 oz H₂O/day, 1hr (M)/month

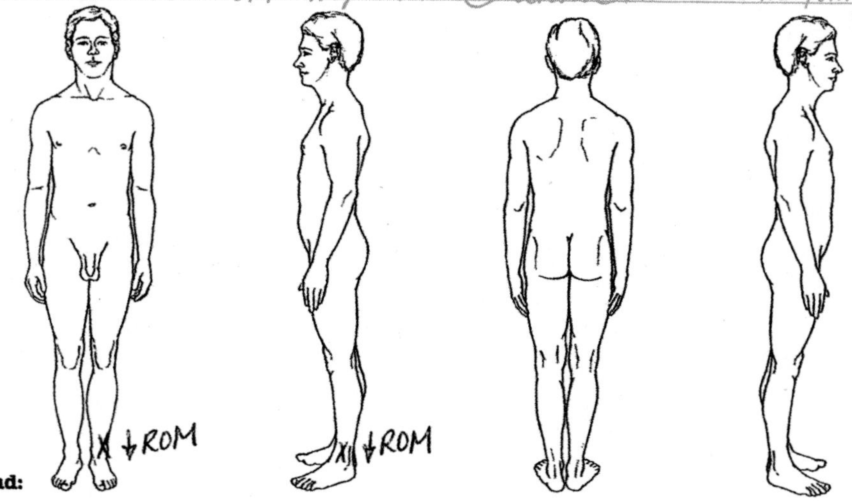

Legend:

℮ TP	● TeP	○ ℗	✳ Infl	≡ HT	≈ SP initials _MH_
✕ Adh	≋ Numb	◯ rot	╱ elev	⊱ Short	↔ Long

Copyright © 2005 Lippincott Williams & Wilkins

Figure 7-12. Client health report for Timothy, highlighting Objective information. (Modified with permission from Thompson DL. Hands Heal: Communication, Documentation, and Insurance Billing for Manual Therapists. 2nd ed. Baltimore: Lippincott Williams & Wilkins, 2002.)

General Assessment Form

Client **Name**: *Kirsten Van Marter*

Standing Postural Assessment (Evaluate level and position of the following)

Cranium (ears)

Shoulder girdle (acromion process)
(BL) rolled forward
Space between body & arm (R) > (L)

Pelvic girdle (ASIS, iliac crest, PSIS)
(L) elevated

Hands and fingers

Knees (patella)

Feet : flat, (normal) high arch
(lateral) or medial deviation
wear pattern on soles of shoes N/A
(new shoes)

Gait Analysis (quantity, quality, fluidity, alignment, arm swing, foot deviation, knee flexion):
wide stance, not much knee flexion, increased arm swing

Range of Motion Evaluation:
Joint: (BL) shoulder   Movement: flexion   Normal or (reduced)
Pain or discomfort with AROM? ✓   PROM? ∅

Joint: _____   Movement: _____   Normal or reduced
Pain or discomfort with AROM? ____   PROM? ____

Joint: _____   Movement: _____   Normal or reduced
Pain or discomfort with AROM? ____   PROM? ____

Joint: _____   Movement: _____   Normal or reduced
Pain or discomfort with AROM? ____   PROM? ____

Appearance of Tissues (color, fullness, bilateral symmetry):
Inflammation (BL) ankles

Palpation Findings (temperature, texture, movement, fullness, rhythms):
Hypertonic - (BL) pecs/rhomb/up trap, (L) QL, TFL
Adhesions - (BL) sup. erector spinae, IT bands
TP - (BL) pec minor
TeP - (BL) traps/rhomb

Therapist's signature: *June Therapist*   Date: 4-9-02

Figure 7-13. General assessment form for Kirsten.

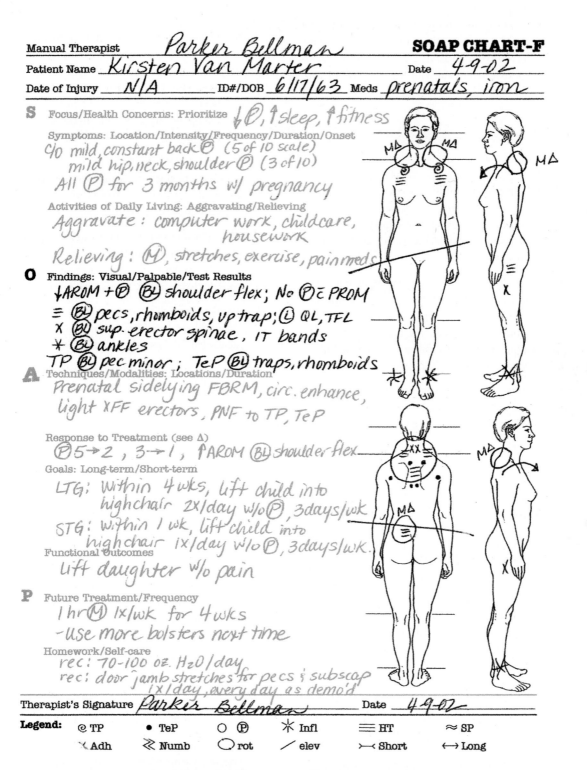

Manual Therapist *Parker Bellman*   **SOAP CHART-F**

Patient Name *Kirsten Van Marter*   Date *4-9-02*

Date of Injury *N/A*   ID#/DOB *6/17/63* Meds *prenatals, iron*

S Focus/Health Concerns: Prioritize ↓℗, ↑sleep, ↑fitness

Symptoms: Location/Intensity/Frequency/Duration/Onset
c/o mild, constant back ℗ (5 of 10 scale)
  mild hip, neck, shoulder ℗ (3 of 10)
All ℗ for 3 months w/ pregnancy

Activities of Daily Living: Aggravating/Relieving
Aggravate: computer work, childcare,
      housework
Relieving: Ⓜ, stretches, exercise, pain meds

O Findings: Visual/Palpable/Test Results
↓AROM + ℗ Ⓑ shoulder flex; No ℗ c̄ PROM
≡ Ⓑ pecs, rhomboids, up trap; Ⓛ QL, TFL
✕ Ⓑ sup. erector spinae, IT bands
✳ Ⓑ ankles
TP Ⓑ pec minor; TeP Ⓑ traps, rhomboids

A Techniques/Modalities: Locations/Duration
Prenatal sidelying FBRM, circ. enhance,
light XFF erectors, PNF to TP, TeP

Response to Treatment (see Δ)
℗ 5→2, 3→1, ↑AROM Ⓑ shoulder flex

Goals: Long-term/Short-term
LTG: Within 4 wks, lift child into
    highchair 2x/day w/o ℗, 3 days/wk
STG: Within 1 wk, lift child into
    highchair 1x/day w/o ℗, 3 days/wk.

Functional Outcomes
Lift daughter w/o pain

P Future Treatment/Frequency
1 hr Ⓜ 1x/wk for 4 wks
-Use more bolsters next time

Homework/Self-care
rec: 70-100 oz. H₂0/day
rec: door jamb stretches for pecs & subscap
    1x/day, every day as demo'd

Therapist's Signature *Parker Bellman*   Date *4-9-02*

Legend: ℮ TP   • TeP   ○ ℗   ✳ Infl   ≡ HT   ≈ SP
ↆ Adh   ≫ Numb   ◯ rot   ╱ elev   ⊱ Short   ↔ Long

Figure 7-14. SOAP note for Kirsten, highlighting Objective information. (Modified with permission from Thompson DL. Hands Heal: Communication, Documentation, and Insurance Billing for Manual Therapists. 2nd ed. Baltimore: Lippincott Williams & Wilkins, 2002.)

The concepts of ethics and professionalism, effective communication and documentation, and assessment skills can be combined with your anatomy and physiology knowledge to develop a treatment plan with the objective of promoting overall health and well-being with a client-centered focus.

CHAPTER EXERCISES

1. Using the procedure outlined in this chapter, perform general assessments on at least five friends or family members. (Try to use the same people who filled out client histories and participated in the intake interview exercises.)

2. Watch people (on television, in a shopping mall, in the break room, at the beach, etc.) to make quick postural assessments and write a list of at least 20 observations. For example, you might notice one shoulder higher than the other, a hunched posture, uneven arm swing, or a tilted head.

3. Demonstrate AROM for each of the movements possible at the following joints, remembering to use a slow, steady speed while keeping your body very still:

   a. Glenohumeral joint
   b. Knee
   c. Elbow
   d. Temporomandibular joint
   e. Ankle
   f. Neck

4. Using flexion of the elbow:

   a. Ask someone to quickly and casually show you the movement, without giving them any specific directions.
   b. Watch the movement and notice where the ROM ends.
   c. Then demonstrate slow and steady elbow flexion, isolating the joint movement.
   d. Ask your partner to perform the movement again, this time using the technique you demonstrated.
   e. Compare the range that was performed quickly to the range that was performed slowly and write down any differences you notice.

5. Practice evaluating body rhythms on at least three different people.

   a. Ask the person to lie in a prone position, on the stomach.
   b. Gently place one hand over the person's lumbar spine and the other over the thoracic spine.

   c. Relax your hands and tune in to their breathing—the rhythm, the amount of movement, the location of the movement.
   d. Try to notice other rhythms, such as the heartbeat or the craniosacral rhythm.
   e. Compare the different rhythms of different people.

6. Perform AROM for elbow flexion. Perform PROM for elbow flexion with your own arm. If they have different end feels or different limits to the ROM, list some reasons why they might differ.

7. Considering the guideline to treat where it hurts, where it is compensated, and at the ends of the fascial restriction, describe how fascia is involved in muscle tissue and compensation patterns.

8. Position yourself in an abnormal standing posture (hips forward, shoulders forward, shoulders shrugged upward, head forward, shoulders backward, etc.).

   a. Walk around with that posture for 2 to 3 minutes and then return to your normal, relaxed posture.
   b. Describe any areas that feel hypertonic or uncomfortable.
   c. Consider the long-term effects of that abnormal posture and identify some of the muscles that might become posturally shortened.

9. Use abbreviations and symbols to document the following objective assessments:

   a. The client's right elbow flexion had a reduced active range of motion.
   b. The client's skin was red and hot over the right quadratus lumborum muscle.
   c. The client's left anterior superior iliac spine was higher than the right anterior superior iliac spine.
   d. Upon active range of motion of the neck rotating to the left, the client shrugged the left shoulder and dropped the chin.
   e. Passive range of motion of neck rotation to the left was greater than the active range of motion of neck rotation to the left.

10. Take several deep breaths while doing the following, and compare how the different postures affect your breathing:

    a. Tighten the muscles in your pelvic floor and squeeze your abdominal muscles.
    b. Hunch forward at the shoulders.
    c. Slump in your chair, rolling your pelvis downward.
    d. Raise your arms over your head.
    e. Stand in your normal, relaxed position.
    f. Sit in your normal, relaxed position.

SUGGESTED READINGS

Biel A. *Trail Guide to the Body.* 2nd ed. Boulder, CO: Books of Discovery, 2001.

Clarkson HM. *Musculoskeletal Assessment Joint Range of Motion and Manual Muscle Strength.* 2nd ed. Philadelphia: Lippincott Williams & Wilkins, 2000.

Dickson FD. *Posture Its Relation to Health.* Philadelphia: JB Lippincott, 1930.

Kendall FP, McCreary EK, Provance PG. *Muscles Testing and Function with Posture and Pain.* 4th ed. Baltimore: Williams & Wilkins, 1993.

Kendall HO, Kendall FP, Boynton DA. *Posture and Pain.* Baltimore: Williams & Wilkins, 1952 (reprinted by Robert E. Krieger Publishing Company, Malabar, FL, 1985).

Lowe W. *Functional Assessment.* Bend, OR: OMERI, 1997.

Rattray F, Ludwig L. *Clinical Massage Therapy: Understanding, Assessing and Treating over 70 Conditions.* Toronto: Talus, 2000.

Souriau P. *The Aesthetics of Movement.* Souriau M, trans-ed. Amherst, MA: The University of Massachusetts Press, 1983.

Thompson DL. *Hands Heal: Communication, Documentation and Insurance Billing for Manual Therapists.* 2nd ed. Baltimore: Lippincott Williams & Wilkins, 2002.

Trager M, Hamond C. *Movement as a Way to Agelessness A Guide to Trager Mentastics.* Barrytown, NY: Station Hill Press, 1995.

http://www.cofc.edu/~futrellm/mmtbasics.html, accessed 3.5.06.

http://www.kinesiologycentral.com/index.html, accessed 3.5.06.

http://www.kinesiology.net, accessed 3.5.06.

http://www.painreleaseclinic.com/muscletest.html, accessed 3.5.06.

http://www.uskinesiology.com/faq.htm, accessed 3.5.06.

8

Treatment Plan

Therapists who understand how to read and write all components of the massage treatment record demonstrate a professional image and, more importantly, can make their treatments more effective. Your **treatment plan** is the intended path you recommend for clients to reach their goals, and the three primary components include your suggestions for future treatment, your suggestions for self-care, and referrals to other healthcare professionals. Future treatment refers to the frequency, duration, expected length of treatment, techniques, and reevaluation tips for future massage sessions. **Self-care** (also called **self-help**) refers to activities that clients can use between massage sessions to help maintain progress made during the massage session and encourage the healing process. Self-care activities are excellent tools for getting clients involved in their own healthcare. If you think clients should see another healthcare professional for further evaluation and diagnosis, you can **refer** them, or recommend that they see a specific healthcare practitioner. This component of the treatment plan is not always included, as it is not always necessary.

Treatment plans can be used for both wellness and therapeutic massage. Even in a spa, where the focus is typically wellness massage, clients occasionally ask for therapeutic massage because of a strained muscle or excessive muscular tension. Writing treatment plans for all clients keeps your documentation consistent, and consistency helps you keep track of your clients' progress toward their goals. Additionally, if you work in a setting where other therapists may be working on clients you have treated, they must be able to use your massage treatment records to design a massage that continues progress toward the treatment goals.

Planning Process

Treatment planning is a process of examining a client's unique information and making an educated guess at the best way to reach the treatment goals. The plan should be flexible, allowing for alterations and changes of course with each massage session because clients sometimes reprioritize the original goals or develop new soft tissue dysfunctions that change the priorities. **The plan is a guide and should be adapted to the client's condition at the time of treatment. Most importantly, the treatment plan should always reflect how to continue progressing toward the prioritized goals.** The components of a plan for client care include:

- Duration of sessions
- Frequency of sessions
- Length of treatment
- Techniques or specific areas to incorporate or avoid
- Self-care recommendations
- Referrals to other healthcare practitioners

Keeping all of these components in mind, you ask a series of questions to develop the treatment plan. Ask leading questions about repetitive motions, sustained positions, and the likelihood of reinjuring the area and determine new compensation patterns. Use that information in conjunction with your assessment of the client's overall health to determine the frequency, duration, and length of treatment as well as techniques, self-care activities, and necessary referrals to other healthcare professionals. Before recording the treatment plan, discuss it briefly with your client to ensure that it is feasible and give the client an opportunity to ask any questions. Then document the specifics in the Plan portion of the SOAP note.

Developing the initial treatment plan is a slightly different process from reevaluating the plan for subsequent massage sessions, since you have more information to use during subsequent sessions.

Initial Session

The first time clients come to you for massage, you have to make an educated guess at your plan for reaching treatment goals. Engage clients in a conversation during the initial session to find out how they typically handle stress, how long it usually takes to recover from illness or injury, or how physically active they tend to be. Determining the goals and designing the treatment plan at an initial massage session is often a collaborative effort in which you make suggestions for future treatment, and the clients decide whether those parameters are reasonable for them. To make initial suggestions and plan effective guidelines for reaching treatment goals, you will need to consider your client's health history, the client interview, general assessments, lifestyle, and their willingness to participate in the process. These are the factors that affect the internal healing environment, or ability for the body to recover from illness and injury (Box 8-1).

For example, a new client comes to you who has a high-pressure job, is going through a divorce, eats fast food, drinks six cups of coffee daily, does not exercise or drink much water, and has had multiple injuries. She has a relatively

> **BOX 8-1**
>
> ## Initial Treatment Plan
>
> 1. Evaluate the internal healing environment.
>   a. Health history
>   i. Injuries
>   ii. Length of time condition has been present
>   iii. What makes condition better or worse
>   b. Client interview
>   c. Accumulated stress factors
>   d. General assessments
>   e. Lifestyle
>   i. How do you typically handle stress?
>   ii. How long does it typically take to recover from illness or injury?
>   iii. How physically active are you?
>   f. Participation
>   i. Generally, do you typically take medications or use lifestyle changes as a remedy?
>   ii. Are you conscientious about leading a healthy lifestyle?
>
> 2. Make an educated guess about the client's ability to heal or recover from illness or injury (the following are just generalities).
>   a. Strong—minimal number of chronic conditions, few injuries, few stress factors, actively manages stress, usually heals within a week or two, daily exercise, uses lifestyle changes instead of medications for treatments, tries to eat balanced meals, drink sufficient water
>
>   b. Weak—several chronic conditions, several injuries, many stress factors, does not dissipate stress, usually takes months to heal, eats fast food, drinks a lot of coffee, smokes cigarettes, no time or energy to lead a healthy lifestyle
>
> 3. Consider the client's treatment goals and ability to heal to suggest a treatment plan.
>   a. Future treatment
>   b. Frequency
>   c. Duration
>   d. Length of treatment
>   e. Techniques or areas to include or avoid
>   f. Reevaluation suggestions
>   g. Self-care
>   h. Specific activities
>   i. Specific frequency, duration, and amounts
>   j. Referrals, if appropriate
>   k. Healthcare practitioner's name
>
> 4. Discuss the plan with clients to make sure it is feasible for them and to address any questions.
>
> 5. Document the treatment plan recommendations in the Plan section of the SOAP note.

good internal healing environment, so you could set treatment goals that are easily attainable and recommend a fairly aggressive treatment plan.

Long-term goal (LTG)—Within 2 months, be able to lift her toddler in and out of the high chair twice a day, three times a week, without pain.

Short-term goal (STG)—Within 2 weeks, be able to put dishes into the above-counter cabinets once a day, three times a week, without pain.

Given those goals, your treatment plan could recommend 60-minute massages, once a week, for 2 months. You might want to try myofascial release work, proprioceptive neuromuscular facilitation work, and vibration for the muscles involved in shoulder flexion. You could mention that if she consumed at least 60 ounces of water each day and applied ice to both shoulders for 20 minutes, at least three times a week, she might be able to reach her goals faster. All of this information is recorded in the Plan section of the SOAP note.

Subsequent Sessions

In each subsequent massage session, ask questions to reevaluate the previous treatment plan and make necessary changes

(Box 8-2). Review the prior session's treatment notes to know how clients responded to the last treatment and follow up on self-care activities and any referrals. Additionally, assess their current stress level by asking them how they feel that day, how they are doing, how life is treating them, and where their body hurts. Record their answers in the Subjective section of the SOAP chart. If there are new areas of pain or discomfort, perform the appropriate assessments to discover new compensation patterns, which muscles might be affected, and any new contraindications. The new assessments are recorded in the Objective portion of the SOAP note.

If clients seem to have continued progress between massage sessions, you can use the treatment plan from the previous session as a springboard, incorporating similar techniques into the current massage. If their condition seems worse or if they express doubt, you can design a massage that is very different from the previous session. Document techniques you use and the clients' responses in the Activity and Analysis section of the SOAP note.

Consider the sample client used to illustrate the initial treatment plan. A year later, she may have delegated some of her work responsibilities, settled the divorce, received massages once a month, and started to exercise and drink at least 50 ounces of water every day. Her healing environment is much better, and she would be able to reach more aggressive treatment goals with less treatment.

BOX 8-2

Session-to-Session Treatment Plan

1. Review the SOAP note from the previous massage session.

2. Ask clients about the self-care recommendations.
   a. Were you able to incorporate the (insert specifics here)?
   b. Did you have any trouble with any of the self-care?
   c. Did any of the self-care make noticeable changes?

3. Ask clients about any referrals.
   a. Were you able to talk with (insert practitioner's name here)?
   b. If so, did the practitioner make any diagnoses, prescribe any treatments, or make any recommendations?

4. Ask clients how they felt after the previous massage.
   a. Better, worse, or no change?
   b. How long did that last?

5. Ask about the client's current condition.
   a. How are you feeling today, in general, or, how is life treating you?
   b. Describe today's pain level or discomfort and the areas of discomfort.

c. Are there any new medications or other new treatments?
d. Are there any new areas of concern, cuts, or bruises?
   • If so, perform the appropriate assessments and record them as Objective information on today's SOAP note.

6. Consider the client's progress toward treatment goals and results of the previous treatment to determine whether you will continue with the original treatment plan or make adjustments to
   a. Future treatment recommendations
   b. Self-care activities
   c. Referrals

7. Discuss the treatment plan with clients to make sure it is feasible for them and to address any questions.

8. Properly document the current treatment plan in the Plan section of your current SOAP note.

9. If the client had an appointment with the referred healthcare practitioner, remember to obtain copies of the medical records, either formally or informally.

LTG—Within 2 months, be able to lift her toddler in and out of the crib twice a day, 5 days a week without pain.

STG—Within 2 weeks, be able to lift her toddler in and out of the high chair three times a day, 3 days a week without pain.

The treatment plan could recommend 60-minute massages, twice a month, for 2 months. Your recommendations for techniques could be primarily relaxation techniques with a little extra attention to the muscles involved in shoulder flexion. You could mention that warm baths at least twice a week could help her relax and that consuming at least 60 ounces of water each day would help maintain the soft tissue work that was accomplished.

Future Treatment

The treatment plan includes your recommendations for future massage treatments. You should refer to the duration and frequency of future sessions, length of treatment, techniques to include or avoid, and specific suggestions for reevaluation. The amount of time a client's body requires to change the condition of soft tissue strongly affects your determination of future treatment. Document the future treatment information in the Plan section of the SOAP chart. To recommend 60-minute massage sessions once a week for 8 weeks, incorporating myofascial release at the left iliotibial band, you could write:

1-hr (M) 1X / wk for 8 wks, try MFR on (L) IT band

These notes help you determine progress and design each massage session. Besides, it is often difficult to remember details for each client, especially when seeing many clients in your practice.

Healing Time

Approximated healing time, or the length of time that may be required to restore normal function, influences the treatment plan. Healing time is affected by the client's internal healing environment, which you evaluate by learning about their physical, emotional, mental, and nutritional stressors in addition to their lifestyle, illness, injuries, and the general length of their recovery or healing times. It takes longer for clients to recover from illness or injury when they lead an unhealthy lifestyle with a lot of stressors than when their life is relatively uncomplicated and they are comfortable and content. Healing time is unique to an individual and can only be estimated as a relative amount of time for that person. You should not compare the healing time of one client to that of another. In other words, your best estimations for healing time are based on information that you accumulate over a period of months or years. A strong healing environment allows a more aggressive treatment plan, with longer or more frequent massages and more aggressive techniques. A weak healing environment is best treated with a conservative plan, including shorter or less frequent massages and less aggressive techniques.

Duration of Future Sessions

How long should the next massage last? The duration of each future massage session is the first consideration when developing a treatment plan. Massage sessions can be 15, 30, 60, or 90 minutes long. Most massage sessions are about an hour, so most treatment plans imply future sessions of 60 minutes. Occasionally, your clients might be better served with a shorter or longer session. A shorter session may be warranted if clients are uncomfortable during the massage, for any reason. Discomfort can outweigh the benefits of the massage, and clients who are uncomfortable throughout the massage, either physically or mentally, can actually feel worse after the massage. Your effective communication skills, especially with nonverbal cues, are critical for determining whether future sessions should be limited in duration.

If clients experience pain, uneasiness, or lack of trust in you or your massage, those feelings can last for days. Thirty-minute sessions give those clients an opportunity to develop trust with you as a professional therapist who understands that everyone has different needs. Some clients, such as elderly clients and chronic pain clients, are uncomfortable lying on your massage table for extended periods of time. Rather than subject them to hour-long sessions, you can try 30-minute sessions to see if there is less discomfort and more overall benefit. Clients who are focusing specifically on healing a soft tissue injury may benefit from shorter sessions to avoid making their condition worse, or exacerbating it. There is a delicate balance between beneficially treating and overtreating an injury.

At the other end of the spectrum, some clients may benefit from a 90-minute massage session. As long as their internal healing environment is good, you might recommend a 90-minute session for clients with multiple compensation patterns or those who need a longer period of time to feel relaxed.

Frequency of Future Sessions

Healing input influences healing output. This concept is a factor in determining the frequency of future sessions for both wellness and therapeutic massage. Massage enhances the healing process by mechanically increasing the circulation of blood and lymph to and around the area of concern. Nutrients and oxygen are brought to the area by the arterial system, and waste products are removed by the lymphatic and venous systems. Massage is also beneficial by mechanically reducing physical tension and reflexively inducing the parasympathetic nervous response, both of which encourage relaxation.

Determining the frequency of massage sessions depends on the condition of your clients' soft tissues and their lifestyle. For clients whose soft tissues are healthy, treatments as frequent as twice a week can be beneficial for maintaining relaxation, reducing muscular tension, and relieving fascial adhesions that cause compensation patterns. On the other hand, you can get too much of a good thing, including massage. The problem with receiving massage too frequently is that it can overwhelm the body and can easily exacerbate the original condition.

There are a number of reasons to recommend at least one massage every few months. Clients can benefit from a regular investment in health maintenance. Occasional massage can help minimize the stressors and reduce the accumulation of stress to improve health and the internal healing environment. Clients who regularly get an occasional massage benefit your practice. Seeing clients once every few months allows you to develop relationships, which can lead to more trust and stronger rapport. It also establishes a regular and dependable client base, which is what you depend on for a financially stable practice.

The benefits of massage are cumulative, and your recommendations are based on how much healing input clients need to restore function and reach their treatment goals. You must balance the frequency of sessions such that you can make steady progress but do not overtreat. Most likely, the frequency of treatment is somewhere between once a week and once every few months. Clients are ultimately responsible for the frequency of their massage treatments, taking into consideration their financial situation, transportation arrangements, schedules, and child care.

Length of Treatment

The length of treatment you recommend should not exceed the time frame of the LTGs, which should be attainable and recognizable within 1 to 2 months. It is relatively easy for clients to commit to this kind of time frame, considering finances, transportation, schedules, and child care.

Techniques and Areas to Include or Avoid

During the massage, you may try specific strokes or techniques that are ineffective or disliked by a client. On the other hand, you may find techniques that are especially effective on a particular client or techniques that a client enjoys. Some clients do not want to be touched in certain areas, such as their abdomen, feet, or face. For a client who does not want abdominal massage, but likes trigger point techniques and responds well to them, you could write:

Cl–avoid abdomen, likes TP work. Use TP next session.

It is a good idea to ask clients prior to their massage session if there is any area of their body that they prefer not to have touched.

There are occasions when you do not have enough time during the session to use all of the techniques you want or you think of a technique that might be good to try during the next session. Sometimes the massage is almost finished when you discover an area of restricted fascia that you suspect could be the primary imbalance causing the client's compensation patterns. Rather than start therapeutic techniques on that area at the end of the massage, you can recommend that these techniques be incorporated into the next session.

Reevaluation

Reevaluation is performed when the original treatment goal has been reached, and it is also important for determining the progress toward STGs and LTGs. You may want a particular area or joint movement reevaluated before the next massage session, especially if the self-care activities were focused on that area. For example, your plan might include a suggestion to reevaluate right shoulder flexion for hesitation upon active range of motion (AROM). While you are continually reevaluating clients during each session, you might use some of the general assessments you performed in their initial visit. Any new assessment findings are documented in the "O" portion of the SOAP note.

Self-Care Recommendations

You typically treat clients for 30 to 90 minutes at a time, which is enough time to make progress. Between massage sessions, clients can help to maintain and advance the progress by using self-care, which is simply homework to support the treatment goals and reduce physical tension. This is not to say that clients will not benefit from the massage treatment alone, but that the benefits usually increase and goals can be reached sooner if clients participate between sessions with self-care techniques. Self-care gives clients an opportunity to participate in the maintenance and improvement of their health. Using the concept that healing input influences healing output, you can educate your clients about participating in their healthcare and following self-care recommendations to progress toward their goals faster.

It is not in the massage therapy scope of practice to prescribe, but there are clients who assume that massage therapists have the same responsibilities and capabilities as medical professionals who are allowed to diagnose and prescribe. Emphasize to clients that self-care activities are suggestions for enhancing the effects of the massage session and improving the health of the soft tissues and not in any way a prescription. Clarify that you treat only soft tissue conditions via massage and emphasize that any other conditions should be diagnosed and treated by the appropriate healthcare professional. It is your responsibility to ensure that clients experience no confusion regarding diagnosis, prescription, or treatment. To avoid any misconceptions, you can offer handouts and a suggested reading list with information about self-care activities you recommend.

Self-care is recorded in the Plan section of the SOAP note. Try to be specific but brief and refer to the specific activities, frequencies, durations, and amounts you recommend. For instance, you recommend a client increase water intake to 60 ounces per day and stretch the left triceps twice a day, five times a week. You demonstrate the stretch by flexing the left shoulder and elbow and, using your right hand to slowly push upward on the distal humerus, increase flexion of the left shoulder. Your notes could say:

rec: H_2O to 60 oz/day, perform (L) triceps stretch
2X/day, 5X/wk, as demonstrated

Considerations for Self-Care

Consider your client's lifestyle and time constraints when making self-care recommendations. If your recommendations do not fit within either of these, clients are not likely to comply or, even worse, their confidence in the treatment process may be diminished. Clients can feel empowered to take responsibility for their health and well-being when they are comfortable with the self-care you suggest, so activities should be added gradually.

Many clients feel burdened with self-care, as if it were a dreaded homework assignment. Limit the number of activities you recommend to minimize the number of things they have to remember and the amount of time and energy they have to commit. Too much too soon can overwhelm the body and even lengthen the healing process. For example, it is beneficial for a client to receive massage treatment, increase water intake, and use one or two stretches for the connective tissue in the affected area. However, adding a vigorous exercise program, using heat and ice therapy, radically changing the diet, and adding five specific stretches on a daily basis could overwhelm the body. The combination of all these activities could add more stress, the body might not be able to distinguish or integrate so many changes, and the client's initial condition could be aggravated.

Nevertheless, massage therapists often see clients resist self-care and resist progress toward their goals. This situation can be very frustrating and you must be aware of this behavior. Many persons have suffered from chronic conditions for so long that they stop paying attention to the discomfort. Their compensation patterns, pain patterns, and coping skills become part of their everyday routine and can even become part of a person's identity. The clients' goals for moving toward a better and more balanced state of health may effectively take away a part of their identity. Life without pain and discomfort may be unknown territory for a person with a chronic condition. Most people are somewhat uncomfortable about change and unfamiliar experiences. This is exactly the situation that may occur when clients start making progress toward their goals. It may seem strange, but it will make sense as you see it occur in your practice. For example, clients who have had a chronic pain condition for years can get attention and concern from friends and family. Losing this attention may deter them from letting go of their pain and from participating in their healing process. You have a professional obligation to support clients in making progress toward their goals, but you must not judge or harbor negative feelings toward a client who is hesitant or does not want to participate in the healing process.

Making self-care recommendations is the massage therapist's responsibility, whether clients choose to participate or not. Some self-care topics include internal and external hydrotherapy, rest and sleep, nutritional awareness, specific stretches for the areas of concern, physical awareness, and ergonomics.

Hydrotherapy

Hydrotherapy is the use of water as a treatment. It can be used internally to support cells and organs, and it can be used externally. Water, the universal solvent, is so inexpensive and readily available that it is often overlooked as a valid therapeutic approach. Because of its simplicity and availability, water is excellent for self-care.

Internal Hydrotherapy

Water has many functions in the body: elimination of waste, delivery of nutrients and oxygen to the cells, maintenance of tissue pliability and function, cushioning of joints, and regulation of body temperature. The muscles are composed of about 75% water, and blood about 90%, and those percentages must be maintained with sufficient water intake or the health of those tissues will suffer. Muscle tissue and fascia can get stuck together and cause fascial adhesions, muscle contractions can become less efficient, blood becomes more viscous, blood volume decreases, the ability of blood to flow decreases, and thus the delivery of oxygen to cells is reduced.

One of the most common self-care recommendations is for clients to drink enough water to stay hydrated. After a massage session, adequate water intake helps flush the waste out of the body that would otherwise sit in the tissues, impeding healing and restoration of function. Hydration further enhances relaxation of the muscles and surrounding soft tissue during the massage session. Encourage clients to drink enough water after a massage and in between sessions as an important self-care activity. Recommendations vary widely, but a general rule is to drink ½ ounce per pound of body weight. The intake should be increased with physical exercise, salty food, alcoholic beverages, exposure to sun or heat, and illness. Any time you discuss or suggest hydrotherapy, provide safe guidelines rather than simply telling clients to drink more water.

To avoid this, find several references for water consumption and create handouts for your clients. Insufficient water intake leads to diminished cellular function, which in turn reduces the body's ability to recover from injury and maintain a healthful state. It makes tissues sticky and more difficult to heal. It is harder to attain STGs when tissues are dehydrated, and it requires more time to reach the LTGs. Dehydration occurs when the body does not get enough water or loses too much fluid, which can result in diminished soft tissue function, muscle cramps, fatigue, headaches, and dizziness.

The average person is typically dehydrated because of insufficient water intake and substances that rob the body of water, such as alcohol and salt. Instead of judging clients' habits and tendencies, you can teach them about the effects of alcohol and salt. Alcohol is a diuretic, meaning that it causes excess amounts of water to be eliminated from the body, and it can actually cause dehydration. As alcohol is consumed, the tissues are prone to dehydration and may require more time to heal. Consuming excessive amounts of salt makes the body shed extra amounts of water in an effort to maintain homeostasis. The negative effects of alcohol and salt can be counteracted to some extent by additional water intake. A common misconception is that caffeine contributes to dehydration, but numerous scientific studies have shown that caffeine has no effect on dehydration. You can educate clients about hydration and health, but it is up to them to decide what they will and will not consume.

The color of urine is a simple and sometimes useful indicator of hydration. Generally, pale yellow or clear urine usually indicates adequate hydration. Although deep yellow or dark coloring can indicate concentrated urine and dehydration, it can also reflect chemicals, vitamins, and minerals that are being eliminated.

Persons who are retaining water tend to drink insufficient amounts of water. They falsely believe that the less water they consume, the less water they retain. Actually, the opposite is true. As a cactus in the desert retains all of its water because of minimal rain, the body retains its precious supply of water when insufficient water is consumed. This is one of the many homeostatic mechanisms that protect and maintain our health. Drinking more than the generally recommended amount of water makes the homeostatic mechanisms eliminate any excess water that was being retained, thus reducing water retention.

External Hydrotherapy

External hydrotherapy refers to applications of cold and heat, because those treatments were initially only provided by water in its solid (ice), liquid (water), and gaseous (steam) states. Today, there are chemical forms of cold and heat, but the original term remains. Hydrotherapy is covered extensively in the Complementary Modalities chapter, but self-care information for clients is summarized here.

Alert

Ice should be avoided for persons with circulatory problems.

Ice and cold applications reduce circulation and nervous system activity. Ice is typically used in acute conditions in which inflammation, spasms, and pain are present. Any time you use deep-fiber friction techniques, you can recommend ice to prevent inflammation and promote healing. Ice, or an equally cold substitute, should be applied for a maximum of 20 minutes.

A plastic bag filled with ice works, and crushed ice conforms nicely to the body. Ice can be used directly on the skin, but a washcloth or towel helps to hold onto the melting ice, and it soaks up the resulting water. Chemical gel packs are available that also conform to the body, and many people have them in their freezers at home. They must be used cautiously because they are colder than 32°F and can damage the skin.

Alert

Use a layer of fabric between a chemical gel pack and the skin.

Heat applications enhance circulation, which can increase healing.

Alert

Heat should be avoided if there are signs of inflammation, heat, or redness.

Heat relaxes people and may be used for acute conditions in the muscles surrounding an injury, muscle spasms, or other forms of pain. For chronic conditions in which techniques other than friction are used, heat may be applied for up to 20 minutes to increase circulation in the affected muscles. Heat may also be used concurrently while the client is applying ice to help maintain the body's core temperature and to distract the client from the unpleasant effects of ice.

Stretches

Stretching the muscles and surrounding connective tissue in the clients' affected areas may be the second most common self-care recommendation. Although massage lengthens muscles and stretches tissues, the body will adapt to the mechanical changes and new positions faster when clients reinforce those changes between massage sessions with additional stretches. Remember, massage therapists do not diagnose nor prescribe treatment, so be careful to educate clients only about how stretches affect soft tissues and enhance the massage treatments. Clients must understand that stretches are not a substitute for treatment from other healthcare professionals that may be necessary. If you recommend stretches to clients for self-care, you should have books and handouts in your office that illustrate specific stretches (see Suggested Readings). To keep from overwhelming clients with "homework," suggest one or two stretches at most.

As with all self-care, thoroughly explain effective stretching to clients. They should understand how to do the stretch properly, the possible contraindications, and the expected results. Ideally, take time to demonstrate the stretch for clients and let them try it while you observe. This way you can ensure that they are stretching the correct area with a safe technique. You can describe the end feel of a stretch and make sure they are not compromising any anatomical structures or triggering the stretch reflex. Always provide specific information about the frequency and duration of stretches and techniques to use.

Rest

Most people underestimate the value of rest for promoting healing and regeneration. Essentially, rest is a period when mental, physical, sensory, and emotional activity slows or ceases, allowing the body to redirect its energy to restoration. People lead very busy lives, often moving from one event to another and taking little time for rest until they fall into bed in the evening, exhausted from the day's events. Taking time for a massage is one way for people to slow down and rest; however, it is most likely not enough to completely rejuvenate the body and mind. Clients should be told that it is good to take time for massage and that adequate rest can maximize the benefits of massage.

Sleep

Sleep is a deep state of rest when tissues regenerate, repair, and prepare the body for new activity. Oftentimes, sleep positions are the cause of pain and discomfort, which may include stiff necks, aching backs, and numbness and tingling in the arms or hands. It can be difficult for people to change their sleep positions, but you can educate clients about sleep positions and leave it up to them to try to incorporate the changes. Sleep positions can cause pain and discomfort, and yet sometimes pain and discomfort cause problems with sleep.

Stomach sleepers tend to develop stiff necks because they have to turn their heads to the side to breathe.

Additionally, stomach sleepers may hyperextend their lumbar spine, which may create pain. They can benefit from sleeping in a different position. Persons who sleep on their side sometimes complain of back pain, which can result from the torque and tension on the pelvis and hip when the top leg drops down to the bed. You can suggest a body pillow to support the top leg and relieve the torque on the pelvis. Sometimes side sleepers complain of numbness and tingling in their arms and hands, which can be caused by nerve impingement from compression on the shoulder they sleep on. They can be relieved by sleeping on their backs. Persons who sleep on their backs sometimes complain of back pain, which can be caused by the lordotic curve of the spine. Supporting the knees with a pillow reduces the lordotic curve and sometimes relieves pain.

Sleep disruption can cause irritability, concentration difficulty, poor muscle coordination, increased sensitivity to pain, fatigue, sluggishness, a diminished sense of well-being, an inability to cope with the physical and mental challenges of life, and, in some cases, depression. Too little sleep creates "sleep debt," which is similar to being overdrawn at a bank. In time, the body will demand that the debt be repaid. Our bodies do not adapt well to getting less sleep than required, and while we may get used to a sleep-depriving schedule, our judgment, reaction time, and other functions are still impaired.

When massage clients discuss their lack of sleep, you can educate them about the importance of sleep for health and healing and offer some self-care recommendations. Sleep can be affected by a number of factors, and you can recommend that clients examine their daily habits to see if any of them are affecting their sleep patterns:

- Eating or drinking too close to bedtime
- Eating or drinking too much caffeine
- Eating or drinking too much sugar
- Smoking cigarettes with nicotine
- Medications or medication schedules
- Lack of physical activity
- Temperature of the bedroom
- Insufficient body support
- Bedtime schedules
- Amount of sleep necessary for optimal daily function
- Other individuals who might be keeping them awake

Clients who are chronically sleep deprived and cannot seem to change their sleep pattern may need to be referred to a medical doctor, who can look for a diagnosis and make a prescription. If you do refer your clients to other healthcare practitioners, you should document the referral in the Plan portion of the SOAP note and follow up by writing a letter to that practitioner.

In addition, clients can be encouraged to take "mini-breaks" during the workday to stretch or walk for a few minutes once every other hour or so. Our body rhythms create a dip in brain activity in the middle of the afternoon, which creates a natural naptime. A short, 15- to 20-minute nap sometime between 1 and 4 pm can be refreshing and is least likely to affect that night's sleep.

Nutrition

Nutritional awareness is another form of self-care a therapist may encourage in a client. Unless you are a properly trained dietitian or nutritionist, you should be very careful not to offer professional advice in this area. With this in mind, massage therapists can make nutritional recommendations from an educational standpoint as they pertain to soft tissue health. Have nutritional references on hand for clients who are interested. Vitamin C is required for tissue repair and thus is important to include in the diet. Nerve cells and muscle cells require sodium and potassium to conduct electrical charges properly, so it is generally recommended that these electrolytes be included in a balanced diet. Calcium and magnesium are critical for proper muscle contraction, making them necessary dietary elements. Nutritional recommendations generally accepted by the public are usually valid, but myths and false information are widespread. Massage therapists can demonstrate professionalism by sorting through nutritional information and guiding clients toward scientifically proven, valid facts with reasonable explanations. There are a number of herbal and "natural" remedies on the market that claim all kinds of benefits, but because many of them have not been scientifically proven, it is best to refer clients with questions about these products to a nutritional or herbal specialist. For specific dietary and nutritional recommendations, however, therapists should practice the rule "When in doubt, refer out."

Body Awareness

Increasing a client's physical awareness is not only a benefit of massage; it can also be recommended to clients as a self-care activity. As mentioned above, many persons with chronic conditions do not remember what it is like to be without pain or to have unlimited function. Some get used to gauging their days by the amount of pain they experience, or they regularly describe their pain to friends and family. Sometimes the pain and discomfort become so much a part of their identity that they do not know how to let go of it. Having lived with tension or pain in an area for so long, they get used to it being there and are generally unaware of times when they do not feel pain. You may encourage clients to shift their focus to

times when the tension or pain is absent, even if it is just for a few moments a day. Another approach is to get clients to periodically check for pain at mealtimes or at other regular intervals during their day. It can help them realize that being without pain is acceptable and can help them look forward to less pain and discomfort and encourage them to participate in the progress toward their goals. You could write:

rec: Cl record (P) every day at mealtimes

Massage therapy can be compared to peeling layers of an onion—the layers of compensation are treated with a series of massage sessions. You must inform clients that the tension or pain may get worse as these layers are removed, that you are addressing the core of their condition, and that this is a normal part of the progress. The old adage "Change is good" applies in this context. Massage treatment that increases or decreases the client's pain and ROM indicates that the body is responding to the work. If significant therapeutic work was done, the mechanical effects can be uncomfortable but not extremely painful. Discomfort resulting from massage usually decreases within 2 to 3 days as the body accommodates the mechanical changes. If it does not, it is possible that you over-treated the client, and you should adjust the massage techniques for the next session. If this is the case, you must look over your documentation notes and reevaluate:

- The client's condition
- Contraindications
- Your treatment
- Possible referral to another healthcare practitioner

You have a responsibility to address your clients' responses to your treatment. A thorough general assessment may be necessary, and you may need to ask more leading questions to elicit information that might suggest contraindications that you did not identify before the previous session. The techniques you used might have been too aggressive or inappropriate for the client's condition and relative tissue health. If you cannot determine how pain resulted and why it did not go away, you may need to refer the client for further evaluation by another healthcare practitioner to maintain a client-centered practice. It is in the client's best interest to be referred out for conditions that you do not understand, which means it is also in your best interest.

When no change occurs after a massage, it suggests that the massage treatments are ineffective. If no change occurs, you should reevaluate the above factors and make adjustments to your treatment.

Ergonomics

Ergonomics is the science that designs and coordinates people's activities with the equipment they use and the conditions of their working environment. Ergonomics focuses on minimizing the mechanical stress placed on the body and soft tissues, which is usually accomplished by maintaining body positions that are as close to our natural and relaxed standing position as possible. For example, chairs with a flat seat and a flat back provide no support for our natural spinal curves. After sitting in that kind of chair for extended periods of time, we tend to slump, which puts mechanical stress on the spine and the nerves that exit the spine, and some persons can suffer nerve impingement as a result. Ergonomic chairs are designed to provide support for our natural spinal curves to reduce the mechanical stress on our body. There are computer keyboards that are ergonomically designed to accommodate the natural resting position of our wrists and hands to reduce

compression of the carpal tunnel in the wrist. This compression is sometimes responsible for impinging the radial nerve and causing neurological symptoms of numbness and tingling in the first few phalanges.

Special equipment is not required to make ergonomic changes. Instead of looking at a computer screen that is above or below your head, which forces your neck into hyperextension or flexion, you can position the screen at eye level. Instead of carrying a purse or backpack on the same shoulder all the time, which can create chronically hypertonic muscles and fascial restrictions, you can occasionally switch the shoulder you carry the bag on. These kinds of ergonomic changes are a good source for self-care recommendations and they tie into body awareness.

Referral to Other Healthcare Professionals

With a few exceptions, massage is a good form of treatment for soft tissue dysfunction, injury recovery, and stress reduction, but it is not a cure for everything. Some conditions require the care of other healthcare professionals, and as a professional massage therapist, you have an ethical responsibility to refer clients to the appropriate healthcare practitioner. You should also be aware of professional etiquette when contacting that practitioner regarding the referral.

Whether you suspect a problem with the client's skin, nervous system, teeth, body temperature, feet, emotional instability, joints, or skeletal structure, if it is not soft tissue, massage therapists *do not* treat it. Generally, you refer clients to their primary caregiver, who further evaluates or diagnoses the condition.

Alert
Even if you feel confident of a diagnosis, it is not in your scope of practice to share that diagnosis in any form of communication, verbal or written.

Again, clients often see their massage therapist as a healthcare professional who can diagnose medical conditions. As a massage professional, you must ethically and legally educate clients that diagnosing medical conditions is in no way a part of a massage therapist's scope of practice.

By referring clients to other healthcare professionals when it is appropriate, you maintain the core principle of client-centered care. Maintaining this principle creates a ripple effect of respect and trust not only with your client

but also with other healthcare professionals. The key to the ripple effect is your ability to recognize when a condition is out of your scope of practice and needs to be addressed by another professional. This is essential for upholding the standards of practice and ethical codes of the massage therapy profession as well as preserving client-centered care. Document your recommendations for referral to other healthcare professionals in the Plan section of the SOAP chart. If you recommend that a client see his or her primary care physician (PCP) for further evaluation of the left shoulder, you could write:

rec: Cl see PCP for further evaluation of (L) shoulder

Follow-up Communication

Professional communication skills and a command of the common professional language facilitate effective communication between you and other healthcare practitioners. Correct pronunciation of anatomical and physiological words, scientific terms, and techniques is required to convey true knowledge. Proper spelling, grammar, and use of terminology are also critical for communicating a sense of understanding, especially when you are trying to develop a respectful working relationship with other healthcare professionals. Working *with* other professionals is always better than working apart from them, because clients generally feel better when everyone is working together, toward the same goal—their health and well-being.

Once a referral is made, you can ask clients to keep you in the communication loop, which makes you part of their cooperative team of healthcare professionals. You should request copies of medical reports and medical updates so you are aware of any medical diagnoses, treatments, and test results. The client-centered focus encourages determination of whether massage treatment is appropriate for the client. Without team communication, you cannot make the best decisions for soft tissue treatment, which can result in over- or undertreating the soft tissues. Conversely, if a healthcare practitioner refers a client to you, you should contact the practitioner to complete the communication loop and start creating a healthcare team.

Keeping the above in mind, there is a protocol for communication between you and other healthcare practitioners. You should keep all communication simple and to the point. Rarely do other healthcare providers have time to sort through pages of information to ascertain what you are requesting or communicating. Essentially, you should summarize the details and state the progress of the client's condition. Familiarize yourself with how to make a written or verbal request for copies of medical reports and updates, how to discuss a client's condition, how the referral process with another healthcare professional works, and how to communicate with insurance companies so you can be reimbursed for massage treatments.

Requesting Copies of Medical Records

You can request copies of medical reports and updates either formally or informally. To request copies of medical information formally, your client must fill out a records release form (see Chapter 2, Fig. 2-3), and you must send a copy to the practitioner along with a cover letter stating your request. Figure 8-1 shows an example of a cover letter. Informally, you can ask clients to request copies from their healthcare practitioner and bring them to you. These forms are kept in the client's file.

Discussing a Client's Conditions

On occasion, you may need to discuss a client's condition with another healthcare practitioner. For example, the healthcare practitioner may need some information about your soft tissue treatment before writing a prescription. Before contacting the healthcare practitioner, you must first get written permission from the client to share the information in the massage treatment records. You can include such a statement in your client history forms rather than use a separate permission form. (See Chapter 2, Fig. 2-3 for a health information form that asks for the client's permission to consult with the referring healthcare professional.)

Communication for Referral and Insurance Reimbursement

Insurance laws vary from state to state, so if you are seeking insurance reimbursement, you must be aware of the insurance laws in your state and research how those laws affect reimbursement for massage. The information presented here is very general and is intended to give you a basic idea of how communication flows in this process.

Currently, clients have direct access to massage therapy, meaning they can seek treatment without a formal referral or prescription from another healthcare practitioner. In spite of direct access, most insurance companies will not reimburse without a medical prescription or formal referral for treatment as well as treatment notes. A prescription is a written order from a medical professional who is legally allowed to prescribe, and it pertains to treatment for a specific condition. A prescription typically includes the referring healthcare practitioner's name and contact information, date, patient's name, diagnosis, diagnosis code, and the prescribed treatment with frequency and duration parameters.

Since massage therapists cannot write prescriptions, you can use a referral form to get a prescription from the physician for initial or additional massage treatment. The form should include space for your contact information and the client's name, and it should be clear that you need to have the physician write the diagnosis, precautions, body areas to treat, frequency and duration of massage treatment, and whether progress updates are requested as well as how the physician wishes to receive them, a reevaluation date, and the physician's signature and contact information. Figure 8-2 is an example of a prescription and referral form. Fill out your contact information and the client's (patient's) name and send the form to the client's physician. The physician can then fill in the treatment protocols and return the form to you. Make a copy to send to the insurance company and keep a copy in the client's file. Notice whether an initial treatment report and/or progress notes are requested in return. Your initial treatment report should include a note of thanks to the physician for referring the client to you for massage in addition to your initial findings and massage treatment plan. Essentially, it summarizes the SOAP notes and general assessment form information. Figure 8-3 shows an example of an initial treatment report. A progress report, basically a summary of the Subjective and Objective sections of the SOAP notes, is often requested by the referring physician. If you are recommending further care, specify the new duration and frequency parameters. Generally, a progress report is sent to the healthcare provider every 30 days or for the length of the prescription (see Fig. 8-4).

MassageWorks!
123 North Main Street
Zionsville, IN 46077
317-555-8734

February 2, 2006

Sam Jones, DC
Family Chiropractic
2222 Healing Way
Indianapolis, IN 46220

RE: Susie Smith

Dear Dr. Jones:

Susie Smith has recently become a client in my massage therapy practice.
I would like a copy of her most recent MRI report to identify any potential
effects on Ms. Smith's soft tissues so that I may provide the most
appropriate massage treatment for her condition.

Please find enclosed a signed release form granting permission to release
Ms. Smith's records.

Thank you for your assistance. Please call me should you have any
questions.

Kindest regards,

Jane Therapist, CMT
Enclosure

Figure 8-1. Cover letter.

MassageWorks!
Jane Therapist, CMT
123 North Main Street
Indianapolis, IN 46220
317.555.1234

Prescription and Referral

Client name _____ Date _____

Date of Injury _____ Insurance ID# _____

Diagnosis (Include Codes)   Condition is related to

_____   □ Automobile Accident
_____   □ Work Injury
_____   □ Other _____
_____   _____

Cautions/Contraindications:

_____

_____

_____

Medically Necessary Treatment: Follow Plan Prescribed

Body areas to be treated: **Treatment Type:**

□ Head _____   □ Discretion of the massage therapist
□ Neck _____   □ Massage Therapy _____
□ Chest _____   □ Hydrotherapy _____
□ Shoulders _____   □ Self-Care Education _____
□ Back _____   □ Other _____
□ Lowback/Hips _____
□ Upper Extremities _____   **Treatment Goals:**
□ Lower Extremities _____   □ Decrease Pain
□ All of the above _____   □ Decrease Muscle Tension/Spasm
□ Other _____   □ Decrease Compensation patterns
                                        □ Increase Mobility
Duration and Frequency   □ Increase Function
□ Daily   □ Other _____
□ ____ x per wk for ____ wks   _____
□ ____ x per month for ____ months
Reevaluation Date: _____

Additional Instructions:

_____

_____

Referring Healthcare Provider (HCP)

Contact Information   **Progress Updates**
Provider Name _____   □ Send Progress Report after Initial Session
Provider No. _____   □ Send at end of Prescription
Address _____   □ Send copies of Treatment Notes at end of Prescription
_____   □ Mail □ Fax □ Email
Phone _____
Fax _____
Email _____
Provider Signature _____ Date _____

Figure 8-2. Prescription and referral form.

MassageWorks!
123 North Main Street
Zionsville, IN 46077
317-555-8734
email: Jane@massageworks.com

February 2, 2006

Sam Jones, DC
Family Chiropractic
2222 Healing Way
Indianapolis, IN 46220

RE: Susie Smith

Dear Dr. Jones:

Thank you for referring Susie Smith to me for massage treatment. Ms. Smith had
her first appointment on February 2, 2006.

Ms. Smith was seeking massage treatment with bilateral neck pain and tension.
Her immediate goal is to get relief from the neck pain and tension, but eventually
she would like to be able to work at her computer for 2 hours a day during her
work week without neck pain and tension. Initially, our treatment goal is to have
her working at the computer for 15 minutes a day with mild pain and tension.

Together, Ms. Smith and I will work toward the treatment goals as follows:
Massage and myofascial release 2X/week for 1 month with specific focus on the
bilateral neck muscles and surrounding soft tissue; hydrotherapy to reduce any
muscle spasm and/or inflammation; self-care recommendations as appropriate.

I will report back to you in 30 days with Ms. Smith's progress. Please contact me
should you have any questions, remarks or concerns.

Kindest regards,

Jane Therapist, CMT
Enclosure

Figure 8-3. Initial treatment report.

MassageWorks!
Jane Therapist, CMT
123 North Main Street
Indianapolis, IN 46220
317.555.1234
email: Jane@massageworks.com

Client name Susie Smith _____ Date 30 September 2003
Date of Injury 15 August 2003 _____ Insurance ID# 123-45-6789

Client's Current Condition
After 8 sessions of Myofascial release, Ms. Smith has reached her initial goals of relief
from her neck pain and tension as well as working 15 minutes a day with moderate neck
pain and tension. _____

Subjective Findings:
Body areas

☐ Head _____
☒ Neck BL neck P and ≡ _____
☐ Chest _____
☐ Shoulders _____
☐ Lowback/Hips _____
☐ Upper Extremities _____
☐ Lower Extremities _____
☐ All of the above _____
☐ Other _____

Objective Findings:

☐ Muscle Spasm _____
☒ Increased mobility _____
☐ Decreased mobility _____
☐ Hypersensitivity _____
☐ Increased Tension _____
☒ Decreased Tension Δ mod
☐ Increased Pain _____
☒ Decreased Pain Δ mod
☐ Other _____

Recommendations for Further Care:
Duration and Frequency
Additional Care Needed
☐ None needed
☐ Daily
☐ _____ x per wk for _____ wks
☐ _____ x per month for _____ months
☐ PRN max visits _____ per _____

Please contact me with any questions, remarks or concerns. Thank you for your referrals.

Jane Therapist _____ Jane Therapist, CMT 30Sept03 Date

Figure 8-4. Progress report.

Presenting the Treatment Plan

The process of developing treatment plans may seem awkward at first, but with practice, you will become very skilled at making recommendations for treatment. In the beginning, you may find it easier to leave out the treatment plan for initial appointments and only consider a treatment plan after subsequent massage sessions. This gives you time to analyze the history and assessment findings and get a feeling for your client's internal healing environment and participation in healthcare. Presenting the plan to clients is a way of educating them about the information that guided your recommendations, essentially telling them why you are making the recommendations. **Clients are more likely to commit and comply with your recommendations if they know why they are doing so.**

Treatment Recommendations

The first question clients typically ask is, "How long it will take to (stop hurting, return to "normal" function, or stay relaxed for longer than a day)?" There is no single answer, much to their disappointment. You can explain that health and healing times are affected by the physical, emotional, mental, and nutritional stress that a person has accumulated and that healing time can be reduced with the help of massage and self-care. Once you educate your clients about the "whys" of your recommendations, you can discuss the treatment plan and use their input to make adjustments to the plan. All of your recommendations for future treatment are documented in the Plan section of the SOAP note.

Referral Recommendations

If your assessment of the client reveals a health condition or the possibility of a health condition that contraindicates massage or is outside the scope of practice, it is in the client's best interest to refer the client to the appropriate healthcare professional. Anything in the client's best interest is in your best interest. Sometimes clients are aware of their conditions and sometimes not. If not, you may need to have a delicate conversation to refer them to a medical professional without making a diagnosis or alarming them.

Remember to be very careful not to suggest that clients may have "XYZ" condition because they could misinterpret your statement as a diagnosis; assume they have it; and tell their friends, family, or healthcare practitioner. For example, if you detect some inflammation at or around a musculotendinous juncture, *do not* say that it might be tendinitis or that you think it could be tendinitis. Instead, you could say, "From my assessment, I have determined that I can effectively treat your soft tissue condition with massage." Conversely, if you suspect clients may need further examination, you could say, "From my assessment, I have determined that massage might not be helpful for you, and before I do any harm, I recommend that you see your primary healthcare practitioner for further examination. Once your doctor has determined that massage is indicated, I would be happy to continue treatment." There are more complex situations, such as rotator cuff injuries, in which clients have one condition that indicates massage and another that presents a contraindication for massage. In this situation, you could say, "After my assessment, I have determined that you have a soft tissue condition that I can treat, and you also might have a condition that I do not treat. I recommend that you see your primary healthcare professional for further evaluation, and when your doctor authorizes massage treatment, I can confidently continue treatment."

Case Studies

The treatment plans for Rob Blackwell, Timothy Roberts, and Kirsten Van Marter are based on the initial treatment plan procedure.

Progressive Case Study 1:
Rob Blackwell

Considering Rob Blackwell's health history, interview, and assessment process, you determine that Rob's internal healing environment is good and that he is

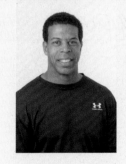

very likely to participate in his healing process. His involvement with sports and his self-employment as a personal trainer suggest that he is moderately likely to repeat the motions that created his neck and shoulder pain or reinjure the affected tissues. Rob's right shoulder is elevated and rolled forward, and there are a number of associated hypertonic muscles. Despite his good internal healing environment, the hypertonic muscles, associated fascial restrictions, and his likelihood to reinjure the tissues could increase the healing time.

Since his musculature is so developed and healthy, his body could withstand 90-minute massages without suffering overtreatment, but his financial situation cannot support them. Rob's initial treatment plan includes 60-minute massages once a week for 6 weeks, at which point the goals will be reevaluated. For the next session, you suggest vibration over the right pectoralis muscles. You mention that there are some self-care activities that he could use to help maintain progress made during the massage and reduce the length of the course of treatment. He could apply ice to his right upper trapezius for 20 minutes, at least once a day, every day. You could demonstrate some specific stretches for the pectoralis major and sternocleidomastoid muscles, explaining that he could use these stretches at least once a day, 5 days a week. He could also increase water intake to 100 ounces per day. You refer Rob to Dr. Christian for an evaluation and current diagnosis of his knees to make sure massage is not contraindicated. These recommendations are highlighted in the Plan section of Rob's SOAP chart in Figure 8-5.

Progressive Case Study 2:
Timothy Roberts

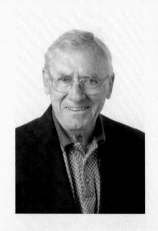

Timothy is only seeking relaxation massage, and he reports no pain, numbness, or stiffness. From the client interview and general assessment, you notice some restrictions in ROM of the left ankle, but you also detect his impatience with the assessments. To strike a balance between gaining his trust and remaining professional, your assessments are brief, primarily looking for any contraindications. For wellness clients like Timothy, you complete the initial treatment plan procedure mostly for consistency in your documentation. Should he seek more therapeutic treatment in the future, you would need to perform a more thorough intake and assessment

as well as use the initial treatment plan procedure to determine a more specific plan. His initial treatment plan is simply to receive 60-minute relaxation massages at least once every 3 months, but you suggest trying cross-fiber friction on the left ankle. You can offer him a glass of water following the massage, briefly mentioning that if he were to drink at least 80 ounces of water a day, it would help his body retain the benefits of the massage. Timothy's treatment plan information is highlighted in his massage treatment record (see Fig. 8-6).

Progressive Case Study 3:
Kirsten Van Marter

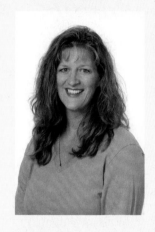

Although she is a new client to you, Kirsten's health information form indicates that she has received regular massage in the past. The information from the history and assessment process lets you know that her internal healing environment is good, but because of her hectic lifestyle of taking care of her child, being pregnant, and working two separate jobs, she may not find time to participate in her healing process. She will probably repeat the motions that created the soft tissue condition as she continues her work and household activities. Both of her shoulders are rolled forward, and her left hip is elevated. Even though she is in her third trimester of pregnancy, the distribution of her weight will continue to change, and her hip pain could get worse. Healing and restoring function may be a challenge until after the baby is born.

Kirsten's muscles and soft tissues are fairly healthy because of her regular exercise and massage. The initial treatment plan suggests 60-minute massages once a week for 4 weeks. Since she is uncomfortable with her pregnancy, it would be good to try more bolsters during massage. You educate Kirsten about the benefits of proper hydration and offer her a glass of water following the massage, asking whether she drinks at least 70 ounces of water a day. You also demonstrate specific stretches for pectoralis major and subscapularis muscles, explaining that if she were to use those stretches at least once a day, every day, it could help her retain the benefits of the current massage. Kirsten's SOAP note highlights the treatment plan information (see Fig. 8-7).

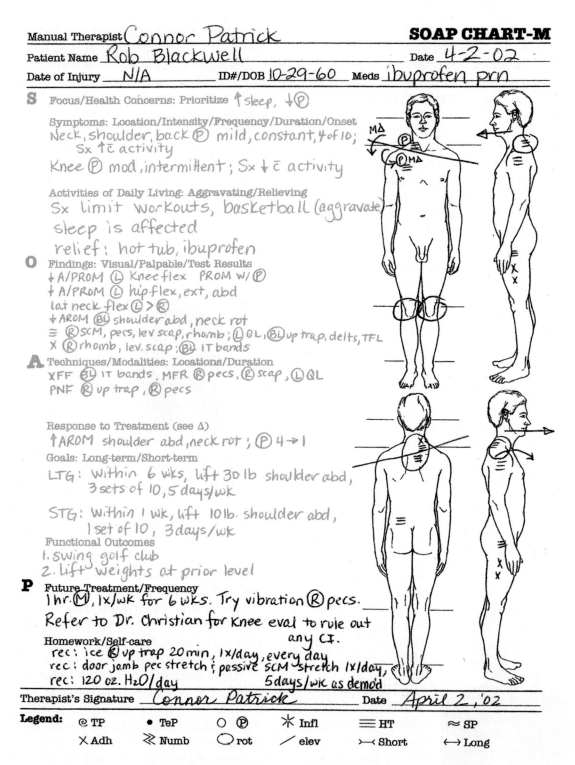

Manual Therapist *Connor Patrick*   **SOAP CHART-M**

Patient Name *Rob Blackwell*   Date *4-2-02*

Date of Injury *N/A*   ID#/DOB *10-29-60*   Meds *ibuprofen prn*

S Focus/Health Concerns: Prioritize ↑sleep, ↓Ⓟ

   Symptoms: Location/Intensity/Frequency/Duration/Onset
   Neck, shoulder, back Ⓟ mild, constant, 4 of 10;
      Sx ↑c̄ activity
   Knee Ⓟ mod, intermittent; Sx ↓ c̄ activity

   Activities of Daily Living: Aggravating/Relieving
   Sx limit workouts, basketball (aggravate)
   sleep is affected
   relief: hot tub, ibuprofen

O Findings: Visual/Palpable/Test Results
   ↓A/PROM Ⓛ Knee flex PROM w/ Ⓟ
   ↓A/PROM Ⓛ hip flex, ext, abd
   lat neck flex Ⓛ > Ⓡ
   ↓AROM ⒷⓁ shoulder abd, neck rot
   ≡ Ⓡ SCM, pecs, lev scap, rhomb; Ⓛ QL, ⒷⓁ up trap, delts, TFL
   ✗ Ⓡ rhomb, lev. scap; ⒷⓁ IT bands

A Techniques/Modalities: Locations/Duration
   XFF ⒷⓁ IT bands, MFR Ⓡ pecs, Ⓡ scap, Ⓛ QL
   PNF Ⓡ up trap, Ⓡ pecs

   Response to Treatment (see Δ)
   ↑AROM shoulder abd, neck rot; Ⓟ 4→1
   Goals: Long-term/Short-term
   LTG: within 6 wks, lift 30 lb shoulder abd,
        3 sets of 10, 5 days/wk

   STG: within 1 wk, lift 10 lb. shoulder abd,
        1 set of 10, 3 days/wk
   Functional Outcomes
   1. swing golf club
   2. lift weights at prior level

P Future Treatment/Frequency
   1 hr. Ⓜ, 1x/wk for 6 wks. Try vibration Ⓡ pecs.
   Refer to Dr. Christian for Knee eval to rule out
                              any CI.
   Homework/Self-care
   rec: ice Ⓡ up trap 20 min, 1x/day, every day
   rec: door jamb pec stretch; passive SCM stretch 1x/day,
   rec: 120 oz. H₂O/day   5 days/wk as demo'd

Therapist's Signature *Connor Patrick*   Date *April 2, '02*

Legend: ℮ TP   • TeP   ○ Ⓟ   ✳ Infl   ≡ HT   ≈ SP
             ✗ Adh   ≷ Numb   ○ rot   ╱ elev   >—< Short ↔ Long

Copyright © 2005 Lippincott Williams & Wilkins

Figure 8-5. Rob's SOAP note, highlighting Plan information. (Modified with permission from Thompson DL. Hands Heal: Communication, Documentation, and Insurance Billing for Manual Therapists. 2nd ed. Baltimore: Lippincott Williams & Wilkins, 2002.)

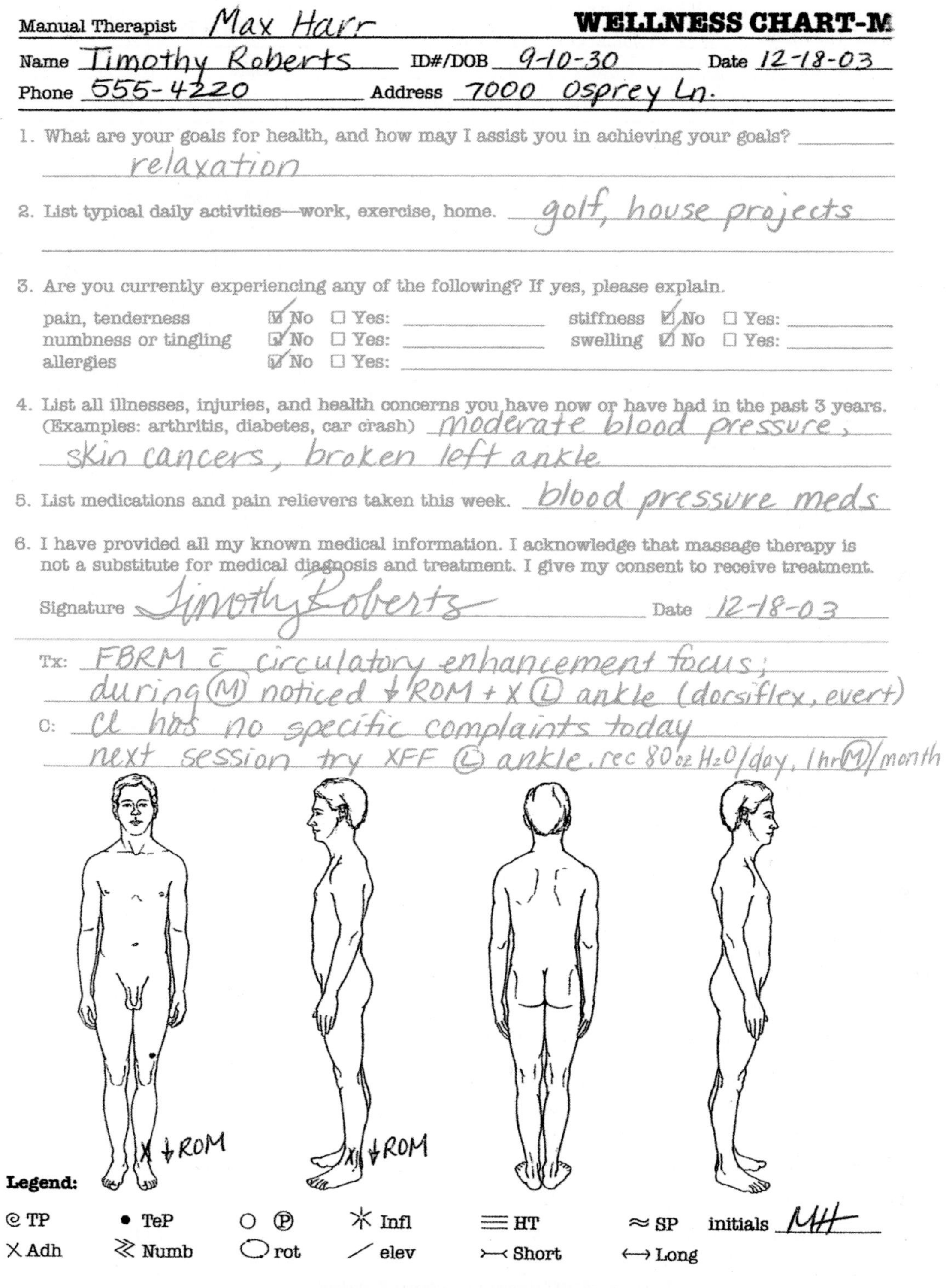

Manual Therapist *Max Harr* **WELLNESS CHART-M**

Name *Timothy Roberts* ID#/DOB *9-10-30* Date *12-18-03*

Phone *555-4220* Address *7000 Osprey Ln.*

1. What are your goals for health, and how may I assist you in achieving your goals? _____
   relaxation

2. List typical daily activities—work, exercise, home. *golf, house projects*

3. Are you currently experiencing any of the following? If yes, please explain.

pain, tenderness	☑ No ☐ Yes: _____	stiffness	☑ No ☐ Yes: _____
numbness or tingling	☑ No ☐ Yes: _____	swelling	☑ No ☐ Yes: _____
allergies	☑ No ☐ Yes: _____		

4. List all illnesses, injuries, and health concerns you have now or have had in the past 3 years. (Examples: arthritis, diabetes, car crash) *moderate blood pressure, skin cancers, broken left ankle*

5. List medications and pain relievers taken this week. *blood pressure meds*

6. I have provided all my known medical information. I acknowledge that massage therapy is not a substitute for medical diagnosis and treatment. I give my consent to receive treatment.

   Signature *Timothy Roberts* Date *12-18-03*

   Tx: *FBRM c̄ circulatory enhancement focus; during Ⓜ noticed ↓ROM + X Ⓛ ankle (dorsiflex, evert)*

   C: *Cl has no specific complaints today next session try XFF Ⓛ ankle. rec 80oz H₂0/day, 1hr Ⓜ/month*

↓ROM *↓ROM*

Legend:

℮ TP	● TeP	○ Ⓟ	✳ Infl	≡ HT	≈ SP	initials *MH*
✕ Adh	≋ Numb	⌒ rot	⁄ elev	⊱⊰ Short	↔ Long	

Figure 8-6. Timothy's HxTxC, highlighting Plan information. (Modified with permission from Thompson DL. Hands Heal: Communication, Documentation, and Insurance Billing for Manual Therapists. 2nd ed. Baltimore: Lippincott Williams & Wilkins, 2002.)

8 Treatment Plan

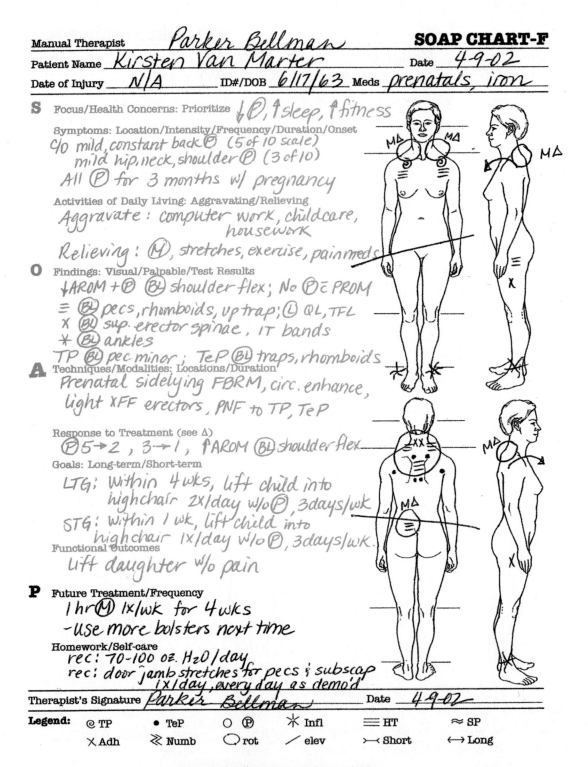

Manual Therapist _Parker Bellman_   **SOAP CHART-F**

Patient Name _Kirsten Van Marter_   Date _4-9-02_

Date of Injury _N/A_   ID#/DOB _6/17/63_ Meds _prenatals, iron_

S Focus/Health Concerns: Prioritize ↓℗, ↑sleep, ↑fitness

Symptoms: Location/Intensity/Frequency/Duration/Onset
c/o mild, constant back ℗ (5 of 10 scale)
mild hip, neck, shoulder ℗ (3 of 10)
All ℗ for 3 months w/ pregnancy

Activities of Daily Living: Aggravating/Relieving
Aggravate: computer work, childcare, housework
Relieving: Ⓜ, stretches, exercise, pain meds

O Findings: Visual/Palpable/Test Results
↓AROM +℗ ⒷⓁ shoulder flex; No ℗ c̄ PROM
≡ ⒷⓁ pecs, rhomboids, up trap; Ⓛ QL, TFL
✗ ⒷⓁ sup. erector spinae, IT bands
✳ ⒷⓁ ankles
TP ⒷⓁ pec minor; TeP ⒷⓁ traps, rhomboids

A Techniques/Modalities: Locations/Duration
Prenatal sidelying FBRM, circ. enhance,
light XFF erectors, PNF to TP, TeP

Response to Treatment (see Δ)
℗5→2, 3→1, ↑AROM ⒷⓁ shoulder flex

Goals: Long-term/Short-term
LTG: Within 4 wks, lift child into
        highchair 2x/day w/o ℗, 3days/wk
STG: Within 1 wk, lift child into
        highchair 1x/day w/o ℗, 3days/wk.

Functional Outcomes
lift daughter w/o pain

P Future Treatment/Frequency
1 hr Ⓜ 1x/wk for 4 wks
- use more bolsters next time

Homework/Self-care
rec: 70-100 oz. H₂O/day
rec: door jamb stretches for pecs & subscap
        1x/day, every day as demo'd

Therapist's Signature _Parker Bellman_   Date _4-9-02_

Legend:

⊙ TP	• TeP	○ ℗	✱ Infl	≡ HT	≈ SP
✗ Adh	≋ Numb	◯ rot	╱ elev	⊱⊰ Short	↔ Long

Figure 8-7. Kirsten's SOAP note, highlighting Plan information. (Modified with permission from Thompson DL. Hands Heal: Communication, Documentation, and Insurance Billing for Manual Therapists. 2nd ed. Baltimore: Lippincott Williams & Wilkins, 2002.)

CHAPTER SUMMARY

Massage therapists should always maintain a client-centered focus for care. The treatment plan for client care is part of that professional focus. With space and time constraints, you can write only brief notes in your massage treatment records, but you still need to document details accurately. Another therapist should be able to read your SOAP note and understand what the treatment plan includes, which self-care activities were recommended between sessions, and any referrals you may have made.

Self-care techniques give you a good topic of discussion for the next session, asking about which self-care techniques clients used or which ones were more effective. Soft tissue health and healing should always be the objective of self-care techniques recommended to clients. The effective and efficient documentation of treatment and self-care are vital aspects of a professional practice.

CHAPTER EXERCISES

1. Use abbreviations and symbols to rewrite the following treatment plans:

    a. Sixty-minute massages, twice a month, for 2 months. Try vibration over the left scapula, and stay away from the client's feet. Reevaluate active range of motion of left shoulder extension to see if the triceps stretches that were demonstrated and recommended once a day, every day, were helpful.

    b. Ninety-minute full body relaxation massages, once a month, for 3 months. Avoid proprioceptive neuromuscular facilitation and active range of motion evaluations, because the client does not like to actively participate during the session. Referred to Dr. Park for pain upon right elbow passive range of motion.

    c. Thirty-minute massages, once a week, for 4 weeks. Only use supine, since client is claustrophobic and does not like to be prone. Discussed use of a bolster under the knees during sleep to relieve low back pain.

2. Develop and properly document treatment plans for the following sample clients:

    a. A 20-year-old man, at least 50 pounds overweight, quietly complains of bilateral knee pain. His physical activity is limited to his walk to and from work, 5 days a week. At work, he sits at a computer all day and drinks diet soft drinks all day long. He eats fast food every day and does not like to drink water. Your general assessments discover bilateral symmetry with a forward posture, rolled shoulders, and knock-knees. He reports pain upon AROM and PROM of his knees, suggesting that some passive structures that are outside the massage scope of practice are involved.

    b. A 50-year-old man who appears in good physical condition explains that his friend got a massage from you and convinced him to try one even though he has no areas of concern. He swims for 30 minutes, at least five times a week, and drinks at least 60 ounces of water a day. He has a wife, three kids, and two dogs and is self-employed in an established and stable business. His posture is bilaterally symmetrical, but his head is forward, and he experiences occasional neck pain and tightness. You found fascial restrictions all around the cervical area, but did not have enough time to address them. He reports that he was able to relax but not until the massage was almost over and asks if massages can be longer than 60 minutes.

    c. A 70-year-old woman has been coming to you regularly, once a month, for over a year. She is retired and enjoys her gardening club activities and worldwide travel. Every day, she drinks a glass of juice, a cup of tea, a glass of water, and a cup of coffee. Every day, she eats a lot of fruits and vegetables, very few carbohydrates, and a small amount of protein. In the past, she has always responded well to a full-body relaxation massage that includes some craniosacral work. She has not incorporated any self-care in the year you have been treating her, but she always asks about what she should do between sessions.

3. Explain the difference between an initial treatment plan and a treatment plan for the subsequent massage sessions.

4. List the six components included in the plan section of the SOAP note.

5. List at least five questions you can use to evaluate clients' internal healing environment to estimate their healing time and length of treatment.

6. Explain why it is not always better to recommend massage sessions that last longer and are more frequent.

7. Explain why it is not always better to recommend a lot of self-care activities.

8. Explain why we encourage clients to participate in self-care activities.

9. Name at least seven factors that can disrupt sleep.

10. Describe at least three different reasons why you need effective communication skills to follow up on your treatment plan.

SUGGESTED READINGS

Batmanghelidj F. *You're Not Sick, You're Thirsty: Water for Health, for Healing, for Life*. New York: Warner Books, 2003.

Bicknell J, Benjamin BE. The importance of water. *American Massage Therapy Association's Massage Therapy Journal* 2003:28–36.

Chopra D. *Restful Sleep: The Complete Mind/Body Program for Overcoming Insomnia*. New York: Three Rivers Press, 1994.

George M. *Learn to Relax: A Practical Guide to Easing Tension & Conquering Stress*. San Francisco: Chronicle Books, 1998.

Kneipp S. *The Kneipp Cure: An Absolutely Verbal and Literal Translation for "Meine Wasserkur" (My Water Cure)*. New York: Nature Cure Publishing, 1949.

Sapolsky RM. *Why Zebras Don't Get Ulcers: An Updated Guide to Stress, Stress-Related Diseases, and Coping*. New York: WH Freeman, 1998.

Thompson D. *Hands Heal: Communication, Documentation, and Insurance Billing for Manual Therapists*. 2nd ed. Baltimore: Lippincott Williams & Wilkins, 2002.

Tobias M, Sullivan JP. *Complete Stretching: A New Exercise Program For Health and Vitality*. New York: Alfred A. Knopf, 1994.

Yee R, with Zolotow N. *Yoga the Poetry of the Body*. New York: Thomas Dunne, 2002.

http://jointhealing.com/pages/productpages/cryotherapy.html, accessed 3.5.06.

http://www.21c-online.com/2001-pickering-sleep.htm, accessed 3.5.06.

http://www.boston.com/globe/search/stories/health/how_and_why/011298.htm, accessed 3.5.06.

http://www.bottledwater.org/public/hydratio.htm, accessed 3.5.06.

http://www.healthyroads.com/mylibrary/data/ash_ref/htm/art_waterrequirementshelpyourbodymaintainnormalfunction.asp?HP=&, accessed 3.5.06.

Massage Strokes and Flow

Objectives

Upon completion of this chapter, the student will be able to:

- Name the three client positions on the massage table
- Demonstrate draping techniques to expose at least three different areas of a partner's body on the massage table
- Name the three stationary massage "strokes"

- Identify and demonstrate the six basic massage strokes
- Explain at least two effects of each basic massage stroke
- Explain the effects of joint movement
- Follow a basic relaxation massage flow
- Demonstrate an abdominal massage
- Identify at least three research-proven benefits of massage in the workplace

Key Terms

Centering: A technique that helps you focus your attention on your clients.

Chair massage: A massage for persons who are fully clothed that is delivered while the client is seated in a specially designed chair, also called seated massage, onsite massage, corporate massage, and event massage.

Compression: A stroke that applies pressure to soft tissues to squeeze them together without any slip.

Deep-fiber friction: A stroke that is applied with deep, localized pressure without any slip on the skin to break up fascial adhesions and separate the muscle fibers.

Effleurage (EF-lur-ahzh): A slow, gliding stroke along the client's skin.

Flow: A routine-like sequence of steps that leads the massage from one body part to the next in a

systematic, fluid pattern that often specifies stroke sequences.

Grounding: A technique you can use to establish an emotional and energetic boundary between you and your clients.

Petrissage (PET-rih-sahzh): A stroke that kneads soft tissues with a grasping and lifting action.

Prone: Lying face down.

Resting stroke: A stroke that requires you to stop moving and lightly rest your relaxed hands, fingers, or arms on your client for several seconds.

Side-lying (laterally recumbent): Lying on one's side.

Slip: The sliding of your skin over the surface of the client's skin.

Superficial friction: A brisk variation of light effleurage that increases circulation in the superficial tissues and dissipates body heat.

Supine: Lying face up, on back or spine.

Tapotement (tuh-POHT-ment): A fast rhythmic stroke that uses both hands, like rapid drumming.

Vibration: A stroke that involves high-frequency shaky hand movements and is capable of deep effects.

The main considerations when performing massage are comfort and safety for both you and your clients. To relax, clients must feel safe, secure, and comfortable. Before clients get on your massage table, you must be familiar with the different body positions clients can use, different ways to drape their bodies to keep them warm and modestly covered, and the different ways to position and support them throughout the massage. Appropriate client positioning, proper bolstering, and secure draping, which must all be considered before and during the session, are the topics discussed in this chapter.

Your own body should remain relaxed and comfortable to deliver massage techniques effectively and efficiently, without injuring yourself. Remember to set up your workspace to allow you to move freely as you work and always incorporate good body mechanics. As you learn, apply, and practice your strokes and techniques, continually monitor your body to make sure that you establish muscle memory that includes good body movement habits.

Once you master how to position your client on the table and how to use your own body during a massage session, you may realize that massage is both art and science. There are individual nuances to every massage that make it impossible to perform the exact same massage twice. This artistic aspect of massage encompasses the personal and unique characteristics of touch:

- The intent of the touch
- The delivery of the touch
- The attitude of the person delivering the touch
- The focus of the person delivering the touch
- The mental condition of the person receiving the touch
- The physical condition of the person receiving the touch
- All of the factors of the massage environment

Touch can be obvious or subtle, significant or meaningless. For example, a very light caring touch is vastly different from an accidental brush against a stranger in a crowded store. As a massage therapist, you have the ability to use the power of touch to affect another human being. The trick, therefore, is to know how to tailor the massage session to the needs and wants of your clients. You must know how to perform the basic massage strokes, but it is equally—if not more—important to know where and when to use them. The scientific aspect of massage includes all of the anatomy and physiology involved in massage as well as the organized approach to assessments and treatment plan. Along with effective communication skills and your academic knowledge of anatomy and physiology, the physiological effects of massage presented in this chapter will help you determine which strokes are appropriate for each individual client. Combining your scientific knowledge with an artistic and individualized approach to touch creates a unique massage every time.

Even though each massage is different, there are many similarities. The massage flow is like an outlined sequence that leads the massage from one body part to the next in a systematic, fluid pattern. Similar to a recipe, a flow can specify the parts of the body you treat, the order in which you treat them, and the strokes you apply. Some flows start with clients in the prone position (face down), whereas others begin with clients in the supine position. Some flows are designed for clients who remain in a laterally recumbent (side-lying) position throughout the entire massage, whereas others are designed for clients in a seated position. With practice, flow will become second nature and you will be able to think about which strokes and techniques to apply instead of which body part to work on next.

Client Positioning

Clients can lie on the massage table in three different positions to receive massage: **supine (face up), prone (face down),** or **laterally recumbent (side-lying).** Seated

massage, an alternative to table massage, is covered later in this chapter as an alternative to table massage. Most therapists develop a preference for starting clients in the

Figure 9-1. Supine with neck and knee bolsters.

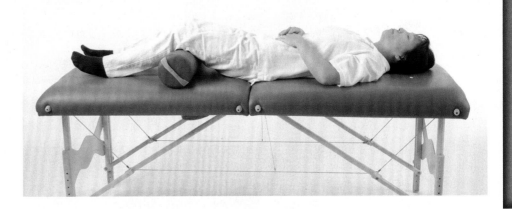

prone or supine position, but most important is maintaining a client-centered focus and modifying your preferences and tendencies to fit your individual client's needs and wants. Some clients determine their own positioning for the massage, asking to turn supine before you are ready for them to turn over or asking to remain in a side-lying (laterally recumbent) position for the duration of the session. Unless there are contraindications associated with the client's requests, it is appropriate to follow the client's lead.

You can make clients more comfortable during the massage by using bolsters and table extensions. These cushions, pillows, and platforms fit under and around clients' bodies for extra support and padding. Bolstering is intended to help clients' bodies relax with the natural curves of their bodies supported, but not all clients like to be bolstered. Position a bolster for support and ask if the client is more comfortable with the bolster in place. If not, remove it. You can use pillows and vinyl-covered retail bolsters or you can fashion your own bolsters out of rolled or folded towels and blankets. Remember to properly disinfect bolsters after every use or place them inside a covering that can be properly disinfected after every use. As an added layer of protection, you can slide bolsters underneath the sheet that covers the table. Proper sanitation and hygiene are as important to your practice as your massage. You will learn more about sanitation and hygiene in Chapter 13.

Several factors govern how you position clients on the massage table, including their preferences, physical condition, and treatment goals and your preferred strokes, techniques, and flow. Flow, covered in more detail later in this chapter, is a routine-like sequence of steps that leads the massage from one body part to the next in a systematic, fluid pattern. A flow often includes directions for specific stroke sequences and techniques to use.

Supine Position

Supine is the term that describes someone lying on the back, or spine, face up. When clients are in the supine position, you have direct access to the anterior surface of their body and you can incorporate a number of joint movements into the massage. A small bolster under the curve of the neck and a larger bolster under the client's knees support the spine in a more natural position (Fig. 9-1). There is a bolster that is specially shaped to elevate the lower legs, ankles, and feet that you can offer as an alternative. The supine position is preferred by clients who do not like confined spaces, whose heads are congested, or who are uneasy and nervous about being on the table.

Some clients like to talk through the duration of the massage. Starting the massage in the supine position allows them to talk freely and use eye contact while speaking. It is easy to get swept into conversation when clients share their experiences and emotions, but your job is to treat the soft tissues, not the emotions. Listen to clients more than you talk, and stay focused on the soft tissues.

Clients with allergy- and cold-related upper respiratory congestion may prefer being supine for the duration of the massage because the prone position can aggravate congestion. In the supine position, gravity enhances the flow of deoxygenated blood and lymph out of the sinuses to reduce sinus congestion.

Along with the advantages of the supine position, there are some considerations to keep in mind. Ceiling light fixtures, especially if they are directly over the massage table, can be bothersome to clients while supine. Turn off or dim the overhead lighting and use floor and table lamps, if possible.

Some physiological conditions can also influence client positioning. Just as the prone position may aggravate a congested head, the supine position may aggravate a congested chest. You can adapt the supine position to clients

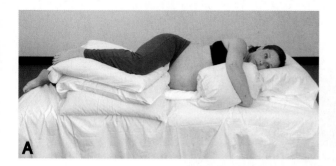

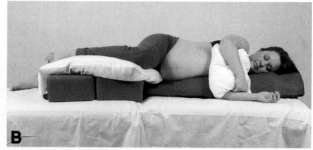

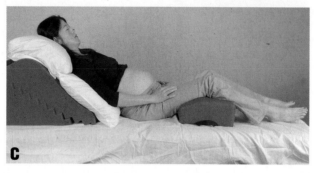

Figure 9-2. **(A–C)** Prenatal bolstering.

with chest congestion by using a bolster or pillow to elevate their head and shoulders. The supine position is contraindicated for women who are in their last few months of pregnancy, because the weight of the fetus can compress the aorta and cut off the mother's circulation. The side-lying (laterally recumbent) position is the least dangerous to the mother and fetus, but some women find it uncomfortable. You can bolster these women in a semireclining position to let them relax comfortably and enjoy massage (see Fig. 9-2).

Prone Position

Prone is the term that describes clients who are lying face down on the massage table. When clients are in this position, the therapist has unrestricted access to clients' backs and gluteal areas and can easily incorporate joint movements into the massage. A face cradle and bolsters provide additional comfort for this position. The face cradle allows the client's neck to remain neutral during the massage. Without the face cradle or a face hole in the table, clients can cross their arms under their chin or they can turn the neck to the side. If clients choose to turn their head to the side, encourage them to switch the direction they are facing once or twice during the prone massage to avoid cramping. Sometimes they naturally turn their head when they get uncomfortable, but if you notice that about 10 minutes have passed without a head turn, you can suggest they change. Most therapists offer clients a small

bolster under the ankles (Fig. 9-3A), but clients with a large chest may be more comfortable with a soft bolster supporting the upper chest (Fig. 9-3B), and clients with low back pain may be more comfortable with a small bolster under the pelvis.

Back pain and tension are among the most common client complaints, making the prone position a good way to start the massage. By treating their back first and spending a lot of time working on it, you reassure clients that you heard them explain their condition and are delivering what they need. Additionally, first-time clients may feel safer and more comfortable if the massage starts with the prone position because the genital areas are more protected.

Sometimes the prone position is not the best for the client. Avoid using the prone position for any clients suffering from head congestion. Massage promotes vasodilation of the blood vessels as well as the release of histamines, which are fluids the body secretes to flush out allergens and foreign particles. Gravity encourages extra fluids to drain into the sinuses and then out through the nose, and clients who are face down will find themselves in need of some tissues. Pressure on the face from the face cradle restricts circulation altogether, aggravating any head congestion that was already present. Clients who are uncomfortable with confined spaces may not like using a face cradle. Clients who are larger in size or who have large chests present a few challenges to using the prone position. First, their bodies are much higher off the table, making it necessary to lower your table for proper body mechanics. Second, you may need to bolster the upper chest to reduce the strain on the neck. And

Figure 9-3. Prone position. **(A)** Prone with ankle bolster. **(B)** Prone with chest bolstering for a large chest and pelvic bolstering for low back pain.

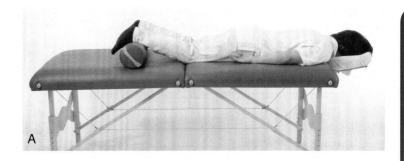

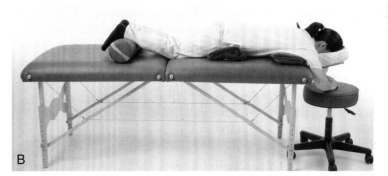

third, they may have to protract the neck an unreasonable amount to use a fixed face cradle. A face cradle with a telescoping mechanism that allows the whole face cradle to be raised can be helpful for a client who is larger or who has a large chest.

Side-Lying (Laterally Recumbent) Position

The **side-lying (laterally recumbent)** position describes when clients lie on their side. This is sometimes the most effective position for treating clients but requires extra bolstering to keep clients positioned comfortably. It is excellent for working on neck and shoulder conditions because it presents all of the tissues and allows many different ranges of neck movement. You need to have bolsters ready and you may need to give the client specific directions such as:

1. Straighten the bottom leg and keep it in line with the rest of the body.
2. Flex the knee and hip of the top leg, bringing it forward in a bent position to rest on a large bolster.
3. Flex the elbow and shoulder of the lower arm, and slide the hand under a pillow that supports the neck and head (Fig. 9-4).

This position may be more comfortable for larger clients, for persons who do not like using a face cradle, or to

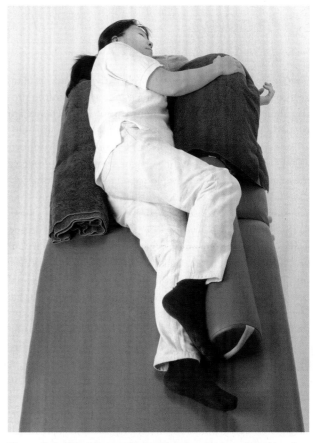

Figure 9-4. Side-lying position with bolsters for neck and head, top arm, top leg, and along back.

give you better access to the side of a client's neck. It is also beneficial for working on women who are in the last few months of pregnancy. When a pregnant woman can no longer lie on her stomach, the side-lying position is appropriate for the entire massage session. More specific information on how to perform massage on pregnant clients is covered in Chapter 12, Special Populations.

The side-lying position is not as popular because it is somewhat awkward to drape and bolster clients properly and access different parts of the body. Since this position can be uncomfortable for clients without sufficient bolstering, you need to make sure that clients feel comfortable and secure when laterally recumbent. Try to keep your client's spine aligned along the midsagittal plane. The bolster under the neck and head should keep the client's head from laterally flexing in either direction. The bolster that supports the top leg should be large enough so that the top leg does not drop down significantly and strain the hip or back. Some clients cannot relax because they feel that they may roll off the table during the massage. You can roll up a towel or blanket and lay it at the base of the back to stabilize them and add a sense of security (see Fig. 9-4).

Determining Client Positioning and Bolstering

Based on the above information, ask yourself the following questions when determining how to position and bolster clients for their massage sessions:

- Does the client have a preferred position?
- What are the treatment goals for today's massage session?
- Does the client have any condition today that requires table adjustment?
- Does the client have any condition today that requires him or her to be in a different position from the one I usually use?
- Does the client have any condition today that requires additional bolstering or support?
- Where do I need bolsters or supports today?
- Does the face cradle need adjusting?

Draping

Draping is the process of using sheets, towels, and/or blankets to keep clients covered during a massage session to protect their modesty and keep them warm. Once clients are properly positioned and supported with bolsters, appropriate and modest draping helps them feel secure and comfortable as you uncover specific parts of their body to receive massage. It may sound simple to keep clients completely covered during a massage, but it is more challenging than you think as you expose different body parts and ask clients to change positions. If you accidentally expose clients during a massage, which commonly happens during the learning process, cover them up, make a simple apology, and carry on. Draping helps you maintain ethical and professional boundaries during a massage session, and it helps clients feel safe and trusting enough to relax, even when they are undressed. Follow sanitation and hygiene standards by using clean, disinfected linens and making sure to properly disinfect them after every use.

A particular amount of draping may be required by law in your locale or state, by the licensure or certification requirements, or as part of the professional standards of care governed by the professional organization with which you are affiliated. You are legally bound to adhere to the regulations, but they represent the minimum. If you feel

that more draping is necessary or if your clients want more draping, you can ethically and professionally accommodate those situations. For example, you discover that under the law and professional standards of care, there are no requirements for draping whatsoever, and a male client wants only a small towel to cover his groin area. If you are not comfortable with that kind of exposure, how do you handle the situation? First, you can put a draping policy in your policy and procedures and/or informed consent as part of your intake process. Second, you can discuss your preference or mandated requirement for more draping as well as educate your client about how massage tends to reduce body temperature. If the client wants to continue with treatment, he can agree to be covered with more draping. If he insists that he is perfectly comfortable with so much skin exposed and is not concerned about body temperature or modesty, you can refer him to another therapist for treatment.

It is easiest to access clients' bodies if they remove most of their clothing, but clients must not feel exposed or vulnerable. Reassure them that they only have to take off the clothing they feel comfortable removing. As you step out of the room you can simply say, "I'll step out while you get undressed and get on the table, under the top sheet. Please leave your underpants on as well as anything else you want to leave on. I'll knock on the door before I walk in to make sure you're covered with the sheet and ready." Even if clients choose to wear shorts, swimsuit, or a sports bra during the massage, you should still use draping. The most important goal of draping is to protect their modesty and comfort level, because clients who feel uncomfortable or compromised in any way may be distracted, they may not be able to relax, and they may not get the best results from the massage session.

The core body temperature drops with the parasympathetic (relaxation) response to massage, making it a good idea to have extra blankets and towels on hand to cover clients who get cold. You can also have a portable heater, heated blanket, or massage table warmer for extra warmth. Being cold during a massage may cause muscles to remain tight, and it can inhibit the client's ability to relax. On the other hand, some clients may get hot during a massage session due to hormonal shifts that occur with pregnancy, menopause, and menstruation or after exercise. You can cool clients down by turning on an overhead or portable fan, or by uncovering their arms or legs to dissipate heat.

Sheet Draping

Sheets are larger than towels and, as long as you cannot see through them, they provide better and more secure coverage of the client's body than towels. This text focuses on the use of simple, two-sheet draping, but there are several different ways to drape with sheets. The examples here are only suggestions; your school or your instructor may have a preferred method of draping.

When clients step into your treatment room, the draping should already be on the massage table. Sheet draping can be less intimidating than towel draping for clients because it is so similar to the way a bed is made. First-time clients may feel familiar with climbing onto the table and covering themselves with the top sheet, just as if they were getting into bed. Before you walk into the room, clients can cover themselves completely with the sheet, which gives them a sense of control and security.

A basic set of linens for two-sheet draping can include a fitted sheet to cover the table, a flat sheet to cover the client, and a pillowcase or fitted covering to cover the face cradle. A prepackaged set of twin sheets and a pillowcase provides the basics for two-sheet draping. Purchase several sets in different colors or patterns, and avoid light, see-through colors. Flannel and jersey sheets may be softer, but they tend to stick to each other, making it a bit challenging when learning the process of sheet draping. You may want to drape the table with differently colored flat and fitted sheets to make it easier to differentiate the top sheet from the bottom sheet.

There is no single acceptable way to arrange your draping fabrics when you expose a body part to work on it, but your school or instructor may have recommendations or requirements. Basically, the goal is to uncover different areas of the body without exposing the genital area, the gluteal cleft, or a woman's breasts. In the process of uncovering parts of the body and redraping them, you can pick up the client's arm or leg so the client can stay relaxed, or you can ask clients to help you by lifting their own limbs. Maintain good body mechanics by using your legs to lift clients instead of your back and shoulders. Box 9-1 leads you through some steps to expose different areas of the body with two-sheet draping techniques.

When you pull the draping aside to expose an area of the body, make sure that the sheet is tucked firmly against the client's skin. You want to give clients the feeling that there is a defined line between what is covered by the sheet and what is exposed. Clients with high levels of modesty may feel that you can see their covered "parts" if they feel a breeze under the sheets.

Sheet Draping for Position Change

Clients typically change position at least once during the massage, and you will need to help them to make sure they turn over safely and that their body remains covered. If clients are in the prone position and need to turn over into the supine position, you can follow the steps in Box 9-2.

The process of turning from the supine position into the prone position is similar; your position is not as critical during the turn. You can use the following sequence of steps:

1. Remove the bolsters.
2. Hold the sheet up like a tent, using both hands, and lean against the table to pin the sheet to the table.
3. Ask the client to turn over, onto the front.
4. If you use a face cradle, ask clients to scoot toward their heads and rest their faces on the face cradle.
5. Pull the sheet down to uncover the head.

Towel Draping

As in sheet draping, a fitted sheet covers the table, but clients are covered with one or more towels. There are various towel arrangements you can use to keep the genital area, gluteal cleft, and women's breasts covered to protect the ethical and professional boundaries of the session while working on different areas of the body. The simplest approach to towel draping is to use one large bath sheet with the same draping techniques you use for sheet draping (Fig. 9-5).

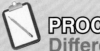 **BOX 9-1** **PROCEDURE** Draping Techniques for Uncovering Different Areas of the Body

A. Supine position, uncovering abdomen

   1. With the client supine, lay a pillowcase on top of the sheet, over the client's chest, with the client's hands on top of the pillowcase.

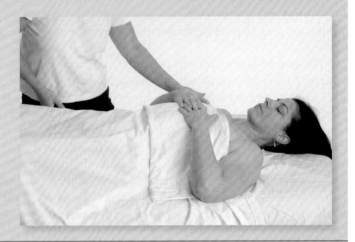

   2. Client holds the pillowcase while therapist pulls the sheet down to expose the abdomen.

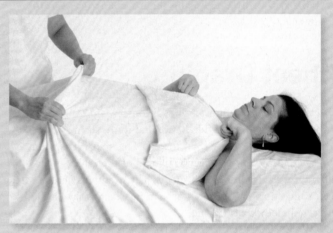

   3. Rest stroke on the client's abdomen.

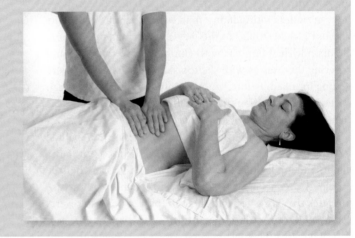

BOX 9-1 PROCEDURE Draping Techniques for Uncovering Different Areas of the Body (continued)

B. Prone position, uncovering leg

1. With the client prone, push drape medial to the leg.

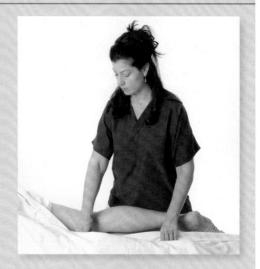

2. Grasp the edge of the sheet and pull laterally with one hand while supporting and lifting the client's knee with the other, and tuck the sheet under the client's hip.

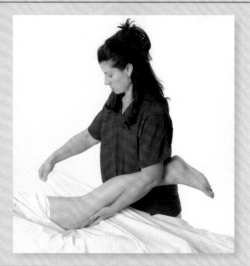

3. Offer the client the edge of the sheet to hold for security, and rest your hands on the client's leg.

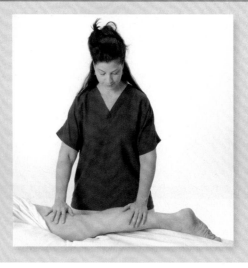

BOX 9-1 **PROCEDURE** Draping Techniques for Uncovering Different Areas of the Body (continued)

C. Side-lying position, uncovering back

1. Standing at the client's back, make sure his or her top arm is on top of the sheet and tuck the drape into the armpit and under the chin to eliminate gaps in draping.

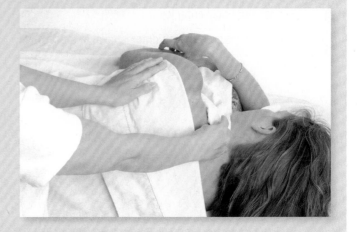

2. Place your hand on the client's low back, around the waistband, while pulling the drape aside to expose the back.

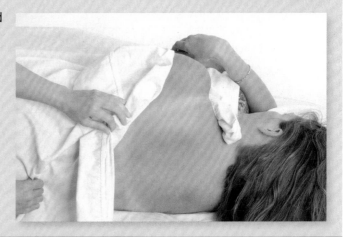

3. Rest your hands on the client's back.

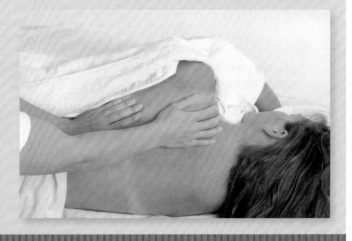

BOX 9-2 **PROCEDURE** Sheet Draping for Changing from Prone to Supine

1. Remove bolsters.

2. If using a face cradle, ask clients to scoot toward their feet, out of the face cradle.

3. Reach across the table, gently scoop your fingers under the client's far shoulder, and lightly pull up on it, saying something like, "I'm going to hold the sheet up while you roll over this way, onto your back."

4. Pick up the sheet with both hands into a tent, stand against the table to pin the sheet to the table, and ask the client to turn over.

5. Pull sheet down to expose the client's face.

Towel Draping for Position Change

Turning clients over with towel draping is a little trickier because towels are smaller, and there is a greater chance of exposing your clients. As an alternative, you can use multiple towels to provide additional coverage. When clients need to turn from prone to supine, you can follow the same steps that you used for sheet draping, but hold the towel(s) firmly to avoid accidental exposure.

Communication for Client Positioning and Draping

As part of promoting safety and comfort, you may want to explain the general positioning, bolstering, and draping of a massage session to clients who have never had a massage. A person who knows what to expect is better able to relax.

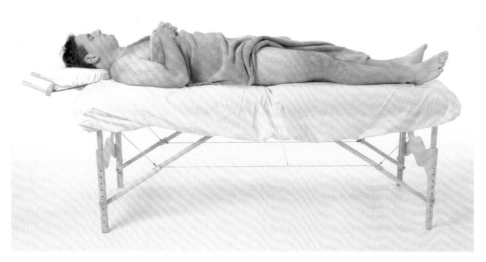

Figure 9-5. Towel draping showing exposed leg.

Even for clients who have had massage before, but are new to you, it is good to clarify the positioning and draping techniques before or during the session. Box 9-3 presents one approach for explaining a massage session to new clients. This is only an example; with practice, you will develop your own way of familiarizing people with your massage session.

On the other hand, the summary of an entire massage session can be too much for clients to comprehend all at once. You may find it more effective to explain your bolstering and draping techniques as you apply them during the massage. For example, as you start to uncover a client's back, you can say, "I am going to pull the sheet down to your waist so I can work on your back now." Or, as you finish working on the client in a supine position, you can say, "I'm going to hold the sheet up like a tent while you roll over onto your front and put your face in the face cradle. If you don't like the face cradle for any reason at any time, just let me know, and we'll continue without it."

When asking clients to change positions or actively participate in the massage, be aware that some directional terms are confusing for clients who are lying on the table. They may not be sure whether "up" means toward the ceiling or toward their head, or whether "down" means toward the floor or toward their feet. Instead of asking clients to move "up" on the table, ask them to move their whole body toward their head. Rather than ask clients to push "down," ask them to push toward the floor. When it is time for a client to switch from prone to supine, you can reach across the table to the client's far shoulder, scoop your fingers under it and gently pull up on it while you say, "Go ahead and roll over this way, onto your back." As clients roll over from prone to supine, it is safer if their back is toward you during the turn to prevent them from accidentally rolling off the table.

BOX 9-3

An Example of How to Describe a Massage Session to a New Client

"My goal is to have you comfortable and safe during your massage session. I will start the session with you lying face down on the table, underneath the top sheet, with your face in the face cradle. There is a hole in the face cradle so you can breathe comfortably. I will leave the room to wash my hands while you get undressed. You only need to take off the clothing you are comfortable removing, but know that your body will be covered by the top sheet throughout the massage, and only the body part I am working on will be exposed. I will knock on the door before I come in, just to make sure you are comfortably situated under the sheet. I will place a bolster under your ankles for comfort, and about halfway through the massage, I will ask you to turn over on your back. I will place bolsters under your knees and your neck for comfort, and I will massage your head and neck last. When I am finished, I will leave the room and give you time to get off the table and get dressed. There is a stool to use as you step down off the table, but if you need my assistance, let me know. Please tell me if you are uncomfortable at any time during the session, and I will make adjustments accordingly. For example, clients commonly feel a little cold during a massage, and I have extra blankets here if you need one. If you have any questions now or during the massage, please feel free to ask."

Assisting Clients on and off the Table

Some clients may need assistance getting on and off the massage table if the table is too high or their physical condition makes it difficult or painful. You can have a footstool available for clients who have trouble with the height of the table, but sometimes that is not enough. Let your clients know that their safety is very important to you and that it is not a problem to help them get on and off the table. You can protect their modesty by showing them how to wrap the folded sheet around their body before you come into the room. If you want them in the prone position to start the massage, the free ends of the sheet should open to the front of their body, with the ends of the sheets overlapped in front. Conversely, if they are starting supine, the free edges of the sheet need to open to the back of their body, with the ends of the sheets overlapped behind them. After you have helped the client onto the table, and he or she is in the proper position, you can open the draping without exposing the client. (See Box 9-4 for an illustration of this process.)

For clients who require assistance off the table, make sure they are in the supine position. If the massage ended in the prone position, ask the client to turn over to the supine position. Once in the supine position, you can use a "diaper drape" technique to help the client off the table while keeping the whole body completely covered. It may not be attractive, but it protects modesty. (See Box 9-5.) There is a simpler alternative to diaper draping, in which you tuck the sheet under the client's armpits, gather the sheet together at the back, and then help the client off the table. The problem with that technique is that the sheet is left to drag on the floor, which could easily trip someone who needs help getting off the table, such as the elderly, the injured, and those with balance problems.

BOX 9-4 **PROCEDURE** Assisting a Draped Client into the Prone Position on the Table

1. Offer the sheet, folded in half, to your client, and demonstrate how you want him to wrap up in the sheet with the fold under his armpits and the free edges opening to the front. Leave the room and let the client undress and wrap himself in the sheet.

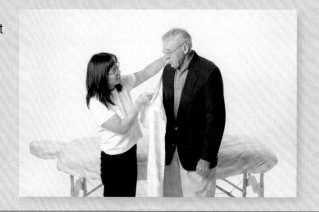

2. Offer the client your hand for support and stabilization while he uses a step stool to get on the table in a prone position.

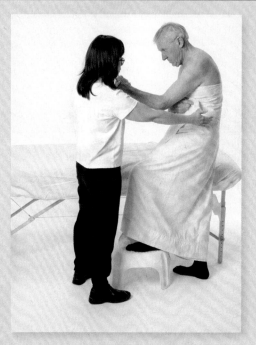

3. With the client prone and wrapped in the sheet, you pull the sheet out from under him.

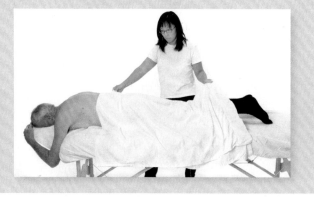

4. Unfold the sheets.

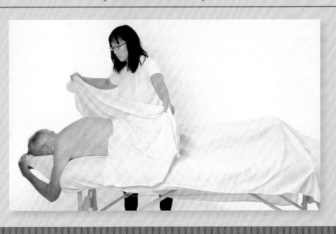

BOX 9-5 **PROCEDURE** Assisting a Draped Client off the Table

1. Tuck the top edge of the sheet tightly under the client's armpits, and push the bottom corners of the sheet under the client's bent knees.

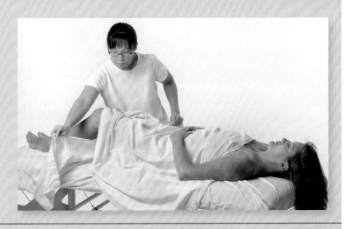

2. Ask your client to grab the bottom corners, lift the hips, and pull the sheet up to the waist.

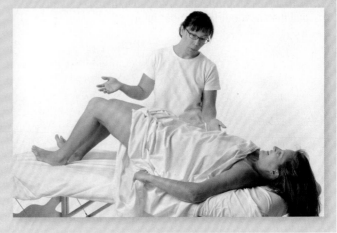

BOX 9-5 **PROCEDURE** Assisting a Draped Client off the Table (continued)

3. Take the corners of the sheet from your client and firmly tie them in front of the client's waist.

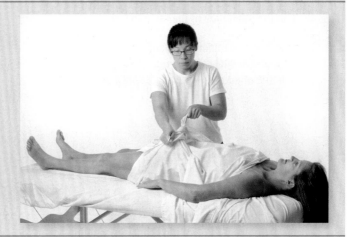

4. Lift the client's shoulder closest to you and tuck the sheet under it, pushing it toward the far shoulder.

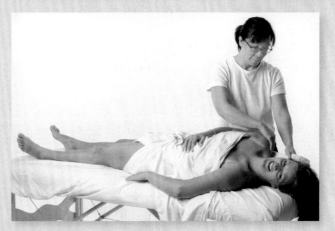

5. Walk to the other side of the table and gently lift upon the client's closest shoulder, ask your client to roll onto the side, and firmly tie the corners behind the client's back.

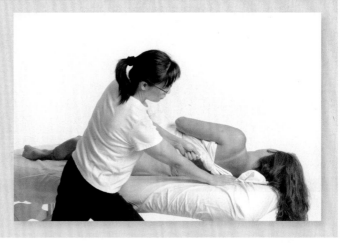

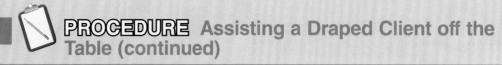

BOX 9-5   **PROCEDURE** Assisting a Draped Client off the Table (continued)

6. Walk to the other side of the table to face the client and
   a. slide one arm under the client's neck and your hand on the back.
   b. slide the other arm under the client's knees.

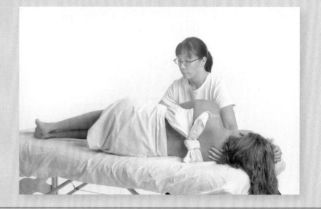

7. Lower your hips and pivot the client into a sitting position.

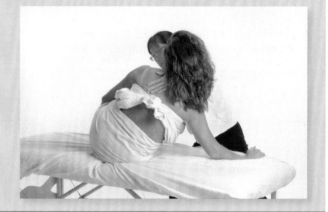

8. Offer your hand for support and stabilization as the client puts on socks and then steps off the table.

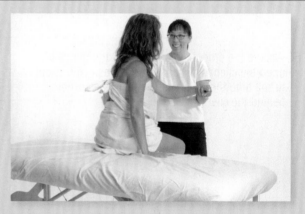

General Effects of Massage

Without question, massage affects the physiology of the human body. You may recall Dr. John Kellogg's determination of the mechanical, reflexive, and metabolic effects of massage (see Chapter 1). Mechanically, massage directly changes the shape or condition of the skin, fascia, muscle, and connective tissues via pressure and manipulation and enhances their movement and pliability. Reflexively, the application of massage strokes stimulates the nervous system to change the shape or condition of the tissues in the areas that were directly addressed as well as in other areas of the body. In other words, a massage stroke on someone's foot can neurologically encourage the hip flexor muscles to flex and pull the foot away from the touch. Metabolic effects are a combination of mechanical and reflexive responses that create a change that affects the whole body. For example, sustained touch on someone's arm can warm the area that is being contacted and can also lower the person's heart rate and blood pressure by stimulating a parasympathetic nervous system response. The metabolic effects of massage are primarily due to the responses of the circulatory and nervous systems, which transport blood, lymph, nutrients, hormones, neurological signals, and neurochemicals to and from all parts of the body.

The effects of massage on the different organ systems are incorporated into the text of Chapter 3 and outlined below in Table 3-6. In addition to the effects on specific organ systems, massage also plays a part in thermoregulation. Even when muscles are "at rest," some of the muscle cells in a muscle are contracting to maintain muscle tone. The primary mechanism for producing body heat is muscle contraction. Heat is similarly produced when muscles are kneaded, but the increased temperature of the muscles does not raise the body temperature significantly. Brisk, superficial massage on the skin, sometimes called superficial friction, creates vasodilation in the blood vessels of the skin. As a result, body heat is dissipated and the core temperature can drop.

Alert

It is possible to create fatigue-like symptoms with massage techniques that are too aggressive.

Although the benefits of massage vary greatly depending on health, lifestyle, stress levels, pathological conditions, or injuries, it can safely be said that massage is beneficial to most people and can have an enormous impact on the body's ability to restore and maintain homeostasis. It is important to remember that you, the massage therapist, function only as a facilitator of this rebalancing. You are not personally making the changes; you are helping the client's body cause these changes to occur. Following are some general benefits of massage:

- Reduces pain (see Box 9-6)
- Reduces edema
- Relieves hypertonic muscles
- Encourages a balance between sympathetic and parasympathetic nervous system activity
- Reduces adhesions in the connective tissue and fascia within and surrounding the muscles
- Restores movement and circulation to soft tissues
- Reduces stress and stress hormones (see Box 9-7)

Massage is generally beneficial for most people. Conditions and situations in which massage is recommended or that are positively affected by massage are called indications for massage (see Table 9-2). Even though massage carries a low risk for injury, a poorly trained therapist can certainly damage tissues and elicit pain. There are some instances where massage should not be applied and some conditions for which you should obtain clearance from a healthcare professional before proceeding with massage. **The most important thing to remember when you are unsure whether to apply massage is "WHEN IN DOUBT, DON'T."** Use the pathology appendix of this text or a thorough massage pathology book if you have any question about whether to proceed with massage. See Table 9-3 for a brief list of contraindications for massage.

Table 9-1 Effects of Massage on Different Organ Systems

Integumentary system	• Mechanically warms the skin with friction • Increases circulation of blood and lymph within the skin • Stimulates sebaceous gland secretions, which make skin more supple and pliable • Stimulates sweat production, which cools the body upon evaporation of sweat • Breaks down fascial adhesions in the subcutaneous layer (superficial fascia) to restore circulation and movement to skin
Skeletal system	• Joint movement stimulates synovial fluid production, which cushions and lubricates synovial joints • Increases the health of skeleton by enhancing circulation of blood and lymph to and from the bones
Muscular system	• Increases nutrition and development of muscles by enhancing circulation of blood and lymph to and from the muscles • Increases the excitability of muscles, making them more sensitive to nerve impulses • Discourages the formation of lactic acid in muscles following physical exertion • Accelerates recovery of fatigued muscles by reducing the lactic acid buildup • Increases heat in and around muscles to loosen fascia and restore movement and circulation to the muscles • Decreases hypertonicity in muscles and tendons
Nervous system	• Increases production of dopamine, a pain-relieving chemical involved in voluntary movement and clear thinking • Increases production of endorphins, strong pain-relieving chemicals • Increases production of enkephalins, strong pain relievers involved in sensory integration • Increases secretion of oxytocin, a chemical that increases the pain threshold, stimulates smooth muscle contractions, decreases sympathetic nervous system activity, and has sedative effects • Increases production of serotonin, which generally diminishes pain and appetite, regulates moods and sleep patterns, and stimulates smooth muscle contractions • Decreases production of cortisol, a natural anti-inflammatory produced in response to stress that can accelerate tissue breakdown and prevent tissue repair • Decreases substance P, a neurotransmitter that triggers the pain response
Circulatory system	• Increases circulation of blood and lymph in and around the area being addressed • Reduces the symptoms of ischemia by increasing circulation to capillaries with poor blood flow • Increases permeability of capillary walls, enhancing delivery of oxygen and nutrients • Sustained percussion can cause vasodilation deep within the area being addressed to increase blood flow • Increases circulation of lymph to help the body fight germs • Increases circulation of lymph, which increases removal of metabolic waste • Reduces edema
Respiratory system	• Encourages slow, deep contractions of the diaphragm, which helps remove carbon dioxide waste via the lungs • Percussive techniques can relieve chest congestion by loosening mucus within lungs
Digestive system	• Enhances the digestive process reflexively by stimulating the parasympathetic nervous response • Mechanically pushes indigestible waste through the intestines

continues on following page

Table 9-1   Effects of Massage on Different Organ Systems *continued*

Urinary system	• Increases cellular and chemical waste excreted via urine • Encourages constriction of the smooth muscle of the urinary bladder to eliminate more urine as a reflexive response of the parasympathetic nervous system
Endocrine system	• Increases delivery of hormones and other chemicals as a result of increased circulation of blood • Reduces levels of cortisol and norepinephrine (noradrenaline), stress-related hormones

---

RESEARCH BOX 9-6

Massage and Pain: The Gate Control Theory of Pain

In 1965, researchers Ronald Melzack and Patrick Wall published the now-famous Gate Control Theory that explained the pain mechanism. Afferent (sensory) nerve fibers transmit sensory nerve impulses from all over the body, through the spinal cord, and up to the brain. According to the theory, once the nerve impulses arrive at the spinal cord, they must pass through a "gate" in order to reach the brain and be recognized. Essentially, if the gate is open, impulses will travel to the brain. But if the gate is closed, no sensory input is transmitted to the brain and no sensation is perceived. The gate opens in response to impulses along the pain-sensitive nerve fibers, and it closes in response to impulses along the larger fibers that detect light touch, temperature, and pressure. Theoretically, light touch or pressure interferes with pain by closing the gate so the pain impulses cannot pass through to the brain, thus reducing the pain and the perception of it. In other words, massage can reduce the sensation of pain. This theory is supported by the natural tendency for people to rub a bumped shin or hold their hand over a sore area.

Melzack R, Wall PD. Pain mechanisms: a new theory. Science 1965; 150: 971.
Dickenson AH. Gate control theory of pain stands the test of time. Br J Anaesth 2002;88:755–757.
Davis P. Pain: opening up the gate control theory. Nurs Stand 1993;7:25–27.
The gate control theory of pain. Br Med J 1978; 2:586–587.
American Journal of Pain Management: www.ajpmonline.com.
Journal of Pain and Symptom Management: www.elsevier.com/locate/jpainsymman
International Journal of Acute Pain Management: www.elsevier.com/wps/product/cws_home/622996

RESEARCH BOX 9-7

Massage and Stress

Cortisol decreases and serotonin and dopamine increase following massage therapy. In this article, the positive effects of massage therapy on biochemistry are reviewed including decreased levels of cortisol and increased levels of serotonin and dopamine. The research reviewed includes studies on depression (including sex abuse and eating disorder studies), pain syndrome studies, research on autoimmune conditions (including asthma and chronic fatigue), immune studies (including human immunodeficiency virus [HIV] and breast cancer), and studies on the reduction of stress on the job, the stress of aging, and pregnancy stress. In studies in which cortisol was assayed either in saliva or in urine, significant decreases were noted in cortisol levels (averaging decreases 31%). In studies in which the activating neurotransmitters (serotonin and dopamine) were assayed in urine, an average increase of 28% was noted for serotonin and an average increase of 31% was noted for dopamine. These studies combined suggest the stress-alleviating effects (decreased cortisol) and the activating effects (increased serotonin and dopamine) of massage therapy on a variety of medical conditions and stressful experiences.

Field T, Hernandez-Reif M, Diego M, et al. Cortisol decreases and serotonin and dopamine increase following massage therapy. Int J Neurosci 2005; 115:1397–1413.

Table 9-2 Indications for Massage

Research has shown that massage is beneficial for the following conditions:	
Anxiety	Immune function
Cancer symptoms	Migraine headaches
Carpal tunnel syndrome	Pain
Chronic fatigue	Posttraumatic stress disorder
Depression	Premenstrual syndrome
Diabetes in children	Preterm (premature) infants
Fibromyalgia	Sleep
Hypertension (high blood pressure)	Stress

Table 9-3 Some Contraindications for Massage

Local Contraindications	Systemic Contraindications	Clearance from a Healthcare Professional
Acute sprains/strains	Acute or contagious viral or bacterial infections	Aneurysm
Blisters	Acute systemic inflammatory processes	Atherosclerosis
Bone fractures	Acute burns	Cancer
Bruises	Acute gout	Burns
Bunions	Aneurysm	Impaired cardiovascular system
Contagious skin conditions	Fever	Traumatic brain injury
Cuts and open wounds	Fungal infections that cover large areas of the body	Recent major surgery
Cysts	Intoxicated clients	
Fungal infections	Recent surgery	
Gouty joints		
Local inflammation		
Moderate to severe varicose veins		
Pitting edema		
Subacute and postacute burns		

Components of a Massage Stroke

As previously stated, the application of massage is as much of an art as it is a science. The evolution of massage into an art occurs gradually, starting when you first learn how to apply the basic massage strokes. Each particular stroke has the following components:

- Direction of movement—the direction the stroke moves in relation to the client's body (toward or away from the heart, across the muscles fibers)
- Excursion—the length of the stroke along the client's skin (a sweeping stroke may travel along 10 to 15 inches)
- Rate of movement—the speed at which a stroke moves along the client's skin (sweeping strokes often travel about 1 to 2 inches per second)
- Rhythm—the pattern and speed of repeated strokes (percussive strokes have a fast, even rhythm of approximately 10 to 20 strokes per second, whereas sweeping strokes are applied at a slower rhythm of 1 stroke every 5 to 10 seconds)
- Pressure—the amount of force applied directly into the client's tissues

The directions of movement and excursion affect the outcome of a stroke. Long, sweeping strokes directed toward the heart tend to decrease edema and encourage relaxation: they mechanically increase movement of lymph and venous blood, and they move generally parallel to the muscle fibers and crowd fibers toward the origins of the muscles, which influences the proprioceptors in the joints and muscles to relax the muscles. In contrast, short, sweeping strokes directed away from the heart tend to have energizing effects. They mechanically increase the flow of arterial blood and they create tension at the origins of muscles, which influences the proprioceptors to tone the muscles. Strokes directed perpendicular to the muscle fibers (cross fiber) or in a circular direction across the fibers reduce soft tissue adhesions and increase mobility of those tissues.

The rate and rhythm of movement also affect the outcome. To achieve relaxation, apply strokes with a slow, even rhythm to promote a parasympathetic nervous response. For a stimulating effect, apply the strokes quickly, at a rate faster than the client's rate of respiration, or with an uneven rhythm.

Diffuse pressure, applied lightly with the whole hand or with a broad surface such as the forearm, is often considered most relaxing. Concentrated pressure applied with supported fingers, thumbs, or the distal end of the elbow may initially have a stimulating effect, but prolonged applications of pressure will have a relaxing effect on the client.

Over time, as you practice and develop comfort with the components of the different strokes, you will focus less on the application of each stroke and more on the integration and combination of strokes to individualize the benefits and outcomes for a particular client. Practice, along with a client-centered focus, will help develop the palpation skills and intuition you need to provide an appropriate and beneficial massage. (Chapter 7 leads you through the assessment process for determining appropriate massage treatment.)

Stationary Massage Strokes

There are several techniques and strokes that you may incorporate into a basic massage. Some do not require any pressure or manipulation of soft tissues, and others do. Grounding, centering, and resting strokes require no lubricant because there is no slip, which is the sliding movement of your skin across the surface of the client's skin.

Grounding

Grounding is a process that is typically used before the massage to create a kind of boundary between yourself and your clients. Massage therapists who regularly give several massages a day sometimes feel drained or exhausted after a particular client, suggesting that some people "take" more of our core energy than others. Instead of thinking that you are "giving" clients your energy, slightly change your frame of mind and think of yourself as a conduit for energy, a mechanism that redirects and refocuses the client's energy. **Think of yourself more as a conductor of energy than as a source of energy.** By changing the perception of your work, you may not feel the exhaustion that results from conceptually giving away your own energy. Grounding is an intangible screen of protection that helps you keep your energy separate from your client's energy.

Spending time with people who are laughing and happy can raise our spirits, just as people who are sad and depressed

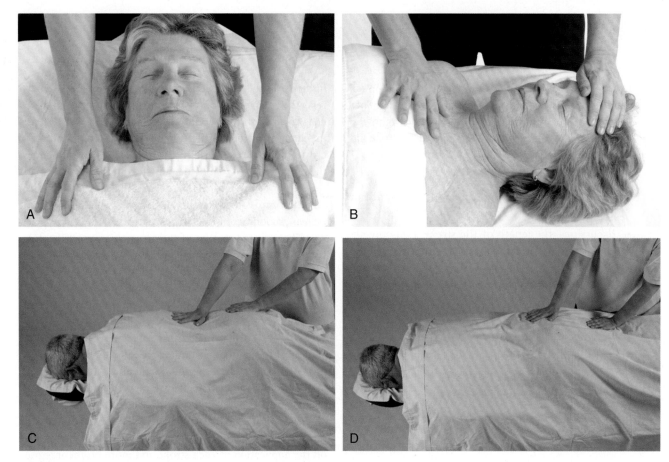

Figure 9-6. Resting strokes. **(A)** Shoulders of supine client. **(B)** Forehead and heart. **(C)** Connecting back to gluteals. **(D)** Connecting gluteals to leg.

can make us feel gloomy. Basically, we are susceptible to other people's emotions. A similar phenomenon sometimes occurs with a client's symptoms. There are occasions when, following a massage, your client's original complaints seemingly manifest themselves in your own body. Although it may sound incredible, it does happen, and the experience can be unsettling and unpleasant. Grounding techniques used before and during a massage can prevent such situations.

Generally, you ground yourself as you establish initial contact with a client at the beginning of the massage. The following visualization technique is an easy way to ground yourself while establishing contact with a fully draped client on the massage table:

1. Stand next to the massage table and direct your thoughts to your feet and their contact with the floor.

2. Imagine your feet as the roots of a tree, giving you stability and acting as a sort of drain for any unwanted tensions or stressful energy.

3. Establish contact by gently resting your hands on top of the sheets, on your client:

   a. If the client is supine, rest your hands on the shoulders or feet.

   b. If the client is prone, rest your hands on the back, shoulders, or feet. (See Fig. 9-6 for different hand positions for resting strokes.)

4. Close your eyes and take a few deep breaths as you clear your mind and focus on your client.

Grounding techniques can be used before the massage, either outside or inside the treatment room, and they can be used during a massage if you feel distracted or if you are running out of energy. You can ground yourself anytime, any day, in your personal life as well as your professional life.

Centering

Centering is the process of focusing your attention on the massage session and being present in the moment. It should be done before every massage session and can be combined with your grounding technique. You may find it challenging to clear your mind. Instead of paying attention to the distractive thoughts you want to forget, such as schedules, grocery lists, errands, finances, or social commitments, you can start centering yourself by focusing on your breath.

Close your eyes and focus on deep breathing in an attempt to quiet your mind and eliminate any stray thoughts or concerns. Listen to the air as it moves through your airway. Feel the expansion of your rib cage while you relax the muscles in your shoulders and your pelvic floor. Focus on a few deep breaths to clear your mind, and as you feel yourself calm down, start turning your attention to your client. Think about the client's concerns and consider how his or her life is being affected. By giving clients your full attention, you can better respond to, and be guided by, their needs and your intuition. The purpose of centering is to put your own concerns aside and focus on the client's needs and wants.

Diaphragmatic Breathing

The process of breathing involves the antagonistic actions of inhalation and exhalation. Inhalation occurs in two phases. In the first phase of proper, natural breathing, the diaphragm contracts and pulls downward until it rests on the abdominal organs. The abdomen expands as the diaphragm pulls air down into the lungs. Once the organs stop the diaphragm, the second phase of inhalation begins. The diaphragm continues to contract and pull air into the lungs, resulting in an upward expansion of the rib cage. With palpation, you can feel your belly expand during the first phase of inhalation and your sternum rise up in the second phase. Normal, natural exhalation occurs in the opposite sequence, with the chest deflating first, and the abdomen contracting second.

To take a full, deep breath, you need to use your diaphragm muscle instead of the scalenes and other accessory muscles. First, make sure your waistband or belt is loose to give your abdomen room to expand. Place one hand on your abdomen, and the other hand on your sternum. Sit or stand up straight, drop your shoulders, and slowly inhale through your nose and feel the expansion of your belly followed by the rise in your rib cage. You can look in the mirror or use a partner to monitor your shoulders while you take a deep breath. Watch to make sure that the shoulders do not elevate significantly and that the scalene muscles do not tense up. Slowly exhale through your mouth, feeling the deflation of your rib cage followed by the contraction of your abdomen. Full, deep diaphragmatic breathing is more efficient than quick, shallow breathing because it provides more oxygen with less energy expenditure. Now try to make yourself yawn while you keep your hands in

position to monitor the expansion and contraction that occurs. Notice how your body naturally breathes properly during a yawn, straightening the back, lifting the head on top of the spine, and using the diaphragm to breathe in and out.

Resting Stroke

The resting stroke involves no movement, no slip, and no application of pressure, but it requires that you touch your client with a therapeutic intent. When you stop moving and lightly rest your relaxed hands, fingers, or arms on clients for several seconds, it is considered a resting stroke. It is a good stroke to use at the beginning of the massage, as a sort of greeting to the client's body, but it can be used just as effectively anytime during the massage.

When applied at the beginning of the massage, a resting stroke establishes your initial contact with the client and lets his or her nervous system recognize your touch as safe and nonthreatening. Figure 9-6 illustrates some different hand positions for resting strokes. Besides using the resting stroke to signal the nervous system that you present no danger, you can use the resting stroke as an initial palpation assessment tool to evaluate body rhythms and temperature, texture, and fullness of the tissues under your relaxed hands.

In addition to using it at the beginning of your massage, you can use the resting stroke periodically throughout the massage. You can use it to ground or center yourself or to reevaluate the client's tissues to help you choose the appropriate technique at any given moment. After you work on a specific area for a long time or use a lot of therapeutic techniques on one area, your touch can be perceived as a source of aggravation that stimulates the sympathetic nervous response. Avoid that situation by using a resting stroke to settle the nervous system and allow relaxation to continue.

Another way to use a resting stroke during the massage is to use it as a connecting stroke. You want to minimize the number of times you break contact with the body because every time you break contact, you have to reinitiate contact, and initial contact can be stimulating. To move from one area of the body to another without breaking contact, you can leave one hand on the area that you have just finished massaging, and place the other hand on the area that you will start working on. Essentially, your resting stroke connects the area that has been massaged with the area that will be massaged.

Basic Massage Strokes

The six basic massage strokes involve the application of pressure in some form, and they all have mechanical and reflexive effects. Some strokes incorporate slip on the client's skin, and others do not. Compression is a variation of a resting stroke, but because

pressure is applied, it is considered a basic massage stroke. The fundamental massage techniques that arise from Per Henrik Ling's Swedish Movements include effleurage (EF-lur-ahzh), petrissage (PET-rih-sahzh), tapotement (tuh-POHT-ment), friction, and vibration. A Swedish massage, also called a relaxation or wellness massage, is one that generally includes these basic strokes and no specific therapeutic techniques.

Compression

The compression stroke applies pressure to soft tissues to squeeze them together without any slip. The tissues can either be pressed against the underlying bone, or they can be manually squeezed together with your own hands or fingers. Compression can be used to increase circulation, warm the tissues, decrease muscular tension, and reduce pain. You can apply compression with your thumbs, finger pads, the palm or heel of your hand, the knuckle portion of a fist, or your forearm. In a special form of bodywork called Shiatsu, therapists also use their feet and knees to apply compression. (Fig. 9-7 shows some examples of compression.)

Effects of Compression

With your knowledge of anatomy and physiology of circulatory vessels, you can understand how compression is useful for increasing circulation and warming tissues. Blood is pushed through the arteries with the forceful contractions of the heart. By compressing the arteries and arterioles and stopping the flow of oxygenated blood, pressure builds behind the blockage as the heart continues to pump blood. When the compressed artery is released, a larger amount of blood rushes forth with a higher force than usual, warming the tissues supplied by that artery.

The veins and lymph vessels are equipped with valves that force their contents to flow in only one direction. Compression strokes force blood out of the veins and through the one-way valves toward the heart. Likewise, compression on the lymph vessels forces lymph toward the lymph ducts that drain into the heart. There are better strokes for enhancing venous and lymph flow, but manual

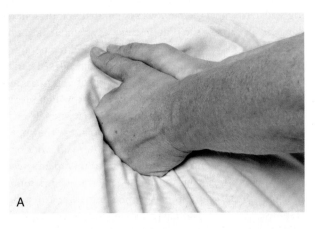
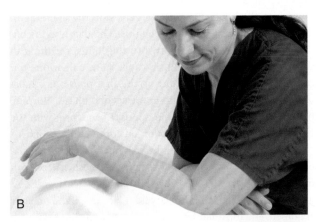
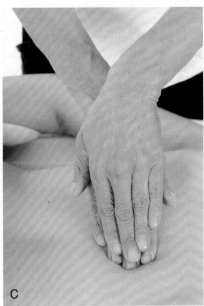
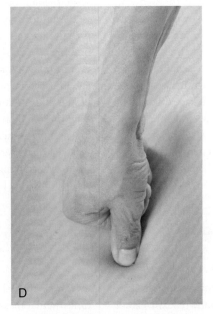
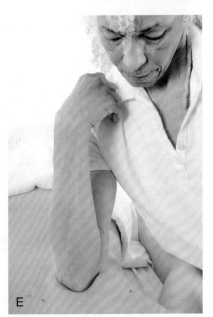

Figure 9-7. Compression strokes. **(A)** Back of knuckles(fist). **(B)** Forearm. **(C)** Fingers. **(D)** Thumbs. **(E)** Palm/heel of hand.

compression works as effectively as the active muscle contractions of the skeletal muscle pump.

Because of the thixotropic property of fascia, compression strokes can soften the fascia to restore movement and circulation to the muscles. Thus, compression can reduce muscular tension.

Muscles are composed of organized groups of muscles cells bundled together with fascia. Nerves and nerve cells travel through that fascia, carrying nerve impulses to and from the skeletal muscles. Compression on the soft tissues puts pressure on the nerves as well as the blood vessels and can reduce the nerve impulses transmitted by pain receptors. Consider the many ways people instinctively use pressure for pain relief:

- People put pressure on their cheek when they have a toothache.
- People press on their temples when they have a headache.
- People press on muscles that are sore.
- People press on their shin when they bump it.
- People squeeze or press on the abdomen when they experience abdominal pain.

Application of Compression

Thumbs, finger pads, the palm or heel of the hand, fists, and forearms can be used to deliver compression. The stroke requires no slip on the skin, making it easier to apply compression without lubricant or on a clothed client. You can squeeze tissues together to compress them, but that form of compression requires muscular work from your hands, which should be avoided when possible. To apply compression with less work, simply touch the client and gradually apply pressure using proper body mechanics such that your compression slowly sinks into the client's tissues. You can use your fingers to press on the tissues of the face or phalanges, but for the larger leg or gluteal muscles, you need to use good body mechanics with a proper lean to compress the tissues against underlying bones. If you are leaning instead of pushing into the large muscles, you will sink farther into the tissues as they soften up, without any extra effort. You can support your hand, finger pad, or thumb with the other hand when you need to maintain the compression for extended periods.

There is a variation of compression called rolling. Like the method you use to roll a pencil back and forth on a table, you can use rolling on the arms, legs, fingers, and toes by applying compression and rolling the structure back and forth under the pressure. There is no slip on the skin, so it does not matter whether there is lubricant on or not. The amount you can roll a body part varies with the size of the body part, the joint structure, and the soft tissue restrictions.

Move slowly enough to sense a joint's end feel and stop the movement.

Compression should not be applied over open skin or contagious skin conditions, bruised areas, moderate to severe varicose veins, or areas of acute injury.

Effleurage

Effleurage is an elongated, slow stroke that slides across the surface of the client's skin with minimal drag. It benefits the skin by warming it with friction and increasing its circulation of blood and lymph, stimulating the sebaceous glands that make the skin soft and pliable. It is used to apply and spread lubricant, assess the client's soft tissues, create heat, increase circulation of blood and lymph, decrease muscle tension, relieve pain, and encourage relaxation and for connecting strokes. Your forearm, the palm or heel of your hand, your knuckles, thumbs, or finger pads can deliver effleurage strokes, but you need to use common sense. It is obviously inappropriate to use a forearm to apply effleurage to someone's face. The pressure varies from superficial to deep, and you need to keep your hands and wrists relaxed so they can gently encompass or mold to the client's body throughout the stroke. During the stroke, make palpation assessments regarding the quality of the client's tissues.

Effects of Effleurage

Most often, effleurage is used to apply and spread lubricant, and it is one of the best strokes for assessing the quality of superficial and deeper layers of tissue. You can feel the movement, fullness, texture, temperature, and body rhythms as your stroke travels across the tissues. When the effleurage stroke is directed toward the heart, it assists the return of blood and lymph through the valve system in the veins and lymph vessels, making it the best stroke for circulatory enhancement. As the effleurage stroke compresses tissues, it increases arterial circulation and cellular metabolism, including glycolysis, the heat-producing chemical reaction that occurs in muscle cells. Additional heat is created with the deformation and softening of the thixotropic fascia, which decreases muscular tension. Ischemic tissues, or tissues that have a poor blood supply, are often painful as they suffer the effects of insufficient oxygen. Effleurage can restore circulation to ischemic tissues to improve the health of those tissues and reduce pain. With less pain, people are better able to relax. Effleurage applied with lighter pressure tends to have reflexive effects, whereas deeper pressure causes more of the mechanical effects on the circulatory system.

Application of Effleurage

You must use lubricant for effleurage because the stroke travels across the surface of the client's skin. The lubricant reduces drag and increases slip to make the stroke more comfortable for clients. Be that as it may, too much slip is disadvantageous. It reduces your ability to assess the movement and texture of tissues, and you may need to compromise your body mechanics to resist the slip. Clients who have a lot of body hair present a special challenge. You can use more lubricant or use lubricants with a lot of slip, such as oil or gel, to keep from pulling their body hair. Some people find it uncomfortable to be rubbed "against the grain" of their body hair, so you may want to move in the same direction the hair lies, but some clients are not bothered if you use enough lubricant. Generally, effleurage strokes are performed at a rate of about 1 to 2 inches per second, and the excursion, or length of the stroke along the client's skin, is about 10 to 15 inches.

The amount of pressure that accompanies the effleurage stroke depends on where and why you apply it. Effleurage on the face typically uses very little pressure; effleurage on the back and shoulders usually requires more pressure. With that in mind, massage is a client-centered art that requires you to be aware of the needs of each client and treat accordingly.

Body mechanics must be incorporated with every stroke, but because effleurage is used so much, it is especially important to learn to use proper body mechanics with effleurage strokes. Keep your wrist and hand as relaxed as possible to minimize your own muscular tension and maximize your palpation sensitivity. Keep your joints stacked as much as possible and use a proper lean. Avoid twisting and bending, and maintain an asymmetric stance. There are a few precautions to take when using your forearm to apply any massage stroke. First, it is especially important to keep your wrist and hand relaxed. A forearm with a relaxed hand and wrist feels better to the person receiving the massage, and it also benefits you. It prevents you from building up excess tension, it helps you conserve your energy, and it increases your sensitivity for palpation assessment. Second, although some recommend using your elbow to deliver pressure, you must use the proximal part of your forearm and not the point of the olecranon process. The ulnar nerve, which is often referred to as the "funny bone," is relatively unprotected as it runs through the cubital tunnel of the elbow, making it susceptible to damage if you use your olecranon process to apply pressure.

Alert

Use the proximal part of your ulna to deliver pressure instead of the olecranon process because it protects the ulnar nerve from damage. Figure 9-8 shows various applications of effleurage, including proper use of the forearm.

Effleurage should not be applied near or on an area of inflammation, infection, or acute or subacute injury. Other local contraindications for effleurage include open wounds, contagious skin conditions, and bruises. Avoid repetitive applications of effleurage on the extremities of clients with high blood pressure, cardiovascular disease, varicose veins, or edema.

Superficial Effleurage

Superficial effleurage strokes, also called nerve strokes, can be performed with short, long, or circular motions with the thumbs, fingertips, or palms of the hands. Short and circular superficial effleurage can be applied to the face and other small areas of the body.

Nerve strokes are very light, feathery effleurage strokes applied in long, sweeping motions that are slow or fast (Fig. 9-9A). You can use them to "brush down" an area of the body after massaging it, giving the client's nervous system an opportunity to recognize that the invasive work is finished and that there is no need to stimulate sympathetic nervous activity.

Massage can cause a client to feel "disconnected" toward the end of the massage because each part of the body receives what can seem like a separate massage. For example, you spend some time massaging the client's back, spend a few minutes on the right arm, spend a few more minutes on the left arm, move to the left leg and devote several minutes to it, and then spend several minutes on the right leg, and so on. Nerve strokes can be used as connecting strokes during the massage, sweeping from the area that you just finished to the area you plan on massaging next. They signal a transition from one area to the next to help the client know what to expect. Remember, more relaxation is possible when the sympathetic nervous response is not stimulated. Clients who are comfortable and who know what to expect are more likely to relax throughout the massage, and nerve strokes are a nonverbal way to let clients know what you are doing.

Slow nerve strokes that run from head to toe can also be used at the end of the massage to conceptually and proprioceptively reconnect all of the separate body parts. The proprioceptors are the sensory receptors responsible for the position and tension of the muscles and joints to tell us where we are in physical space and to help us coordinate our movements. Nerve strokes that run the length of the body serve as gentle proprioceptive reminders of the position of all the body parts in space. The head-to-toe nerve stroke should last between 5 and 10 seconds, and as you move toward the client's feet, you take steps as necessary to maintain proper body mechanics:

1. Stand next to the massage table, at the client's shoulder, facing the client's head.
2. Gently rest the fingertips of both hands on the top of the client's head.

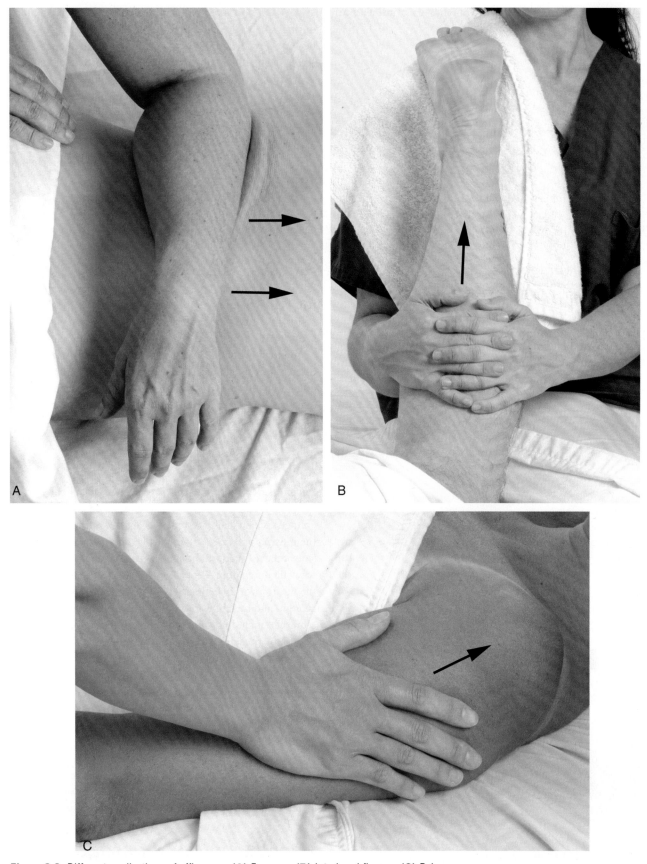

Figure 9-8. Different applications of effleurage. **(A)** Forearm. **(B)** Interlaced fingers. **(C)** Palm.

3. Apply a nerve stroke with your fingers from head to toe, moving lightly from:

   a. Top of the head

   b. Shoulders

   c. Elbows

   d. Hands

   e. From the hands onto the client's legs

   f. Knees

   g. Feet

If you always end massages with this full-body nerve stroke, your returning clients will learn that this stroke signals the completion of the massage.

Deep Effleurage

The deeper strokes are often applied with your thumb, your knuckles, the heel of your hand, interlaced fingers, or forearm. (Fig. 9-9B shows deep effleurage strokes.) You want the client's body to relax during deep effleurage so you can assess and treat the deeper tissues; therefore, you *must* apply the stroke slowly to avoid triggering protective muscular tension.

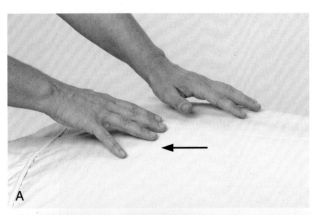

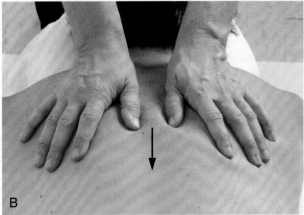

Figure 9-9. Types of effleurage. **(A)** Superficial effleurage, also called nerve strokes. **(B)** Deep effleurage.

Again, you need to maintain proper body mechanics during effleurage. The asymmetric stance is usually better because the stroke tends to travel along the client's skin. Apply deep effleurage strokes by leaning into tissues so that your stroke runs uphill rather than downhill. The compression is more effective when you lean into uphill tissues, and you tend to move more slowly and carefully. Gravity can accelerate a downhill stroke, and you may have to hold your body back to avoid sliding too fast. Resisting gravity requires unnecessary work and can create excess stress, so direct your deep effleurage strokes uphill.

Petrissage

Petrissage is directly translated from French as "the act of kneading." It is delivered as a rhythmic series of intermittent compressions combined with a grasping and lifting action that pulls the tissues away from the bones. The tissues can either be compressed against the underlying bones or manually squeezed with your hands, but you must use proper body mechanics in either application. The benefits of effleurage also pertain to petrissage, but petrissage is more effective at improving muscle tone, increasing the elasticity of muscle tissue, and increasing muscle contractility.

Effects of Petrissage

The pressure of petrissage strokes increases the circulation of blood and lymph, stimulates sebaceous gland activity to soften the skin and keep it supple, warms the soft tissues, makes the muscles and fascia more pliable, decreases muscular tension, relieves pain, and encourages relaxation in the same way effleurage does. Petrissage is very effective at improving the health of muscle tissue. The deep kneading increases circulation and metabolism of all of the cells and tissues within a muscle, including the blood vessels, lymph vessels, nerve cells, and muscle cells. Studies have shown that muscles respond to massage with better muscle tone, more elasticity and pliability, and greater sensitivity to nerve impulses for contraction or contractility. Muscles also demonstrate faster reaction times and more coordinated movements.

The focus of superficial petrissage is to soften the thixotropic fascia and increase circulation to the superficial fascia. Deep petrissage focuses on the muscle tissues and deep fascia. It deforms the deep fascia and improves the circulation of blood and lymph to the deepest layers of muscles, which increases the elasticity and health of the muscle tissue.

Application of Petrissage

The amount of force you put into your petrissage varies, but generally thicker tissues take more pressure. Superficial applications of petrissage are very much like skin pinches and require little or no lubricant because the strokes only treat the superficial fascia and subcutaneous fat. The strokes can be effective when applied to general areas of the body, both localized and broad, because the focus is on the continuous sheet of superficial fascia.

Because of the effects of deep petrissage on the muscle tissues, these strokes are often applied to an individual muscle or a group of synergistic muscles rather than a general area of the body. For deeper applications of petrissage, you may need a small amount of lubricant to prevent the stroke from pinching, to ensure that the strokes are comfortable, and to help put the muscle or group of muscles into passive contraction. When muscles are stretched out, the aligned muscle fibers get closer together and become taut, like the way a rubber band acts when it is pulled tight. In a passive contraction, the therapist brings the origin and insertion of a client's muscle closer together while the client relaxes. Again, like a rubber band, the muscle fibers are more flexible and pliable in this position, allowing you to work deeper with less effort. If you attempt to resolve deep muscle tension in muscles that are stretched tight, you waste energy and can hurt the client.

The petrissage stroke has no true excursion; you apply a series of individual strokes all over the area you are treating. Each stroke should move to a slightly different spot so that you do not grasp the same exact tissues twice in succession. As you apply petrissage in an attempt to reach the deeper tissues, slowly increase your pressure to allow the tissues time to adjust and soften enough to let you in. Petrissage is generally applied with soft hands that squeeze, lift, and release the client's tissues in an alternating rhythm of left and right hands. A typical rhythm for petrissage is about 1 stroke per second, but the rhythm is faster for smaller or thinner tissues such as the face and hand, and slower for the thicker or larger tissues like the thigh and scapular area.

Try to keep your fingers together and use them as one large surface to scoop the tissues into the fleshy part at the base of the thumb called the thenar eminence (THEH-nahr EHM-ih-nents), grasp and squeeze those tissues gradually, and then release them. By pulling the tissues up and away from the bone, you mechanically deform and separate the layers of superficial and deep fascia more than you can with rhythmic compression or effleurage strokes. Some variations of petrissage use your thumb and finger pads, whereas others use a soft fist to push the tissues into the relaxed, cupped palm of the other hand. (Fig. 9-10 illustrates different forms of petrissage.)

Petrissage is one of the more challenging strokes when it comes to maintaining good body mechanics. The hand muscles are required to work harder than normal to squeeze and lift tissues. Also, excessive strain occurs in the muscles that move the forearm and wrist because you use so much active supination, pronation, and wrist extension. As you repeatedly compress and lift the tissues, it is easy to forget about leaning properly. To avoid stress on your low back, make sure you maintain the straight line between your head and back toe when you lean and lift. Try to minimize the amount of petrissage you use because it requires so much muscular work, and when you do use it, watch your body mechanics.

Avoid petrissage on open or contagious skin conditions; bruises; moderate to severe varicose veins; and areas of acute injury, inflammation, or infection.

Variations of Petrissage

Deep petrissage is occasionally applied without the grasping and lifting component, which makes it resemble circular deep effleurage. Because the focus is still on intermittent and rhythmic compression of the tissues, the stroke is still considered petrissage. There is minimal slip on the skin, just as with standard petrissage, but instead of grasping the tissues, you push them aside and out of the way, which causes them to lift up to some extent.

During a massage, you may cross an area of restricted superficial fascia, which can feel as if your massage stroke is skidding along the client's skin or has come to a stop. In other words, the slip turns into drag. There are several forms of petrissage that you can use to loosen these restrictions. Wringing is a slow application of petrissage that does not include the lifting component. The hand movement of this stroke mimics the act of wringing out a wet towel and is very similar to an "Indian burn" that children give each other, except there is no friction or slip on the client's skin. You grasp a limb with both hands and simultaneously rotate your hands in opposite directions without any slip on the skin. One stroke lasts 2 seconds, making it more like a very slow moving compression stroke that primarily deforms the superficial fascia.

Skin rolling is a variation of petrissage that primarily lifts the superficial fascia to deform and loosen it.

Alert

Skin rolling may be uncomfortable to clients, so move slowly, pay attention to their response to this stroke, and make adjustments to your technique.

Grasp a large section of skin and superficial fascia with your thumbs and finger pads. Pinch it together and lift it up, away from the body. With the roll of tissue in your grasp, *very slowly* walk your fingertips and thumbs away from you while keeping the roll of tissue elevated (Fig. 9-11). The rate of movement tends to be about 1 cm per second, but looser fascia can be rolled faster, and more restricted fascia must be rolled more slowly. The excursion of the skin roll should

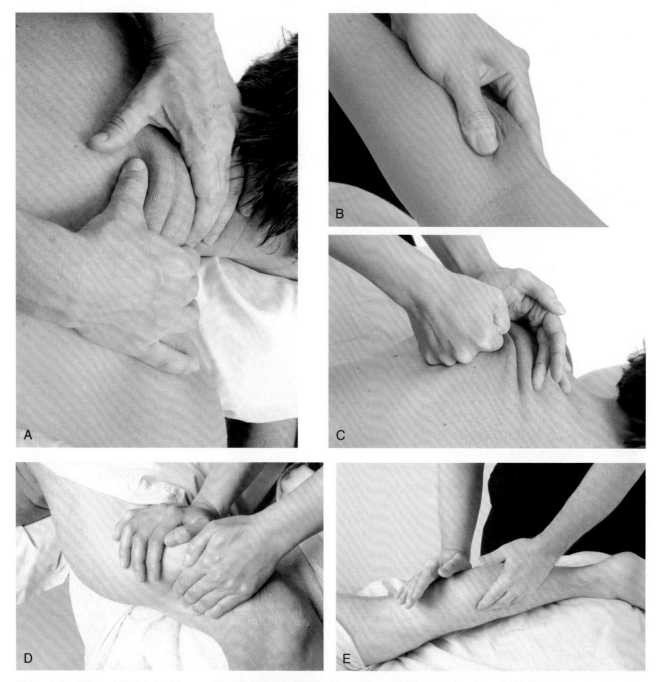

Figure 9-10. Different kinds of petrissage. **(A)** Whole hand. **(B)** Thumb and fingers. **(C)** Into cupped hand. **(D)** Heel of one hand and pads of fingers on other hand. **(E)** Heel of one hand and pads of fingers on other hand.

travel across the area of the restriction, which can be anywhere between 3 and 12 inches or longer. Make sure that there is no lubricant on the skin because you need to have a firm hold on the tissues, which is impossible with lubricant. If you find an area of restricted superficial fascia in the middle of a massage and have already applied lubricant, you can use a towel to wipe off the excess. This technique can be applied therapeutically if you perform specific assessments prior to using a skin roll. (See Chapter 10, Therapeutic Applications, for more detail.)

Tapotement

Tapotement is a fast rhythmic stroke in which you use both hands, like rapid drumming. In fact, sometimes tapotement is referred to as percussion, and it can be applied with cupped hands, flat hands, the medial side of open hands, the medial side of the relaxed fists, or the fingertips. See Figure 9-12 for different examples of tapotement. Initial and very light tapotement strokes stimulate

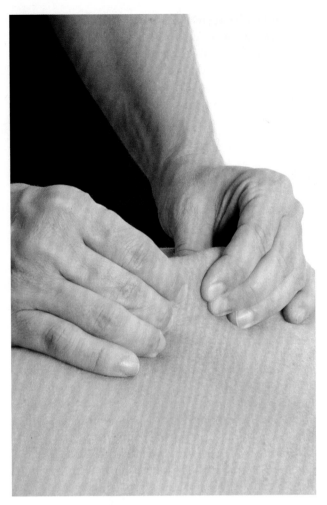

Figure 9-11. Skin rolling.

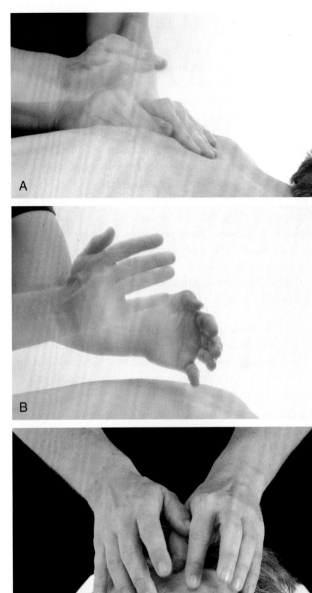

Figure 9-12. Tapotement. **(A)** Cupping. **(B)** Hacking. **(C)** Tapping.

the sympathetic nervous system and cause superficial vasoconstriction. Conversely, sustained and heavy tapotement results in superficial vasodilation, pain relief, and relaxation.

Effects of Tapotement

The different effects of tapotement are determined by its application. Consistent with the general physiological effects of touch, initially tapotement is more stimulating than relaxing, whereas prolonged applications encourage relaxation. In addition to stimulating the parasympathetic nervous response, research shows that performing several minutes of tapotement has an anesthetic effect on hypersensitive nerve endings.[1] When applied with more force, the effects of tapotement are similar to those of compression, including vasodilation, increased circulation, and increased tissue temperature. Firm, abrupt applications of tapotement, especially when applied near the musculotendinous junction, stimulate muscle contractions with

the tendon reflex. The response to very light fingertip tapotement is quite different, however, as the body reacts with a more protective mechanism. Vasoconstriction of the superficial blood vessels pulls them away from the surface of the skin to keep them from being damaged. Therapeutically, tapotement with cupped hands can be used to break up congestion in the lungs of people with cystic fibrosis. This stroke can be very effective, but you need a thorough understanding of the pathological condition, you need to know the specific technique, and the client will benefit more if you can work with the client's physician.

Application of Tapotement

There is no slip with any form of tapotement, so you can perform the stroke with or without lubricant. The rhythmic percussive strokes are delivered very quickly, somewhere around five beats per second, but they can be applied faster with the fingertips and more slowly with the fists. There is a critical elastic component of tapotement that allows the stroke to affect the deeper layers of tissue without damaging the more superficial layers, and it can only be accomplished by keeping your wrists and hands relaxed. In addition to being safer for the client's tissues and being less stressful for your body, tapotement delivered with a relaxed, springy rebound feels better. As in petrissage, there is no excursion with the stroke. You apply a series of individual strokes over the area you are treating.

The different variations of tapotement can be applied as follows (Fig. 9-12):

- To use cupped hands (cupping), your wrists must stay relaxed, but you need to hold your fingers loosely in the cupped position. When you strike the client's skin, the cupped hand should make a resounding kind of hollow noise.

- To use the flat surface of your finger pads (slapping), keep your fingers together but keep your wrists and fingers relaxed and loose. When your hand strikes the client's skin, it should sound and feel like a light smack.

- If you use the medial edge of your open hands for tapotement (hacking), keep your hands relaxed so that your fingers are comfortably spread apart. Upon striking the client's skin, your relaxed fingers "squish" together to absorb some of the shock.

- To use your fists for tapotement (pummeling or beating), keep your fists and wrists loose, and only use this stroke on the fleshy areas of the body such as the hips, thighs, and gluteal areas. There is almost no sound when your fist strikes the client's skin.

- If you use your fingertips for tapotement (tapping), the superficial fascia should be thin to create the appropriate effect. No sound occurs with fingertip tapotement because you use hardly any pressure, and you keep your fingers relaxed to absorb what little rebound there is.

As you apply tapotement, constantly move around to avoid striking the same spot repeatedly and be careful of areas where nerves and organs are relatively unprotected.

Do not use tapotement directly over the spine, bruised areas, or varicose veins, and use caution when applying it to the back in the kidney region.

The kidneys are relatively unprotected and are suspended in a fatty mass called the adipose capsule, and although it is not likely that you will shake them loose with tapotement, you need to ensure that you do not traumatize or injure them. The kidneys are located on either side of the spine, at the level of the superior lumbar vertebrae, just beneath the rib cage.

As with the other strokes, avoid tapotement over open or contagious skin conditions, bruises, varicose veins, injuries, inflammation, or infection.

Watch your body mechanics when you use tapotement. Besides keeping your wrists and hands relaxed, use your legs with your knees slightly bent as you move around to apply tapotement instead of bending and twisting at the waist.

Friction

Friction is a multidirectional stroke that you can apply superficially or deep with completely different methods and effects. **Superficial friction** is a brisk variation of light effleurage intended to increase circulation in the superficial tissues and dissipate body heat. The application of **deep-fiber friction** (also called **cross-fiber friction** and **transverse friction**) resembles the variation of compression called rolling. It is a deep, localized application of pressure, without any slip on the skin, primarily used to break up fascial adhesions and separate the muscle fibers.

Effects of Friction

Heat is created by friction, which is the physical resistance between two surfaces as they rub against each other. The massage stroke called superficial friction is applied by briskly rubbing the client's skin to create heat. It mechanically enhances the flow of blood and lymph and reflexively causes vasodilation in the skin, which increases circulation in the skin, increases the temperature of the skin and superficial fascia, and dissipates body heat from the skin. The general purpose of superficial friction is to create heat and increase the blood flow to the treated area, or local hyperemia (HAHY-per-EE-mee-ah).

Deep-fiber friction is quite different from superficial friction. The pressure of the stroke increases circulation in the deep fascia and muscle tissues, breaks up fascial adhesions and scar tissue, and separates the different components within a muscle. Chronically hypertonic muscle tissue is often accompanied by restrictions in the deep fascia. When people "stretch" their connective tissues, the elongation of the tissues also causes the muscle fibers and surrounding fascia to get closer together. Deep-fiber friction, especially when applied perpendicular to the relaxed muscle fibers of a passive contraction, is uniquely able to separate those fibers, increase local circulation, and restore movement.

Application of Friction

More heat is created when there is more resistance between your skin and the client's skin, so if you are applying superficial friction to warm the tissues, less lubricant is better. The rate of the strokes is moderately fast, somewhere around 1 to 3 strokes per second, and the length of the stroke along the skin, or excursion, is a few inches. You can use your thumbs, finger pads, or palms to apply superficial friction with just enough pressure to feel the surface resistance as you briskly rub the client's skin. When you vigorously rub your palms together to warm them up, you are using superficial friction. To maintain proper body mechanics for superficial friction, keep your arms, wrists, and hands as relaxed as possible and minimize the use of superficial friction because it requires vigorous activity on your part.

Deep-fiber friction is applied without any slip on the skin, so again, little or no lubricant is better. It can be applied perpendicular to the length of the muscle fibers with a strumming action, or it can be applied in a circular motion over the muscle fibers. Typically, deep-fiber friction strokes take about 3 seconds to travel across 1 inch of muscle tissue, without any slip on the skin. You can use your thumbs, finger pads, the knuckle portion of a fist, or your forearm, but it is wise to always remember the body mechanics rules of keeping your joints stacked, keeping your shoulders down, and maintaining a proper lean. See Figure 9-13 for deep-fiber friction over the erector spinae muscles. Because deep-fiber friction can be perceived as an invasive technique, you must prevent the guarding response by warming up the tissue with other techniques prior to applying it.

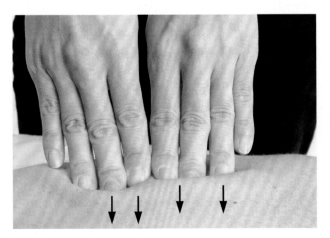

Figure 9-13. Deep-fiber friction.

Contraindications for friction include open or contagious skin conditions, bruised areas, moderate to severe varicose veins, acute injuries, inflammation, and infection.

Vibration

Vibration is a stroke that involves high-frequency shaky hand movements. Vibrations can travel through our bodies, affecting everything from the surface of the skin to the deepest organs. A common misconception in massage is that deep tissue work requires a lot of pressure or manipulation, but vibration demonstrates just how incorrect that is. Consider how the ground shakes when a large trailer truck rumbles by or how you feel the booming bass of a nearby car stereo sometimes more than you hear it. Vibration can be used to stimulate the nerves, muscles, and organs; to increase circulation and temperature of local tissues; and as a form of anesthesia. Some variations of vibration, including rocking and jostling, are generally used for relaxation.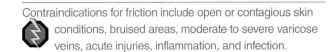

Effects of Vibration

Muscle contractions can be sustained when the muscle receives 10 to 20 nerve impulses per second. Vibration can stimulate muscle contractions when the frequency of the vibratory movements matches or exceeds the frequency of the nerve impulses for muscle contraction. Unfortunately, our hands can move at a rate of about 10 to 12 movements per second, which is not usually fast enough to stimulate muscle contraction. If you or your clients want the stimulating effects of vibration, you can consider using a machine that is more effective at delivering the necessary high frequencies. Like the other initial reflexive effects of touch, vibration initially stimulates the nervous system and organ activity. The effect is very similar to being shaken awake or shaken to pay attention. After several minutes of vibration, the reflexive effects of relaxation begin: pain sensitivity is decreased, circulation increases, the temperature of the tissues increases, and muscle tension decreases.

Application of Vibration

Some people find it difficult to learn how to apply vibration because you have to keep your shoulder, arm, wrist, and hand very relaxed while moving them very fast. Without loose joints and muscles, you will create excessive strain on your muscles and you lose the effectiveness of the stroke. Rest your relaxed fingertips or finger pads on the client's skin and start moving your wrist and hand with a gentle, nervous trembling motion. Again, maintain proper body mechanics by staying as relaxed as possible, from your shoulders through your fingertips. Your fingers can remain stationary on the client's skin or you can lightly slide your fingertips along the surface of the client's skin while applying vibration.

> Do not apply vibration over open or contagious skin conditions, bruises, varicose veins, acute injuries, inflammation, or infection.

Variations of Vibration

Rocking is a technique in which you use smooth, rhythmic, intermittent pushes to slowly rock a client's limb or entire body. Slow and gentle rocking movement is a well-known way to soothe and relax babies and adults alike. Rocking is accomplished by maintaining the back-and-forth rhythm of the client's body with well-timed series of pushes and releases. You can put pressure on the client's arm, leg, or pelvis to create the rocking motion. You must tune into the client's natural rhythm when rocking to allow the body to relax. Once you start rocking the client, make sure that you push at exactly the same time the client's body is starting to roll away from you. If you push while the body is still rolling toward you, there will be an irregularity and awkwardness to the rocking that is more bothersome than relaxing. The main purpose of rocking is to encourage relaxation.

Jostling moves the client's limbs back and forth in a wave-like snaking motion. The purpose of jostling is to confuse the nervous system and induce relaxation. It is applied by grasping an arm or leg, providing a small amount of traction, and then moving the extremity by wiggling it side to side (Fig. 9-14).

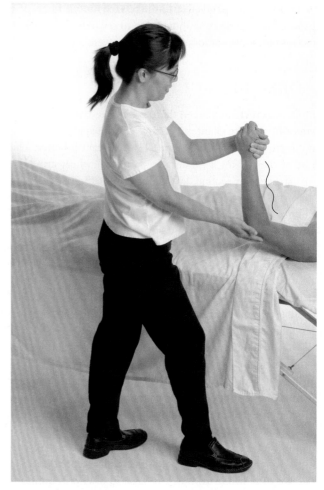

Figure 9-14. Jostling.

Joint Movement

All of the movements of the synovial joints are listed in the special muscle section at the end of Chapter 4, Kinesiology and Body Mechanics. Movement of the synovial joints, whether active or passive, encourages the production of synovial fluid, which nourishes and protects the joint structures. Joint movement also encourages the circulation of lymph by activating the skeletal muscle pump mechanism. Joint movements are easily incorporated into a massage and are very beneficial for the client. Passive movements require that you hold and move your clients gently and securely. Figure 9-15 illustrates passive lateral flexion of the neck. It takes more work on your part but allows clients to relax while you evaluate the quality and quantity of the movement. Active movements allow you to save your own energy because the client does the work while you visually evaluate the quality and quantity of the movement. Some clients do not like to participate during the massage session, but you can still incorporate active joint movements during the pretreatment and posttreatment assessments.

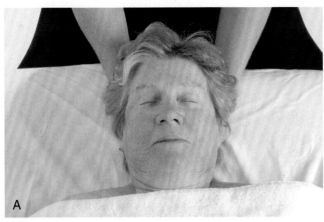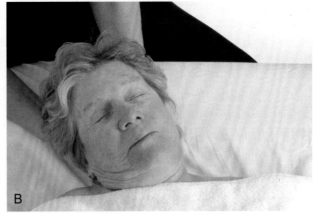

Figure 9-15. Passive lateral flexion of the neck. **(A)** Starting position. **(B)** Final position: at limit.

Endangerment Sites

There are some areas of the body for which you may need to adjust your speed and/or pressure in order to prevent damage to your client's body when applying massage techniques. Generally, deep, direct, and/or compressive pressure should be avoided in these vulnerable areas of the body, such as where the nerves, blood vessels, bony structures, organs, and lymph nodes are more superficial or unprotected:

- Nerves—Compressed nerves may result in sensations such as "pins and needles," tingling, numbness, or burning or shooting pain. If a client tells you that he or she is experiencing any of the aforementioned sensations, immediately adjust your pressure or move to another area of the body. Check with your client to see if the sensation has subsided to ensure he or she is comfortable. Prolonged compression may cause injury, bruising, or irritation to the nerves.

- Blood vessels—Compression on superficial arteries and veins affects circulation. Prolonged compression to an artery will cut off the flow of oxygenated blood to everything distal of the point of compression, potentially causing numbness, discomfort, panic, or blackouts. Veins, which are weaker than arteries, may be injured by excessive compression, possibly resulting in varicose veins or blood clots. Because arteries and veins are located very close together, massage techniques will typically affect both, so be cautious and avoid prolonged pressure to superficial blood vessels.

- Bony structures—Compressive massage or sustained, direct pressure on or near small, fragile, or prominent bony structures can cause pain, bruising

to the surrounding tissue, and in some cases, fracture of the bone.

- Organs—Some organs are located or anchored in a way that makes them vulnerable to some types of bodywork. Deep pressure, compressive techniques, or tapotement on or around the kidneys, just below ribs on posterior back, or to the abdominal area may cause pain, nausea, bruising, or diminished function.

- Lymph nodes—The functions of the lymph nodes are to produce lymphocytes and filter and clean lymph. These oval, bean-shaped structures are located superficially in several areas of the body (see Fig. 3-65). When lymph nodes are working overtime to filter excess toxins or fight an infection, they are generally enlarged and inflamed. Avoid massaging lymph nodes as their function could be impaired.

In the field of massage therapy, **endangerment sites** are specific areas on the body where the nerves, blood vessels, bony structures, organs, and lymph nodes are more superficial or unprotected that should be avoided (see Fig. 9-16):

- Eyes—Eyes are very sensitive structures, especially if the client wears contact lenses. There are nerves in this area that supply the face with feeling and motor control. Exercise caution when applying massage around the eyes.

- Temporomandibular joint (TMJ)—Located immediately anterior to the ear, the TMJ (jaw) is the only bilateral joint of the body and is susceptible to alignment problems. Avoid deep pressure to the bony projection itself as well as to the facial arteries and nerves located just anterior to the ear and along

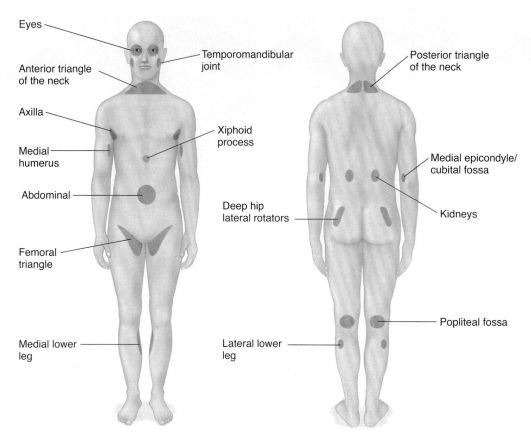

Figure 9-16. Endangerment sites.

the edge of the jaw inferior to the TMJ. There are specific techniques that may alleviate symptoms associated with TMJ tension and/or pain, but they require specialized knowledge and training so as not to cause injury or make the client's condition worse.

- Anterior triangle of the neck—Located just inferior to the chin, the anterior triangle contains structures that may be injured by invasive or deep pressure techniques: carotid artery, jugular vein, vagus nerve, hyoid bone, trachea, thyroid cartilage, and glands. Applying massage in this area requires advanced training and skill.

- Axilla—The soft area of the client's armpit holds the axillary and brachial arteries and multiple nerves: axial, median, musculocutaneous, radial and ulnar nerves, and the brachial plexus. If, when applying massage to this area, the client feels tingling, "pins and needles," or burning, sharp, or shooting pain, you are compressing the blood vessels and/or nerves and should adjust your pressure or move to a different area.

- Medial humerus—Located on the soft, medial side of the upper arm, the brachial plexus and the cephalic and basilic veins are located here and should be avoided.

- Abdominal area—Many susceptible structures are located in this area: abdominal aorta, inferior vena cava, ovaries in a female client, liver, spleen, and intestines. Light pressure applied in this area can enhance blood flow and digestion, but too much may diminish the function of these structures or cause injury.

- Xiphoid process—This spear-like, bony projection is the inferior portion of the sternum and should be avoided.

- Femoral triangle—Bilaterally located toward the medial side of the upper leg, just inferior to the pelvis, this area contains the femoral artery and vein, the femoral nerve, and the inguinal lymph nodes.

- Medial lower leg—Located on the medial side of the lower leg, this area contains the unprotected great saphenous vein.

- Posterior triangle of the neck—Located at the posterior base of the neck, the spinous processes are sensitive areas.

- Medial epicondyle/cubital fossa—Located between the olecranon process of the ulna and the medial epicondyle of the humerus, this area contains the radial nerve. Sustained compression may cause injury to the nerve. This endangerment site is especially important for a massage therapist's self-care regime. Applying compression with your elbow can be an effective technique, but you must use the area that is distal to the olecranon process. If you use the pointy part of the olecranon process, you will be putting pressure on your cubital fossa and possibly endangering the radial nerve.

- Kidneys—Located posteriorly and superficially, just deep to the inferior rib cage, the kidneys are unprotected and held in place by soft tissue. Avoid deep, direct, or compressive pressure and heavy tapotement to this area.

- Deep lateral hip rotator muscles—The sciatic nerve runs through these muscles, just deep to the gluteal muscles. The thickest nerve in the body, the sciatic nerve may be irritated by massage to these if it is compressed in any way.

- Popliteal fossa—Located on the posterior of the knee, this soft area contains the common peroneal

and tibial nerves as well as the popliteal artery and vein and small saphenous vein.

- Lateral lower leg—The common peroneal nerve is unprotected on the lateral side of the lower leg, just inferior to the head of the fibula.

If your assessment of a client's condition leads you to believe that the client may benefit from work to these areas, special training in some energy techniques that require little or no pressure or off-the-body work will allow you to facilitate healing within the area.

Any time a client has reduced pain sensitivity, massage therapists must be especially cautious about moving the client's joints through their range of motion. There are different kinds of barriers that limit joint movement, and some of them involve hypertonic muscle or restricted fascia. Pushing the tissues past their barriers can injure anatomical structures. With experience, you can learn to feel the barriers to avoid hurting clients; however, as a beginner, you may need input from your clients. Generally, clients feel discomfort when the limits of joint movement are being approached, but with reduced pain sensitivity, they may not.

Flow

You are now faced with the challenge of putting all of your academic knowledge and artistic skill into a massage. The first time you stand beside a client who is lying on a massage table, waiting for a massage, you may wonder whether it is possible to spend an hour massaging one body. Where do you start? What strokes do you use? Should the client start supine or prone? What position should the client be in? You will find the answers to these questions by learning and understanding massage flow, which is a routine-like sequence of steps that leads the massage from one body part to the next in a systematic, fluid pattern. Table 9-4 summarizes the strokes, their purposes and effects, and contraindications.

Similar to a cooking recipe, a flow is a set of step-by-step directions for your massage. It usually specifies the client's position on the table and tells you which body parts to work on and in what order. A flow can also suggest massage strokes to use on the different areas of the body. With practice, a flow becomes second nature and lets you evaluate the tissues throughout the massage instead of focusing on which body part to work on and what strokes to use. Good cooking recipes present their directions in a logical order that can be followed easily and efficiently. In the same way, a good massage flow guides therapists through a fluid, logical order from body part to body part without a lot of wasted time or energy. For instance, a good flow might direct you to massage the client's right hand, work up the right arm to

the right shoulder, connect the right and left shoulder with a resting stroke in which one hand is on each shoulder, and with a nerve stroke, move down to the client's left hand to begin work there. A bad flow might instruct you to massage the client's right hand, then move to the left hand, then the right shoulder, and then to the client's left shoulder. As a recipe is written to help us prepare edible and presentable food that people enjoy and does not make people sick, the massage flow is designed to accomplish the long-term treatment goal without endangering the client's health.

Flow Sequences for Different Client Positions

There are general flows for clients in the supine position, prone position, laterally recumbent (side-lying) position, and seated position. Each position limits your access to some part of the client's body, which is why most therapists prefer asking a client to assume two or three different body positions during the massage. The flow sequences for these different positions outlined below are very general directions that guide your movement around the client's body to

Table 9-4 Strokes: Purposes, Effects, and Contraindications

Stroke	Purposes and Effects	Contraindications
Grounding	Establishes boundary between therapist and client Helps massage therapist conserve energy	None
Centering	Helps massage therapist clear mind and focus attention on client	None
Resting	Establish contact with the client Assess the client's tissues Connect areas of the client's body throughout the flow of the massage	None
Compression	Enhances arterial circulation Enhances lymph and venous blood flow Warms tissues via increased arterial circulation Decreases muscular hypertonicity (tension) Softens fascia Decreases pain	Application over open or contagious skin conditions Application over bruised areas Application over moderate to severe varicose veins Application over areas of acute injury
Effleurage	Apply lubricant Assess muscle and soft tissue Light pressure has a reflexive effect on circulation Deep pressure has a mechanical effect on circulation Enhances venous and lymph circulation Enhances arterial circulation Enhances cellular metabolism Decreases muscular hypertonicity/tension Decreases ischemia and pain	Application over open or contagious skin conditions Application over bruised areas Application over moderate to severe varicose veins Application over areas of acute or subacute injury, inflammation, infection Repetitive application for clients with high blood pressure, cardiovascular disease, varicose veins or edema
Petrissage	Increases circulation of blood and lymph Softens skin by stimulating sebaceous gland activity Warms the soft tissues Enhances pliability of muscles and fascia Decreases muscular hypertonicity Relieves pain Encourages relaxation	Application over open or contagious skin conditions Application over bruised areas Application over moderate to severe varicose veins Application over areas of acute injury, inflammation, infection
Tapotement	Brief applications are stimulating Prolonged applications encourage relaxation Prolonged applications have anesthetic effects on hypersensitive nerve endings Increased circulation of blood Increases temperature of tissues Stimulates muscle contractions Breaks up lung congestion	Applications over the spine Applications on client's back over the kidney area Application over open or contagious skin conditions Application over bruised areas Application over moderate to severe varicose veins Application over areas of acute injury, inflammation, infection
Friction	Increases temperature of tissues Enhances flow of blood and lymph Dissipates body heat from the skin Breaks up fascial adhesions	Application over open or contagious skin conditions Application over bruised areas Application over moderate to severe varicose veins Application over areas of acute injury, inflammation, infection

continues on following page

Table 9-4 Strokes: Purposes, Effects, and Contraindications *continued*

Stroke	Purposes and Effects	Contraindications
Vibration	Brief applications stimulate nervous system and organ activity Prolonged applications are relaxing Decreases pain sensitivity Increases circulation of blood Increases temperature of tissues Decreases muscle hypertonicity	Application over open or contagious skin conditions Application over bruised areas Application over moderate to severe varicose veins Application over areas of acute injury, inflammation, infection

access all the different body parts smoothly and efficiently. As you gain experience, you will develop your own combination of strokes and techniques, but as a place to begin, the following section includes suggestions for sample flows for specific body parts.

Supine Position Flow

The supine position allows for direct access to the anterior side of the body—the face, the chest, the abdomen, and the anterior aspect of the legs. Persons with sinus congestion, those who do not like confined spaces, and those who are very talkative during a massage may prefer the supine position. Box 9-8 includes an illustrated series of steps for a general supine massage flow.

Prone Position Flow

Clients who are not very conversational or who are suffering back pain may prefer the prone, or face down, position. In this position, you have particularly good access to a client's back, gluteal muscles, and the posterior aspects of the legs, but your access to the anterior aspect of the body is limited. If a client uses the face cradle to maintain a neutral neck position while lying in the prone position, the entire neck and shoulder region is easily accessible to you. Box 9-9 shows a sample flow for massaging clients in the prone position.

Side-Lying (Laterally Recumbent) Position Flow

The side-lying (laterally recumbent) position is not as popular as the others because it requires additional bolstering and because the draping can be awkward and a bit challenging to learn. Many therapists do not incorporate this position into their massages, but there are times when a client

is better served in the side-lying position. For example, it is dangerous to keep a pregnant woman supine during her last few months of pregnancy because the fetus can put excessive pressure on her descending aorta. Massage is very beneficial during pregnancy, though, and pregnant clients can safely receive massage in the side-lying position as long as there are no systemic contraindications. Prenatal or pregnancy massage is covered in more detail in Chapter 12, Special Populations.

When a client has a lot of neck and shoulder restrictions, the side-lying position provides excellent access to the entire region. It also gives you a unique ability to maneuver the client's neck and shoulders through all of the possible joint movements, so if you find that many of your clients are complaining of neck and shoulder problems, you should incorporate the side-lying position. Box 9-10 includes an example of a massage flow for a client who is lying on her left side, properly positioned and bolstered.

Seated Position Flow

You may need to give a complete relaxation massage to a client who is seated. If someone is unable to climb onto your table, is not comfortable lying down, or is bound to a wheelchair, a seated massage may be the most appropriate position. This seated flow is designed for relaxation, making it different from the stimulating focus of chair and corporate massages with a short duration. Because clients remain clothed for the massage, there are no draping considerations, but if they wear shorts and tank tops or short sleeves, you have better access to their tissues and can apply more strokes that offer clients more benefits. You can easily apply compression, tapotement, and vibration through clothing, and possibly some petrissage or deep-fiber friction. Effleurage, which is such a good stroke for assessing the condition of the client's tissues, is not appropriate for clients who are clothed. You can deliver a seated massage to a client in a chair by following the steps in Box 9-11.

BOX 9-8 **PROCEDURE** **Supine Position Massage Flow**

1. Stand or sit at the head of the massage table, facing the client to massage the:
   - Face
   - Ears
   - Scalp
   - Neck
   - Upper chest
   - Shoulders

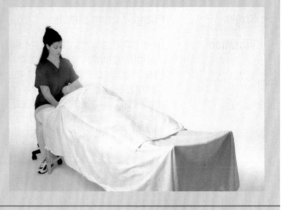

2. Walk to the client's left side, undrape the left arm and massage the client's left hand, forearm, upper arm, and shoulder, and redrape the arm.

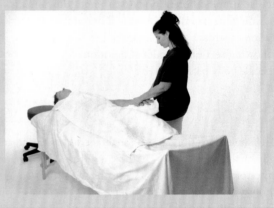

3. Use connecting strokes to walk toward the client's left foot.

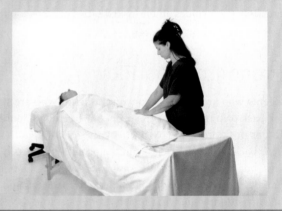

4. Sit or stand at the client's feet, undrape the left foot and massage the:
   - Sole
   - Ball of the foot
   - Toes
   - Top of the metatarsals
   - All around the ankle and heel

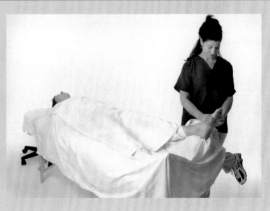

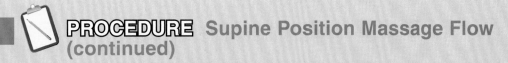

BOX 9-8 **PROCEDURE** (continued) Supine Position Massage Flow

5. Stand at the client's left side, expose the left leg, and massage the:
   - Lower leg
   - Upper leg

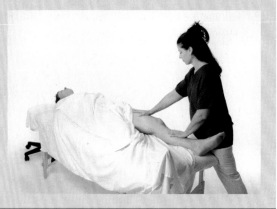

6. Redrape the left leg and move to the client's feet.

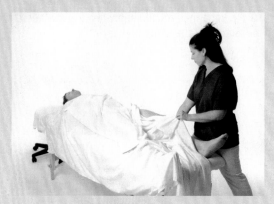

7. Undrape the client's right foot and massage the sole of the foot, ball of the foot, toes, and all around the ankle and heel.

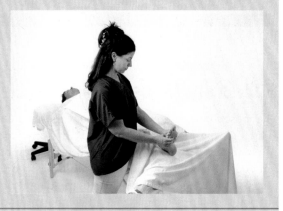

8. Stand at the client's right side. Expose the right leg and massage the lower leg and upper leg.

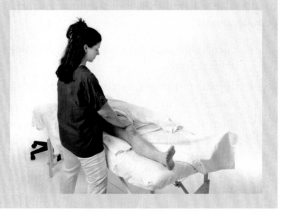

BOX 9-8　**PROCEDURE** (continued)　Supine Position Massage Flow

9. Redrape the right leg, undrape the right arm, and massage the:
   * Hand
   * Forearm
   * Upper arm
   * Shoulder

10. Redrape the arm and apply head-to-toe nerve strokes to reconnect the entire body.

Full-Body Massage Flows

The most common flow for a full-body massage utilizes at least one position change during the massage. You can combine the sample flows in any order to accomplish a full-body or partial-body massage. Most massage therapists use the prone and supine positions, in either order, but you should try several different combinations to get comfortable with the change of positions and the draping considerations:

* Clients start supine, then turn over, finishing in the prone position

* Clients start prone, then turn over to finish in the supine position

* Clients start prone, assume a side-lying position on their right side, turn to lie on their left side, then turn onto their back, finishing in the supine position

* Clients start supine, lie on their left side, turn over to their right side, then flip once more to finish in the prone position

* Clients start in the side-lying position on one side, then flip over to finish in the side-lying position on the other side

It takes time for clients to change positions during a massage, so you may want to minimize the position changes. Also, some clients do not like to have to move during the massage and do not appreciate having to flip over more than once during the massage. On the other hand, therapeutic massage is intended to treat soft tissue conditions that you discover before and during treatment, and it may serve the client best to use more than two positions during a massage. If you discover that the client will benefit from multiple positions, educate him or her on your plan and why you will be moving him or her around during the session. The sample flows do not provide directions for a full-body massage because we believe that an individualized massage is best.

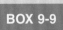

BOX 9-9 **PROCEDURE** Prone Position Massage Flow

1. Standing at the client's left side in an asymmetric stance, place your hands on top of the drape and apply a resting stroke to the client's low back.

2. Expose the client's back and, working only on the client's left side, massage the:
   • Back
   • Scapular area
   • Shoulder area
   • Neck area

3. Use connecting strokes to walk around the client's head to the client's right side and massage the right side of the client's back, scapular area, shoulder area, and neck area.

4. Redrape the back and use connecting strokes to move to the client's right gluteal area.

5. Massage the right gluteal muscles on top of the sheet, with compression and possibly some petrissage.

6. Expose the client's right leg and massage the:
   • Upper leg
   • Lower leg

7. Redrape the right leg, leaving the right foot exposed, and sit or stand at the end of the table to massage the client's right foot.

8. Redrape the right foot and use connecting strokes to walk around the table to the client's left gluteal area.

9. Massage the left gluteal muscles on top of the sheet with compression and possibly some petrissage.

10. Expose the client's left leg and massage the upper leg and lower leg.

11. Redrape the left leg, leaving the left foot exposed, and sit or stand at the end of the table to massage the client's left foot.

12. Redrape the left foot, and place one hand on each of the client's feet as a resting stroke.

BOX 9-10 **PROCEDURE** Side-Lying Massage Flow
(Client Positioned as in Fig. 9-4)

1. Stand at the side of the table, facing the client's back, and rest your hands on the client's right shoulder and hip.

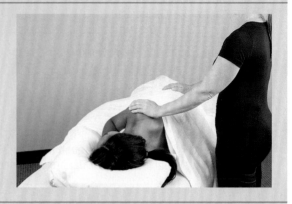

2. Expose the client's back and massage the right side of the:
   - Back
   - Scapular area
   - Shoulder
   - Neck

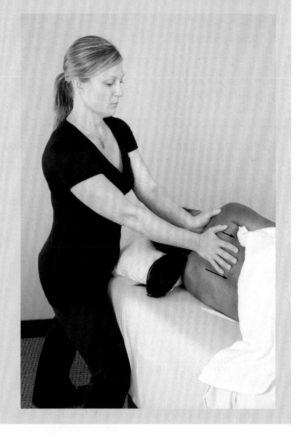

BOX 9-10 **PROCEDURE** Side-Lying Massage Flow (Client Positioned as in Fig. 9-4) (continued)

3. Redrape the back and maintain contact with your client as you walk around his or her head to the other side of the table.

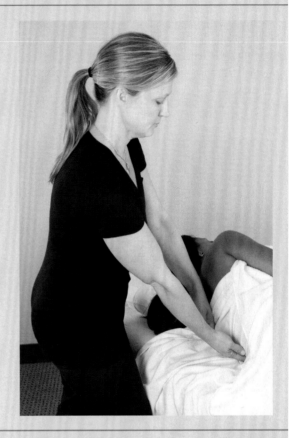

4. Facing your client, expose the right arm and massage the:
   - Hand
   - Forearm
   - Upper arm
   - Shoulder
   - Neck

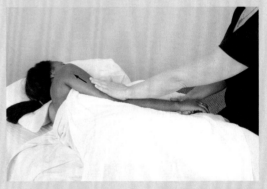

5. Redrape the right arm, and use connecting strokes to move to the legs.

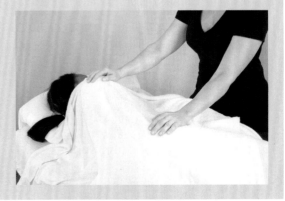

BOX 9-10

PROCEDURE Side-Lying Massage Flow
(Client Positioned as in Fig. 9-4) (continued)

6. Expose the right leg (top leg) and massage the:
   • Upper leg
   • Lower leg
   • Foot

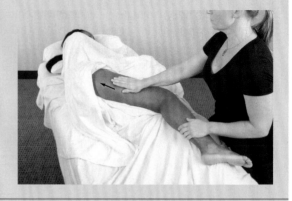

7. Redrape the right leg and use connecting strokes as you move around the client's feet to the other side of the table and stand beside the left leg.

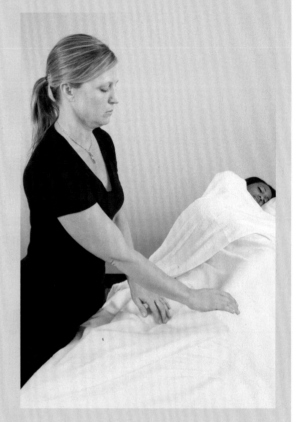

BOX 9-10	**PROCEDURE** Side-Lying Massage Flow (Client Positioned as in Fig. 9-4) (continued)

8. Expose the left leg and massage the:
   - Upper leg
   - Lower leg
   - Foot

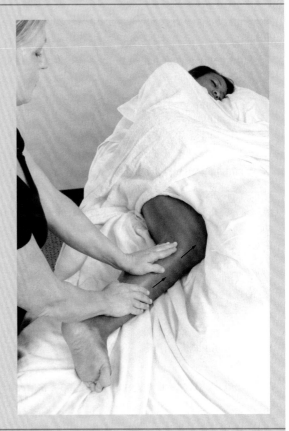

9. Redrape the left leg and use a head-to-toe nerve stroke to reconnect the body.

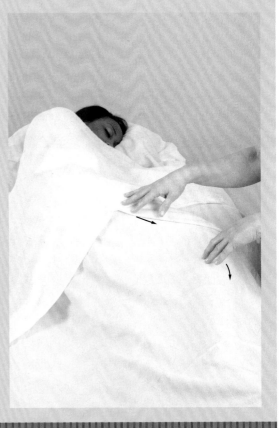

BOX 9-11   📋 **PROCEDURE** Seated Relaxation Massage Flow (Client Fully Clothed)

1. Stand behind the client's chair, and gently rest your hands on the client's shoulders.

2. Slowly move your hands to the top of the client's head and massage the:
   - Scalp
   - Neck
   - Shoulders
   - Scapular areas
   - Any areas of the back you can access easily, which depends on the chair

3. Maintain contact with the client as you move to the client's left side.

4. Sit or kneel next to the client to massage the left hand.

5. Stand up to massage the:
   - Forearm
   - Upper arm
   - Shoulder

6. Use connecting strokes as you move around to the client's right side and sit or kneel next to the client to massage the right hand.

7. Stand up to massage the forearm, upper arm, and shoulder.

8. Sit or kneel next to the client's right foot and massage the:
   - Right foot
   - Right lower leg
   - Right thigh

9. Move to the client's left foot and massage the left foot, left lower leg, and left thigh.

10. Stand up, facing the client, and use a head-to-toe nerve stroke to reconnect the body.

Sample Flow Sequences for Specific Areas

Below are some suggested flows to familiarize you with the process of combining basic massage strokes with resting strokes and connecting strokes. These flows are only a guide to get you started. Once you are comfortable holding and touching clients and you can use different massage strokes effectively, use the strokes you think are most appropriate and treat the client's body parts in the order that makes sense to you. In all of the following flows, clients start fully draped in the position indicated, and you have already performed your grounding and centering techniques. There are no specific directions for lubricant application because it is up to you to determine how much is necessary to make your strokes comfortable with the right amount of slip.

Supine: Chest, Neck, and Head

A supine client's chest, neck, and head can all be accessed from one position, as you stand at the head of the massage table.

 When massaging the chest and neck area, do not put pressure over the endangerment sites of the anterior triangle of the neck, the jugular vein, or the brachial plexus.

Box 9-12 illustrates a massage sequence for a supine client's chest, neck, and head.

BOX 9-12 **PROCEDURE** Massage Flow for a Supine Client's Chest, Neck, and Head

1. Standing at the client's head, uncover the client's upper chest, tuck the drape underneath the client's armpits, and perform a resting stroke with one hand on each shoulder.

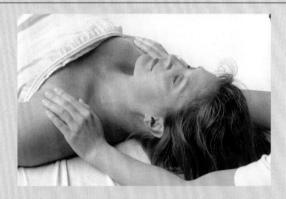

2. Effleurage the client's chest, from the sternum to the shoulders, with both palms simultaneously, two to three times.

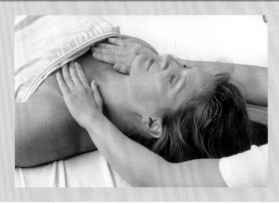

3. Effleurage the back of the client's shoulders, from the deltoids to the neck, using both palms simultaneously, two to three times.

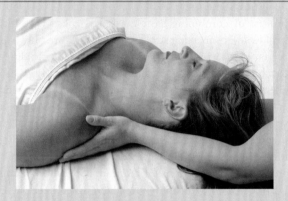

4. Redrape the upper chest and slide both hands under the shoulders to cradle the client's upper thoracic spine with both hands. Using your finger pads, effleurage and petrissage the muscles just lateral to the spine, all the way up to the occipital ridge, about 20 seconds.

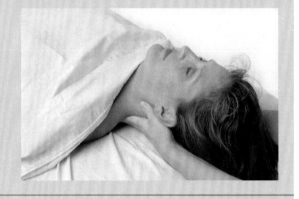

5. Cradle the client's head and perform passive joint movements:
   • Neck flexion
   • Neck rotation to the left and to the right
   • Lateral neck flexion to the left and to the right

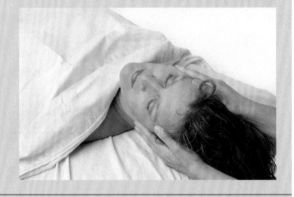

6. Petrissage the entire scalp and external parts of the ear with your fingertips and thumbs, 20 seconds.

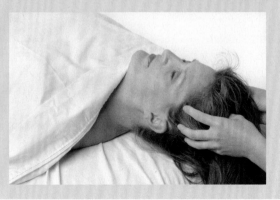

BOX 9-12 **PROCEDURE** Massage Flow for a Supine Client's Chest, Neck, and Head (continued)

7. Starting medial and moving laterally, use your thumbs and fingertips to effleurage once or twice each:
   - Along mandible
   - Along maxilla
   - Along inferior surface of zygomatic process to temples
   - Along eyebrow ridge
   - Along the top of the forehead

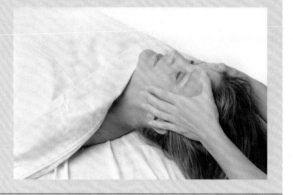

8. Use your fingertips to apply tapotement lightly to the face, 10 seconds.

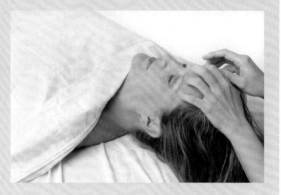

9. Apply nerve strokes from the chin to the temples, twice.

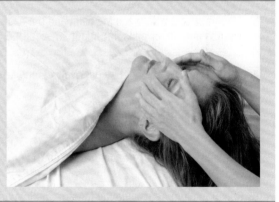

10. Loosely cradle the client's head.

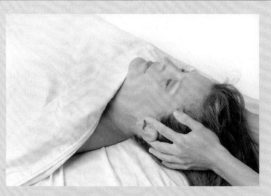

Massage Strokes and Flow

9

Supine: Arm

It is possible to massage the client's arm in both the prone and supine positions. The shoulder, however, is capable of more joint movements when clients are supine. The massage sequence in Box 9-13 describes how you can massage the arm of a client who is in the supine position.

Supine: Abdomen

The abdomen is often left untreated during a massage session for different reasons. Many people are uncomfortable with abdominal massage, but it is beneficial for the digestive system and is worth learning. Scientific research has shown that abdominal massage provides relief from constipation as well as intestinal discomfort and pain. The parasympathetic nervous response, induced by relaxation massage, stimulates digestive activity. When pressure is exerted on the abdomen, underlying structures are compressed and pushed out of the way. An effleurage stroke can mechanically push intestinal contents through the intestines. Massage may also stimulate peristaltic contractions of the intestines, which is the body's natural mechanism for pushing contents through the digestive tract toward the rectum. The individual effleurage strokes must be applied in the same direction as peristalsis to enhance digestive progress.

Because clients are often unfamiliar with abdominal work, always ask them if they want the work done. With their permission, you can proceed. The abdomen is best accessed via the supine position. The client's knees must be bent to keep the abdominal area soft enough to let you apply pressure, so a bolster is particularly helpful under the knees. Draping requires at least one extra blanket or large towel, if not two, in addition to the standard sheets. Properly draping the abdomen is slightly more complicated than draping the

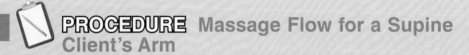

BOX 9-13   PROCEDURE Massage Flow for a Supine Client's Arm

1. Stand at your client's right side, facing your client.

2. Push the drape aside to take hold of the client's right hand and expose the arm, tucking the edge of the sheet under the client's arm and under the armpit, and place the arm on top of the sheet.

3. Effleurage and petrissage the palm and the back of the client's hand and each finger individually, using your thumbs and finger pads, for about 20 seconds.

4. Perform joint movement by passively extending client's wrist and fingers in pairs:
   • Pinky and thumb
   • Ring finger and index finger
   • Middle finger and wrist

5. Jostle the client's arm while grasping the client's hand and supporting the elbow.

6. Effleurage and petrissage the forearm, maintaining your grasp of the client's wrist with one hand for stability while you apply a stroke with your other hand, and then alternate hands to apply strokes, proximally from wrist to elbow, for about 20 seconds.

7. Rest your client's arm on the table for support while you apply effleurage and petrissage with alternating hands, proximally from elbow to shoulder and over the deltoids, for about 20 seconds. You can abduct your client's arm to put the deltoids into passive contraction, which allows you to get deeper into the tissues with less work.

8. Apply nerve strokes from shoulder to wrist.

9. Redrape the arm and apply nerve strokes from shoulder to hand.

10. Connect the client's wrist and shoulder with a resting stroke.

rest of the body. The draping process described in Box 9-1 maintains the client's modesty and warmth.

Abdominal massage for digestive enhancement uses an approach similar to that for venous enhancement and lymphatic drainage, in which you start closest to the outlet or drain and progressively move farther away from it. The sequence of strokes is a counterclockwise pattern, but the individual strokes move clockwise along the large intestine (Fig. 9-17). These directions are determined as if the client is holding a clock on his or her abdomen so that you can read the face of the clock. Strokes should be slow and firm rather than quick and light. The abdominal massage backtracks through the large intestine, starting with the rectal area and moving counterclockwise toward the cecum. Clearing the exit end first is more effective than pushing from the other end, which could compact the contents in the passage.

Having the abdomen exposed often makes a person feel vulnerable and unsure. Be careful to help maintain the client's physical and mental safety, and be especially sensitive to the client's

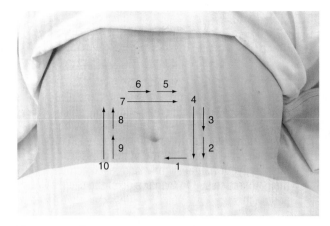

Figure 9-17. Abdominal massage stroke sequence.

acceptance or discomfort with the work. Stay attuned to the client's verbal or nonverbal communication to be aware of the client's comfort level throughout the abdominal massage. Box 9-14 includes a suggested flow for massaging a client's abdomen.

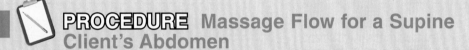

BOX 9-14   📋 **PROCEDURE** Massage Flow for a Supine Client's Abdomen

1. Position your fully draped client supine, with both knees bent to soften the abdomen, and place a towel across the chest, on top of the draping.

2. Ask your client to rest the hands on the chest. Explain that the hands act as a physical barrier to stop you from touching the abdomen any higher than the hands. (Some clients will rest their hands close to their navel, while others may not need a barrier. Whatever your client's modesty, keep your work inferior to the xiphoid process.)

3. Establish the inferior limit for your work by tucking the sheet tightly under the client's hips, just inferior to the ASIS. You can place a second towel over the client's pelvis to cover the area inferior to the ASIS for additional modesty or warmth.

4. With the superior and inferior borders determined, ask the client to firmly hold onto the towel on the chest.

5. Gently pull the draping sheet out from under the towel to expose the abdomen down to the pelvis, stopping at the inferior barrier.

6. Stand at your client's side in a symmetric stance and apply effleurage with both hands crossing the abdomen in an alternating pattern to spread the lubricant and help the client get used to abdominal contact, 8 strokes.

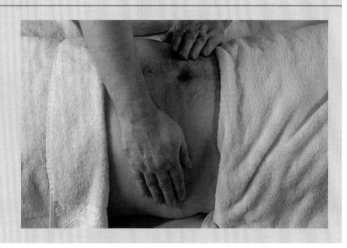

BOX 9-14   **PROCEDURE** Massage Flow for a Supine
Client's Abdomen (continued)

7. Place the palms of both hands against the near side of your client's abdomen and firmly effleurage across the abdomen, your hands moving away from you. Before your fingertips reach the client's midline, relieve some of the pressure by lifting your hands slightly, and reach across the gathered tissue to the far side of the client's abdomen.

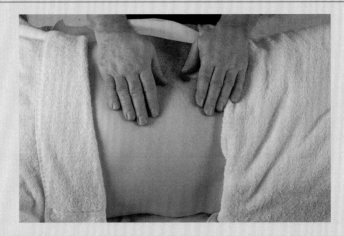

8. Use both of your flat hands to slowly and firmly effleurage the abdomen toward you. Repeat steps 7 and 8 several times with slow, rhythmic, wavelike strokes across the abdomen.

9. Change to an asymmetric stance beside the client's femur, angled toward the client's head, and effleurage with the flats of your alternating hands in a clockwise pattern to enhance peristaltic activity, as in Figure 9-17.

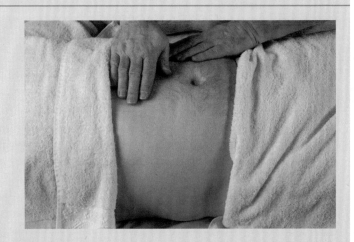

10. Apply a resting stroke with both palms on the client's abdomen.

11. Redrape the abdomen by pulling the sheet up, leaving the chest drape in place underneath the sheet. Apply a resting stroke on top of the drape, connecting the abdomen to the upper part of the client's sternum.

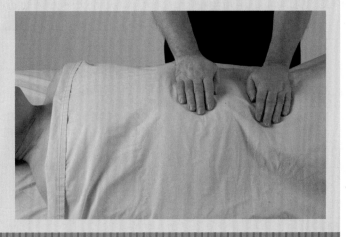

Indications and Contraindications for Abdominal Massage

Abdominal massage is beneficial for enhancing digestion and relief from intestinal discomfort, constipation, diarrhea, colic, gas, and nausea. It also helps the uterus return to its normal size during the postpartum period. For clients who are generally healthy, it is unnecessary to obtain a healthcare professional's consult before doing abdominal massage. If, on the other hand, the client is pregnant; has a history of diverticular disease or pelvic disorders such as endometriosis or pelvic inflammatory disease; or fits the profile for aneurysm (history of heart disease, atherosclerosis, and high blood pressure), you should encourage that client to get clearance from his or her healthcare professional.

Supine: Leg and Foot

Feet are especially ticklish, but slow movements and firm pressure can minimize or prevent the ticklish sensation. The legs and feet can be treated in both the supine and prone positions, and whether you use one or both positions in your massage depends on your client's treatment goals, your preference, the amount of time you have, and your instructor's or school's recommendations. Applying massage to the leg when your client is supine can be done as shown in Box 9-15.

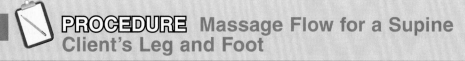

BOX 9-15 **PROCEDURE** **Massage Flow for a Supine Client's Leg and Foot**

1. Stand, kneel, or sit at the foot of the table, or sit on the end of the table, expose the client's foot, and apply compression by squeezing both sides of the client's foot, about five times.

2. Deep effleurage the sole of the foot, distally with your thumbs, three times.

3. Apply circular friction to the ball of the foot with your thumbs, about 20 seconds.

4. Apply deep effleurage with your thumbs or finger pads around the ankles, and along the tops of the metatarsals and each toe, moving distally, two to three times.

5. Perform joint movements by passively:
   - Extending each toe
   - Moving the ankle through a circular motion from dorsiflexion, to eversion, to plantarflexion, to inversion

6. Hold the client's foot for a resting stroke.

7. Expose the leg and stand near the client's foot in an asymmetric stance, facing the client's head.

8. Effleurage and petrissage the anterior and lateral aspects of the lower leg, in a proximal direction, using your thumbs and the heels of your hands, for about 30 seconds.

9. Effleurage and petrissage the anterior, medial, and lateral aspects of the client's thigh, using your palms, the heels of your hands, or your fists, for about 30 seconds.

10. Redrape the leg and apply nerve strokes from the client's hip to toes, two times.

Prone: Back

The prone position allows you access to the entire back, and also gives you a good opportunity to make visual assessments. As you massage the back, remember that the kidneys are relatively unprotected.

> ⚠ Use light applications of tapotement over the kidneys to avoid traumatizing or injuring them.

Prone clients are easily startled when you establish initial contact. To minimize the stimulation, you can tighten the draping near the area where you will contact the body, and use that sensory input to ease clients into your touch. You can apply massage to the back as illustrated in Box 9-16.

Prone: Leg and Foot

By using both the prone and supine positions to massage a client's legs and feet, you can easily access all the soft tissues of the legs.

> ⚠ Do not apply direct pressure over the endangerment site at the popliteal fossa behind the knee.

The steps in Box 9-17 can be used to apply massage to the client's legs and feet in the prone position.

Closing Sequence

One way to finish a massage is to reconnect all the parts of the body and apply a last resting stroke to signal the end of the physical contact. Whether a client is supine, prone, or side-lying, the following steps can be used as a closing sequence:

1. Apply one or two slow nerve strokes from head to toe.
2. Apply a series of resting strokes:
   a. Both feet
   b. Both knees
   c. Both hips (anterior superior iliac spine [ASIS] if supine, posterior superior iliac spine if prone, or the protruding greater trochanter if side-lying)
   d. Head

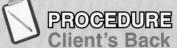

BOX 9-16 **PROCEDURE** **Massage Flow for a Prone Client's Back**

1. Stand with an asymmetric foot position at the client's left side, facing the client's head, and expose the client's back.

2. As you tuck the sheet near the hips, leave your hand on the sheet and transition onto the client's skin to minimize the stimulation of initial contact. Apply effleurage to the left side of the client's back, using flat hands or the heels of your hands, first to spread lubricant and then progressively deeper, about six times.

3. Apply effleurage and petrissage, using the heel of your hand or your thumbs all over the left side of the client's back, from the iliac crest to the occipital ridge and from the spine all the way out to the muscular attachments at the proximal humerus.

4. Use the hacking form of tapotement over the left rhomboids, for 10 seconds.

5. Apply gentle effleurage over the left side of the client's back, using flat hands in a superior direction, about four times.

6. Maintain contact with client's left shoulder as you walk around the client's head to the client's right side, and repeat steps 2 to 5 on the right side of the client's back.

7. Redrape the back and apply a resting stroke on top of the sheet with one hand on the middle of the client's back, and the other hand over the sacrum.

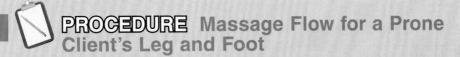

BOX 9-17 PROCEDURE Massage Flow for a Prone Client's Leg and Foot

1. Stand beside the client's leg, undrape the leg, and give a little tug on the sheet at the client's hip as sensory input to minimize the stimulation of your initial contact as you apply a resting stroke to the client's thigh.

2. Apply effleurage strokes in a proximal direction, first to spread lubricant on the client's thigh, and progressively deeper, for about 20 seconds.

3. Effleurage and petrissage the upper leg, using your fists and the heels and palms of your hands, from the knee to the ischial tuberosity, making sure to address the lateral and medial aspects of the thigh, about 30 seconds.

4. Support the client's ankle on a bolster and apply effleurage and petrissage to the lower leg in a proximal direction, using your palms and thumbs, making sure to address the lateral aspects of the lower leg and the entire gastrocnemius muscle, which goes past the knee joint, for 20 seconds.

5. Redrape the leg and apply nerve strokes, hip to heel, two times.

6. With the bolster still supporting the client's foot, expose the foot and apply compression to the sole of the foot.

7. Apply deep effleurage to the sole of the foot in a distal direction, using your thumbs or the heel of your hand, three times.

8. Redrape the foot and apply a resting stroke to the sole of the client's foot.

Chair Massage

Chair massage, also called seated massage, event massage, onsite massage, or corporate massage, gives people an opportunity to receive massage during the workday or at an event. Although some people think that getting a massage at work may slow them down and make them sleepy for the rest of the day, this is not the case. Research has found that massage in the workplace increases productivity and employee job satisfaction. One of the leading researchers in the field of massage is Tiffany M. Field, PhD, of the Touch Research Institute at the University of Miami's School of Medicine. Dr. Field's work is well received by the medical and scientific communities because her studies incorporate critical scientific methods, using control groups and objectively measured responses. By measuring hormone levels, blood pressure, brain wave activity, and math test performance, she showed that after a massage, employees were more alert, felt less job stress and anxiety, could perform more efficiently, and were more accurate with math calculations. After chair massage, most people feel more relaxed and less anxious, feel that they can think more clearly, and have increased energy. (Box 9-18 identifies some highlights of chair massage.)

When clients are at work, they can be comfortably and modestly supported in a seated position using a massage chair (Fig. 9-18). They remain fully clothed, which means the massage is applied through their clothing. You typically use no lubricant. You work primarily on the client's posterior neck and shoulder muscles, the back muscles, and the arms and hands. This massage usually lasts only 10 to 15 minutes, the general pace of the massage is faster and brisker, and the flow follows somewhat of a routine. Often performed in a well-lit, open area, with upbeat or no music, the strokes used are quick and brisk to keep the client awake and invigorated. (See Box 9-19 for a sample chair massage flow.)

BOX 9-18
Highlights of Chair Massage

- Clients are fully clothed
- Clients receive massage in the seated position, usually in a massage chair
- 10- to 15-minute treatment
- Fast-paced, brisk compression and tapotement are the major strokes
- Focus on the neck, shoulders, upper back, arms, and hands
- No lubricant
- No draping

A massage chair is a great piece of equipment to use to market your skills and gain access to persons who may not otherwise experience massage. It is a good first exposure for persons who are hesitant or have misconceptions regarding massage therapy, and it is a good vehicle for educating clients about the benefits of regular massage.

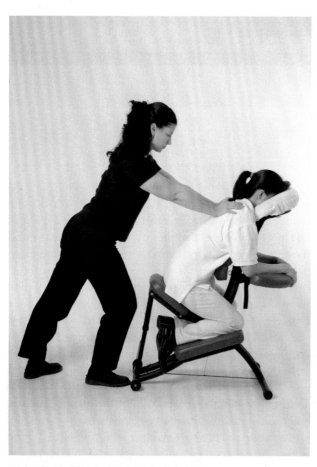

Figure 9-18. Chair massage client positioning.

Safety and Sanitation for Chair Massage

You must be sure to consider safety and sanitation as part of performing chair massage. Safety considerations include transporting equipment safely, adjusting the equipment properly, and inspecting the chair with each use. You should follow the universal precautions and guidelines for hygiene and sanitation as covered in Chapter 13.

Alert

When carrying your massage chair, you should be sure to use proper lifting procedures to avoid injuring yourself.

Keep your back as vertical as possible and bend your knees until your arms can grab whatever you want to lift. With a firm grip on the item you are lifting, straighten your knees while keeping your back as vertical as possible. If you use your massage chair frequently, you might consider buying a chair or a cart that has wheels for easier mobility. Once you have determined where your chair will be set up, make sure that all adjustments are securely tightened to prevent the chair from shifting during the massage. It is also a good idea to periodically check for cracks in the wood and damaged hinges.

There are three primary sanitation considerations with chair massage:

- Chair surfaces
- Client's face
- Massage therapist's hands and forearms

All of the chair's surfaces that contact the client's skin must be properly sanitized with every use. Because clients are often in the middle of their workday, it is especially important to keep the face cradle clean and sanitary. You should sanitize the face cradle before each chair massage session and use a covering of some kind. Examples include paper towels, bouffant caps, and washable fabric covers (Fig. 9-19). Finally, your hands and forearms must be properly disinfected using proper handwashing procedures between each client as well as immediately prior to beginning the massage (see Chapter 13). In a corporate or event setting where handwashing is not available to you, gel hand sanitizer is a convenient option to consider as long as you follow the product's directions. If you or your client has a cut, wound, or open skin, you may choose or the client may request you to use gloves.

BOX 9-19 | **PROCEDURE** Sample Chair Massage Flow

1. Welcome the client:
   a. Greet the client.
   b. Inquire about spine or neck injuries or conditions, wrist and shoulder issues, or recent surgeries.
   c. Orient the client to the massage chair and demonstrate how to sit in it.
   d. Ask client to sit in the chair, and adjust the chair to the client's body.

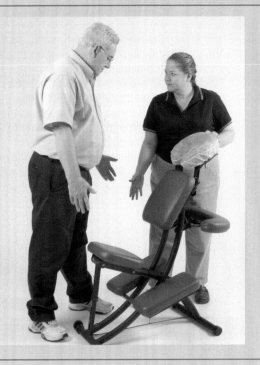

2. Apply a resting stroke to both of the client's shoulders.

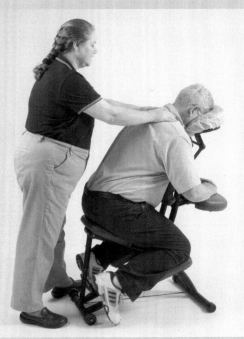

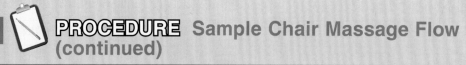

BOX 9-19   **PROCEDURE** (continued)   Sample Chair Massage Flow

3. Stand behind the client in an asymmetric position and warm up the shoulder and back muscles by applying compression and pétrissage:
   a. With loose fists on either side of the spine, from shoulder to sacrum, two to three times
   b. With the heel of the hand, compressing the erector spinae muscles laterally, from shoulder to iliac crest, on one side of the spine at a time
   c. With the thumb, down the erector spinae muscles, working into the intercostal spaces, one side of the spine at a time

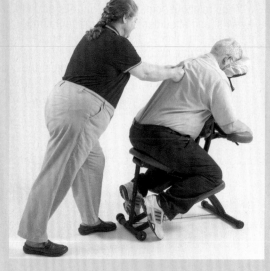

   d. With the forearm, into the upper trapezius and levator scapulae, one side at a time

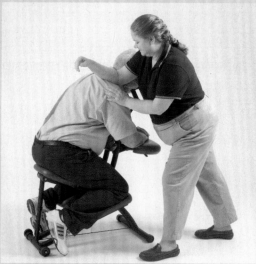

4. Apply 8 seconds of moderate hacking over the whole upper back.

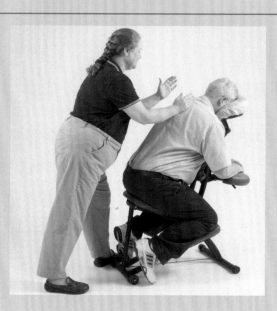

BOX 9-19 **PROCEDURE** Sample Chair Massage Flow (continued)

5. Stand by the client's right side, and apply compression to the right arm, from the deltoids to the hand, two to three times.

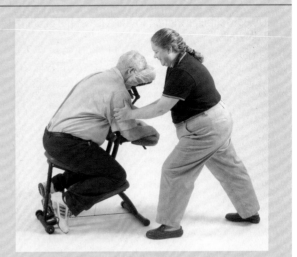

6. Apply compression and pétrissage to the right hand, paying extra attention to the thenar eminence, and passively extend and stretch the hand and finger flexors.

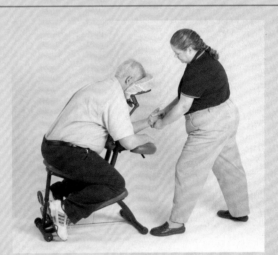

7. Move to the client's left side and repeat steps 4 to 7 on the left arm.

8. Move to face the client and apply compression and petrissage strokes with both hands, moving medially from the shoulders toward the neck.

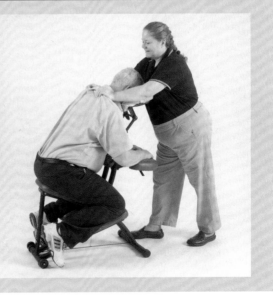

BOX 9-19 **PROCEDURE** Sample Chair Massage Flow
(continued)

9. Apply circular friction to the base of the occiput, moving
   laterally.

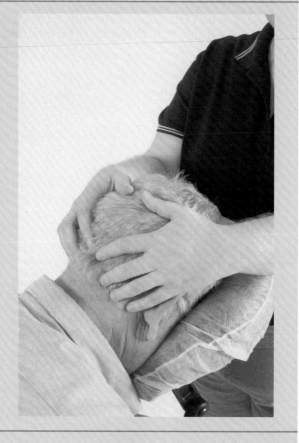

10. Apply brisk effleurage strokes:
    a. Starting at the neck and brushing off the shoulders

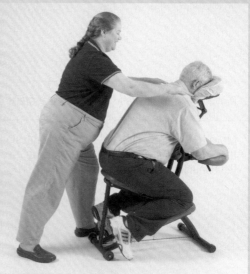

BOX 9-19 **PROCEDURE** Sample Chair Massage Flow
(continued)

b. Starting at the shoulders and brushing down, toward the sacrum

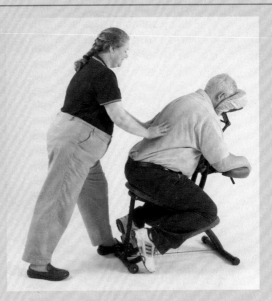

11. Stretch the client's pectoral muscles:
   a. Ask client to sit up and take a deep breath.

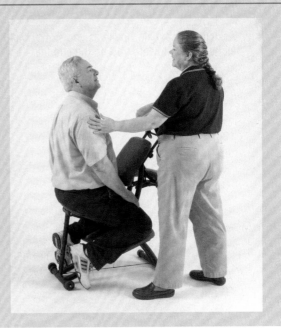

BOX 9-19 **PROCEDURE** Sample Chair Massage Flow (continued)

b. Ask client to place both hands behind the head and inhale slowly.

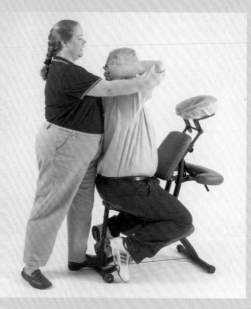

c. Ask client to exhale slowly as you slowly pull the elbows back, toward you, to the end feel.

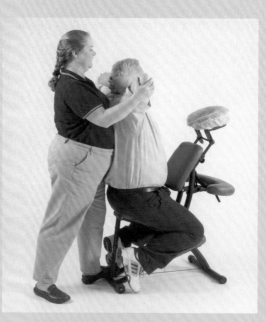

d. Repeat two to three times.

12. Apply a resting stroke to the client's shoulders.

Courtesy of Kathy Latimer, RRT, NCTMB.

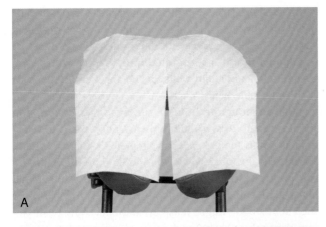

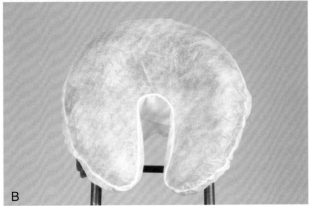

Figure 9-19. Face cradle coverings. **(A)** Paper towel. **(B)** Bouffant cap.

> **Alert**
>
> *Some people are allergic to latex, so be sure to have gloves that are made from a nonlatex material.*

Corporate Chair Accounts

Acquiring an account to provide corporate chair massage may be as simple as contacting local companies, educating them on the benefits of massage, and setting up an initial session for their employees. Corporations can justify the financial cost of massage therapy in the workplace with increased productivity and the ability to attract and retain high-quality employees, and improve employees' health and thereby minimize health insurance premiums. Many hospitals, doctors' offices, pain clinics, regional conference gatherings, and schools provide chair massage.

Corporations and business organizations generally schedule your visits on a weekly or monthly basis with a contractual agreement, and they typically pay you directly, rather than requiring their employees to pay you individually. Make sure that you and the business both understand each other's expectations and accommodations:

- Your time commitment
- Specific location and space you will use
- Length of each appointment
- Appointment scheduling responsibility
- Payment arrangements
- Fee schedule
- Who is responsible for payment
- When payments must be made
- Sound system, or music
- Your parking arrangements
- Missed appointments
- Your tardiness or inability to meet the schedule

If you and the organization establish and clarify these responsibilities at the beginning, you can avoid potential complications and misunderstandings in the future.

Indications and Contraindications for Chair Massage

The indications and contraindications for massage are generally the same as those for chair massage, but there are pain patterns in the lumbar, thoracic, shoulder, and cervical (neck) regions for which chair massage is indicated (Box 9-20).

CHAPTER SUMMARY

A routine massage that strictly follows a given flow applies the same number of strokes in the same order and treats the body parts in the same order for every client. Although a routine is easier in that you do not need to think about what to incorporate into the session, a routine also seriously limits your capability to provide a client-centered massage. Going back to the recipe analogy, people commonly substitute ingredients or alter the directions of a recipe with excellent results. Consider a good cook who can make delicious food without a recipe, using everyday cooking tools and whatever ingredients are in the house. Those creations allow the cook

BOX 9-20
Indications and Contraindications for Chair Massage

Indications
- Cervical
  - Muscle pain and tension
  - Decreased ranges of neck motion
  - Tension headaches
- Shoulder
  - Decreased ranges of shoulder motion
  - Subacute shoulder strain
  - Subacute or chronic shoulder pain and muscle tension
  - Carpal tunnel syndrome
- Thoracic area
  - Pain between scapulae
  - Decreased range of motion of scapula
- Lumbar area
  - Subacute low back strain
  - Decreased flexibility
  - Subacute or chronic low back pain and muscle tension

Contraindications
- Systemic
  - Acute stage of contagious disease
  - Fever
- Local
  - Acute inflammation
  - Swollen lymph glands
  - Acute injuries (24 to 72 hours after injury)
  - Recent surgery (24 to 72 hours after surgery)
  - Open wounds, blisters, burns, and abrasions
  - Bruises/contusions
  - Skin infections
  - Rash

is provided in Table 9-5 to help you evaluate the individual needs of your client and to decide what course of treatment would be most appropriate for him or her. (Please note that this model is also incorporated into chapter exercises in Chapters 10 and 11, and will help you apply critical thinking skills to realistic client scenarios.)

Throughout the flow of the massage session, you should "listen" and respond to the client's tissues, traveling only as fast as the tissues allow. In general, the more tense the muscle, the more slowly you should move. If you move too quickly or with too much pressure, the client might hold his or her breath, the client's body might resist the work, or the client's body might tense up and effectively push you out. When there are any indications that the body is tensing up, you need to adjust your stroke, the pace, or the intention of the massage. You must remain psychologically flexible about the flow instead of approaching your massage with a determined and uncompromising attitude.

By combining techniques and strokes and applying them to different body parts in different orders, you can create thousands of different flows. As a result, therapists often develop their own unique general flow for a massage session. The key to a good massage lies in blending rhythm and pressure with continuity and focused contact. Once you have learned the basic massage strokes and are comfortable applying them, your flow will become natural and effortless.

There will be situations when you are practicing massage that will require you to make modifications to your treatment. Whether a client is coming in for his or her first or fifteenth massage, you must assess your client before every session to know whether there are any health conditions that are local or systemic contraindications. If a client has a systemic contraindication, such as a fever or viral infection, you should reschedule the appointment. You may have to modify the direction or rate of movement, excursion, rhythm, or pressure in response to the current condition of the client's tissues and pain tolerance.

Client comfort and relaxation as well as the long-term success of your practice depend on your use of client positioning, draping, and body mechanics. Once you are adept at simple draping, you can explore adaptations and supplemental draping options with extra blankets, towels, or an additional sheet. It can be an awkward process at first, but with practice, you will develop your own draping techniques. The outcome will be good if the client's comfort level remains your primary intention.

Massage has many physiological benefits, but you must assess your clients before and during treatment to make sure there are no contraindications. You can educate clients about their conditions and how massage might benefit them. Massage that lasts for 10 minutes or longer can improve circulation of blood and lymph, increase the warmth of the tissues, decrease pain, induce the relaxation

to add special ingredients or combine the ingredients in interesting ways to make the dish more successful than a standard recipe. In the same manner, you can make adjustments to a massage flow by tailoring the session to each client with different strokes or techniques. Your artistic combination of strokes and techniques, the speed at which you apply them, and the length of time you keep the client in any one position creates a unique massage every time. Flow can be varied to accommodate your equipment, the client's body position, or the condition of the client's soft tissues. For example, a client who complains of excessive shoulder pain may want you to spend extra time working on the shoulder area with therapeutic techniques. Follow a flow loosely to allow the massage to fit the needs of the client. A critical thinking model

Table 9-5 Critical Thinking Format for Designing a Therapeutic Massage

Review client information	Condition	What current soft tissue or pathological conditions is the client experiencing? • What are the functional limitations associated with this condition? • Is massage indicated or contraindicated for this condition? If contraindicated, refer client to appropriate healthcare professional. (See pathology quick reference in Appendix for specific conditions.) • Has the client undergone any other treatment for this condition? If so, what have the results been? • How long has this condition been present and how long does it typically last?
Interview	Pain	Using open-ended questions and reflective listening, what are the past or present conditions that might be causing pain or compensation patterns (pay attention to nonverbal communication)? • Qualify the pain as sharp, dull, or radiating (radiating pain may indicate nerve involvement and possible referral to another healthcare professional, whereas sharp pain may indicate a recent injury). • Quantify the pain on a scale of 1–10. • Does the pain increase or decrease during the day? • What tends to aggravate or reduce the pain?
	Sleep	If sleep seems to be affected by the condition, compare the client's past sleep patterns with the present: • Bedtime and amount of time it takes to fall asleep • Number of consecutive hours of sleep • Number of times client awakens during the night • Pain/discomfort level upon waking • Anything the client thinks might be affecting sleep
	Hydration	How much water does the client tend to drink during the day? (Insufficient water levels can result in thickened fascia, increasing friction between tissues and increasing pain.)
	Physical activity	What are the client's physical activity habits? • Duration/frequency of physical activity/exercise • Does the client tend to warm up and/or stretch prior to or after exercise? (This is an opportunity to educate clients.) • Does the client tend to increase water consumption following exercise?
Assessment	Determine which muscles are involved	What movements are involved, causing pain or are restricted? • Consulting the special muscle section in Chapter 4, what muscles are involved in the movement(s)? • Consulting Table 10-1, what are the antagonists to the involved muscles? • Consulting Box 7-2, identify any compensation patterns.
	Determine which areas to treat	Given the muscles involved and compensation patterns revealed, choose only two or three areas to address (to minimize the body's recovery after treatment). • Avoid treating areas that elicit pain upon passive contraction (outside the scope of practice).

continues on following page

Table 9-5 Critical Thinking Format for Designing a Therapeutic Massage *continued*

	Goals	Based on the client's input, the physician diagnosis and treatment, and massage therapy assessment, what are some appropriate short-term and long-term goals?
Design the massage	Determine techniques to use during the massage	Consider the history, interview, and assessment to decide which techniques to use: • If the client's goal is general relaxation, and massage is not contraindicated, use one or a combination of the basic massage strokes. • Clients who rub or knead their shoulder when describing shoulder pain might respond well to effleurage and petrissage on the shoulder. • A client with chest congestion might benefit from tapotement on the upper back area. • Friction can be beneficial for scar tissue and fascial adhesions. • People involved in sports tend to respond well to proprioceptive neuromuscular facilitation techniques. • Long-term conditions and compensation patterns may have fascial restrictions that can benefit from myofascial work. • A hypertonic area that refers pain and may have been activated by overuse may respond well to trigger point work.
	Treatment adaptation	Are there any adaptations that should be made to a standard massage flow? • Are there any conditions that require positioning or bolstering considerations (pain, sinus congestion, low back pain)? • Are there any local contraindications that you must avoid during the massage? • Are there any sensitivities or allergies to consider? • Does the client have any special needs such as assistance on or off the table (visual impairment, physical impairment)?

response, decrease muscular tension, and normalize the activity of the nervous system.

Practice massage strokes and flows and get constructive feedback as you learn. Receive massage from others; it helps you understand how much one person's touch differs from another's. By experiencing different therapists' flows, you will also understand how a flow can influence the response to the massage. The basic techniques are much more effective when applied appropriately. With a lot of experience, the distinct differences between the individual strokes become less defined. For instance, you could be applying an effleurage stroke when you come across a fascial restriction, and instantly turn the effleurage stroke into a compression stroke. The compression may lead you into an application of vibration or any one of the therapeutic techniques. As you get more comfortable with applying the different strokes and knowing when to use them, they will run together and your massage will become more fluid and efficient.

CHAPTER EXERCISES

1. Describe the following terms:

   a. Laterally recumbent

   b. Prone

   c. Supine

2. Practice client positioning with a fully clothed partner on the massage table in the prone, supine, and side-lying positions, with and without a face cradle, and with and without the following bolsters:

   a. Neck (prone, supine, and side-lying)

   b. Chest (prone)

   c. Pelvis (prone)

   d. Ankles (prone)

e. Knees (supine)

f. Top leg (side-lying)

g. Along the length of the back (side-lying)

3. Practice draping with a partner on the massage table (the partner should be undressed and underneath the drape) to expose different areas of the body:

a. Prone position—back, leg, foot, arm

b. Supine position—arm, upper chest, abdomen, leg, foot

c. Side-lying position—back, top arm, top leg, bottom leg

4. Practice helping undressed clients on and off the massage table, maintaining modesty by keeping them covered with the drape.

5. There are circumstances for which certain client positions are recommended. Identify at least two reasons to put a client in each of the three positions: prone, supine, and side-lying.

6. Name the two primary reasons for draping clients during a massage.

7. Explain the importance of grounding and centering before a massage session.

8. Lead a partner through diaphragmatic breathing by describing the process of taking a deep breath using the diaphragm.

9. Explain the purpose of using a resting stroke.

10. List and describe the six basic massage strokes.

11. Practice each of the six strokes on a partner. Ask your partner to watch your shoulder, elbow, wrist, and hand as well as your head-to-heel line while you apply the strokes. Ask your partner to let you know if any part of your arm looks tight and tense or if you have abandoned the head-to-heel line.

12. Describe the difference between superficial and deep effleurage.

13. Describe at least one effect of each basic massage stroke:

a. Compression

b. Effleurage

c. Petrissage

d. Tapotement

e. Friction

f. Vibration

14. Describe the benefits of using joint movement during a massage session.

15. Write a flow for a relaxation massage, including step-by-step instructions for client positioning, bolstering, draping and redraping of specific areas of the body, and specific strokes and techniques.

REFERENCES

1. Russell WR. Percussion and vibration. In: Licht S, ed. *Massage, Manipulation and Traction.* Huntington, NY: Robert E. Krieger Publishing, 1976.

SUGGESTED READINGS

Aslani M. *Massage for Beginners.* New York: Carroll & Brown, 1997.

Bruder L. Navigating the pathway to phenomenal touch: 10 steps to transform your massage. *Massage Magazine* 2002: March–April.

Claire T. *Bodywork: What Type of Massage to Get—and How to Make the Most of It.* New York: William Morrow, 1995.

Cyriax JH. Clinical applications of massage. In: Licht S, ed. *Massage, Manipulation and Traction.* Huntington, NY: Robert E. Krieger Publishing, 1976.

David S. Benefits of massage therapy should not be overlooked. *Am J Hosp Palliat Care.* 2005;22:257–258.

DeVane CL. *Substance P: A New Era, A New Role.* http://fmscommunity.org/subp.htm, accessed 9.2.03.

Dickson FD. *Posture: Its Relation to Health.* Philadelphia: JB Lippincott, 1930.

Françon F. Classical massage technique. In: Licht S, ed. *Massage, Manipulation and Traction.* Huntington, NY: Robert E. Krieger Publishing, 1976.

Frye B. *Body Mechanics for Manual Therapists: A Functional Approach to Self-Care and Injury Prevention.* Seattle, WA: Consolidated Press, 2000.

Greenman PE. *Principles of Manual Medicine.* 3rd ed. Philadelphia: Lippincott Williams & Wilkins, 2003.

Kellogg JH. *The Art of Massage.* Reprinted. Mokelumne Hill, CA: Health Research, 1975.

Latchaw M, Egstrom G. *Human Movement with Concepts Applied to Children's Movement Activities.* Englewood Cliffs, NJ: Prentice-Hall, 1969.

Licht S. Mechanical methods of massage. In: Licht S, ed. *Massage, Manipulation and Traction.* Huntington, NY: Robert E. Krieger Publishing, 1976.

Lidell L, Thomas S, Cooke CB, et al. *The Book of Massage.* New York: Simon & Schuster, 1984.

Lindsey R, Jones BJ, Whitley A. *Body Mechanics, Posture, Figure and Fitness.* 4th ed. Dubuque, IA: Wm. C. Brown, 1979.

Maxwell-Hudson C. *Complete Massage.* New York: Dorling Kindersley, 2001.

Rattray F, Ludwig L. *Clinical Massage Therapy: Understanding, Assessing and Treating over 70 Conditions.* Toronto, Ontario: Talus Incorporated, 2006.

Russell WR. Percussion and vibration. In: Licht S, ed. *Massage, Manipulation and Traction.* Huntington, NY: Robert E. Krieger Publishing, 1976.

Seedor MM. *Body Mechanics and Patient Positioning.* New York: Teachers College Press, 1977.

Souriau P. *The Aesthetics of Movement.* Amherst, MA: The University of Massachusetts Press, 1983.

Stephens R. *Therapeutic Chair Massage.* Baltimore: Lippincott Williams & Wilkins, 2006.

Stryer L. *Biochemistry*. 2nd ed. New York: WH Freeman, 1981.

Trager M, Hamond C. *Movement as a Way to Agelessness: A Guide to Trager Mentastics*. Barrytown, NY: Station Hill Press, 1995.

Wakim KG. Physiologic effects of massage. In: Licht S, ed. *Massage, Manipulation and Traction*. Huntington, NY: Robert E. Krieger Publishing, 1976.

Werner R. *A Massage Therapist's Guide to Pathology*. 3rd ed. Baltimore: Lippincott Williams & Wilkins, 2005.

http://members.aol.com/thelucid1/Page12.html, accessed 3.5.06.

http://music.osu.edu/Ethnomus/EMW/EntrainNetwork.html, accessed 3.5.06.

http://stress.about.com/cs/relaxation/a/aa090900_p.htm, accessed 3.5.06.

http://www.cochrane.org/colloquia/abstracts/amsterdam/Amsterdam97P229.htm, accessed 3.5.06.

http://www.harcourt-international.com/journals/jbmt/, accessed 3.5.06.

http://www.holistic-online.com/massage/mas_home.htm, accessed 3.5.06.

http://www.icnr.com/articles/thenatureofstress.html, accessed 3.5.06.

http://www.increasebrainpower.com/brain-wave-entrainment.html, accessed 3.5.06.

http://www.magazine.ucla.edu/year1997/fall97_01_3.html, accessed 3.5.06.

http://www.massage-research.com/blog/?p=520, accessed 12.30.11.

https://www.mhn.com/static/pdfs/Details_Evolving_Theory_Pain_Mgt.pdf, accessed 3.5.06.

http://www.miami.edu/touch-research/references.html, accessed 3.5.06.

http://www.ncbi.nlm.nih.gov/pubmed/19283590, accessed 12.29.11.

http://www.ncbi.nlm.nih.gov/pubmed/19888909, accessed 12.29.11.

http://www.ncbi.nlm.nih.gov/pubmed?term=15788892, accessed 4.5.12.

http://www.nu.ac.za/undphil/collier/papers/20140.pdf, accessed 3.5.06.

http://www.nursingtimes.net/nursing-practice/clinical-specialisms/continence/does-abdominal-massage-relieve-constipation/5027718.article, accessed 12.30.11.

http://www.painbustersclinic.com.au/causes-pain/gate-control-theory.htm, accessed 3.5.06.

http://www.painezer.com/info/gatecontrol.html, accessed 3.5.06.

http://www.phas.ubc.ca/berciu/TEACHING/PHYS349/alex.pdf, accessed 3.5.06.

http://www.rmtao.com/home, accessed 4.5.12.

http://www.scienceofmassage.com/dnn/som/journal/1107/therapeutic.aspx, accessed 12.29.11.

http://www.scientificacupuncture.com/modernresearch/scientifictheory.htm, accessed 3.5.06.

http://www.soundfeelings.com/products/alternative_medicine/music_therapy/entrainment.htm, accessed 3.5.06.

http://www.transparentcorp.com/products/np/brainwaves.php, accessed 3.5.06.

http://www.transparentcorp.com/products/np/entrainment.php, accessed 3.5.06.

http://www.whonamedit.com/doctor.cfm/2538.html, accessed 3.5.06.

Therapeutic Applications

Objectives

Upon completion of this chapter, the student will be able to:

- Describe what happens in each of the three phases of healing
- Explain the three stages of the pain cycle
- Identify the four signs of inflammation
- Explain the difference between lengthening and stretching
- Name the three types of circulatory enhancement massage

- Describe at least three ways to enhance the flow of lymph
- Name and locate the major lymphatic ducts on an illustration of the skeleton
- Correctly perform at least three proprioceptive neuromuscular facilitation techniques on a partner
- Correctly perform at least one connective tissue technique
- Correctly perform at least one trigger point release technique

Key Terms

Direct manipulation (DM): A proprioceptive neuromuscular facilitation (PNF) technique in which you use the muscle spindles and Golgi tendon organs to relax a hypertonic muscle.

Direction of restriction: The direction in which tissues resist movement the most.

Hypertonic (HAHY-per-TAHN-ik): Excessively tense or tight.

Lengthening: The neurological process that lengthens myofibrils and results in a longer muscle.

Lymph: The fluid that started out as blood plasma, leaked out through the capillaries to become interstitial fluid, and is picked up by the very delicate ends of the lymphatic vessels from tissues all over the body.

Muscle energy techniques (METs): Bodywork applications that use the nervous system to change a

muscle's resting length, also called proprioceptive neuromuscular facilitation.

Muscle guarding: Hypertonic muscles stabilizing or splinting an injured area.

Positional release (PR): A PNF technique that relieves hypertonicity by holding the body in a painless position and waiting for the nervous system to trigger relaxation, also called strain/counterstrain.

Post-isometric relaxation (PIR): A PNF technique that uses active contraction and relaxation of the target muscle to lengthen the muscle.

Proprioceptive neuromuscular facilitation (PROH-pree-oh-SEP-tive NOO-roh-MUSS-kyoo-lar fah-SIHL-ih-TAY-shun) (PNF): Bodywork applications that use the nervous system to change a muscle's resting length, also called muscle energy techniques.

Reciprocal inhibition (RI): A PNF technique in which the client contracts a target muscle's antagonists to reflexively relax the target muscle.

Resting length: The length to which a relaxed, inactive muscle can be safely extended.

Right lymphatic duct: A major drain that collects all of the lymph from the upper right quadrant of the body, including everything on the right side of the body above the diaphragm, and empties it into the right subclavian vein.

Strain/counterstrain (SCS): A PNF technique that relieves hypertonicity by holding the body in a painless position and waiting for the nervous system to trigger relaxation, also called positional release.

Stretching: An elastic deformation of the fascia that extends its length.

Target muscle: The muscle being treated in a therapeutic technique.

Tender point: A small, painful area of hypertonicity, also called a tender spot.

Thoracic duct: A major drain that collects the lymph from everywhere in the body, except the right side of the head and thorax, and empties it into the left subclavian vein.

Trigger point (TrP): A localized area of hypertonicity at the motor end unit, or neuromuscular junction, that refers symptoms to other areas of the body.

Unwinding (myofascial unwinding): The process in which soft tissues move in different directions, circles, or wavy lines as the collagen fibers change shape and the fascia softens.

This chapter focuses on therapeutic and rehabilitative massage applications. In addition to providing the general benefits of the basic massage strokes such as relaxation, pain relief, enhanced circulation, and decreased muscular tension, therapeutic applications treat soft tissue conditions more efficiently. Clients often complain of tightness in a particular muscle, a "knot" or localized area of tight muscle tissue, pain or discomfort in a specific muscle, restricted movement, and specific soft tissue injuries. By understanding the body's tissue repair mechanism, you will know how to prevent further injury to the area and you will appreciate how massage promotes the healing process.

There are principles for applying therapeutic techniques that can maximize the efficiency of your work. It makes sense to want to work with the body rather than against it, but sometimes that means you accentuate the client's problem before you resolve it. Second, you must incorporate both lengthening and stretching of soft tissues into therapeutic massage because without both, the results of the massage could be short lived. If your treatment does not improve their condition, clients can lose interest or question your skills.

Four main categories of therapeutic applications are introduced in this chapter: circulatory enhancement, neuromuscular techniques, myofascial techniques, and trigger point (TrP) techniques. Circulatory enhancement is a way of using massage techniques to mechanically manipulate the flow of blood and lymph. Neuromuscular techniques utilize the nervous system to create reflexive changes in the length of muscles. Myofascial techniques concentrate on manipulating the fascia in and around the muscles, mechanically changing the shape or structure of the muscles and other soft tissues. TrPs, localized areas of hypertonicity that occur at the neuromuscular junction, can be treated with both mechanical and reflexive techniques.

Another difference between wellness massage and therapeutic massage is the depth of the treatment plan. Sometimes therapeutic massage is referred to as treatment-oriented massage. For professional consistency, include a treatment plan for all of your clients, but when clients are looking for specific results for a particular condition, incorporate more details in your plan for future treatment. Specify the duration and frequency of future sessions, suggested techniques, client likes and dislikes, self-help suggestions, and, when appropriate, professional healthcare referrals. With all of the specific information in a therapeutic treatment plan, a standard SOAP note or other medical charting method is more appropriate than a shortened health form or history form.

Therapeutic techniques are nothing more than the basic massage strokes. Compression, effleurage, petrissage, tapotement, friction, joint movements, palpation skills, and the principles of proper body mechanics are your foundations for therapeutic applications.

Mechanisms of Injury and Tissue Repair

When tissues are injured, the body automatically repairs the damage with regeneration, the process of replacing destroyed cells, and with fibrosis, the production of fibrous connective tissue (CT). Bones, epidermis, and mucous membranes can successfully regenerate and be repaired with CT. Muscle cells and nerve cells, however, cannot be replaced. Injured muscle tissues and nervous tissues can only be repaired with CT. The extent to which any given tissue undergoes regeneration or fibrosis depends on the types of cells, the severity of the injury, and the local supply of blood via the circulatory vessels. The healing process occurs in three physiological phases, as described below for a typical skin wound. In phase I, the bleeding stops and inflammation occurs. During phase II, tissue regeneration occurs, if possible, and in phase III, the remodeling of tissues is completed. **While each phase is described with its approximate duration, it is important to understand that the phases are not mutually exclusive and may overlap as the body heals the injury.**

Healing: Phase I

When tissues are torn, the first phase of injury repair begins immediately and usually lasts a few days. Phase I is also known as the inflammatory phase, as it involves inflammation. The process starts with hemostasis (HEE-moh-STAY-sis), which forms a blood clot and stops the bleeding. Inflammation occurs next, flooding the area with oxygen-rich blood and neutrophils and constructing a framework for tissue repair. Finally, macrophages, attracted by the neutrophils, help digest and eliminate debris and then attract fibroblasts to synthesize collagen fibers.

Hemostasis

The body's first line of defense to tissue injury is hemostasis, an automatic response to stop blood loss. As discussed in the cardiovascular system section of Chapter 3, the process of hemostasis starts when the blood vessels within a tissue are injured. Blood platelets that contact the injured tissue burst open, releasing chemicals that:

1. Attract more platelets to the area. The platelets clump together to form a platelet plug or clot to seal the hole in the blood vessel.

2. Convert fibrinogen, a protein suspended in the blood, into strands of fibrin, which tangle together at the injury site. As circulation continues, red blood cells and platelets are caught in the tangle, further reducing blood flow in the area. Leukocytes, which remove cellular debris and fight infection, also get caught.

3. Cause the blood vessels to narrow, resulting in localized vasoconstriction (VAY-zoh-kuhn-STRIHK-shun) that restricts blood flow to the area.

As the platelet plug shrinks, the fibrin strands contract and pull the edges of the wound together to provide a framework for tissue repair.

Inflammation

After blood loss has been stopped, inflammation occurs, increasing circulation to the injured area, preventing further damage to the injured area and the immediate surroundings, and setting the stage for repair processes. **Without inflammation, healing will not occur.** After hemostasis, inflammation is the body's second line of defense and can be identified by the following characteristics:

- Redness
- Swelling
- Heat
- Pain

Chemicals in the blood cause vasodilation (VAY-zoh-dahy-LAY-shun); the blood vessels widen and flood the area with red blood cells that carry oxygen and white blood cells that fight infection. The increased amount of blood circulating through the area increases the temperature of the skin and creates redness in the area that is healing. Increased circulation transports platelets, red and white blood cells, macrophages, and proteins to the area.

The capillaries become thinner and leaky, allowing extra interstitial fluid to seep into the surrounding tissues as lymph. The resultant edema (eh-DEE-muh), or swelling, puts extra pressure on the nerves, causing pain. When persons experience swelling and pain, the natural response is to minimize movement of that area or minimize any movements that increase the pain. Not only does reduced movement prevent further damage to the original injury, but it also keeps the surrounding areas from being flooded with the chemicals that induce vasodilation and leaky capillaries.

Phagocytosis

Swelling restricts circulation, and the body's third line of defense, the immune response, is activated. The increased temperature of the area amplifies chemical reactions for increased immune activity that destroys pathogens and that breaks down cellular debris. Neutrophils, which are special white blood cells, pass through the capillaries more easily to destroy any pathogens that might have entered the wound. Neutrophils attract even more leukocytes to the area. Macrophages gravitate toward the neutrophils to destroy and digest cellular debris and pathogens.

Finally, fibrin protein strands tangle together at the injury site and trap other blood cells with a platelet plug, further decreasing blood flow and blood loss. The platelet plug, or scab, shrinks and pulls the edges of the wound together, creating a framework for tissue repair.

Inflammation subsides, leading to the next phase of the healing mechanism. Since the many factors of a person's healing environment influence the speed at which the body accomplishes each phase of healing, phase I can last anywhere from 2 days to 3 weeks.

Healing: Phase II

The second phase of healing, also called the proliferation phase, typically begins 2 to 3 days after the injury and lasts about 6 weeks. During this process, many new blood vessels and capillaries develop, bringing nutritious, oxygenated blood to the area. The macrophages continue to remove damaged tissue, pathogens, and other cellular debris, and they attract fibroblasts, which serve as precursors for collagen fibers. The first strands of collagen are laid down randomly, forming a tangled web of fibers that serves as the foundation for replacement tissues.

Fibroblasts continue to migrate across the injury to provide the collagen framework for replacement tissue. Once the fibroblasts have covered the entire wound and epithelial cells have grown into the framework to create a layer of epithelial tissue, tension gradually pulls the edges of the wound together.

When the cells cannot be regenerated, as occurs with nervous and muscle tissue, only CT is produced. When a lot of fibrous CT is deposited without the appropriate replacement cells, the result is scar tissue. The problem with scar tissue is that as it is laid down, it can attach to overlying tissues. These CT adhesions, or fascial restrictions, can interfere with normal function of the tissue. **A fascial restriction in one area of the body can restrict movement in other parts of the body, depending on how long the restriction has existed.** Massage therapists *must* understand the development of scar tissue because of its impact on muscle tissues and skeletal movement.

Healing: Phase III

The third phase of healing, also called the remodeling phase, starts about 6 weeks after the original injury, and it can last a year or longer. The collagen fibers that were laid down in the previous stages of healing are steadily replaced with another, more organized form of collagen. The blood vessels that developed during phase II are no longer necessary, and little by little, they break down. As they recede, the scar loses some of its redness.

Remodeling is a dynamic process in which the replacement tissue gradually gains tensile strength and the collagen

fibers can be rearranged until they are aligned like the fibers of the surrounding tissue. You must understand this process because muscle tissue is repaired primarily with collagen and CT. During this phase, you must use either active and passive ranges of motion without weights or electrical stimulation to keep the collagen fibers from adhering to surrounding tissues.

> ### Alert
> *Using weights or electric stimulation is generally not in the scope of practice for a massage therapist; however, the client may be under concurrent treatment with another healthcare professional. You must know what kind of treatment is being administered so you do not overtreat the client.*

As long as the scar remains mobile, the fibers can still be realigned. Gentle movement of the healing muscle tissues also encourages the collagen fibers into the same alignment as the original muscle fibers. This functional linear alignment provides greater strength and flexibility to the healing tissue. Without mobility, the repair process can result in tough, nonelastic scar tissue that is more easily reinjured.

The permanence of scars depends on the individual's healing capacity as well as the kind of movement the scar is subjected to. Several factors can increase or decrease the effectiveness of the body's natural healing mechanism:

- Injury—the extent and location of tissue damage
- Client—time lapse before treatment, general health, smoking habit, age, prior injuries, cooperation with self-help suggestions, nutrition, amount of rest/sleep, stress levels
- Treatment—improper self-care, inactivity, excessive activity, medicine, therapeutic interactions

Because the tissue repair process requires additional resources from the body, adequate amounts of rest, hydration, nutritional protein, and vitamins are necessary to facilitate healing. For example, vitamin C is needed for fibroblasts to be converted into collagen fibers, which is why vitamin C is so critical to health and healing. The speed of healing varies with the individual's age, health, nutrition, emotional and environmental stressors, and self-care. Massage can facilitate the healing process by restoring movement, creating functional scar tissue, and increasing the circulation of blood and lymph, which delivers nutrients and removes waste from the cells and tissues.

Pain

One of the primary reasons people seek massage therapy is in response to pain that resulted from illness, emotional or muscle tension, injury, or repetitive motion. In practical terms, pain is a subjective and sensory perception that something is wrong in the body. More specifically, pain is a complex feedback mechanism that involves receptors in the skin and soft tissue called nociceptors. The nociceptors receive information from the skin and soft tissue, send it to the spinal cord and brain, and the person perceives pain. The speed of transmission varies according to the severity of the malady and the health of the body. For example, if the person experiences severe injury or trauma, the impulses usually travel rapidly. On the other hand, if the trauma is mild or tension has built up over time, the impulses travel more slowly. Repetition of the transmissions will also affect the experience of pain in the body. **The physiologic law of facilitation states that when impulses pass through the same set of nerves, those signals will tend to take that same path on future transmissions.** This explains the tendency of the body to experience pain in the same place when the body is under increased stress or tension. It also explains why receiving regular massage helps the body relax.

One of the effects of massage is a reduction in actual or perceived pain. In 1965, Melzack and Wall's research found that before pain impulses reach the brain, they must pass through a "gate" in order to be recognized. If the gate is open, the impulses reach the brain and pain is perceived. The gate opens if the nerve fibers detect pain from the impulses transmitted from the nociceptors, and closes when the larger fibers that detect light touch, temperature, and pressure are activated (see earlier Box 9-6, on the Gate Control Theory of pain). Simply, the light touch or slow, sustained pressure of massage will interrupt the impulses and close the gate, resulting in a diminished perception of pain.

While it is out of your scope of practice to diagnose or treat emotional conditions, it is important to keep in mind that pain or other symptoms may result from or be enhanced by emotional tension. It is important to take formal notes regarding what type of pain clients are experiencing as well as how long they have had it, and reassess from session to session so you can adjust your techniques accordingly. If the client is experiencing acute or severe symptoms, you may use lighter techniques. Conversely, if the client is experiencing chronic symptoms, you may want to try using deeper pressure techniques. Both light and deep techniques will interrupt the pain impulses. Generally, if the client has an acute condition, it will take a few sessions

to resolve; if the condition is severe or chronic, it will take more sessions. Understanding the client's pain will help you recommend appropriate further treatment.

Pain–Spasm Cycle

Pain can occur in a vicious circle that involves the muscles and circulation. A **hypertonic** (HAHY-per-TAHN-ik) muscle is an excessively tight muscle. Hypertonicity results when many of the muscle's individual muscle cells remain in a contracted, shortened state and do not relax, even when the muscle is inactive. Even when a hypertonic muscle is relaxed, it has a shorter **resting length**, or the length to which a relaxed, inactive muscle can be extended, because so many of its muscle cells are shortened. Like a spring that has been wound tighter and gets shorter, a muscle that becomes hypertonic develops a shorter resting length. The myofibrils within a muscle cell are tightly packed together, reducing circulation within a hypertonic muscle. **Insufficient oxygen supply can result in pain, discomfort, compensation patterns, and restricted functional movement.** Restricted movement then leads to reduced circulation, reducing the amount of oxygen available to cells, and so on. This is an interconnected pattern called the pain–spasm cycle, also known as the pain cycle (see earlier Fig. 5-4):

1. Pain causes a person to tense up, resulting in hypertonicity.

2. Hypertonicity causes decreased movement and also reduces local circulation of oxygen and other nutrients.

3. Reduced amounts of oxygen, or ischemia, can cause tissue degeneration and pain, returning the person to step 1.

A variation of this cycle begins with an injury. The body responds to an injury by minimizing movement of the injured area in an effort to minimize pain. The decreased activity requires less oxygen and nutrition, so local circulation is reduced. Nerve impingement may occur as well. When the blood supply to a localized area is insufficient, the supply of oxygen is decreased. The condition, called ischemia (iss-KEE-mee-uh), prevents efficient healing of an injury and causes more pain. **Without oxygen, cells suffer and eventually die.** The resulting pain often causes a person to tense up or reduce movement of the injured area, and the cycle keeps repeating.

Being caught in the pain cycle can have significant effects, such as muscle imbalance, joint stress, muscular and skeletal compensation patterns, chronic ischemia, and tissue degeneration. Fortunately, the cycle can be broken anywhere along the way, using several different methods of intervention. The first step is to recognize this pattern and intervene to break it. Then, methods involving pain reduction, increased circulation, and increased exercise and stretching can all help break the cycle. Massage can relieve pain, reduce hypertonicity, and increase circulation. Better yet, specific therapeutic massage techniques can reflexively trigger the shortened muscles to lengthen.

Principles of Therapeutic Techniques

Sometimes called rehabilitative or treatment-oriented massage, therapeutic massage is based on the assessment, palpation, and treatment of specific injuries or compensation patterns in soft tissue structures of the body with therapeutic techniques. When using a therapeutic technique to change the length of a muscle, the muscle you are addressing is called the target muscle. In other words, if a client complains of pain and tension in the calf, one of your target muscles is the gastrocnemius, and you could apply one or more therapeutic techniques to relax and lengthen it. Applications of therapeutic techniques are based on the core principles listed in Box 10-1. The pain and swelling that occur in the process of injury repair can develop into a compensation pattern. To protect itself from further injury, the body sometimes develops muscle guarding to stabilize or splint the injured area with hypertonic muscles. The decreased mobility is exaggerated further when people hold their body in positions that ease the pain and/or avoid moving a body part that hurts. The combination of the muscle guarding, reduced mobility, and abnormal positions people hold their bodies in to correct an imbalance or protect a primary dysfunction or injury is called a compensation pattern. In the third phase of injury repair, the client's compensation patterns or movements can establish nerve tracks that cause those unnatural positions to develop into a bad habit.

When a client has developed compensation patterns because of an injury, always be aware of tissue resistance and acceptance. The longer a person has held the pattern, the more it will resist change. If your technique exceeds the tissue's tolerance, the client's body may react adversely by increasing the muscle guarding, which reinforces the compensation patterns and can cause further injury. Use good body mechanics, including the proper leaning technique, to avoid pushing into tissues that are resistant, so you can better follow the tissue's lead. With practice, you will be able to feel the difference between when tissues are resistant and when the client's tissues soften up to allow deeper or more invasive work.

Treating soft tissue injuries and compensation patterns is like peeling the layers of an onion. You begin treatment with the outside layer, making necessary changes and adjustments according to the client's condition. Then move, layer by layer, to the core, treating tissue layers appropriately along the way and encouraging the body to restore itself to its most functional state. Go slowly, pay attention to the tissue's resistance, and wait for tissues to accept your work. This allows the client's tissues to lead the treatment.

Following the tissues' lead is not the only way to use massage therapy, but it will help you work with the body instead of against it, using an approach that is gentle instead of forced. The technique that uses the least energy from both client and therapist is more effective than one that uses more energy and creates more pain.

Several other principles, some of which may seem illogical, are equally important. **Too often, when it comes to massage treatment, people think that more is better. In reality, more is usually not better; more treatment can create more inflammation, more injury, or more compensation. Follow the principle that less is more.** Slowly and carefully palpate tissues

---

BOX 10-1
Principles of Therapeutic Massage

- Respect the client and the client's body.
- Work within the client's tolerance.
- Follow the tissue's lead.
- SLOW DOWN . . . and wait for the tissues to respond.
- Less is more.
- Overtreating can be worse than not treating at all.
- Sometimes the lightest work can create the deepest effect.
- Massage is essentially the application of pressure moving across the skin.

to make your way through "the layers of the onion" with the appropriate amount of treatment to facilitate healing and restore normal structure and function. Overtreatment is not optimal, and the same is true for undertreatment. Always remember that each client is unique and that a technique that was effective for one client with a particular condition may not work on another with the same condition.

Another concept to keep in mind is the antagonistic activity of muscles and muscle groups. To create movement, one group of muscles contracts and gets shorter while the antagonistic muscles relax and get longer. If there is a restriction in either muscle or muscle group that prevents a length change, movement will be limited in varying degrees. Both lengthening and stretching are critical to therapeutic massage, and although the terms are mistakenly interchanged, they are very different techniques with very different results. This is explained in detail later in this section.

Fascia

It is important to understand that when movement occurs, the whole body is involved via the seamless web of CT called fascia. Fascia is pervasive, wrapping around and running between all the organs, muscles, and layers of tissue. (See earlier Fig. 3-17 of deep fascia surrounding muscle.) Its tough, pliable, plastic structure forms a sort of spider web throughout the body that functions as a support, protection, and communication network within the body. As it receives input from physical pressure or stressors, the fascia responds and remodels itself. The protein fibers in fascia can get crumpled, kinked, or stuck together, making it difficult for muscle fibers to slide back and forth for smooth contraction and movement. These **fascial adhesions**, also called **fascial restrictions**, are disruptions in the smooth fascia that can result from:

- Insufficient hydration
- Injury
- Accumulated scar tissue
- Tissue dehydration
- Repetitive motions
- Sustained positions
- Postural deviations

In addition to the local restrictions and tightness, fascial adhesions have far-reaching effects on other soft tissues because of the intertwined three-dimensionality of fascia.

It is particularly important for massage therapists to understand fascial adhesions because fascia's involvement with muscle tissues can cause the location of your clients' pain to differ from where the pain originates. In concrete terms, fascia

is much like a sheet of plastic wrap. When a sheet of plastic wrap is pulled on at one corner, the tension creates deformities that extend across the plastic in lines. When a section in the middle of a sheet of plastic is crumpled, it creates several lines of tension that radiate out from the crumpled area. If there is a local restriction in the muscle and soft tissues, there will be similar lines of tension called fascial lines that extend out to other areas of the body. (Earlier Fig. 7-1 illustrates lines of tension that reach out from a restriction to other areas, similar to the way a fascial adhesion can pull on structures far away.) Restricted movement, compensation patterns, reduced circulation, muscular tension, and pain in seemingly unrelated areas can all result from fascial tension. Generally, the longer the restriction exists, the more the fascia will be deformed and the longer it will take for the client's tissues to return to normal. The length of time the pain and restriction have existed, in addition to stress factors and client participation, will determine the best treatment techniques and the amount of time it could take to "unwind" the restriction.

Direction of Ease

The direction of ease concept can be applied to massage by working with the body instead of against it. If you accentuate a compensation pattern and then slowly lead the client's body out of the compromised position, you are working in the direction of ease. For example, a client's right sternocleidomastoid muscle could be hypertonic, giving the client a stiff neck that is slightly flexed and slightly rotated to the right. To relax and lengthen the sternocleidomastoid muscle, you can move in the direction of ease by first shortening the muscle even further with a passive contraction that increases the client's neck flexion and rotation to the right. Accentuating the body's compensation pattern usually reduces the pain. By assuming the position slowly and safely without endangering the tissues, the nervous system perceives no threat or danger and can neurologically allow the sternocleidomastoid muscle to relax.

The following is a different example of using the direction of ease in therapeutic massage, illustrating how to work with the body rather than against it. A client who has right shoulder pain may find it uncomfortable to flex the right shoulder. Your assessment determines that the coracobrachialis muscle, which is partially responsible for flexing the shoulder, is hypertonic. To treat it, you want to put the coracobrachialis into passive contraction, but flexion is painful for the client. Rather than making the client uncomfortable by moving the shoulder directly into flexion, you can work in the direction of ease and position the coracobrachialis in a passive contraction from a different, less painful direction. You could try abducting the shoulder to bring the client's arm overhead, and then lower the client's arm to the position of passive contraction of the coracobrachialis.

Lengthening and Stretching

You must understand the difference between lengthening and stretching in treatment-oriented massage. These are two very distinct and different mechanisms and involve different structures. Lengthening, the technical term for muscle relaxation, is a neurological process that elongates myofibrils and results in a longer muscle. Stretching is an elastic deformation of the fascia that extends its length. When muscles are stretched, the elastic CTs in and around the muscle cells are pulled into a longer form. As with a rubber band, though, the stretch is temporary, and the resting length of those muscles is basically unchanged. Both lengthening of the muscle and stretching of the fascia must be accomplished to create an effective and lasting change in muscle length.

Lengthening

Each muscle has a normal resting length. When it is too short or too long, there is an imbalance that leads to dysfunction. The resting length can be shortened actively with excessive, repetitive, or atypical kinds of muscular activity. The resting length can also be shortened passively if the muscle is held in a contracted state for an extended time. For example, a person who sits for long periods is putting the psoas major in passive contraction. Eventually, the psoas major will have a shorter resting length, which may cause low back pain and other symptoms.

With the appropriate techniques, the muscle's resting length can be reset through the body's neurological system. Lengthening restores a muscle to its normal resting length or to the most functional resting length for the individual client. Simply, lengthening is a true, neurological relaxation of the muscle.

Stretching

The elastin proteins in soft tissues allow soft tissues to be stretched without being torn, but the elasticity also returns those tissues to their original length. A stretch pulls the fascia, the muscles, and their tendinous attachments. A stretch does not change the resting length of a muscle, but once a muscle has been neurologically lengthened, a stretch can help maintain the new length, increase flexibility, and enhance the fluidity of movement. The proprioceptors that sense tension in the muscle or tendons can trigger the stretch reflex, which is a protective muscle contraction that occurs when the tissues are stretched too far and/or too fast. The stretch reflex defeats the purpose of a stretch and can even put the muscle farther into spasm. The tendon reflex, on the other hand, is triggered when the proprioceptors sense a slow, gradual, sustained stretch at the musculotendinous junction. When a stretch does not threaten the muscle's integrity, the nervous system responds by allowing the muscle to relax and lengthen. Therefore, it is recommended that stretches be performed slowly and gradually rather than quickly or with a bouncing action, and that stretches be held for at least 5 to 10 seconds to achieve the tendon reflex.

The concept of lengthening and stretching can be likened to a loaf of bread (the muscle) in a plastic bag (the fascia). The individual pieces of the loaf of bread are like the myofibrils of the entire muscle. When myofibrils are lengthened, the entire muscle becomes longer than it used to be, just as thicker pieces of bread make a longer loaf. Fitting the longer loaf into its old, short bag would require "squishing" the bread into a shorter loaf. But if the longer loaf is put into a bag that has been stretched, it could retain its new length. The same is true of muscles. If the muscle is lengthened but the fascia is not stretched, the muscle will cramp back down to fit within the contracted fascia. First, the muscle must be lengthened, and then the fascia must be stretched. This lengthening can be accomplished effectively by many of the therapeutic techniques in this chapter.

Circulatory Enhancement

Within the circulatory system, oxygenated blood, deoxygenated blood, and lymph circulate throughout the body in a network of vessels. Oxygenated blood is pumped from the heart, through the arteries, and out to the rest of the body. As the arteries get farther from the heart, they decrease in diameter and branch out until they become tiny capillaries. Oxygen molecules pass through the walls of the capillaries and diffuse from the blood to the body cells. From the capillaries, the deoxygenated blood is transported back to the heart through the veins. Lymph is the fluid that started out as blood plasma, leaked out through the capillaries to become interstitial fluid, and is picked up by the very delicate ends of the lymphatic vessels from tissues all over the body. From there, lymph travels toward the heart through the lymphatic vessels, eventually entering the heart through the subclavian vein and being added back to the blood. To prevent a backflow of the fluids, the veins and lymphatic vessels are supplied with valves.

One of the primary benefits of massage is the increased circulation of blood and lymph. Compression strokes applied distally over the arteries, and light effleurage strokes applied proximally over the veins and lymphatic vessels mechanically encourage the movement of fluids through the circulatory vessels. Please note that effleurage strokes applied to affect the lymph must be very light and superficial or the very delicate lymph vessels could be compressed, effectively diminishing the flow of lymph. By taking advantage of the mechanical pump behind the arterial system and the valves in the venous and lymphatic systems, a therapist can intentionally increase circulation to a specific area of the body.

◇ Alert

Remember, however, that the massage therapist's scope of practice encompasses treating the soft tissues of the body, not the circulatory system. If you are trying to encourage circulation in an effort to facilitate a change in the client's muscles and CT, it is acceptable to incorporate circulatory enhancement into a session.

Your intent and knowledge base will determine how effective your circulatory enhancement work will be. With increased circulation, there is an increased oxygenated blood supply, along with cellular and chemical waste removal. The health of the tissues, including the musculature, is promoted with enhanced circulation.

Arterial Enhancement

Fresh, oxygenated blood is pushed through the arteries by the forceful muscular contractions of the heart and continues with the help of gravity to flow to the cells and tissues throughout the body. The heart, as long as it is contracting, will continue to push blood into the arteries. Using the mechanical concept of pressure building behind a dam, a massage therapist can intentionally encourage arterial blood flow. In a massage session, the therapist can apply rhythmic, manual compression strokes that progressively move away from the heart along an artery. These compression strokes need moderate pressure to pinch off the blood supply without damaging the blood vessels. When you release the compression, blood will flow back into the vessels and increase the flow of blood to the local area. Box 10-2 describes the steps for arterial circulation enhancement.

Venous Enhancement

Deoxygenated blood returns, often against gravity, to the heart through the veins at the so-called end of the circulatory path. Many of the veins have a series of valves in them to prevent blood from flowing away from the heart. They are more prevalent where blood has a longer distance to travel back to the heart and are especially numerous in the veins of

10   Therapeutic Applications

BOX 10-2   📋 **PROCEDURE** Arterial Circulation Enhancement

1. Use the heel of your hand to apply moderate compression to the client's upper arm for about 3 seconds, giving the heart a chance to pump some more blood down the artery to build pressure.

◇ Alert

Pay attention to your wrist position because it is easy to overextend the wrist while applying compression.

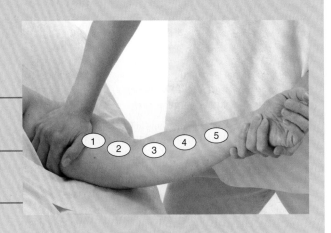

2. Release the compression to allow the arterial blood to rush forward.

3. Move the heel of your hand a couple of inches distally and apply another 3-second compression stroke.

4. Repeat steps 1 to 3 until you reach the client's wrist, using less pressure as you move toward the wrist.

the lower extremities, where blood must be pumped against gravity. Remember, the heart does not pump blood through the veins. Instead, contraction of nearby muscles compresses the veins and squeezes the blood in the only direction the valves allow—toward the heart. Movement of deoxygenated blood occurs via gravity, the skeletal muscle pump, and very weak peristaltic action of the tunica layers of circulatory vessels.

A massage therapist can enhance a client's venous return during a session by active or passive contraction of the client's muscles. By applying effleurage, you can also encourage blood movement through the veins. Because veins are more superficial than arteries, a massage that addresses venous flow does not require deep pressure. Light effleurage strokes directed toward the heart encourage the blood to move through the veins. Gravity can also assist venous flow toward the heart. As long as the client is positioned with the heart inferior to the body part, gravity helps return blood to the heart. For example, elevating the arm or leg during a massage can enhance venous return. Box 10-3 describes techniques for venous circulation enhancement.

BOX 10-3
Venous Circulation Enhancement

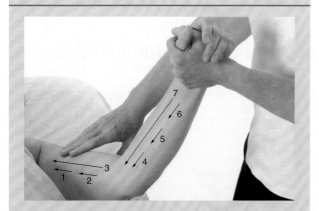

- The individual effleurage strokes sweep proximally, toward the heart, but the series of strokes start progressively farther from the heart.
- Closer to the heart, use long effleurage strokes to encourage the blood to move through a series of valves.
- In the distal portions of the arms and legs, where there are more valves, use short, 1- to 2-inch effleurage strokes.
- Periodically use 1 long effleurage stroke that covers the area treated by the 2 or 3 previous effleurage strokes, ensuring that the blood still flows freely along the path.

Lymph Drainage

The lymphatic system, first identified in 1622, is a component of the circulatory system that transports nutrients and immune cells, and cleans and filters cellular waste, debris, and pathogens from the interstitial fluid (fluid between the cells and within the tissues). The flow of interstitial fluid and lymph is vital to the health of the body; without it, blood becomes thicker, blood volume decreases, and blood pressure falls.

The pressure of blood as it moves through the arterial capillaries is high enough that fluid, proteins, nutrients, and gases pass through the capillary walls into the interstitial spaces. There, the fluid and all of its components, including the waste products from the cells, is called interstitial fluid. Some of the proteins, cellular waste, and other ingredients cannot move back into the capillaries and must be removed from the interstitial spaces. The very delicate ends of the lymphatic vessels pick up interstitial fluid and the larger constituents. Once the fluid enters the lymphatic vessels, it is called lymph. The lymphatic vessels form a drainage system that leads to the main veins that empty into the heart. Along the way, the lymph passes through lymph nodes, which house immune cells that engulf and neutralize the pathogens. Eventually, the system of lymphatic vessels ends at one of two ducts, right or thoracic, that drain the cleaned and filtered lymph directly into the bloodstream and into the heart. (Fig. 10-1 illustrates the lymphatic drainage pathways.)

There are two separate "drains" for the lymph. The **right lymphatic duct** drains all of the lymph from the upper right quadrant of the body, including the right arm, anterior and posterior shoulder region, and the right side of the head, into the right subclavian vein. The **thoracic duct** drains lymph collected from everywhere else on the body into the left subclavian vein (see Fig. 10-1B). Because lymph collection is divided into two separate paths, you must understand the direction of the lymph flow before attempting to enhance it.

Lymphatic vessels are like veins in several ways. They have valves that prevent lymph from flowing away from the heart, and the lymphatic system lacks a true mechanical pump to push lymph through the vessels. Instead, it moves via gravity and the skeletal muscle pump mechanism, in which muscles and surrounding tissues put pressure on the lymphatic vessels and squeeze the lymph in the only direction the valves allow—toward the heart. A variation of lymph flow via the skeletal muscle pump occurs upon deep breathing, in which contraction of the diaphragm puts pressure on many lymph vessels and encourages the flow through the vessels. The very weak peristaltic action of the tunica layers of circulatory vessels contributes only minimally to the flow of lymph.

Emil Vodder, PhD, a Danish physiotherapist, developed a system of lymphatic drainage in 1936, which is commonly called manual lymphatic drainage. The Vodder method uses

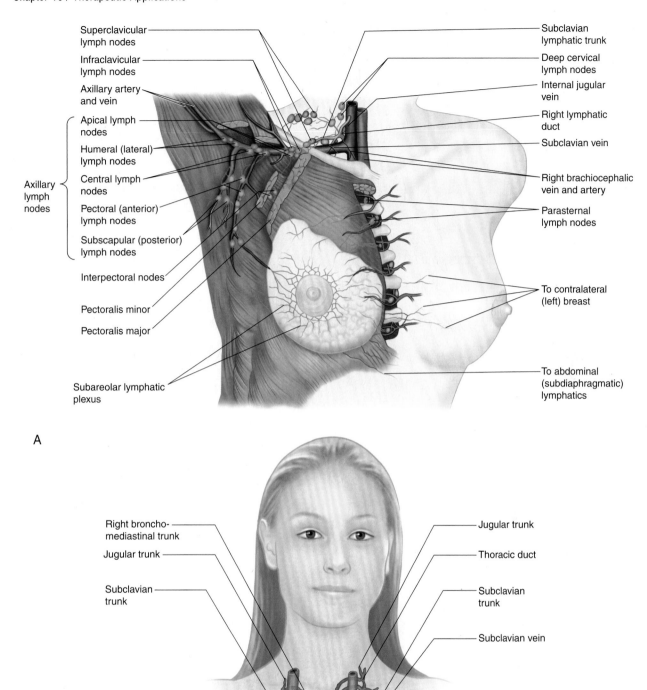

Figure 10-1. Lymphatic drainage. **(A)** Anatomy of right axillary lymphatic duct. **(B)** Anatomy of lymphatic drainage pathways.

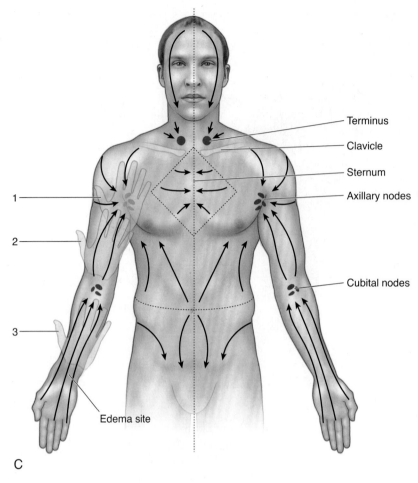

C

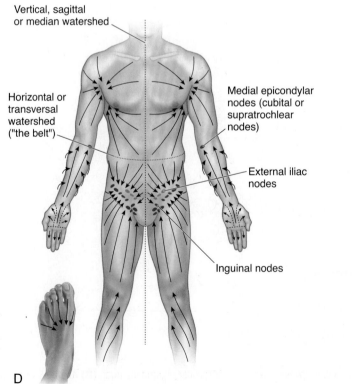

D

Figure 10-1. (*continued*) **(C)** Application of lymphatic drainage. **(D)** Superficial lymph circulation of the anterior body.

light, rhythmic, spiral-like movements to encourage the flow of lymph. More recently, Dr. Bruno Chikly developed and currently teaches Lymph Drainage Therapy (LDT), a technique based on the work of Dr. Vodder, and many other physicians throughout history. LDT teaches therapists an anatomical approach that allows them to map the vessels, assess the quality and depth of overall circulation, and determine the best alternative pathways for draining stagnant body fluids. Therapists use all of the finger pads to simulate gentle, specific wavelike movements that activate lymph and interstitial fluid circulation and stimulate immune function and parasympathetic nervous system activity.

The main purpose of using lymphatic drainage is to reduce edema by draining excess fluid from the body's cells and tissues. Lymphatic drainage is indicated for edema that is the result of an injury such as a strain, sprain, or repetitive overuse syndrome. As the excess lymph is removed from interstitial spaces, the pressure it was exerting on pain receptors is reduced, and thus, pain decreases. See Box 10-4 for a list of benefits and contraindications for enhanced lymph drainage.

Although the methods of Drs. Vodder and Chikly require advanced training, the beginning massage therapist can enhance lymph drainage with techniques similar to venous enhancement. The movement of lymph is encouraged by deep breathing, gravity, joint movement, muscular contraction, and general massage.

Deep Breathing

Full, deep breaths enhance lymphatic flow. Not only do full breaths bring more oxygen into the lungs to be delivered to the blood, but when the diaphragm contracts for inhalation, it also puts pressure on the lymphatic vessels and organs in the thorax to encourage the flow of lymph. **Lymphatic vessels are concentrated near the diaphragm, and the full contraction and relaxation of the diaphragm during deep breathing significantly enhances lymph drainage.**

BOX 10-4

Benefits and Contraindications for Enhanced Lymph Drainage

BENEFITS

Enhanced lymph drainage can be beneficial for the following:

- Reducing edema
- Relieving pain by relieving fluid pressure on nerve endings
- Stimulating immune function
- Relieving tension headache and migraine headache pain
- Minimizing scarring
- Minimizing connective tissue restrictions following surgery
- Accelerating healing time from burns and wounds
- Relieving sinus congestion
- Reducing symptoms of fibromyalgia and chronic fatigue syndromes
- Reducing muscle hypertonicity
- Relieving some forms of gastrointestinal distress such as constipation, colitis, irritable bowel syndrome
- Improving relaxation to aid insomnia, stress, and loss of vitality

CONTRAINDICATIONS

Below are some contraindications for enhanced lymph drainage:

- Systemic
  - Edema not related to soft tissue injury, which could indicate an overtaxed heart
  - Liver and/or kidney congestion
  - Chronic heart failure
  - Angina
  - Thrombosis (blood clot)
  - Acute stage of contagious viral or bacterial infection
  - Fever
  - Toxoplasmosis (a parasitic disease)
- Local
  - Local infection or signs of local infection (pain, redness, heat and swelling)
  - Swollen lymph glands
  - Red streaks from an infection site to the nearest lymph nodes
  - Acute inflammation
  - Acute injuries (24 to 72 hours after injury)
  - Recent surgery (24 to 72 hours after surgery)
  - Open wounds, blisters, burns, and abrasions
  - Contusions (bruises)
  - Skin infections
  - Rash

Gravity

You can use gravity by elevating your client's extremities during the session.

Alert

Be sure to maintain proper body mechanics while you are holding and lifting the client's extremities.

Because lymph nodes are more concentrated near joints, movement of the joints also encourages lymph flow. When the nodes are squeezed, as occurs with active and passive muscle movement, their valves force lymph toward the heart even more effectively than when the lymphatic vessels are squeezed. Joint movement goes hand in hand with muscle contraction, and isotonic contractions that create movement are more effective than isometric contractions.

Massage Strokes

Lymphatic drainage involves the application of very light and repetitive compression and effleurage strokes, generally repeated five to seven times. The general rule for the application of pressure is around 5 grams, or in more practical terms, the weight of a nickel resting on your skin. There are different approaches to lymph enhancement, but 0.5- to 1-inch effleurage strokes or circular effleurage strokes are generally considered acceptable. Because the application is very light, it is important for you to be comfortable and to keep your body and hands relaxed. If you find yourself tensing up, take a deep breath, ground yourself, and lighten your touch.

Deep pressure can damage lymphatic vessels, and damaged lymphatic vessels cannot drain lymph properly, which is why massage is contraindicated over areas of inflammation.

Some of the specialized lymph techniques include nodal pumping, stationary circles, and local technique. Nodal pumping involves compression to the lymph nodes at the most proximal part of the limb. Stationary circles can be used for larger areas of limb. These are modified compression strokes, in which there is no slip on the skin and the therapist moves one or both palms in circles in a rotational or spiral form. Local technique is applied with either the ulnar border of your hand, the web between the index finger and thumb, or with the broad surface of your thumbs. Figure 10-2 illustrates the different specialized lymph techniques. Regardless of which technique you choose, be sure not to apply any technique to

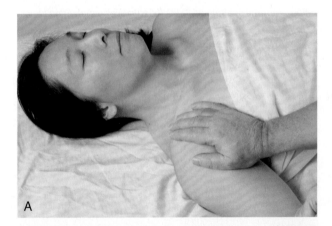
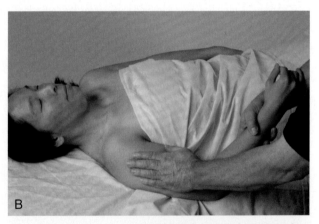
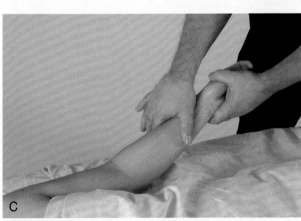
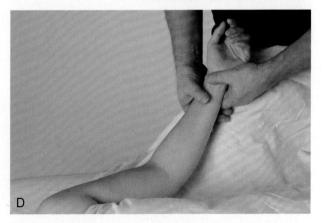

Figure 10-2. Specialized lymphatic drainage techniques. **(A)** Axillary nodal pumping. **(B)** Stationary circles. **(C)** Local technique using web between thumb and index finger. **(D)** Local technique using broad surface of the thumbs.

BOX 10-5 PROCEDURE Basic Lymph Drainage Enhancement

- Pumping—3 rhythmic compression strokes

- Sweeping—a series of short, superficial effleurage strokes that sweep proximally

Supine Position—Neck and Head Drainage

1. Place your relaxed, flat hands on the client's chest, just inferior to the client's clavicles, and apply 3 light compression strokes with a pumping rhythm.

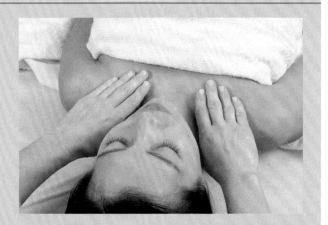

2. Rotate the client's neck to the left, support the head with your left hand, and use your right hand to apply several sets of very light pumping and sweeping to the neck, starting at the client's right clavicle and gradually moving up to the occiput.

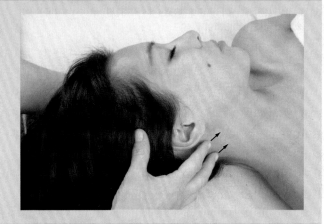

3. Rotate the client's neck to the right, supporting the head with your right hand, and use your left hand to apply several sets of very light pumping and sweeping to the neck, starting at the client's left clavicle and gradually moving up to the occiput.

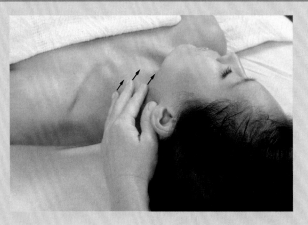

10 Therapeutic Applications

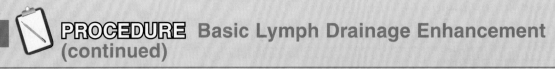

BOX 10-5   **PROCEDURE**   **Basic Lymph Drainage Enhancement**
(continued)

4. Apply several sets of pumping and sweeping to the client's face, starting near the chin and gradually moving out and up to the client's forehead.

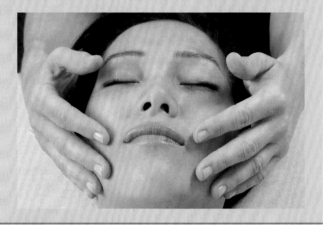

Supine Position—Arm Drainage

1. Use flat fingers to sweep the chest, starting near the client's sternum and gradually moving to the right axilla (armpit area).

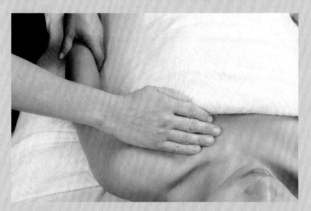

2. Gently but firmly grasp your client's left hand, interlocking your thumb with theirs, support the client's elbow, and rhythmically flex and extend the client's left shoulder and elbow several times.

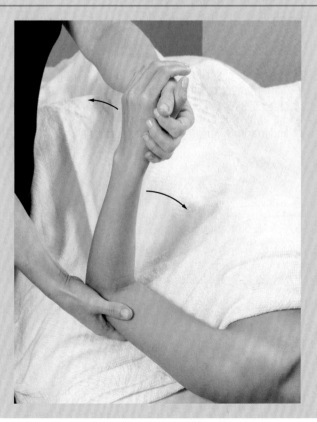

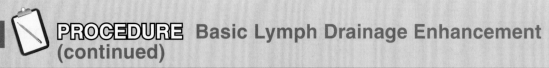

BOX 10-5 **PROCEDURE** Basic Lymph Drainage Enhancement (continued)

3. Use flat fingers to sweep the left arm, starting at the axilla and gradually moving to the hand.

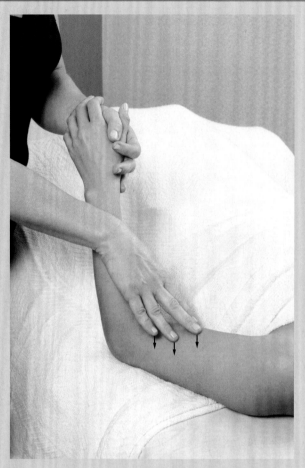

4. Use flat fingers to sweep the thorax, starting at the left axilla and moving down the left side of the rib cage.

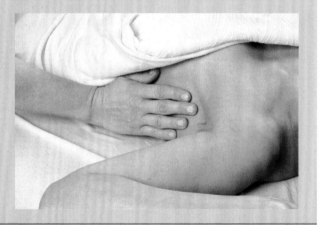

5. Repeat steps 1 to 4 on the right side.

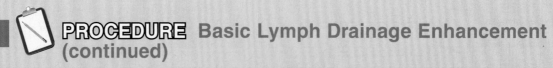

BOX 10-5 📋 **PROCEDURE** (continued) **Basic Lymph Drainage Enhancement**

Supine Position—Leg Drainage

1. Elevate the client's left leg with bolsters or, if possible, gently hold and support the client's left foot and lower leg to rhythmically flex the hip and knee several times.

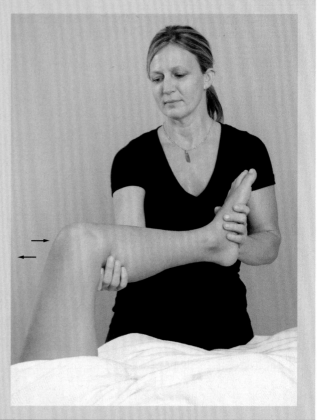

2. Use your palms or flat fingers to pump and sweep the client's left leg, starting at the medial thigh and gradually moving to the ankle.

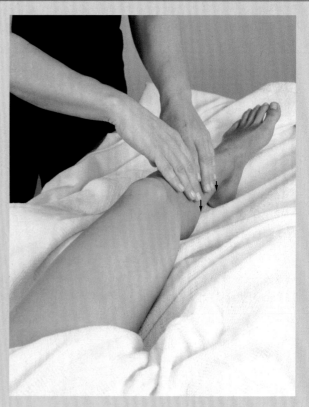

BOX 10-5 **PROCEDURE** **Basic Lymph Drainage Enhancement (continued)**

3. Repeat for the client's right leg.

Prone Position—Leg Drainage

Alert

Do not put pressure on the popliteal fossa at the back of knee because it is an endangerment site.

1. Elevate the client's ankles with a small bolster.

2. Gently and firmly grasp the client's left ankle and rhythmically flex the knee several times.

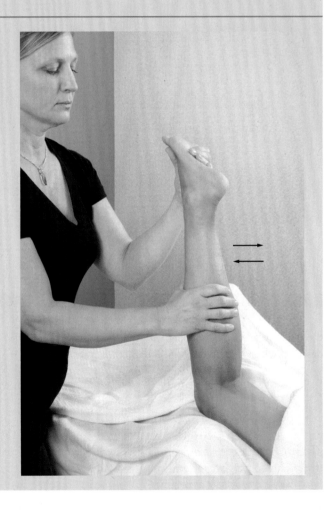

BOX 10-5 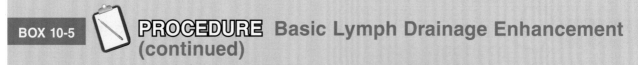 **PROCEDURE** (continued)   **Basic Lymph Drainage Enhancement**

3. Use your palms or flat fingers to pump and sweep the client's right leg, starting at the right iliac crest and gradually moving to the ankle.

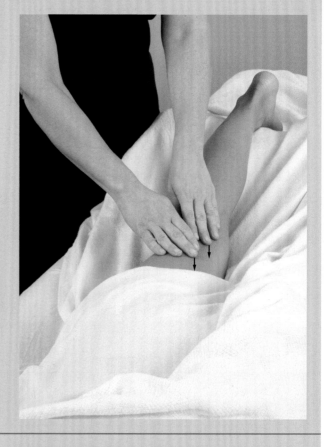

4. Repeat for the client's left leg.

the tissue distal to a developing scar or acute injury. Box 10-5 describes a basic lymph drainage enhancement procedure.

Alert

You should be aware that application of lymph drainage may cause medications to metabolize in the client's system more quickly than expected. Be sure to inform clients that this may occur and that they should seek advice from their healthcare professional before adjusting their medications.

Before applying any of these techniques, make sure there are no contraindications for lymph drainage enhancement (see earlier Box 10-4 for some of the more common contraindications).

Be sure not to apply lymphatic drainage directly on the site of or distally to an acute or subacute injury as it can increase congestion and pain in the area of injury.

Do not push fluids toward a developing scar because the proteins in the interstitial fluid can agglomerate at the scar and form keloids. Instead, you should only enhance lymph drainage in areas *proximal* to the developing scar. If edema is present, it is important to determine whether soft tissue injury is the cause. If not, you should avoid lymph drainage enhancement in that area.

Alert

If you are uncertain whether you should apply lymphatic techniques, do not proceed, and refer clients to their primary healthcare provider.

This section is meant to be an introduction to lymphatic drainage; if you are particularly interested in developing your skills in this area, you must take additional training. To find quality training programs, consult fellow massage therapists, reputable massage schools, or your professional massage organization.

Neuromuscular Techniques

Neuromuscular techniques use a comprehensive system of identifying causative factors and performing soft tissue manipulation to achieve balance between the nervous and musculoskeletal system, thus alleviating pain. There are advanced courses of neuromuscular therapies that have their own levels of certification.

At the introductory level, the two laws of neuromuscular therapy to understand are the law of cause and effect and the law of facilitation. The law of cause and effect states that for every action there is an equal and opposite reaction. Applied to massage therapy, it is the idea that when you affect the body in one area, the whole body responds. This could be due to the body's response to stressors and injury and/or the application of pressure via massage techniques. Dr. Ida Rolf, founder of the structural integration system called Rolfing, simplifies this concept in her timeless statement, "Where you think it is, it ain't." The law of facilitation states that when a nerve impulse has followed a specific pathway of nerves, it will tend to take the same path on future occasions. The law of facilitation explains why a client may experience a familiar pain pattern after aggravating an old injury or reinjuring an area. Essentially, the nervous system trains itself to take the path of least resistance.

Neuromuscular therapy is indicated for hypertonic muscle conditions such as muscle strains, whiplash, repetitive stress injuries, temporomandibular joint dysfunction, headaches, and back or neck pain. Conversely, neuromuscular work is contraindicated for bruised areas, phlebitis, varicose veins, open wounds, skin infections, and broken bones. If you are unsure whether this type of therapy is indicated, consult a massage-specific pathology book or follow the rule, "When in doubt, don't."

What follows in this section is an introduction to the concepts and some practical applications that you can master as a student and beginning massage therapist, including proprioceptive neuromuscular facilitation (PNF) techniques, myofascial techniques, and TrP release techniques.

Proprioceptive Neuromuscular Facilitation Techniques

Proprioceptive neuromuscular facilitation (PROH-pree-oh-SEP-tive NOO-roh-MUSS-kyoo-lar fah-SIHL-ih-TAY-shun), commonly called **PNF**, uses the nervous system to reset a muscle's resting length. PNF is a general term for a set of techniques. Remember, the muscle spindles and Golgi tendon organs are proprioceptors of the nervous system that recognize stretch and tension in the muscles and tendons. These massage techniques manipulate the *proprioceptors* of the *nervous* and the *muscular* systems to *facilitate* a reflexive change in the resting length of a muscle. These techniques are also called **muscle energy techniques**, or **METs**. The terms PNF and MET are often interchanged. PNF techniques can reduce pain, relax a hypertonic muscle, realign postural deviations, and restore range of motion. Some of the more common PNF techniques are direct manipulation (DM), positional release (PR), post-isometric relaxation (PIR), and reciprocal inhibition (RI).

Some people respond well to PNF, and others do not. Some respond better to one particular PNF technique than to another. The results depend on the length of time the target muscle has been affected, the synergists that are involved, any compensation patterns that are present, and the factors that influence the client's health and healing. Sometimes the results can be immediate and permanent, and other times, PNF can be unsuccessful. Most of the time, PNF is an effective and efficient approach to specific areas of hypertonicity that plainly demonstrates some of the benefits of massage.

Muscle Movement and Stability

Performing PNF requires a basic understanding of muscle movement and stability. In addition to creating movement, muscles also function to stop movement and to stabilize joints. The muscle or group of muscles that creates a certain movement is called the agonist (prime mover). The muscle or group of muscles that performs the opposite work is called the antagonist. **In normal, concentric movements, the antagonist must relax for the agonist to contract.** For example, when the biceps brachii muscle contracts and shortens to create flexion, the triceps brachii muscle must neurologically relax and lengthen. PNF techniques often use the antagonistic mechanism of muscle contraction to create reflexive changes in muscle length. Muscles called synergists assist the agonist to create the desired motion. The synergists help by contracting in the same direction as the agonist or by stabilizing the joint to prevent another motion from occurring during movement.

If you are trying to relax and lengthen the biceps brachii muscle, the biceps brachii is your target (agonist) muscle. You can use a contraction of its antagonist, the triceps brachii muscle, to neurologically relax the biceps brachii. Knowing the major skeletal muscles of the body and their actions, antagonists, and synergists is important for using therapeutic techniques. For that reason, massage students must learn antagonistic muscle movements and the muscles responsible for those movements (Table 10-1).

Table 10-1 Antagonistic Actions

Muscles	Antagonistic Actions		Muscles
Levator scapula, rhomboid major, upper trapezius, middle trapezius	Elevation	Depression	Serratus anterior, subclavius, lower trapezius, pectoralis minor
Scapula			
Serratus anterior, pectoralis minor	Protraction	Retraction	Rhomboid major, middle trapezius, lower trapezius
Serratus anterior, upper trapezius, lower trapezius	Upward rotation	Downward rotation	Levator scapula, pectoralis minor, rhomboid major
Shoulder			
Coracobrachialis, anterior deltoid, pectoralis major, biceps brachii	Flexion	Extension	Posterior deltoid, latissimus dorsi, teres major, triceps brachii
Deltoid, supraspinatus, biceps brachii	Abduction	Adduction	Latissimus dorsi, pectoralis major, teres major, triceps brachii, coracobrachialis, pectoralis minor
Posterior deltoid, infraspinatus, teres minor	Lateral rotation	Medial rotation	Anterior deltoid, latissimus dorsi, pectoralis major, subscapularis, teres major
Medial deltoid, posterior deltoid, teres minor, infraspinatus	Transverse abduction (laterally rotated humerus moves horizontally out to sides)	Transverse adduction (laterally rotated humerus moves across chest)	Pectoralis major, coracobrachialis
Pectoralis major, deltoids, coracobrachialis, biceps brachii	Transverse flexion (medially rotated humerus moves across chest)	Transverse extension (medially rotated humerus moves horizontally out to sides)	Posterior deltoid, infraspinatus, latissimus dorsi, teres minor
Elbow			
Biceps brachii, brachialis, brachioradialis	Flexion	Extension	Triceps brachii, anconeus
Pronator teres, pronator quadratus, anconeus, brachioradialis	Pronation	Supination	Biceps brachii, supinator
Wrist			
Flexor carpi radialis, flexor carpi ulnaris, palmaris longus, flexor digitorum superficialis, flexor digitorum profundus	Flexion	Extension	Extensor carpi radialis brevis, extensor carpi radialis longus, extensor carpi ulnaris, extensor digitorum, extensor pollicis longus, extensor indicis
Extensor carpi radialis brevis, extensor carpi radialis longus, flexor carpi radialis, extensor pollicis brevis	Abduction (radial deviation)	Adduction (ulnar deviation)	Extensor carpi ulnaris, flexor carpi ulnaris

continues on following page

Table 10-1 Antagonistic Actions *continued*

Muscles	Antagonistic Actions		Muscles
Fingers			
Flexor digitorum profundus, flexor digitorum superficialis, flexor digiti minimi	Flexion	Extension	Extensor digiti minimi, extensor digitorum, extensor indicis
Dorsal interossei, abductor digiti minimi, extensor digitorum, extensor digiti minimi, extensor indicis	Abduction	Adduction	Palmar interossei, flexor digitorum superficialis, flexor digitorum profundus
Thumb			
Abductor pollicis brevis	Abduction	Adduction	Adductor pollicis
Flexor pollicis brevis, flexor pollicis longus	Flexion	Extension	Extensor pollicis brevis, extensor pollicis longus
Hip			
Adductor brevis, adductor longus, iliacus, pectineus, psoas major, rectus femoris, sartorius, tensor fascia latae	Flexion	Extension	Adductor magnus, biceps femoris, gluteus maximus, semimembranosus, semitendinosus
Gemellus inferior, gemellus superior, gluteus maximus, gluteus medius, gluteus minimus, piriformis, tensor fascia latae	Abduction	Abduction	Adductor brevis, adductor longus, adductor magnus, biceps femoris, gluteus maximus, gracilis, pectineus, psoas major
Gluteus medius, gluteus minimus, tensor fascia latae	Medial rotation	Lateral rotation	Adductor brevis, adductor longus, adductor magnus, biceps femoris, gemellus inferior, gemellus superior, gluteus maximus, gluteus medius, obturator externus, obturator internus, piriformis, quadratus femoris, sartorius
Knee			
Biceps femoris, gastrocnemius, gracilis, popliteus, sartorius, semimembranosus, semitendinosus	Flexion	Extension	Rectus femoris, tensor fascia latae, vastus intermedius, vastus lateralis, vastus medialis
Gracilis, popliteus, sartorius, semimembranosus, semitendinosus	Medial rotation	Lateral rotation	Biceps femoris

continues on following page

Table 10-1 Antagonistic Actions *continued*

Muscles	Antagonistic Actions		Muscles
	Ankle		
Extensor digitorum longus, extensor hallucis longus, peroneus tertius, tibialis anterior	Dorsiflexion	Plantarflexion	Flexor digitorum longus, flexor hallucis longus, gastrocnemius, peroneus brevis, peroneus longus, plantaris, soleus, tibialis posterior
Extensor digitorum longus, peroneus brevis, peroneus longus, peroneus tertius	Eversion	Inversion	Flexor digitorum longus, tibialis anterior, tibialis posterior
	Spine		
External obliques, internal obliques, rectus abdominis	Flexion	Extension	Iliocostalis, longissimus, multifidi, rotatores, spinalis
Multifidi, quadratus lumborum, rotators	Lateral flexion		
External obliques, iliocostalis, internal obliques, multifidi, quadratus lumborum, rotators	Rotation		
	Diaphragm		
External obliques, internal intercostals, internal obliques, rectus abdominis, transversus abdominis	Exhalation	Inhalation	Diaphragm, external intercostals, internal intercostals, scalenus anterior, scalenus medius, scalenus posterior
	Neck		
Scalenus anterior, scalenus medius, scalenus posterior, sternocleidomastoid	Flexion	Extension	Iliocostalis, levator scapulae longissimus, multifidi, rotatores, semispinalis, spinalis, splenius capitis, splenius cervicis, upper trapezius
Levator scapulae, longissimus, semispinalis, splenius capitis, sternocleidomastoid, middle trapezius	Lateral flexion		
Multifidi, rotatores, splenius capitis, splenius cervicis, sternocleidomastoid	Rotation		
	Temporomandibular Joint (or Jaw)		
Masseter, medial pterygoid, temporalis	Elevation	Depression	Lateral pterygoid, platysma, suprahyoids
Lateral pterygoid, masseter, medial pterygoid	Protraction	Retraction	Temporalis

Direct Manipulation

Direct manipulation (DM) is a PNF technique in which your fingers *directly manipulate* the muscle spindles and Golgi tendon organs of a hypertonic muscle to trigger relaxation. The muscle spindles are found between the muscle fibers and respond to tension in the muscles. The Golgi tendon organs are located between collagen fibers in the tendons and also respond to tension. These proprioceptors are components of such reflex arcs as the stretch reflex and the tendon reflex, which are protective mechanisms that help us to avoid injury. You can use these proprioceptors to fool the body into thinking that a muscle is too short or too long. If the proprioceptors sense that a muscle is too short, the nervous system can stimulate muscle lengthening, or relaxation. You can accomplish this with the following steps:

1. Determine the target muscle. Position the target muscle in a partial passive contraction.

2. Use your thumb and fingers to effleurage the target muscle with a pinching or gathering action, which addresses the muscle spindles.

3. Effleurage the tendons toward their bony attachments, which addresses the Golgi tendon organs.

4. Slowly extend the target muscle to its new length, stopping at the end feel. Hold the new length for at least 5 to 10 seconds. During this period, be prepared for a possible tendon reflex that allows the muscle to lengthen a bit further. If so, hold it at its new length.

Box 10-6 illustrates these steps with the biceps brachii as the target muscle.

This technique leads the nervous system's proprioceptors into perceiving that the muscle is dangerously hypertonic. When a muscle is strongly contracted and too short, it is in danger of being torn. Pushing the muscle spindles together sends a message that the muscle fibers are too close, or that the muscle is contracted too much. Pushing the Golgi tendon organs away from the muscle conveys a message that the musculotendinous junctions are being stressed, or that the muscle is contracted too much. The nervous system will respond by protectively relaxing and lengthening that muscle.

These are reflexive responses in which the massage application causes the nervous system to create a physical change. Once the muscle has been lengthened by the nervous system, the surrounding fascia must be stretched for the treatment to retain its effect. The extended hold at the end of the DM procedure provides the stretch for the fascia at the same time it allows the proprioceptors to recognize the new length that should be maintained. All stretching must be done carefully to avoid a protective spasm.

DM is a good technique to use on painful muscles and muscles that are not attached to the limbs, such as the trapezius or rhomboids. Clients who hurt with any kind of movement and clients who are not interested in actively moving or participating in the massage may prefer DM to some of the other PNF techniques.

Positional Release

To perform **positional release**, also called **PR** and **strain/counterstrain (SCS)**, you hold the client's body in a position that reduces the hypertonic muscle pain and wait for the nervous system to trigger relaxation. This technique takes advantage of the body's inherent ability to reduce pain and release hypertonic muscles. When a muscle develops a shortened resting length, the body finds a position that relieves the associated discomfort. Unfortunately, the hypertonicity that reduces the movement and use of a muscle can start the pain cycle. Using the direction of ease concept, you can follow the body's lead rather than work against it. To perform PR, you apply pressure to a localized hypertonic or painful spot and move the client's body into a position that reduces or eliminates that pain. Basically, PR puts the client's body into a position that it may have been in before a protective spasm resulted from stress or strain. When the body senses that the position is nonthreatening, the nervous system may respond by relaxing the protective spasm. Physical therapists, osteopaths, and chiropractors frequently use this technique.

The very small area of pain or hypertonicity is referred to as a **tender point**, tender spot, or knot. It is often found during the massage in the midst of an effleurage stroke. Sometimes the client will express discomfort as you pass over it; other times you may feel a difference in the tissue quality and should ask the client if there is any associated discomfort. With enough experience, you will be able to find tender points without any input from the client, but until then, verbally communicate with the client.

Monitoring the Tender Point

The tender point is monitored with your finger, forearm, or thumb throughout the process, so you need to use good body mechanics while you maintain pressure on it. You should put enough pressure on the tender spot that clients notice the discomfort, but not so much that they are distracted by it. You can ask clients to rate the pain or discomfort on a scale of 0 to 3, where 0 indicates no pain and 3 indicates severe pain, or a scale of 0 to 10, where 0 indicates no pain and 10 indicates severe pain. For clients who do not like to use a rating scale, you can ask them to indicate whether the discomfort is absent, mild, moderate, or severe. With experience, you will be able to feel resistant tissues soften up when you apply the appropriate

BOX 10-6

Direct Manipulation of the Biceps Brachii

1. Determine the target muscle: biceps brachii.
2. Put the biceps brachii into a partial passive contraction.

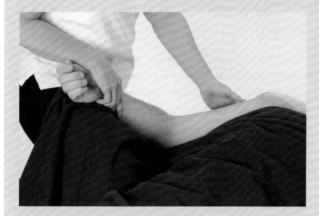

4. Effleurage the tendons toward their bony attachments at the radial tuberosity and the glenohumeral joint.

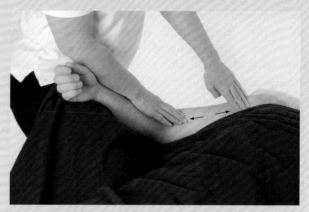

3. Use your thumb and fingers to effleurage the biceps brachii with a pinching or gathering action.

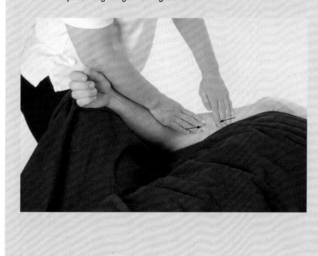

5. Slowly extend the biceps brachii to its new length by extending the elbow and the shoulder, stopping at the end feel. Hold the new length for at least 5 to 10 seconds. During this period, be prepared for a possible tendon reflex that allows the muscle to lengthen a bit further. If so, hold it at its new length.

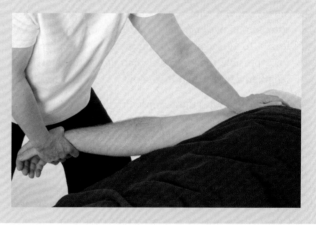

amount of pressure with proper body mechanics and palpation skills.

Positioning the Body

Once the correct pressure and body mechanics have been found, start moving the client's body to minimize the discomfort. Based on your knowledge of the major skeletal muscles and their attachments and actions, you can begin positioning the client by putting the target muscle into a passive contraction. Occasionally, this passive contraction of the target muscle eliminates the pain, but most of the time, you have to fine-tune the position by moving other body parts or changing the position slightly. Since the three-dimensional

fascial pulling can be a component of the client's discomfort, the process of positioning can sometimes require you to move a part of the client's body that is seemingly unrelated to the target muscle. For example, you may flex the client's other elbow, laterally rotate a leg, or rotate the neck to reduce the pain further.

When moving in the primary direction of ease does not decrease the discomfort, continue to adjust the position until the pain diminishes. Since the body has an inherent tendency to find the most comfortable position in any given situation, you can also ask the client to try to find the right position. At times, however, the pain does not seem to diminish in any position. In these cases, another PNF technique may be the better option.

Once you find a position that significantly diminishes or eliminates the pain, hold the client's body in that position for at least 90 seconds. It is not critical to maintain the same amount of pressure with your monitoring finger, but this is a good practice. If you vary the pressure, the client may suspect the pain is gone because you are not pressing as hard. Because you must hold the client's body in position, you *must* maintain good body mechanics.

Releasing the Tender Point

During the hold, your monitoring finger may feel a difference in the tissues as the tender point is released. It can feel like the tissues are melting or softening under your pressure. Sometimes the release is accompanied by a change in the client's breathing pattern or a sigh. Whether or not you notice the release, you need to hold the position for 90 seconds.

After the 90-second hold, slowly and gently return the client's body to the anatomical position. With your monitoring finger on the tender point, ask the client to rate the discomfort level following PR. If the tender spot has been released, there will be no discomfort. If pain is still present but is reduced, you may want to repeat the process. If there is no change, you can try PR with a different position or you can try another technique.

Once the target has been satisfactorily relaxed, the fascia in and around the target muscle needs to be stretched. Slowly extend the target muscle until you reach the end feel. You will sense the end feel better with good body mechanics and proper lean technique. Were you to push the client's body with your own strength, you would be more likely to pass through the client's comfort barrier and the end feel, possibly causing injury. Once you reach the barrier, hold the extension for at least 5 seconds, waiting for a possible tendon reflex to relax the target even farther.

PR is a good technique to use with clients who are not interested in actively moving or participating during the massage. As always, use good body mechanics with PR—especially if your clients are large or heavy—because of the physical work required to lift and hold their limbs or body parts. The PR process is described in Box 10-7.

Post-isometric Relaxation

Post-isometric relaxation (PIR) is a PNF technique that can reduce hypertonicity in a muscle by actively contracting and relaxing the target muscle. Also known as tense and relax, it requires work from the client and is often more effective and longer lasting than DM or PR. PIR uses an *isometric* contraction of the target muscle *followed by* slow *relaxation* and elongation. Isometric contractions use active muscle contraction without producing any movement. For example, if you squeeze your knees together, the adductor muscles are all actively contracting, but no movement occurs because the

opposite knee acts as a physical barrier. The PIR technique involves the following steps:

1. Determine the target muscle and its action.
2. Extend the muscle to its end feel.
3. Pull back from the barrier by a few degrees, or a small amount.
   a. Stabilize the client's body in that position to provide a physical, immovable barrier to the target muscle's contraction.
   b. Ask the client to gently push against the barrier, using only about 10% of his or her strength, and hold the push.
4. After 5 seconds, clearly explain that you want the client to *slowly* relax and let go of the push.
   a. Gently extend the target muscle to the muscle's new length.
   b. Hold the position for at least 5 to 10 seconds, waiting for a tendon reflex to lengthen the muscle further. If it does, hold it at its new length.

Box 10-8 demonstrates PIR applied to the gastrocnemius.

Positioning the Body

Because a fully extended muscle has very little leverage and cannot contract efficiently, synergists are often recruited to perform the desired movement. In an effort to isolate the muscular contraction for PIR, the target muscle is positioned with a slight contraction. To position the target muscle for PIR, you passively extend it, stretching the muscle to its end feel, and then relieve some of your pressure and back away from the end feel, allowing the muscle to rest just short of full extension.

Stabilizing the client's body requires some practice to incorporate good body mechanics. Use a solid lean, either into or away from the client's body, with as little arm or back strength as possible. You may need to remind clients that this technique is not a strength contest, and tell them simply to "hold against my pressure" or to use only 10% of their strength during the contraction—just enough to signal some of the muscle fibers to contract. If you do not, you may get pushed or pulled off balance. Then ask the client to push or pull against the physical barrier and hold the isometric contraction.

Relaxing the Target Muscle

After the client activates the muscle for about 5 seconds, ask the client to slowly relax. This works best if you slowly relieve the counterpressure. As the client relaxes the target muscle, the nervous system relaxes and lengthens the muscle. Slowly take the target muscle into extension, using good body mechanics, and stop at the end feel. Hold the stretch for at least 5 seconds, allowing the proprioceptors to integrate the new muscle length while you wait for a possible tendon

BOX 10-7

Positional Release of the Lower Trapezius

1. Apply a small amount of pressure to a tender point or small knot in the trapezius muscle. Ask the client to rate the discomfort on a scale of 0 to 3 (where 0 is pain free and 3 is very painful). Adjust the pressure of your monitoring finger using good body mechanics until the pressure elicits a pain rating of 1 or 2.

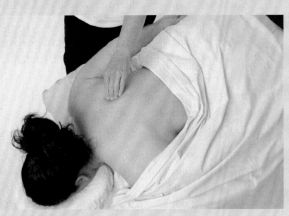

2. Maintain the contact and pressure on the tender point and move the client's body into a position that eliminates or significantly reduces the discomfort.
3. Hold the client's body in this position for at least 90 seconds with your monitoring finger still in place. Ask the client to take a few deep breaths.

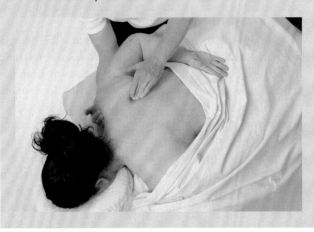

4. Slowly return the client's body to the original position, maintaining contact with your monitoring finger. Ask the client to rate the discomfort again, using the same scale.

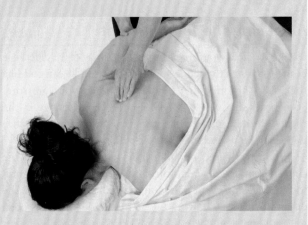

5. After the tender point has been relieved, extend the target muscle to its new length. Hold the new length for at least 5 to 10 seconds to see if the tendon reflex will allow the muscle to lengthen a bit farther. If so, hold it at its new length.

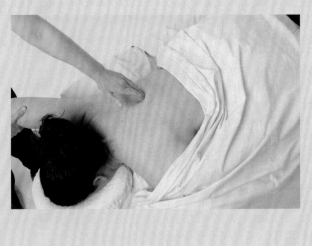

reflex. The tendon reflex will lengthen the muscle even more, and the increased extension provides the CT stretch.

The client must relax the target muscle slowly to prevent a sudden, complete absence of muscular tension. Abrupt relaxation may cause your counterpressure to quickly push the muscle into a stretch, activating the stretch reflex and a protective spasm.

This technique requires the target muscle to contract. By using the neuromuscular communication path for contraction and relaxation of the target muscle, PIR can be very effective for muscles that have been hypertonic for more than 3 weeks. Contracting a muscle involved in a situation

of protective muscle guarding or splinting may be painful or make the original condition worse.

 Any time there is muscle guarding, which often happens with conditions that have been present for less than 3 weeks, or any time there is pain upon contraction of the target muscle, you should avoid PIR.

Reciprocal Inhibition

The PNF technique called **reciprocal inhibition (RI)** is based on the agonist/antagonist principle. Movement

BOX 10-8

Post-isometric Relaxation of the Gastrocnemius

1. Determine the target muscle and its action: the gastrocnemius is responsible for plantarflexion.

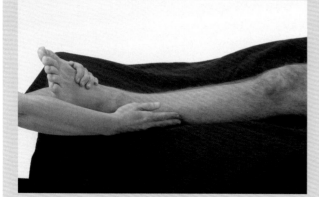

2. Extend the gastrocnemius to its end feel. Stabilize the ankle. Client and therapist push; no movement occurs.

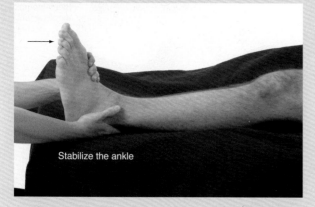

Stabilize the ankle

3. Pull back from the end feel by a few degrees, or a small amount.
   a. Stabilize the client's body in that position and provide a physical, immovable barrier to plantarflexion.
   b. Ask the client to gently plantarflex against the barrier, using only about 10% of his or her strength, and hold the push.

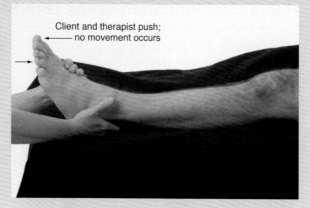

Client and therapist push; no movement occurs

4. After 5 seconds, clearly explain that you want the client to slowly relax and let go of the push. Gently extend the target muscle to the muscle's new length. Hold the position for at least 5 to10 seconds, waiting for a tendon reflex to lengthen the muscle farther. If it does, hold it at its new length.

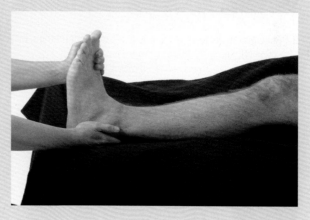

can only be created by the agonist, or prime mover, if its antagonists relax to some degree. During the process of RI, the client contracts the opposing or antagonistic muscles to reflexively relax the target muscle. In other words, by using the reciprocal muscle action, the target muscle's contraction can be inhibited. RI is performed as follows:

1. Determine the target muscle, its action, and the antagonistic action.

2. Position the target muscle in a partial contraction.

3. Stabilize the client's body in that position.

   a. Provide a physical, immovable barrier to the antagonistic action.

   b. Ask the client to gently push against the barrier, contracting the antagonist muscle and using only about 10% of his or her strength, and hold the push.

4. After 5 seconds, tell the client to slowly relax and let go of the push.

   a. Gently extend the target muscle to the end feel at its new length.

b. Hold the stretch for 5 to 10 seconds, waiting for a possible tendon reflex that lengthens the muscle a bit farther. If so, hold it at its new length.

Box 10-9 illustrates how to apply RI to the quadriceps femoris.

Positioning the target muscle for RI is not a precise step. As long as the muscle is held toward the end of its range of motion, the position should be adequate for RI. Understanding the action of the target muscle and its antagonistic action is important. Often, if you can determine the target's action, the antagonistic action is second nature.

BOX 10-9
Reciprocal Inhibition of the Quadriceps Femoris

1. Determine the target muscle, its action, and the antagonistic action: the quadriceps femoris is responsible for hip flexion and knee extension. Antagonistic actions are hip extension and knee flexion.

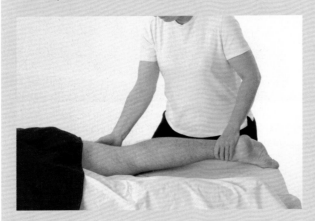

2. Position the quadriceps femoris in a partial contraction.

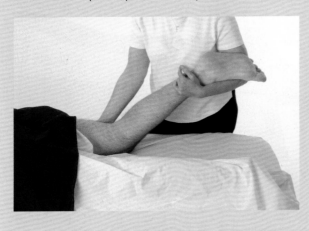

3. Stabilize the client's body in that position by placing a hand near the knee.
    a. Provide a physical, immovable barrier to the antagonistic action of knee flexion by leaning into the client's Achilles tendon.

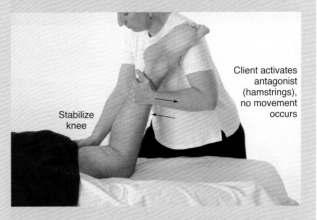

Stabilize knee

Client activates antagonist (hamstrings), no movement occurs

    b. Ask the client to gently flex the knee, pushing against the barrier, using only about 10% of his or her strength, and hold the push.
4. After 5 seconds, ask the client to slowly relax and let go of the push.
    a. Gently extend the quadriceps to the end feel at its new length by flexing the client's knee.

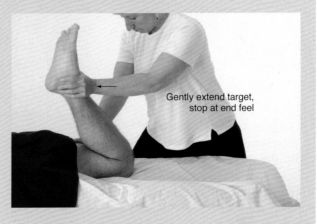

Gently extend target, stop at end feel

    b. Hold the stretch for 5 to 10 seconds, waiting for a possible tendon reflex that lengthens the quadriceps femoris a bit farther. If so, hold it at its new length.

Stabilizing the client's body and providing a physical barrier to the antagonistic action requires good body mechanics. The barrier must not move when pushed by the client, because the muscle contraction must be isometric. With experience, you will develop techniques that work well. As with PIR, ask clients to push against the resistance using only about 10% of their strength and hold the isometric contraction. Ask clients to slowly relax the muscle after about 5 seconds. Once the neurological lengthening (relaxation) has occurred, the surrounding CTs must be stretched to maintain the change in length. Relieve the counterpressure slowly to facilitate smooth relaxation and avoid the protective spasm of a stretch reflex.

RI requires the client to actively participate in the massage but does not require the target muscle to do the work. In conditions that involve an extremely hypertonic or painful target muscle, RI is particularly useful. As with all other PNF techniques, there is a wide variation in the amount of neurological relaxation that occurs as a result of RI. Chronically hypertonic muscles generally require more time and treatment to be restored to their normal resting length because of the fascial restrictions that develop, the compensation patterns that develop, and the nerve tracks that make the compensation patterns habitual. Stretching is important for reinforcing and maintaining RI work on chronically hypertonic muscles.

Myofascial Techniques

Myofascial techniques manipulate the fascia that runs throughout the musculature. Fascia is so pervasive that any restrictions, adhesions, or buildups of fascia can create problems for the musculature. Fascial restriction can often be felt during an effleurage stroke because it causes an irregularity in the speed or quality of the stroke. Sometimes the effleurage stroke will seem to skid across the tissue or get stuck and be difficult to move across the tissue.

Fascia is thixotropic (THIK-soh-TROH-pihk), which means that with deformation and mechanical manipulation, fascia becomes warmer and more liquid. This is primarily a result of the piezoelectric (pee-AY-zoh-ee-LEHK-trihk) quality of collagen. When collagen is mechanically compressed or squeezed, it develops an electric charge on its surface that liquefies the collagen to some degree, and the components of the tissue are rearranged. Recall that CT is made of living cells suspended in a matrix of proteins that are secreted by those cells. The proteins, including collagen, elastin, and reticular fibers, provide strength, elasticity, and structural support. **Without sufficient movement, nutrition, and hydration, fascia stiffens and dries out.**

Myofascial techniques take advantage of the thixotropic nature of fascia to mechanically change the shape and position of restricted tissues. Due to the three-dimensional structure of fascia, the tissues might move in different directions, circles, or wavy lines as the collagen fibers change shape and get rearranged. This slow process is sometimes referred to as unwinding or myofascial unwinding. These techniques require that you maintain your original point of contact on the client's skin without slipping, so little or no lubrication is used. Because these techniques are sometimes uncomfortable, you should perform them slowly and with care. Myofascial techniques include general CT applications as well as specific techniques, including scar release, craniosacral therapy (CST), and friction techniques.

Connective Tissue Techniques

CT techniques make the fascia more fluid, break up fascial adhesions, and can reduce scar tissue. **CT techniques specifically soften the fascia to create more space and allow more movement within the tissues.** You can feel the resistance of the tissues slowly melt away as the fascia softens. CT techniques include the 45° stroke, skin rolling, and variations of skin rolling.

45° Stroke

The most general CT stroke is called the 45° stroke. The degree indicates the direction of pressure applied to the client's skin. The effleurage stroke, which moves along the surface of the client's skin, is considered to be applied at 0°. Compression, which pushes directly into the client's tissues, is considered a 90° stroke. The 45° stroke uses a pressure midway between that of effleurage and compression.

Once a restriction is found, you can alter your body position slightly to change the direction of your stroke to apply pressure at 45°. As you contact the client at this angle, the slip across the client's skin will almost disappear (Fig. 10-3). Maintain your contact point, continue the 45° pressure, and wait for the client's CT to soften and unwind. In a variation of the stroke, you use one hand to stabilize tissue with compression while the other hand applies the 45° stroke.

This general 45° CT stroke can be applied with the fingers, thumbs, heel/s of the hand/s, whole hand, or even forearm. The restricted area on the client's body determines whether you use your fingers or forearms. For a large area, you may use your forearms, but to release a localized point, the fingers may work better.

Skin Rolling

Skin rolling is used mainly to break up adhesions in the superficial fascia. Restrictions in the fascia may be felt during an effleurage stroke as a skidding motion across the tissue or resistance to the stroke moving across the skin. When a large area of fascial restriction is found, skin rolling can be effective. Establish a contact point in the restricted area and palpate the tissues for restricted movement. Without

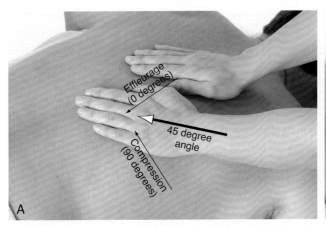
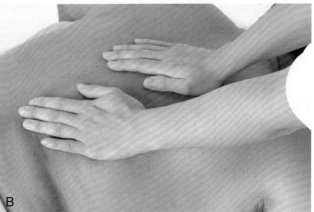

Figure 10-3. 45° stroke. **(A)** Establish contact points and direct pressure at a 45° angle to the client's tissues without any slip on the skin. **(B)** Maintain pressure as the connective tissue softens and spreads out.

any slip on the client's skin, push the tissues away from you, toward you, to your left, and to your right to determine the direction of restriction, which is the direction in which the tissues resist movement the most.

First, you work in the direction of ease, grasping and lifting the client's tissues into a roll, gently pulling it in the direction that it moves easily. Slowly, you change directions to pull the roll of tissues in the direction of restriction. **Going along with the body's tendencies and then slowly moving in a therapeutic direction is usually more effective than immediately pushing the body in the direction of restriction.** Tissues that are more restricted or dehydrated are more difficult to pick up, roll, and move. Skin rolling is especially uncomfortable when the client has considerable fascial restriction and therefore must be performed slowly and carefully, paying close attention to the client's body language. You may tell clients that if the work becomes too uncomfortable, you can slow down or back off a bit. Encourage clients to tell you if the work is beyond their tolerance. People can manage pain better when they can breathe easily without bracing, recoiling, or wincing.

After the skin has been rolled for some distance, the tissues will feel less resistant. At that point, you can slowly release the roll. Use a resting stroke to allow the body a moment to relax and readjust to the reorganized tissues. Then return to the close vicinity of the original contact point and reevaluate the restriction by pushing the tissue in various directions to determine whether a change has occurred. Box 10-10 demonstrates the skin rolling technique.

C-Stroke, S-Stroke

You may find it difficult to lift the tissues enough to grasp them in a roll and even more difficult to keep the roll elevated while transporting it across the client's body. In these situations, you can try one of the variations of skin rolling, such as the C-stroke or the S-stroke.

The C-stroke is a variation of skin rolling in which you still lift a roll of tissue, but instead of transporting the elevated roll, you bend the rolled tissue into the shape of a C. The S-stroke is yet another variation in which you deform the roll of tissue into the shape of an S (Fig. 10-4).

Scar Release

When soft tissues are compromised or injured, the body automatically responds to repair the damage. In phase II of the healing mechanism, collagen fibers are produced to splint the area and prevent further damage. New collagen fibers are relatively easy to align with the fibers of the original tissue, given gentle movement throughout phase III. Collagen fibers continue to be produced during phase III, and without sufficient movement, they become sticky and hard. As a result, the collagen fibers are difficult to realign and they easily develop into CT adhesions, or scars, with far-reaching effects. The scars are visible when the integument is injured, but tissues beneath the surface of the skin can also develop scars. Invisible scars are equally capable of affecting structures in other areas of the body.

Once a scar or adhesion is created in one area, it begins to pull on the fascia throughout the body. The quicker the adhesion is treated, the less likely it is to affect the rest of the body. Because of its patch-like nature, there is a tendency for all other tissues to pull in the direction of the scar, which can lead to more compensation patterns and fascial restrictions.

The above CT techniques are appropriate if the scar is not sensitive. If the client's scar tissue is sensitive, use a gentler technique that promotes the body's self-correcting mechanism and unraveling of the scar tissue. Although it is very similar to the other CT strokes, the scar release technique uniquely combines palpation, CT deformation, and direction of ease. You anchor one end of the scar with a finger, knuckle, or palm, hold another point on the scar, and apply a gentle 45° pressure in the

BOX 10-10

Skin Rolling

1. Establish the contact point and check the tissue for the direction of restriction while maintaining contact.

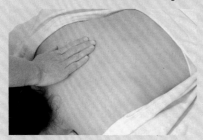

  a. Push the tissue away from you.

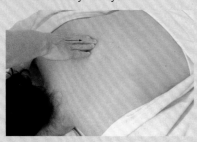

  b. Pull the tissue toward you.

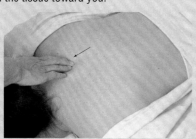

  c. Push the tissue to your left.

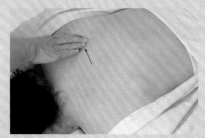

  d. Push the tissue to your right. Tissues do not move easily in this direction, making this the direction of restriction.

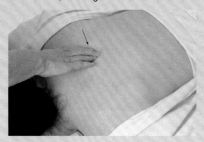

2. Grasp the tissue in a roll, pulling it slightly in the direction of ease, away from the client's spine.

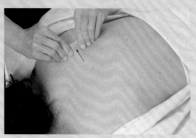

3. Gently change direction, pulling the rolled tissue into the direction of restriction.

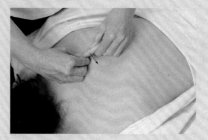

4. Slowly transport the rolled tissue in the direction of restriction by gathering the tissue with your fingers and feeding it into your thumbs, keeping the roll of tissue elevated. Continue the skin roll for several inches, or until the restriction diminishes.

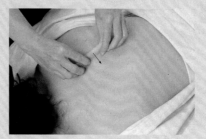

5. Release the roll of tissue carefully. Apply a resting stroke to allow tissues to reorganize. Return to the original contact area and reevaluate the tissue for restriction.

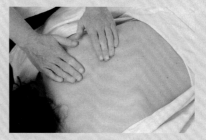

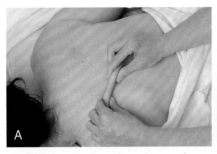
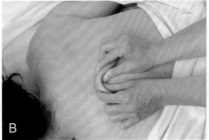
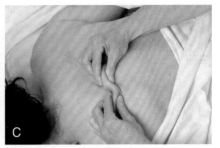

Figure 10-4. Variations of skin rolling: C-stroke and S-stroke. **(A)** Lift tissue into a roll. **(B)** Then deform it into a C-stroke or **(C)** an S-stroke.

direction of restriction. The scar, held in a passive stretch, may start to deform as the tissues are loosened and collagen rearranged.

Maintain your contact point and avoid slipping on the client's skin while you apply sustained 45° pressure. You may feel your finger start to move as the underlying tissues soften and spread out. Massage can help create more functional and mobile scar tissue, but the number of treatments depends on how severe the scarring is and how long the client has had the scar. Box 10-11 illustrates the steps of scar release.

BOX 10-11
Scar Release

1. Palpate the scar to determine the direction of restriction. Anchor one end of the scar with a finger or thumb.

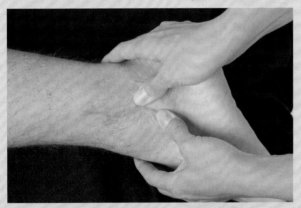

2. Using your other hand, apply 45° pressure with a finger or thumb in the direction of restriction while maintaining the pressure and your contact point. Follow the tissue as it softens and deforms.

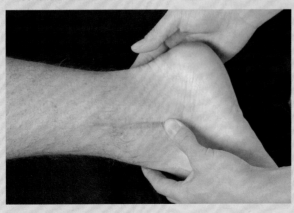

3. Continue to follow the tissue as the fascial adhesions release.

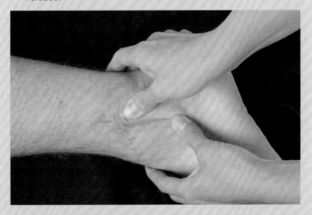

4. Slowly relieve your pressure when you feel the resistance fade away.

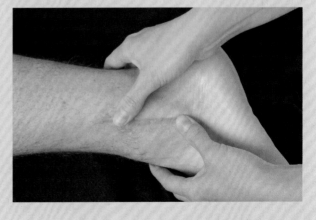

Craniosacral Therapy

Craniosacral therapy (sometimes called cranial sacral therapy and abbreviated CST) is a gentle technique that uses about 5 g of pressure, the weight of a nickel, to evaluate and enhance the craniosacral (KRAY-nee-oh-SAY-kruhl) system in which cerebrospinal fluid (CSF) bathes the brain and spinal cord. By improving the flow of CSF throughout the craniosacral system, overall health can be improved.

In the 1940s, William G. Sutherland, DO, developed a technique he called cranial osteopathy. It is based on his observations of cranial bones moving very slightly in a unique rhythm, distinct from the pulse or breathing pattern. He suggested that restrictions of the cranial movement can negatively affect a person's health. Cranial osteopathy treats an imbalance or interrupted rhythm by manipulating the cranial bones.

John E. Upledger, DO, OMM, born in 1932, further advanced the practice and developed his own form of CST. Using the same basic theory and principles as cranial osteopathy, CST works more with the fascial component of the dura mater and dural tube that encase the brain and spinal cord. From 1975 to 1983, Dr. Upledger performed research at Michigan State University that confirmed the rhythmic movement of the cranial bones and clarified the craniosacral mechanism as the cause for the CSF pulse. His theory suggests that restrictions in the flow of the CSF can cause dysfunctions of the central nervous system, such as sensory and motor dysfunctions and neurological disabilities.

The rhythmic flow of CSF is conducted throughout the body via the three-dimensional fascia, making it possible to feel the movement almost anywhere on the body. Like the cardiac pulse, it is very subtle and difficult or nearly impossible to feel when you apply too much pressure. Although some persons learn to see this slow and very slight movement, most persons can learn to feel it using a very light touch, with no more force than the pressure applied by a nickel resting on your skin. The rate is much slower than the breathing rate, as it generally takes about 10 seconds to complete a cycle. It can be felt as a 4-second outward expansion of the body, followed by a 2-second pause, and then about a 4-second inward contraction or shrinking of the body.

CST practitioners first evaluate the craniosacral rhythm at different key points on the body for smoothness, amplitude, and bilateral evenness. Restricted movement can indicate an obstruction of the CSF flow. By applying very small amounts of pressure to the cranial bones or other areas on the body, you can manipulate the movement, which helps the body restore and regulate the flow of CSF. Theoretically, improving the flow of CSF can relieve a number of associated health conditions such as headaches, autism, tinnitus, poor eye–hand coordination, and vertigo.

The techniques are taught at clinics and workshops worldwide. The Upledger Institute, located in Florida, is one of the foremost authorities on CST and offers courses and certification programs for massage therapists, osteopaths, chiropractors, physical therapists, and other healthcare professionals. See the Upledger Institute web site (www.upledger.com) for more information.

Myofascial Friction Techniques

The fascial layer surrounding the muscles can become sticky or adhesive for several reasons, primarily insufficient hydration, poor nutrition, and inadequate activity. When an adhesion or scar tissue forms, collagen fibers are deposited in a random pattern with the fibers going in multiple directions. Friction is the main form of myofascial work specifically intended to disrupt and break down adhesions and scar tissue in soft tissue structures with linear fiber alignment such as muscles, tendons, and ligaments. The three basic types of friction are cross-fiber friction (XFF), circular friction (CF), and longitudinal friction (LF). The mechanism of friction actually reinjures the affected tissue to initiate phases II and III of the healing mechanism, which involve the production and proper alignment of collagen fibers. Understanding the process of collagen fiber alignment in phase III, you can help the original injury heal with a more mobile and functional scar.

The recovery period following a friction treatment is as important as the treatment itself. Make sure that the client uses the frictioned muscle regularly and without resistance or weight. The activity should be slow and careful, and it should move through the full range of motion to create a functional scar. Without this gentle activity, a CT adhesion is likely to return.

James H. Cyriax, MD, MRCP, was an orthopedic doctor whose approach to musculoskeletal disorders included three principles:

1. Every pain has a source.
2. Treatment must reach the source.
3. Treatment must benefit the source to relieve the pain.

Starting at the location of a person's pain, he followed the myofascial lines of tension back to the site of the initial adhesion and was able to treat the pain by applying **XFF** to the adhesion. His work was so successful that Dr. Cyriax is credited with reintroducing manual therapy to the medical community. Because XFF can be very intense and uncomfortable, take great care to stay within the client's tolerance. Figure 10-5 illustrates XFF.

CF is applied in small, circular motions to the affected tissue. It can be a very useful technique for addressing deep adhesions and scars (Fig. 10-6).

LF can help separate the randomly arranged fibers, freeing them up to allow more muscle movement. It differs from the other friction techniques because it is applied in the direction of the muscle fibers with a quicker and more superficial stroke. Figure 10-7 shows the application of LF.

Several principles guide the use of any type of friction (Box 10-12).

10 Therapeutic Applications

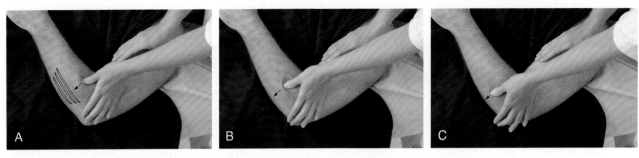

Figure 10-5. Cross-fiber friction. (**A–C**) The stroke runs perpendicular to the muscle fibers.

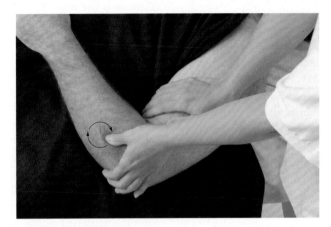

Figure 10-6. Circular friction.

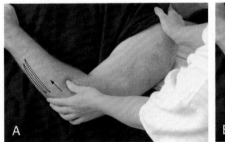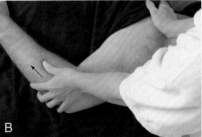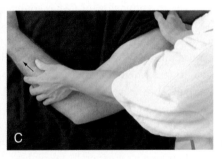

Figure 10-7. Longitudinal friction. (**A–C**) The stroke runs parallel to the muscle fibers.

BOX 10-12

Principles for Applying Friction

- Educate the client about the technique. The therapist should explain that friction is a deep treatment designed to provide a controlled reinjury of the tissue and may induce pain. The therapist can explain that reinjury will allow the body to heal the tissue in a more functional manner.
- Obtain the client's consent to receive friction treatment.
- Fingernails must be short to apply this technique.
- The tissue must be warm prior to application.
- No lubricant is used, to allow the therapist to maintain the contact point.

- The client must be in a comfortable position that gives the therapist access to the affected tissues.
- Pressure is applied in one or more directions based on the objective of the treatment.
- The pressure should be deep enough to penetrate the tissue and be annoying to the client yet remain within the client's pain tolerance.
- The therapist must tell the client that ice is recommended following treatment to reduce inflammation.

Trigger Point Techniques

Usually activated by acute or repetitive overuse, a **trigger point (TrP)** is a localized area of hypertonicity. TrPs occur at the motor end unit, which is the neuromuscular junction, or meeting point between a nerve cell and the muscle cell it controls. TrP techniques are sometimes considered a subcategory of myofascial release and sometimes a form of neuromuscular (NOO-roh-MUSS-kyoo-lahr) therapy. In addition to treating fascial restrictions, TrP techniques address hypertonic areas of muscle tissue. Janet Travell, MD (1901–1997) developed TrP therapy, and her research continues to be the most widely referenced in this type of treatment. Putting pressure directly on top of a TrP is usually painful for the client, and because of the nerve involvement, it refers vague, aching discomfort or an itchy sensation to the surrounding areas, in a specific pattern. It is usually painful for the client to actively move a muscle with a TrP, and the pain tends to limit the range of motion before reaching the end feel.

The difference between a tender point and a TrP is the involvement of a motor end unit. Tender points are areas of hypertonicity that do not refer pain. TrPs are so named because the malfunctioning neuromuscular junction triggers pain in specific patterns elsewhere on the body. Maps and charts of specific TrPs and their referred pain patterns are available for many muscles and can be very helpful. Figure 10-8 is a TrP map for the latissimus dorsi muscle.

A TrP is not a pathologic disease, but it does result from a hypertonic muscle. The decreased circulation in a hypertonic area reduces nutritional exchange to the area, causing

it to be hypersensitive and hyperirritable. This is another example of the pain cycle in action. Several factors can create or perpetuate TrPs:

- Mechanical stresses, including skeletal misalignment
- Poor posture
- Long-term muscle constriction, such as compression by a purse or backpack
- Nutritional inadequacies
- Insufficient hydration
- Psychological factors, such as stress or the sympathetic nervous system response
- Inadequate sleep

TrPs that have existed longer than 3 weeks are considered chronic, and they can cause numbness and tingling along their specific referral patterns. They can also cause satellite TrPs in the synergistic muscles, created as a result of the original muscle being shortened and pulling the synergists into shortened positions.

The general benefits of wellness massage offer relief to clients suffering from TrPs, but specific TrP techniques can provide relief to the localized and referred pain, tingling, numbness, sensation of heat or cold, and itching. A TrP can feel like a nodule or localized area of hypertonicity amid a taut band of tissue running parallel to the muscle fibers. According to Dr. Travell, several methods can be used to release the hypertonicity at these troublesome neuromuscular junctions: PNF and friction techniques (discussed above), TrP pressure release, and strumming. A combination of techniques can also release a TrP.

Trigger Point Pressure Release

In the trigger point pressure release (also the direct pressure release) technique, you first extend the target muscle to its comfort barrier and palpate the TrP. Figure 10-9 illustrates the techniques for palpating TrPs. Increase your finger pressure on the TrP until you feel tissue resistance and maintain that pressure until the tissues release. This may take between 30 and 45 seconds. The release will feel like the nodule is melting as it lets go. Keep your contact finger on the original contact point on the client's skin and follow the release. The tissues may soften to allow your finger to sink deeper or the tissues may move in an irregular path at an irregular speed with fascial unwinding. There is a delicate balance between applying enough pressure to release the TrP and applying so much pressure that it worsens. The completion of the release is similar to the feeling you get at the bottom of a slide; initially, there is a force that pulls you, and then the pull slowly fades away.

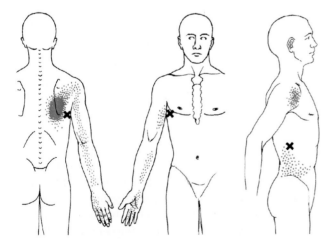

Figure 10-8. Trigger point map for the latissimus dorsi. (MediClip image copyright © 2003 Lippincott Williams & Wilkins. All rights reserved.)

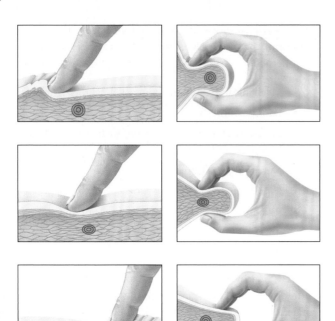

Figure 10-9. Techniques for palpating trigger points. (Reprinted with permission from Bucci C. Condition-Specific Massage Therapy. Baltimore: Lippincott Williams & Wilkins, 2012.)

The release is effectively a neurological lengthening of the muscle fibers. To maintain the new length, the muscle and fascia must then be stretched for 5 to 10 seconds while you wait for a tendon reflex to relax the muscle further. Lengthening without stretching may cause the muscle to revert to its shortened position. Think of the longer loaf of bread in the shorter bag.

The more severe the TrP, the more it refers pain, so apply only minimal pressure to release the TrP. When spasm and muscle guarding are accompanied by satellite TrPs, release the satellite TrPs first. Your initial pressure on the TrP may be uncomfortable for the client but should not register as pain. As you continue to hold the point, the discomfort will diminish as the TrP releases. After circulation and nutrition are restored to the area, you may feel the area heat up. This TrP technique requires very little physical work and is a good approach to use when PNF is unsuccessful.

Strumming

If PNF and the pressure release technique do not release TrPs, you may need to try a more aggressive approach. Dr. Travell's strumming technique is very much like XFF. It is most effective when the TrP is located near the center of the muscle belly. When you find a TrP, strum your finger perpendicular to the muscle fibers, at the level of the TrP

until you come in contact with the TrP. Maintain light pressure on the TrP until it releases and melts under your finger. Following the release, continue the strum across the rest of the muscle's fibers. Finally, the tissues need to be elongated and stretched.

Trigger Point Release Using Combined Techniques

Sometimes a TrP is particularly persistent, and you will have to try several different approaches to facilitate its release. Using a combination of techniques in a single application can sometimes be the gentlest, quickest, most effective choice:

- TrP pressure and PR
- TrP pressure and RI
- TrP pressure and PIR
- TrP pressure and CT strokes
- CT strokes and CST

To combine TrP pressure with a PNF technique, apply pressure to the TrP with a monitoring finger (or knuckle or thumb) and use the pressure release technique while concurrently using the PNF technique. The combinations that use PNF along with the pressure release are very effective and typically last longer.

Combining TrP pressure release and CT strokes often comes naturally. The primary difference between the 45° stroke and TrP pressure release is simply the monitoring finger. In both techniques, you apply pressure and wait for the client's tissues to deform, become more liquid, and release. The combination of these techniques requires maintaining contact with the TrP with a monitoring finger while the CT is being rearranged.

The combination of CT strokes and CST is not used as much as the other combinations, because there is no monitoring finger on the TrP. Either technique can release a TrP using slow, steady pressure to facilitate a myofascial change. Basically, CT strokes, craniosacral techniques, and TrP pressure release are variations of each other, the difference being the monitoring finger.

As with all PNF techniques and TrP release techniques, the target muscle and its CTs should be elongated and stretched following treatment. TrP release is a versatile addition to your toolbox of techniques. It is important to remember from the pain section in this chapter that light pressure is also effective for "closing the gate" of impulses to the brain. Incorporate this concept by finishing your work with a resting stroke, thus reducing the perception of pain. Additionally, following the law of facilitation, consistent massage with either light or therapeutic pressure will help clients reduce their chronic pain patterns.

Trigger Point Techniques for Specific Conditions

While no single technique is a cure-all, TrP therapy can often do a lot to alleviate pain and tension in a particular area or with a particular condition. What follows are common areas or conditions that clients complain of when they seek massage therapy for treatment.

Chronic Neck Pain

There are many causes of neck pain: trauma, injury, or postural distortions such as the forward head posture so often seen in clients who sit at a computer for work. It is important to know which muscles may be involved in the neck pain, so the first step is to identify them using assessment skills. Some of the muscles involved in the neck pain may include:

- Levator scapula
- Trapezius
- Rhomboids
- Subclavius
- Pectoralis major
- Sternocleidomastoid
- Scalenes
- Masseter
- Temporalis
- Medial and lateral pterygoid
- Splenius capitus and splenius cervicis
- Semispinalis
- Suboccipitals

Once the muscles are identified, TrP maps may help you locate a starting point when looking for TrPs. Figure 10-10 shows TrP maps for the muscles that may be involved in neck pain.

When treating chronic neck pain, first prepare the tissue with general effleurage to increase the circulation to the area. If you choose the direct pressure release technique, locate the TrPs in the target muscles and follow the steps below:

- Palpate the TrP and gently increase your finger pressure until you feel resistance.
- Hold for approximately 30 to 45 seconds until you feel a melting of the tissue.
- Stretch the affected area.
- Perform a resting stroke.
- Reassess the client.

Chronic Low Back Pain

As in neck pain, the causes of chronic low back pain are trauma, injury, overuse or repetitive stress, or postural distortions. Compensation patterns may be part of the postural distortions, possibly resulting from ongoing postural strain such as daily heavy lifting or tight hamstrings. Perform an adequate assessment to determine which muscles are involved in your client's low back pain. The following muscles may be involved:

- Quadratus lumborum
- Iliacus
- Psoas major, psoas minor
- Rectus femoris
- Tensor fascia latae
- Gluteus maximus, gluteus medius, gluteus minimus
- Deep hip rotators (piriformis, gemellus superior, gemellus inferior, obturator internus, obturator externus, quadratus femoris)
- Hamstrings

Figure 10-11 illustrates the TrPs and referral patterns for some of the muscles involved in chronic low back pain.

When treating chronic low back pain, start by warming the area with effleurage. If you choose the direct pressure release technique, locate the TrPs in the target muscles and follow the steps below:

- Palpate the TrP and gently increase your finger pressure until you feel resistance.
- Hold for approximately 30 to 45 seconds until you feel a melting of the tissue.
- Stretch the affected area.
- Perform a resting stroke.
- Reassess the client.

CHAPTER SUMMARY

The responses to therapeutic massage vary widely, but these more advanced techniques give you the opportunity to treat specific soft tissue conditions efficiently and effectively. Massage students and massage therapists who understand the mechanisms of injury and tissue repair and the pain cycle can use one or a combination of these techniques when a client is looking for more than a wellness massage. The therapeutic applications in this chapter can easily be added to a wellness massage session. Techniques based on the concepts of lengthening muscles, stretching CT, and going in the direction of ease will minimize the

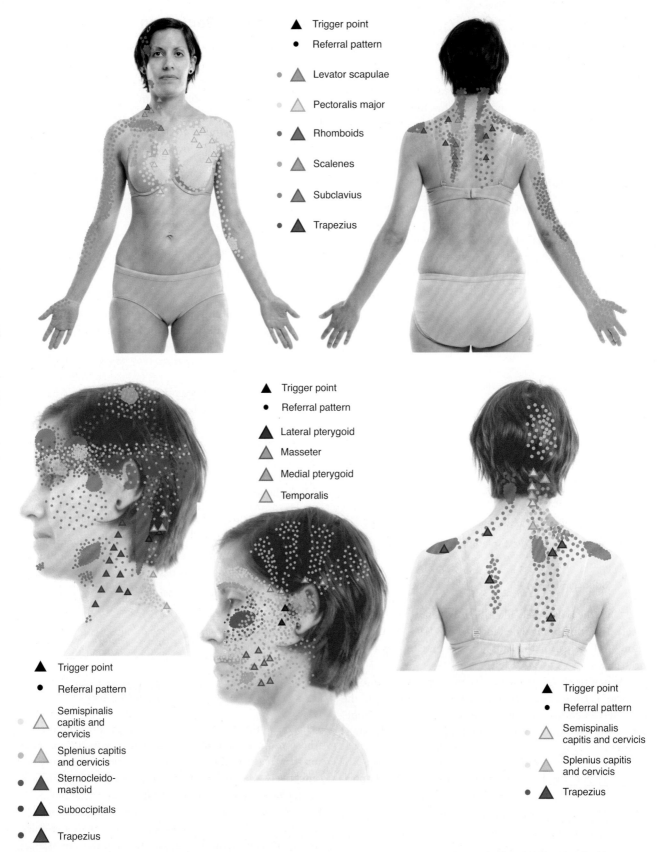

Figure 10-10. Trigger point maps showing trigger points and referral patterns for muscles involved in neck pain. (Reprinted with permission from Bucci C. Condition-Specific Massage Therapy. Baltimore: Lippincott Williams & Wilkins, 2012.)

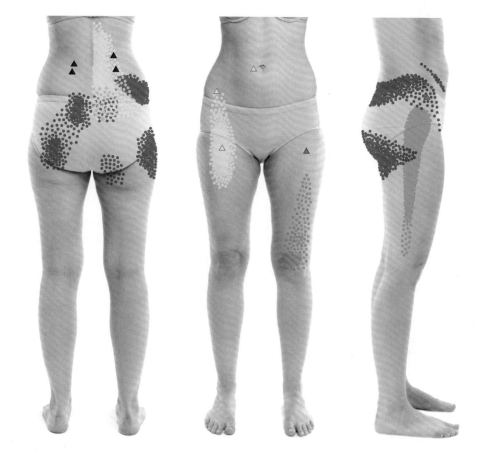

- ▲ Trigger point
- ● Referral pattern
- ○ △ Iliopsoas
- ● ▲ Quadratus lumborum
- ● ▲ Rectus femoris
- ● ▲ Tensor fasciae latae

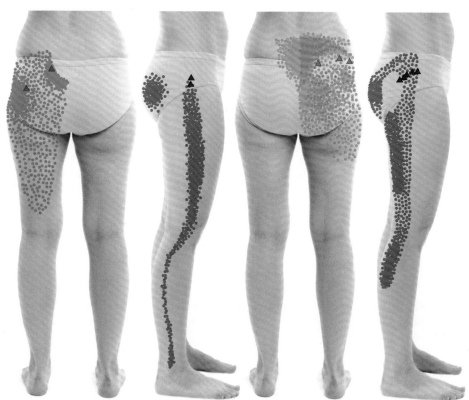

- ▲ Trigger point
- ● Referral pattern
- ● ▲ Gluteus medius
- ● ▲ Gluteus minimus
- ● ▲ Piriformis

Figure 10-11. Trigger points and referral patterns for some of the muscles involved in chronic low back pain. (Reprinted with permission from Bucci C. Condition-Specific Massage Therapy. Baltimore: Lippincott Williams & Wilkins, 2012.)

Therapeutic Applications

10

amount of effort needed to change the musculature while increasing the effectiveness and permanence of changes. Clearly, it is important to address fascia when treating the muscles.

Your knowledge of medical terminology, anatomy, physiology, ethics, professionalism, documentation, and business practices as provided throughout this text are especially important for practicing therapeutic massage, because you are more likely to be communicating with persons in the medical, legal, and insurance fields. Also, the use of professional documentation, assessment, and treatment plans elevate a simple massage to a legitimate form of healthcare.

Documentation keeps all the details straight, so stay on top of your SOAP notes. Remember to include self-care recommendations that are relevant to the client's goals, simple, specific, and easy to follow. Clients who want to restore function and return to a healthier condition will be more likely to participate in their own healthcare and will appreciate your pre- and posttreatment assessment and self-care recommendations. On the other hand, some clients will seemingly resist improvement. You cannot force a client to accomplish a goal. In reality, you are not directly making the changes to a client's tissues—you are helping the client's own body make the changes. Keep in mind that you are only a facilitator, and try to not get frustrated with clients who do not work toward their treatment goals.

Most clients respond well to these therapeutic techniques, and some will be interested in knowing how the techniques work. Any time clients are interested in your work, you have the opportunity to educate them about massage. The more people know about the benefits of massage, the better.

CHAPTER EXERCISES

1. Describe the events that occur in each of the three phases of healing.

2. Provide a real-life example of the pain cycle, including specific muscles or injuries for each stage of the cycle.

3. List at least five of the principles of therapeutic massage.

4. Define the following:

   a. Muscle guarding

   b. Target muscle

   c. Stretching

   d. Direction of restriction

   e. Tender point

   f. Unwinding

   g. Trigger point

   h. Lengthening

5. Practice the PNF procedures on a partner. First assess the joint range of motion moved by your target muscle, then perform each of the following techniques, and finish with a posttreatment assessment to determine whether any changes in muscle length occurred:

   a. Direct manipulation

   b. Positional release

   c. Post-isometric relaxation

   d. Reciprocal inhibition

6. Describe the difference between the stretch reflex and the tendon reflex.

7. Practice each of the following connective tissue techniques on a partner, and ask your partner for feedback regarding discomfort, sensations, and responses:

   a. 45° stroke

   b. Skin rolling

   c. C-stroke

   d. S-stroke

8. Practice your palpation skills by trying to feel the craniosacral rhythm on several different people. With your "client" in a supine position, use a very light touch (the weight of a nickel) on the cranium, anterior superior iliac spines, the knees, and the toes.

9. List at least five of the principles for applying friction.

10. Practice the two different TrP release techniques (direct pressure and strumming) on a partner. If your partner does not have a TrP, pretend that you found one and proceed with the techniques.

CRITICAL THINKING ▪ EXERCISE #1

Using the client information provided, complete the following two critical thinking scenarios, developing a treatment plan appropriate for each client.

Profile of Client

A 35-year-old female complains of stiffness and deep, constant aching primarily in her right knee and also in her right hip. Her symptoms increase with activity, preventing her from running for more than 10 minutes. The discomfort interrupts her sleep, sometimes waking her up two to three times a night. She reports her stiffness is most noticeable when she stands still for more than 15 minutes.

Her health information form indicates that she works as a surgical nurse 3 days a week and normally runs 5 days a week for 60 minutes, but her exercise is now limited by the pain. She has sprained her knee twice in the past: 15 years ago when she twisted her knee stepping off a curb with roller blades on and once about 8 years ago, when she slipped on the ice. The right knee pain has been bothering her for years, but since being diagnosed with a sprain, she has not sought evaluation or treatment from a medical professional. The right hip pain has developed over the past year. She takes ibuprofen as needed for the pain and applies ice to her right knee after running. She drinks about 4 glasses of water and 1 cup of coffee daily, and is fairly health conscious. Monthly massage has been a regular part of her healthcare for several years.

Upon initial assessment, both of the client's feet have low arches and her ankles are slightly everted. Her right hip is medially rotated, and AROM testing of the right hip reveals moderately painful and limited lateral rotation. Her left hip is laterally rotated and exhibits mildly painful and limited medial rotation. Active and passive ROM for bilateral ankle inversion is limited but not painful. There is pain upon AROM of right knee flexion and medial rotation, but no joint movements are accompanied by pain upon PROM. The client had an imbalanced, somewhat irregular gait, but no specific abnormality could be pinpointed.

Functional assessments can help determine whether passive joint structures may be involved in the client's condition and whether the client needs to be referred to another healthcare professional for evaluation. In the case of a ligament sprain, massage is a local contraindication only during the acute phase. After the acute phase, systemic massage encourages the healing process and prevents scar tissue and fascial restrictions from developing.

Compensation patterns commonly accompany knee pain because the knee is such an active joint. This client is on her feet most of her workday and frequently runs for exercise, so it is important to address any muscles that are working to compensate for the pain.

Review Client Information

Condition

What current soft tissue or pathological conditions is the client experiencing?

- What are the functional limitations associated with this condition?
- What are the treatment options for this condition?
- Is massage indicated or contraindicated for this condition?
- Has the client undergone any other treatment for this condition? If so, what have the results been?
- How long has this condition been present and how long does it typically last?

Interview

Pain

What are the past or present conditions that might be causing pain or compensation patterns?

- Qualify the pain as sharp, dull, or radiating (radiating pain may indicate nerve involvement and possible referral to another healthcare professional, whereas sharp pain may indicate a recent injury).
- Quantify the pain on a scale of 1–10.
- Does the pain increase or decrease during the day?
- What aggravates the pain?
- What tends to reduce the pain?

Sleep

If sleep seems to be affected by the condition, compare the client's past sleep patterns with the present:

- Bedtime
- Amount of time it takes to fall asleep
- Number of consecutive hours of sleep
- Number of times client awakens during the night
- Wake-up time
- Pain/discomfort upon waking
- Anything the client thinks might be affecting sleep

Hydration

How much water does the client tend to drink during the day? (Insufficient water levels can result in thickened fascia, which increases friction between tissues and can increase pain.)

Physical Activity

What are the client's physical activity habits?
- Duration/frequency of physical activity/exercise
- Does the client tend to warm up and/or stretch prior to exercise? (This is an opportunity to educate clients about the importance of warming up before exercising and the difference between stretching and lengthening.)
- Does the client tend to increase water consumption following exercise?

Design the Massage

Determine which muscles to treat

What movements are involved, causing pain or are restricted?

Consulting the special muscle section in Chapter 4, what muscles are involved in the movement(s)?

Consulting Table 10-1, what are the antagonists to the involved muscles?

Consulting Box 7-2, identify any compensation patterns.

Given the muscles involved and compensation patterns revealed, choose only two or three areas to address (to minimize the body's recovery after treatment).
- Avoid treating areas that elicit pain upon passive contraction (outside the scope of practice).

Determine techniques to use during the massage

Consider the client's history and interview to decide which techniques to use:
- People involved in sports tend to respond well to PNF techniques.
- Avoid techniques that elicit pain.
- Long-term conditions and compensation patterns may have fascial restrictions that can benefit from myofascial release (MFR).
- Are there any adaptations that should be made to a standard massage flow?
- Are there any conditions such as pain or sinus trouble that require positioning considerations?
- Are there any local contraindications that you must avoid during the massage?
- Are there any sensitivities or allergies to consider?

Develop treatment plan

Based on the client's input, the physician diagnosis and treatment, and the massage therapy assessment, what are some appropriate short-term and long-term goals?

Treatment

With the client's input and all of the information you have regarding the condition, what is a reasonable future treatment plan for achieving those objectives/goals?

CRITICAL THINKING ▪ EXERCISE #2

Profile of Client

A 45-year-old male complains of constant, moderate low back pain that resulted from shoveling snow about 3 months ago. He typically runs 3 miles, five times per week, and bicycles 5 miles to work at least 2 days a week. The pain, which increases after exercising, has forced him to cut back on his regular exercise. His job as a corporate vice president requires him to sit through meetings and conference calls every day, and he has trouble sitting at work all day without taking 400 mg of ibuprofen to relieve the pain. The client drinks at least 8 cups of water per day, but he also eats a lot of fast food and tends to drink alcohol nightly.

Upon initial visual assessment, the left side of his pelvis is higher than the right, and his head is slightly forward. His gait was normal, and ROM evaluations revealed no pain upon limited active lateral flexion of the spine to the right, and pain upon limited AROM of flexion of the left hip.

Functional assessments can help determine whether the pain pattern results from nerve involvement, in which case the client needs to be referred to another healthcare professional for evaluation. In the case of an intervertebral disc herniation, massage is a local contraindication. Systemic massage is beneficial for the client's general health and can keep compensation patterns from developing into fascial restrictions.

Review Client Information

Condition

What current soft tissue or pathological conditions is the client experiencing?
- What are the functional limitations associated with this condition?
- What are the treatment options for this condition?
- Is massage indicated or contraindicated for this condition?
- Has the client undergone any other treatment for this condition? If so, what have the results been?
- How long has this condition been present and how long does it typically last?

Interview

Pain

What are the past or present conditions that might be causing pain or compensation patterns?

- Qualify the pain as sharp, dull, or radiating (radiating pain may indicate nerve involvement and possible referral to another healthcare professional, whereas sharp pain may indicate a recent injury).
- Quantify the pain on a scale of 1–10.
- Does the pain increase or decrease during the day?
- What aggravates the pain?
- What tends to reduce the pain?

Sleep
If sleep seems to be affected by the condition, compare the client's past sleep patterns with the present:
- Bedtime
- Amount of time it takes to fall asleep
- Number of consecutive hours of sleep
- Number of times client awakens during the night
- Wake-up time
- Pain/discomfort upon waking
- Anything the client thinks might be affecting sleep

Hydration
How much water does the client tend to drink during the day? (Insufficient water levels can result in thickened fascia, which increases friction between tissues and can increase pain.)

Physical Activity
What are the client's physical activity habits?
- Duration/frequency of physical activity/exercise
- Does the client tend to warm up and/or stretch prior to exercise? (This is an opportunity to educate clients about the importance of warming up before exercising and the difference between stretching and lengthening.)
- Does the client tend to increase water consumption following exercise?

Design the Massage

Determine which muscles to treat
What movements are involved, causing pain or are restricted?

Consulting the special muscle section in Chapter 4, what muscles are involved in the movement(s)?

Consulting Table 10-1, what are the antagonists to the involved muscles?

Consulting Box 7-2, identify any compensation patterns.

Given the muscles involved and compensation patterns revealed, choose only two or three areas to address (to minimize the body's recovery after treatment)
- Avoid treating areas that elicit pain upon passive contraction (outside the scope of practice).

Determine techniques to use during the massage
Consider the client's history and interview to decide which techniques to use:
- People involved in sports tend to respond well to PNF techniques.
- Avoid techniques that elicit pain.
- Long-term conditions and compensation patterns may have fascial restrictions that can benefit from MFR.
- Are there any adaptations that should be made to a standard massage flow?
- Are there any conditions such as pain or sinus trouble that require positioning considerations?
- Are there any local contraindications that you must avoid during the massage?
- Are there any sensitivities or allergies to consider?

Develop treatment plan
Based on the client's input, the physician diagnosis and treatment, and the massage therapy assessment, what are some appropriate short-term and long-term goals?

Treatment
With the client's input and all of the information you have regarding the condition, what is a reasonable future treatment plan for achieving those objectives/goals?

Find a partner who can be a "sample client" and follow the critical thinking format below to design a therapeutic massage treatment that is appropriate for the client's condition.

CRITICAL THINKING ▪ FORMAT FOR DESIGNING A THERAPEUTIC MASSAGE

Review Client Information

Condition
What current soft tissue or pathological conditions is the client experiencing?
- What are the functional limitations associated with this condition?

- What are the treatment options for this condition?
- Is massage indicated or contraindicated for this condition?
- Has the client undergone any other treatment for this condition? If so, what have the results been?

- How long has this condition been present and how long does it typically last?

Pain
What are the past or present conditions that might be causing pain or compensation patterns?
- Qualify the pain as sharp, dull, or radiating (radiating pain may indicate nerve involvement and possible referral to another healthcare professional, whereas sharp pain may indicate a recent injury).
- Quantify the pain on a scale of 1–10.
- Does the pain increase or decrease during the day?
- What aggravates the pain?
- What tends to reduce the pain?

Sleep
If sleep seems to be affected by the condition, compare the client's past sleep patterns with the present:
- Bedtime
- Amount of time it takes to fall asleep
- Number of consecutive hours of sleep
- Number of times client awakens during the night
- Wake-up time
- Pain/discomfort upon waking
- Anything the client thinks might be affecting sleep

Hydration
How much water does the client tend to drink during the day? (Insufficient water levels can result in thickened fascia, which increases friction between tissues and can increase pain.)

Physical Activity
What are the client's physical activity habits?
- Duration/frequency of physical activity/exercise
- Does the client tend to warm up and/or stretch prior to exercise? (This is an opportunity to educate clients about the importance of warming up before exercising and the difference between stretching and lengthening.)
- Does the client tend to increase water consumption following exercise?

Determine which muscles to treat
What movements are involved, causing pain or are restricted?

Consulting the special muscle section in Chapter 4, what muscles are involved in the movement(s)?

Consulting Table 10-1, what are the antagonists to the involved muscles?

Consulting Box 7-2, identify any compensation patterns.

Given the muscles involved and compensation patterns revealed, choose only two or three areas to address (to minimize the body's recovery after treatment).
- Avoid treating areas that elicit pain upon passive contraction (outside the scope of practice).

Determine techniques to use during the massage
Consider the client's history and interview to decide which techniques to use:
- People involved in sports tend to respond well to PNF techniques.
- Avoid techniques that elicit pain.
- Long-term conditions and compensation patterns may have fascial restrictions that can benefit from MFR.
- Are there any adaptations that should be made to a standard massage flow?
- Are there any conditions such as pain or sinus trouble that require positioning considerations?
- Are there any local contraindications that you must avoid during the massage?
- Are there any sensitivities or allergies to consider?

Develop treatment plan
Based on the client's input, the physician diagnosis and treatment, and massage therapy assessment, what are some appropriate short-term and long-term goals?

Treatment
With the client's input and all of the information you have regarding the condition, what is a reasonable future treatment plan for achieving those objectives/goals? ∎

SUGGESTED READINGS

Chaitow L. *Modern Neuromuscular Techniques*. London: Churchill Livingstone, 1996.

Chaitow L, DeLany JW. *Clinical Application of Neuromuscular Techniques*. Vol 1. London: Churchill Livingstone, 2000.

Chikly B. *Silent Waves: Theory and Practice of Lymph Drainage Therapy: An Osteopathic Lymphatic Technique*. 2nd ed. Scottsdale, AZ: I.H.H. Publishing, 2004.

Chikly B, Welfley S. Lymphedema and lymph-drainage techniques. *AMTA Massage Ther J* 2001; Fall:80–88.

Cohen BJ, Wood DL. *Memmler's Structure and Function of the Human Body*. 7th ed. Philadelphia: Lippincott Williams & Wilkins, 2000.

Dixon MW. *Myofascial Massage*. Baltimore: Lippincott Williams & Wilkins, 2007.

Fritz S. *Fundamentals of Therapeutic Massage*. 2nd ed. St. Louis: Mosby, 2000.

Granger J. *Neuromuscular Therapy Manual*. Baltimore: Lippincott Williams & Wilkins, 2011.

Gray H, Lewis WH. *Anatomy of the Human Body*. 23rd ed. Philadelphia: Lea & Febiger, 1936.

Kneipp S. *The Kneipp Cure*. New York: The Nature Cure Publishing Company, 1949.

Lidell L, Thomas S, Cook CB, et al. *The Book of Massage*. New York: Gaia Books Limited/Simon and Schuster, 1984.

Maxwell-Hudson C. *K.I.S.S. Guide to Massage*. New York: DK Publishing, 2001.

Myers TW. *Anatomy Trains: Myofascial Meridians for Manual and Movement Therapists*. 2nd ed. New York: Churchill Livingstone Elsevier, 2009.

Persad RS. *Massage Therapy and Medications General Treatment Principles*. Toronto: Curties-Overzet, 2001.

Salvo SG. *Massage Therapy: Principles and Practice*. 2nd ed. St. Louis: Saunders/Elsevier Science, 2003.

Schuemann DW. *The Balanced Body: A Guide to Deep Tissue and Neuromuscular Therapy*. 2nd ed. Baltimore: Lippincott Williams & Wilkins, 2002.

Simons DG, Travell JG, Simons LS. *Travell and Simons' Myofascial Pain and Dysfunction: The Trigger Point Manual*. Vol 1. 2nd ed. Baltimore: Lippincott Williams & Wilkins, 1999.

Sjøvold T, et al. *Der Mann im Eis*. Berlin: Springer, 1995:279–286.

Spindler K. *The Man in the Ice*. London: Weidenfeld & Nicolson, 1994.

Thompson D. *Hands Heal: Communication, Documentation, and Insurance Billing for Manual Therapists*. 2nd ed. Baltimore: Lippincott Williams & Wilkins, 2002.

Werner R. *A Massage Therapist's Guide to Pathology*. Philadelphia: Lippincott Williams & Wilkins, 1998.

http://aaomed.org/about/index.php, accessed 3.5.06.

http://erikdalton.com/media/published-articles/pain-game-part-1/, accessed 5.27.12.

http://erikdalton.com/media/published-articles/pain-game-part-2/, accessed 5.27.12.

http://medweb.bham.ac.uk/http/depts/path/teaching/foundat/repair/healing.html, accessed 3.5.06.

http://www.amtamassage.org/articles/2/PressRelease/detail/2545, accessed 5.30.12.

http://www.chiroweb.com/archives/19/08/21.html, accessed 3.5.06.

http://www.cityhealthcentre.nildram.co.uk/cranial.htm, accessed 3.5.06.

http://www.csha.net/advanced/spa.html, accessed 4.11.05.

http://www.cyriax.com/default.html, accessed 3.5.06.

http://www.dayspaassociation.com/mainpages/spaglossary.htm, accessed 4.16.05.

http://www.e-antiinflammatory.com/, accessed 3.5.06.

http://www.efunda.com/materials/piezo/general_info/gen_info_index.cfm, accessed 3.5.06.

http://www.esomc.com/orthopaedic_medicine.htm, accessed 3.5.06.

http://www.exrx.net/Lists/Articulations.html, accessed 3.5.06.

http://www.hendrickhealth.org/rehab/strain.htm, accessed 3.5.06.

http://www.iahe.com/html/therapies/ldt.php, accessed 6.23.12.

http://www.jdaross.cwc.net/inflammatory_response.htm, accessed 3.5.06.

http://www.lymphatics.net, accessed 3.5.06.

http://www.massagemag.com/spa/body/mud.html, accessed 4.21.05.

http://www.m-w.com/cgi-bin/dictionary?thixotropic, accessed 3.5.06.

http://www.myotherapy1.com/myotherapy_faq.htm, accessed 3.5.06.

http://www.pathwaysmag.com/cranios.html, accessed 3.5.06.

http://www.ptcentral.com/muscles/, accessed 3.5.06.

http://www.qub.ac.uk/cm/pat/education/Inflamm/tsld004.htm, accessed 3.5.06.

http://www.stjohnseminars.com/phil.html, accessed 6.11.12.

http://www.thespacenter.com/gscframeset.html, accessed 8.5.05.

http://www.time.com/time/innovators_v2/alt_medicine/profile_upledger.html, accessed 3.5.06.

http://www.upledger.com/therapies/cst_faq.htm, accessed 3.5.06.

http://www.upledgerinstitute.com, accessed 3.10.06.

http://www.woundcare.org/newsvol4n1/ar2.htm, accessed 3.5.06.

11

Complementary Modalities

(with contributions from Marybetts Sinclair, LMT, and Debra C. Howard, AOBTA-Certified Instructor, Dipl. ABT [NCCAOM], LMT)

Objectives

Upon completion of this chapter, the student will be able to:

- Describe how hydrotherapy can enhance a massage session
- Describe how Qi and the Oriental concept of energy meridians relate to each other
- Name the five vital substances in Chinese medicine
- Name the five elements of nature in Ayurveda
- Describe the concept of a chakra
- Name at least four benefits of reflexology
- Demonstrate a basic reflexology treatment
- Describe the concept of polarity therapy

Key Terms

Acupoints: Specifically located points on the body that influence, and are influenced by, body energies.

Acupressure (AK-yoo-preh-sher): A bodywork modality in which firm fingertip pressure is applied to acupoints along the energy meridians to regulate the flow of Qi.

Asian Bodywork Therapy (ABT): The term used to encompass all bodywork modalities that have their theoretical roots in Chinese medicine.

Bioenergy: The electrical, electromagnetic, and/or bioelectromagnetic qualities of living tissue.

Contrast therapy: Heat application followed by cold application, also called alternating therapy.

Deficiency: The term used to describe a depleted condition in Chinese medicine.

Excess: The term used to describe an overly strong condition in Chinese medicine.

Five Vital Substances: Defined by Chinese medicine as the five basic substances that supplement the tissues in a human body: Qi, Blood, Essence, body fluids, and Shen (consciousness).

Hydrotherapy: The external or internal use of water for therapeutic use.

Meridians: Precise and orderly channels or pathways through which Qi flows.

Meridian therapy: The art of working to open and move the joints, release blockages in tissue, balance the Qi moving in the meridians, and stimulate the actions of acupoints as needed.

Polarity (poh-LAIR-ih-tee) therapy: A modality in which very light massage strokes and energy movements are applied on and off the client's body to balance electromagnetic fields, energy nutrition, and develop a higher consciousness.

Qi (C'hi, Ki) (pronounced CHEE): Life force or vital energy; the bioenergy of living things.

Reflexology (REE-fleks-AH-loh-jee): A modality in which fingertip compression is applied to reflex points on the hand, foot, or ear that affect other parts of the body.

Yang (YAHNG): Energy that flows down from the sun and is associated with the active, bright, warm, consumptive, and outward activities of the body.

Yin (YIHN): Energy that flows upward from the earth and is associated with the passive, dark, cool, supportive, and inward activities of the body.

Many complementary therapies can be incorporated into massage sessions. These bodywork modalities have a specific intent and are applied for a specific purpose. Some of these complementary therapies may use massage strokes, but others may not.

Hydrotherapy (HAHY-droh-THAIR-ah-pee) uses water of different temperatures and in various forms to aid in the treatment of soft tissue, and it can easily be used by massage therapists. A number of complementary modalities manipulate energy in and around the body. The concepts of Oriental medicine, including the philosophy of life force energy that flows through orderly patterns, can be incorporated into massage therapy via acupressure (AK-yoo-preh-sher) and Shiatsu (shee-AHT-soo). Ayurveda is a holistic approach to wellness that incorporates bodywork, nutrition, meditation, and exercise.

It teaches that the energies of things in and around us influence our health by affecting the energy balance of our body. **Reflexology** (REE-fleks-AH-loh-jee) is a modality in which you apply fingertip compression to specific reflex points on the hand, foot, or ear to affect other parts of the body. **Polarity** (poh-LAIR-ih-tee) **therapy** uses very light massage strokes, both on and off the client's body, to balance electromagnetic fields. There are too many specialized forms of energy therapy to introduce them all in this text, but they are certainly worth discovering.

Many complementary modalities require advanced study; this chapter only serves as an introduction to some that are commonly used in massage practices. Before applying any new or complementary modality to a client, make sure the client has no pathological conditions for which the particular modality may be contraindicated.

Hydrotherapy

Hydrotherapy utilizes water internally or externally for therapeutic treatment. "Taking the waters" is a phrase that describes the ancient practice of using water to heal. Since the beginning of time, ancient cultures revered water as a gift from the gods and used it for bathing and healing. In Oriental cultures, water was considered a source of Qi (life energy). Similarly, in Indian and Vedic cultures, water was used as a source for the same life energy, referred to as prana. The ancient Romans discovered the mineral springs in Spa, Belgium; the springs were so well known for healing various health conditions that "spa" became synonymous with healing waters. Greek and Roman cultures used water for bathing as well as medicinal purposes from then on. As civilizations evolved, water became a foundation for classic medical philosophy linking physical, spiritual, mental, emotional, and energetic health of the human body.

Water is considered sacred in many religious traditions. It is used in the Christian tradition of Baptism, which is the universal symbol of purification and regeneration. The Judaic tradition uses ritual cleansing baths for spiritual healing. Millions of people every year visit the sacred basilica in Lourdes, France, in hopes of being healed from the water pools there. The modern use of water for hydrotherapy is often attributed to Father Sebastian Kneipp (1821–1897) and his Water Cure (Fig. 11-1). During his training to become a priest, he came across a small book by a German physician, Johann Siegmund Hahn (1696–1773), called *Instructions on the Wonderful Curative Powers of Fresh Water*. Kneipp was able to cure himself from pulmonary tuberculosis by using Hahn's teachings and immersing himself in the icy cold waters of the Danube River. He believed that God had provided the book of treatments that he then refined over time, enabling him to heal hundreds of people. He divided his water applications into the following:

- Wet sheets
- Baths
- Vapor baths
- Gushes

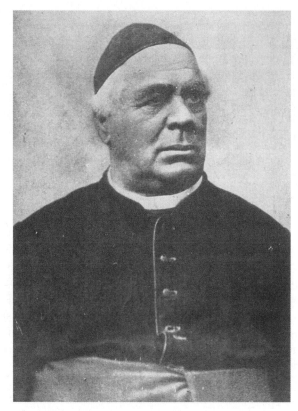

Figure 11-1. Father Sebastian Kneipp. (Reprinted with permission from Kneipp S. The Kneipp Cure. New York: The Nature Cure Publishing Company, 1949.)

Table 11-1 General Categories of Water Temperatures

Category	Temperature Range	Description
Very cold	32° to 55°F	Painfully cold
Cold	55° to 65°F	Uncomfortable
Cool	65° to 92°F	Slightly below skin temperature, goose flesh
Neutral	92° to 98°F	Skin temperature, comfortable
Warm to hot	98° to 104°F	Tolerable, reddens skin
Very hot	104° to 110°F	Tolerable for very short periods
Painfully hot	Over 110°F	Possibly injurious, contraindicated

- Ablutions
- Wet bandages (packages)
- Drinking of water

These treatments had a threefold goal: to dissolve, to evacuate the morbid matters, and to strengthen the organism. Essentially, the Water Cure would diminish disease by removing the diseased substances from the body as well as by cleansing and returning the blood to the cells and tissues while maximizing circulation.

This section focuses on hydrotherapy applications you can use during massage sessions and in spa work, and those you can recommend as self-care activities, including applications of cold or heat, chemical substitutes that provide cold or heat, contrast therapy, or neutral baths. Table 11-1 describes the general categories of water temperatures. You must understand how the different temperatures affect a person's physiology so you can use hydrotherapy safely and effectively. Box 11-1 outlines the physiological effects of cold and heat.

Effects of Hydrotherapy

Before turning to the specific applications of hydrotherapy that you may consider incorporating into your massage

practice, it is important to know some of the general effects of hydrotherapy on the body. These include the effects of cold, heat, contrast, and neutral treatments, which are addressed below.

Effects of Cold Hydrotherapy

Temperatures between 55° and 65°F are generally considered cold, and temperatures between 32° and 55°F are considered very cold. Cold and very cold temperatures applied for a short duration (1 minute or less) cause vasoconstriction, or a narrowing of the blood vessels. When the cold is removed, vasodilation occurs, opening up the blood vessels and allowing arterial blood to rush into the blood vessels and supply the tissues with oxygen. Short applications of cold ultimately increase circulation.

The same mechanism occurs when cold temperatures are applied longer than a minute, but during the extended application, swelling (edema) decreases due to reduced circulation, muscle spasms relax because of the reduced chemical activity of muscle contraction, and pain decreases because of the reduced chemical activity of nerve transmission.

BOX 11-1
Physiological Effects of Cold and Heat

COLD
Reduces

- Circulation (with prolonged use)
- Acute inflammation
- Swelling (edema)
- Muscle spasm via reduction of muscle spindle activity
- Nerve sensation and pain
- Metabolism
- Tissue damage
- Local oxygen supply (temporarily)

Increases

- Circulation and vasodilation (with short use)
- Urine production

HEAT
Reduces

- Pain
- Stiffness and soreness
- Superficial fascia tightness

Increases

- Vasodilation
- Local blood flow/circulation (facilitates healing)
- Oxygen absorption
- Metabolism
- Relaxation
- Joint range of motion
- Sweating, creating a cooling effect on the body

HEAT APPLICATIONS BETWEEN 102° AND 104°F
Increase

- Immune function via inhibition of bacterial and viral growth
- White blood cell count via creating an "artificial" fever

Very cold temperatures (think ice packs) are particularly beneficial following an injury. Applications of very cold temperatures reduce capillary permeability and the amount of inflammatory substances produced, relieve muscle spasms, and decrease pain. As a result, very cold temperatures prevent swelling and encourage movement of the injured area to enhance circulation to the area. To successfully anesthetize or numb the tissues, ice or very cold temperatures must be applied for 20 to 30 minutes. Because of all these effects, ice is one of the most beneficial treatments during the acute phase of an injury (24 to 72 hours following the injury). The reason ice is so much more beneficial than heat at treating injuries is because of our body's natural homeostatic mechanism for maintaining body temperature. The difference between normal core body temperature and ice is somewhere around 65°F, whereas the difference between normal core body temperature and heat is only about 10°F. To restore normal core body temperature, a longer duration of increased circulation is required in an area that has had ice applied than in an area that has had heat applied. In addition to increased circulation, the delivery of oxygen and nutrients, as well as removal of waste products, also increases.

Ice is cold and initially uncomfortable, and the discomfort often becomes worse before numbness sets in. As a result, many people avoid ice applications. If the body part to be iced can be submersed in a bucket or bowl of water, you can reduce the shock of the cold by starting the water at room temperature and gradually adding ice cubes to drop the temperature. Other ways to minimize the shock and discomfort of very cold temperatures are to take a warm bath or shower while applying the ice pack, or to apply a hot pack on another area of the body for distraction and to move blood flow to another area of the body. Although there are many benefits and indications for the use of cold applications, there are some contraindications as well. Box 11-2 lists indications and contraindications of cold and very cold applications.

Alert

When using a chemical gel pack, you must use a layer of fabric between the pack and the skin to avoid damage to the skin and nerves.

Postinjury treatments such as RICE (rest, ice, compression, and elevation) and MICE (mobilization, ice, compression, and elevation) facilitate healing using the same ICE:

- **Ice** causes vasoconstriction, reduces blood flow, prevents further inflammation, and creates an analgesic (pain-relieving) effect.

- **Compression** prevents lymph from accumulating, thus minimizing edema.

- **Elevation** of the injured area encourages lymph to return to the heart, which decreases inflammation.

BOX 11-2
Indications and Contraindications of Cold and Very Cold Applications

INDICATIONS

- Acute or chronic muscle spasm
- Acute or chronic pain
- Acute inflammation or injury
- Muscle strain
- Ligament sprains
- Tissue that has received any kind of myofascial work
- Bursitis, rheumatoid arthritis, osteoarthritis (unless cold aggravates the pain)
- Minor burns
- Fever

CONTRAINDICATIONS

- Decreased cold sensitivity or hypersensitivity
- Compromised local circulation
- Circulatory or sensory impairment
- Spasm of the blood vessels (vasospastic disease)
- Cardiac disorders
- Respiratory disorders
- Use over chest during acute asthma
- Raynaud's syndrome
- Hypertension
- Uncovered open wounds, infections, or rash

RICE and MICE are similar treatments, but the "R" in RICE refers to the "rest" or restricted activity that prevents further injury, and the "M" in MICE refers to the "mobilization" or gentle, non–weight-bearing range-of-motion exercises recommended to prevent connective tissue adhesion.

Effects of Heat Hydrotherapy

Temperatures between 98° and 104°F are considered warm to hot, they are usually tolerable, and they redden the skin. Very hot temperatures are generally between 104° and 110°F and are tolerable only for very short periods. Temperatures above 110°F are dangerous and should be avoided for hydrotherapy purposes.

Heat applied for 5 minutes or less stimulates circulation by promoting vasodilation, which brings more oxygen and nutrients to the tissue and carries away lymphatic fluid and cellular waste. The increased oxygen can reduce muscle spasms, relieve muscle tension, and provide pain relief by breaking the pain cycle. Collagen fibers soften with heat, which increases tissue flexibility and range of motion. Heat applications used in the subacute phase of an injury (72 hours to 6 weeks following the injury) increase blood flow and promote healing in the injured area. In the chronic phase, which occurs between 6 weeks and 1 year after the injury, heat can be applied to tissues as long as the tissues are not swollen because heat can increase edema. As the heat increases the temperature of the underlying tissues, cellular activity increases and immune functions can be enhanced.

Alert

Any client who is being treated with temperatures above 99°F should be watched for nausea, splotchy discoloration developing on the skin, lightheadedness, dizziness, and headache. If any of those symptoms develop during heat application, stop the treatment immediately and monitor the client for improvement.

Despite the many benefits and indications for heat therapy, there are some important contraindications to consider before applying it (Box 11-3).

Effects of Contrast Therapy

Interestingly, when heat is applied longer than 5 minutes, circulation decreases. The tissues get congested with prolonged exposure to heat because although vasodilation delivers more blood to an area, the venous and lymphatic flows are not equally enhanced. Unless there is enough muscular activity to encourage these flows toward the heart, you must use a cold application after long applications of heat. The cold temperatures help the blood and lymphatic vessels constrict to their normal size and return circulation to normal. **Contrast therapy**, sometimes called alternating therapy, involves the application of heat followed by the application of cold or very cold temperatures. By alternating vasodilation and vasoconstriction (and the associated benefits of each), contrast therapy is beneficial for reducing pain, promoting healing, and enhancing immune function. As long as you take into account the client's sensitivity and overall health and make sure there are no contraindications for applications of either heat or cold, you can safely apply and recommend contrast therapy.

Effects of Neutral Hydrotherapy

Neutral baths use water at 92° to 98°F (body temperature) to increase relaxation and sedate the nervous system.

BOX 11-3

Indications and Contraindications for Heat Applications

INDICATIONS

- Muscle spasm
- Pain relief
- Increase range of motion
- Facilitate tissue healing in subacute and chronic injuries (3 days to 3 weeks after injury)
- Enhance immune function
- Increase mobility of tissues—benefits osteoarthritis and rheumatoid arthritis

CONTRAINDICATIONS

- Acute inflammation or injuries (24 to 72 hours after injury), including open wounds, blisters, burns, and abrasions
- Area of a newly developed bruise
- Skin infections or rash
- Fever
- Impaired or poor circulation, including cardiac impairment and phlebitis
- Stroke, also called cerebrovascular accident (CVA)
- Impaired or poor sensation
- Impaired thermal regulation
- Area over implants, joint prosthetics, or pacemakers
- Tumor, cyst, or malignancy
- Autoimmune conditions

Neutral baths are beneficial for reducing stress and anxiety and relieving chronic pain and insomnia. They are contraindicated for a client who has cardiac disease or skin conditions that react badly to water.

Applications of Hydrotherapy

Choosing which treatments to give your client during a massage session can be a creative process. Taking a good history at the first session, listening carefully to your client's concerns, and getting feedback on the treatments make it easy to pick the right one. **Hydrotherapy applications should always complement the massage and work toward the same goals.** For example, when your client arrives, be sure you know whether he or she is more interested in relief from stress, help with a musculoskeletal issue, or simply needs

touch. If relief from stress is the help he or she needs, ice massage is probably not called for; a more soothing treatment would be a warm bath or warming body wrap. If the client does have a musculoskeletal injury, ice massage or a contrast bath may be the best treatment to increase circulation to the injured area before you use massage for the same purpose. If the person needs to be touched, perhaps a friction treatment such as a local salt glow will help to stimulate the skin before massage. Boxes 11-4 to 11-6 give specific hydrotherapy recommendations for three common problems. Also, Table 11-2 presents a glossary of hydrotherapy treatments for the spa. Discussed below are some of the most common whole-body and local hydrotherapy applications.

Whole-Body Applications

A whole-body hydrotherapy treatment can take many forms, from various types of baths and showers to whole-body frictions and wraps. A whole-body treatment that is relatively new

BOX 11-4

Hydrotherapy Treatments for Chronic Low Back Pain

Both hydrotherapy treatments and massage are recommended for chronic low back pain. They are relaxing and nurturing, enhance circulation, ease muscle tension, and may be the best nondrug approach for this condition. Any massage techniques that relieve muscle tension, including circulatory, myofascial, and trigger point, can also address chronic low back pain. Of course, if there is an underlying perpetuating factor that is the cause of chronic low back pain, the best approach is to address the cause. However, even as a symptomatic treatment, massage can be tremendously comforting, and hydrotherapy treatments can make massage more effective. Moist heat applications, salt glows, contrast showers, percussion douches, and ice massage all may help relieve pain and enhance massage. For some clients, both heat and ice may have to be tried to determine which works better.

Here are some different hydrotherapy strategies to use in combination with massage:

1. Moist heat application, followed by salt glow of the entire back, followed by massage.
   Both the moist heat and the salt glow increase circulation to the back.

2. Contrast shower directed to the lower back, followed by massage.
   At home, a client whose back is hurting may take a contrast shower as often as once every hour.

3. Ice massage of the lower back, followed by hands-on massage.

4. Percussion douche to the lower back, followed by massage.

BOX 11-5
Hydrotherapy Treatments for Muscle Spasms

Skeletal muscle spasms are a common occurrence. They can cause much discomfort and are the source of many visits to massage therapists. There are many factors that contribute to muscle cramps and spasms, including tightness of the affected muscle, overstretching of cold muscles, emotional stress, poor local circulation, vitamin and mineral deficiency, sudden movement or chilling of a tight muscle, inactivity, dehydration, and some medical conditions, such as hyperthyroidism. Hydrotherapy treatments can relieve pain, deeply relax skeletal muscles, and increase local blood flow. Ice massage can dull associated pain. Deep heating of acute muscle spasms can relax them, but occasionally, a spasm will respond better to the cold of ice massage or an ice water compress. Deep massage and stretching will be easier to do after performing any of these treatments.

LOWER BACK
To treat muscle spasm in the lower back, here are some different hydrotherapy strategies to use in combination with massage:

1. Moist heat application to the lower back muscles, followed by back massage.

2. Full hot bath, followed by moist heat application to the lower back, then followed by back massage.

3. Ice massage of the lower back, followed by back massage.

4. Ice pack over the lower back, followed by back massage.

5. Contrast treatment to the lower back area, consisting of moist heat application to the lower back muscles followed by ice massage or cold compress, and followed by back massage.

NECK
To treat spasm of neck muscles (stiff neck or crick in the neck), here are some different hydrotherapy strategies to use in combination with massage:

1. Hot moist application to the neck, followed by neck massage.

2. Full hot bath, followed by local moist heat application, followed by massage.

3. Ice massage of the posterior and lateral neck muscles, followed by massage.

---

for massage therapists is Watsu, which is a type of Shiatsu massage performed in a swimming pool. All whole-body treatments apply water, steam, hot air, friction, or wrapping to the entire body, not just one part as in the local applications.

Baths

A full-body bath is defined as the immersion of the entire body in water. Steam baths also fall into the bath category, because when a client sits in a cabinet or room filled with steam, his or her skin is completely coated with warm steamy air.

Whole-body water baths are one of the most ancient of all medical treatments. They can be hot, cold, neutral, or warm, and the different water temperatures will have different, distinct effects on the body. A neutral temperature bath is a classic hydrotherapy treatment in which the temperature has no effect on the body, but the mechanical pressure of being surrounded entirely by water has a tremendously soothing effect. Baths can also have chemical effects if different substances are added to bathwater, such as herbs, salts, oatmeal, baking soda, or essential oils.

Showers

A shower is a stream (or streams) of water from a showerhead that is directed on one or more parts of the body. Showers can be performed with one showerhead or with multiple showerheads, and many specialty showers have been developed by hydrotherapists. Showers can be used to give hot, warm, cold, or contrast treatments.

BOX 11-6
Hydrotherapy for Strain and Fatigue of Upper Extremity Muscles

Those who perform forceful work with their hands, including massage therapists, gardeners, surgeons, office workers, and carpenters, are at greater risk for repetitive strain injuries. To relieve fatigue in upper extremity muscles as well as to treat repetitive strain injuries, here are some different hydrotherapy strategies:

1. Apply moist heat over the area of concern, followed by massage.

2. Daily paraffin bath for both hands, followed by a brief cold dip, followed by massage.

3. Contrast bath for the hands and arms, followed by massage.

4. Ice massage for sharp localized pain, followed by massage.

5. Hot soak for hands while performing stretching exercises in the water, followed by massage.

Table 11-2 Spa Glossary

Algotherapy	The use of algaes in baths, body scrubs, facials, and wraps
Aroma bath	(See Herbal wrap)
Balneotherapy	Hydrotherapies that traditionally use hot springs, mineral water, or seawater to improve circulation, strengthen the immune system, analgesia, and reduce stress
Brine (saltwater) baths	Baths in which the water comes from a sea or an ocean or has been saturated with large amounts of a salt, usually sodium chloride
Brossage	A body polishing treatment using a series of brushes to apply salicylic salt
Brush and tone	An exfoliation treatment that uses a dry brush and is often followed by a moisturizing treatment to hydrate skin
Cold plunge	A deep pool of cold water in which all or part of the body is submerged, originally developed to rapidly contract capillaries and stimulate circulation after the use of a sauna
Crenotherapy (crounotherapy)	Generic term for treatments that use mineral water, mud, or vapor
Dead Sea mud treatment	Mineral-rich mud from the Dead Sea in Israel applied to detoxify skin and relieve arthritis pain
Douche massage	(See Scotch hose)
Dulse scrub	An exfoliation technique especially good for sensitive skin that uses a combination of powdered dulse seaweed and essential oils or water to exfoliate while replenishing lost minerals and vitamins to the skin
Fango (fango treatment, fango therapy, fango bath, parafango)	Fango is a slimy combination of a claylike substance, warm water and/or oil, and a specific kind of algae. Many spas refer to any kind of mud treatment as a fango treatment. The mud mixture can be applied over parts or all of the body as a heat pack to detoxify and soften skin, as an analgesic, to encourage relaxation, and to relieve muscular pain. Parafango treatments apply a mixture of mud and paraffin.

Alert

Radioactivity is present in the mud at several spas, so pregnant women and women in their reproductive years should be cautious about fango treatments to avoid possible exposure to radioactivity.

Finnish sauna (sauna)	A simple technique utilizing perspiration as a way to cleanse the body. Generally, saunas are small, hot (150° to 200°F), low humidity (less than 10%), enclosed rooms. Inside are wooden benches to sit on and a pile of heated stones that you can throw water on to generate steam.
Haysack wrap	Kneipp treatment with steamed hay intended to detoxify the body
Herbal wrap (herbal bath, aroma bath, thermal wrap)	The client is wrapped in layers of warm cotton or linen that has been steeped in a variety of aromatic herbs, and then is covered with blankets and/or towels. To avoid feeling claustrophobic, the client may keep her arms outside of the wrap.
Hydromassage (hydrotub)	Underwater massage in a deep tub equipped with high-pressure jets and a handheld hose

continues on following page

11 Complementary Modalities

Table 11-2 Spa Glossary *continued*

Japanese enzyme bath	A treatment that starts with the client drinking a hot enzyme tea, then submerging in a dry bath of evergreen shavings, grains, and/or fruit and vegetable enzymes. The fermentation process of the enzymes creates heat that stimulates circulation and metabolism and promotes relaxation.
Kneipp (baths, therapy, treatments)	Baths infused with herbs and minerals such as chamomile, eucalyptus, lavender, or rosemary created in Germany by Father Sebastian Kneipp in the mid-1800s. Traditionally, Kneipp baths are used alongside nutrition and exercise programs to comfort body and mind as a component of healthcare.
Loofah body scrub	A full body exfoliation treatment that uses a loofah sponge to massage a mixture of sea salt and warm almond or avocado oil into the skin
Marine hydrotherapy	The use of water jets to massage the body in a pool of salt water to stimulate circulation and reduce pain and inflammation (a form of thalassotherapy)
Mineral water (baths)	Hot or cold water from natural springs and wells that contains a small percentage of minerals and elements. Mineral baths involve submerging all or part of the body in water from thermal springs.
Moor baths (Peat baths)	An application that contains natural peat rich in organic matter, proteins, vitamins, and trace minerals to relieve sore muscle and joint pain, purify and exfoliate
Onsen	Japanese natural mineral hot springs
Ozonized baths	A tub of thermal water or sea water with jetted streams of ozonized bubbles that encourage relaxation, stimulate circulation, and relieve pain
Parafango	(See Fango)
Peat bath	(See Moor bath)
Peloid therapy	Therapeutic uses and applications of muds
Repaichage (repechage) massage/facial	A combination of herbs, seaweed, clay, and/or mud masks to deeply cleanse and moisturize the face or the entire body
Roman bath (pool)	The term usually refers to a hot whirlpool in which one or more persons sit
Russian bath (steam bath)	A steam bath
Salt glow (salt rub)	The body is vigorously rubbed with an abrasive mixture of coarse salt, essential oils and/or water as an exfoliation treatment
Saltwater bath	(See Brine bath)
Sauna	(See Finnish sauna)
Scotch hose (Swiss shower, douche massage)	A standing body massage delivered with high-pressure hoses and alternates from hot to cold water, each for several seconds at a time. This treatment stimulates circulation and relieves pain and tension.
Seaweed wrap	A variation of an herbal wrap that incorporates seawater and seaweed. The minerals, trace elements, and vitamins of the seawater and seaweed nourish the skin and are absorbed by the bloodstream.
Skin glow rub	Often following a sauna, mineral water and sometimes salt are massaged into the skin to soften skin and encourage circulation

continues on following page

Table 11-2 Spa Glossary *continued*

Slenesium wrap (slenisium, slenisuim)	A treatment in which the body is covered in oils and wrapped with cloth to promote relaxation and eliminate toxins and excess fluids.
Steam room	A ceramic-tiled room with wet heat generated by temperatures of 110° to 130°F designed to soften the skin, cleanse the pores, calm the nervous system, and relieve tension. A room that utilizes the principles of wet, hot steam to eliminate the body of toxins through sweating.
Swiss shower	(See Scotch hose)
Thalassotherapy (thalasso is Greek for seaweed)	Treatments that use seawater, seaweed, and algae for the healing and invigorating properties of their vitamins, minerals, and trace elements. Examples include jetted baths of fresh seawater for deep massage, therapist-applied showers and sprays, and body wraps using seaweed or sea algae paste.
Thermal wrap	(See Herbal wrap)
Tonalastil wrap	A thermal wrap that uses oils instead of herbs to eliminate toxins and excess fluids as well as tone and firm the body
Vichy shower	A device that is suspended over a wet table and has multiple water jets that spray water it is frequently used after dulce scrubs or salt glows.
Whirlpool	A pool of heated water (105° to 115°F) with high-pressure jets that circulate the water and can target pressure points on the client's body.

Almost everyone finds showers appealing because they are an efficient method of cleansing the body and the feeling of water running over the skin is soothing and stimulating. If you have a standard shower in your office, clients can use them for many purposes: to relax, warm up on a cold day, cool down on a hot day, receive a contrast treatment either before or after a massage, or to wash off massage oil or lotion.

Sauna

A sauna is a hot, dry air "bath" that is given in a heated cabinet, room, or other enclosure that prevents heat from escaping. Sauna temperatures range from 145° to 200°F, the average temperature being about 160°F. Sauna air is kept very dry, about 6% to 8% humidity. By contrast, the humidity in a steam room is 100%. Saunas have had different forms over the millennia and have been heated in a variety of ways. What we think of as a typical sauna today, however, is modeled on a Finnish sauna: a specially constructed, wood-lined, almost airtight cabinet or room with benches and a heater inside. That heat may be created by wood, gas, infrared, or electricity. Saunas are usually constructed of soft aromatic woods such as cedar, redwood, or white spruce: these porous woods can readily absorb and eliminate

moisture. Saunas are popular in health clubs, wellness centers, spas, and private homes; small ready-made sauna kits are available. Saunas are used for relaxation, cleansing, and detoxification and are a wonderful complement to a massage session.

Friction

Friction treatments are a small but unique part of traditional hydrotherapy and include cold mitten frictions, salt glows, loofah scrubs, Swedish shampoos, and dry brushing. Friction or brisk rubbing of the skin causes it to redden as blood vessels under the skin dilate. Early hydrotherapists, who were deeply involved in manipulating blood flow to different parts of the body, discovered that chafing or rubbing parts of the body would stimulate local blood flow and make their treatments more effective. Frictions were used to encourage warmth in a cold area, to radiate heat from an overheated area, to bring water applications into closer contact with the skin, and to stimulate lymphatic flow and other vital functions. All the friction treatments use a coarse-textured agent and all have the same goal: to vigorously stimulate the skin and its underlying blood vessels, which improves the circulation of blood and lymph, increases uptake of nutrients and excretion of wastes, and stimulates the immune system. Friction treatments are relaxing as well, and salt glows in particular may leave the client feeling euphoric. Friction treatments also remove dead skin cells that remain on the surface of the skin, which is known as exfoliation. In spas, a wide variety of frictioning agents—including cornmeal, sugar, or salts—are also used for beauty effects because exfoliation leaves the skin smoother, brighter, and better able to absorb creams and cosmetics.

Body Wraps

Body wraps are hydrotherapy treatments in which hot or cold water is applied to the client's skin with wet sheets, towels, or steam packs, and then the client is wrapped in layers of additional sheets or blankets. All body wraps use the client's own body heat to advantage, trapping the heat that would normally be lost through radiation. Although sometimes cumbersome to assemble, body wraps are snug and cozy feeling for many people and can be performed where there are no showers, baths, or elaborate hydrotherapy equipment. Sometimes the desired effect of the wrap is achieved through using very cold water, very hot water, or various chemicals mixed with the water: for example, many different herbs, salts, clays, essential oils, and other substances have been added to the water that is used in the wrap.

Local Applications

Any hydrotherapy treatment that is placed on only one part of the body is a local application. These tend to be easier to perform, require less equipment than whole-body treatments, and can be used almost anywhere.

Local Baths: Foot, Hand, Sitz, and Paraffin

Local or partial baths, which immerse only one part of the body, are one of the most ancient of all medical treatments. They have been used for everything from warming and cooling to applying substances to the skin such as herbs, salts, clays, essential oils, vinegar, and seaweed to cleanse and soften the skin and underlying tissue. Partial baths can be hot, warm, cold, or contrast (hot alternated with cold), depending on what they are used for. Depending on the area which is going to be immersed, partial baths can be taken in all sorts of containers, from large bowls and plastic tubs to stainless steel whirlpools. Types of local baths include scalp, eye, sinus, throat, hand, arm, sitz, foot, and leg baths. Steam inhalations also fall into this category. See Box 11-7 for a basic contrast foot bath routine.

BOX 11-7 **PROCEDURE** Contrast Foot Bath Routine

You will need two containers, one for hot water and one for cold water; a water thermometer; and one large towel. Have the client either seated in a chair or lying on a massage table. If the client is seated, put a towel on the floor, and if the client is lying down, drape the bottom end of the table with a large bath towel.

1. Prepare one container of hot water and one container of cold water. Use a water thermometer to be sure that the hot water is at 110°F and the cold water is about 55°F. Ice cubes are usually required to cool tap water down to that temperature. If this is hard for the client to tolerate, begin with warmer water and gradually add ice cubes a few at a time.

2. Put the container of hot water on the towel, rest the client's feet in the container, and cover him or her with a sheet if desired.

3. Leave the client's feet in the hot water for 2 minutes.

4. Replace hot foot bath with the cold, soaking the feet for 30 seconds only.

5. Repeat steps 2 and 3. Make sure hot water continues to be at 110°F: add more hot water if it cools.

6. Repeat steps 2 and 3, for a total of 3 rounds.

7. Dry the feet, which will now be bright red, and proceed with massage if desired.

Moist Heat Applications: Hot Packs, Fomentations, and Moist Heating Pads

Almost everyone loves the application of moist heat during a massage. Moist heat warms tissue, increases local circulation, relieves muscle stiffness and soreness, softens tissue to make it more pliable and stretchable, and perhaps most important to the client, feels deeply relaxing and nurturing. Moist heat can be used before an area is massaged or afterward to keep muscles relaxed and warm. Local heat applications are also portable, unlike such whole-body applications as hot baths or saunas, and are useful when only a small area of the body needs to be treated. Although dry heat such as heating pads, hot-water bottles, or rice-filled microwaveable bags have many of the same effects, they do not penetrate as well as moist heat, nor do they have its soothing "watery" quality. The advantages of any type of hot application, however, must be weighed against two major disadvantages: hot applications can burn and prolonged application of heat to the body surface can raise body temperature.

Alert

Clients with poor sensation are particularly at risk of burns.

Because heat applications are so soothing and relaxing, they are used not only in almost every kind of medical setting but also in spas that offer creative and enjoyable ways to integrate them into massage sessions. It is even possible to use moist heat packs to perform a whole-body heating treatment by applying multiple packs. Moist heat applications are more similar than different, but each has advantages and disadvantages. Hot fomentations can provide intense heat but can also burn the client as well as cool off fast. Silica gel or hydrocollator packs also provide intense heat and cool off relatively fast, but in addition to the danger of burns, they cannot be placed underneath the body and do not conform to body curves. Moist heating pads provide more moderate heat and conform well to body curves, but care must be taken that the client does not fall asleep on them. See Box 11-8 for a description of a moist hot pack application to the lower back.

Compresses

Hot compresses, which are cloths wrung out of hot water, are a milder form of the intense moist heat of the silica gel pack or the hot fomentation. One advantage of hot compresses is that they may be easily and inexpensively made, requiring only hot water, cloths, and gloves to protect the hands when wringing out the cloths. Water for compresses can be heated on a stovetop, in a crockpot, or in a microwave, or even drawn from a tap if the water gets hot enough. Wet washcloths can also be placed in a resealable bag in a microwave oven for a short time.

Cold compresses are cloths wrung out of icy water and applied to various parts of the body. They generally provide less intense cold than ice packs. They may be used to keep the forehead cool during whole-body heating treatments as part of a simple contrast treatment along with hot compresses, and to treat clients who cannot tolerate applications of ice.

Alert

It is important to realize that if more than one-fifth of the body is covered by a cold compress, the core temperature will begin to fall.

This might be desirable for overheated clients on a hot day, but otherwise it could chill clients and make them tense or uncomfortable. In the past, many different chemical solutions have been added to cold compresses for special purposes, such as anti-inflammatory herbs, activated charcoal, or Epsom salts over bruises and sprains; antiseptic herbs or essential oils over wounds; and essential oils for scenting compresses.

Ice Applications: Ice Massage, Ice Pack, Ice Water Bath, and Iced Compress

Ice is an inexpensive and readily available tool for the massage therapist. Whether you are working at a private office, a physical therapy clinic, an athletic event, or a private home, you are almost sure to have ice within easy reach. Ice is useful in massage therapy because it has five important effects on the body:

1. Ice reduces sensations, including pain sensations, by slowing the transmission of sensory messages from local nerve fibers to the brain. This numbing effect is used in medicine for everything from reducing discomfort right after injuries (such as bruises, burns, muscle strains, joint sprains, hematomas, and fractures), to reducing pain after orthopedic surgery, to numbing areas that are going to be injected with anesthetic or stung by bees in bee sting therapy. After an area is cooled, it may take a long time to return to normal temperature, depending on the temperature of the application and the health of the tissues being treated.

2. Ice reduces inflammation by decreasing circulation: as blood vessels constrict, blood supply to the area decreases drastically. This anti-inflammatory effect is used in medicine for many conditions including the itching and oozing of mild poison ivy, swelling from certain cancer chemotherapeutic medications and cancer itself, arresting herpes blisters when they first begin to erupt, and reducing swelling after orthopedic

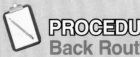

BOX 11-8 **PROCEDURE** Moist Hot Pack Application to Lower Back Routine

You will need a silica gel pack heated either in a special hot water tank, in a container of hot water on a stovetop, or in a bowl of water in a microwave oven, along with tongs or gloves and four to six towels. A heated silica gel pack is used here, but many other types of moist heat packs are available and useful to apply moist heat. Begin with the client in the prone position.

1. Explain use of local heat to the client and get his or her consent, then check the area visually before putting on the moist hot pack.

2. Remove the silica gel pack from the hot water with tongs, or put on gloves and pick the pack up by the loops on the edges.

3. Wrap the hot pack in plenty of towels, which will both protect the client's skin from burning and prevent the pack from cooling off too fast. Silica gel packs generally require four to six layers of towels, but keep extra towels on hand to use if needed. More towels may be needed for an elderly person or a child.

4. Check to make sure the hot pack is not too hot by feeling it with your own hand or wrist.

5. Warn the client before you apply the hot pack and then say, "Be sure to let me know if this ever feels too hot."

6. Place the hot pack on the client's lower back.

7. Check the skin every 2 or 3 minutes at first: simply lift up the pack and check the person's tissue. It is normal for the skin to be bright pink due to increased blood flow. Check for any signs of blistering or burning. Also ask the client how the hot pack feels. Add more towels to protect the skin if needed.

8. Although the hot pack will stay warm for about 20 minutes, it will begin to lose heat right away, which means that danger of burning decreases as time goes on. As the hot pack cools off, you may wish to remove a layer of towels to keep the area warm, but then you will need to keep checking the skin.

9. Remove the hot pack if there are any signs of damage to the skin or if the client tells you the area is too hot. Otherwise, wait 15 to 20 minutes and then remove it.

10. Dry the skin, apply oil or lotion, and begin massage. You will find the client's tissue warm, pink, and pliable, and the client will have a greater feeling of relaxation in the heated area.

surgery. As massage therapists, we can use ice to treat swelling from bruises, sprains, strains, and pulled muscles.

Alert

Massage therapists should not treat bruises or swelling from unknown causes, and other more serious injuries should be treated with ice only with a doctor's permission.

3. Ice can stop bleeding in a local area under the ice application. In an emergency situation such as an impact injury, shutting off the flow of blood into an area can be accomplished very quickly. In one study, an ice wrap applied to one knee was compared to a room temperature wrap applied to the opposite knee. Researchers found that the ice wrap caused a 38% decrease in arterial blood flow, a 26% decrease in soft tissue blood flow, and a 19% reduction in blood flow to the bone itself.[1] As little as 5 minutes of icing a knee can decrease blood flow to soft tissue and bone in the

knee.[2] Ice applications generally should be limited to 15 to 30 minutes because the tissues under the ice may become so ischemic that they are damaged: frostbite and nerve palsy have resulted from longer applications.

4. Ice decreases muscle spasm. Drs. Janet Travell and David Simons, authors of *Myofascial Pain and Dysfunction,* recommend ice stroking of muscles to deactivate trigger points and release muscle tension long enough for individual muscles to be gently but thoroughly stretched.

5. Ice slows the transmission of motor messages from the brain to local nerve fibers. Known as cryostretch, the use of ice massage before stretching can increase range of motion dramatically.

For a sample ice massage routine, see Box 11-9.

BOX 11-9   **PROCEDURE** Ice Massage Routine

Begin by positioning the client prone or supine so that the area to be iced is easy to reach. Drape towels around the area that will be treated. Have ready the ice cup and two towels to drape around the area.

1. Explain the ice massage procedure to the client. It is important that he or she realizes that ice massage will continue until the area is numb. This means the client may experience some burning or aching before numbness sets in.

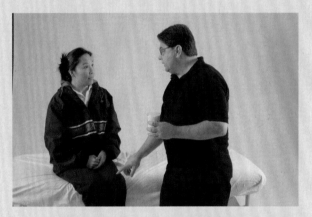

2. Drape towels around the area that will be treated.

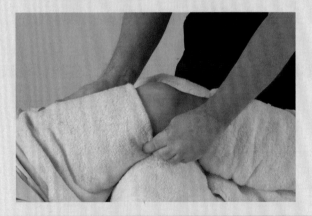

3. Hold the cup of ice in one hand and gently rub it in a circular motion over the area you are treating and a few inches above and below the area as well.

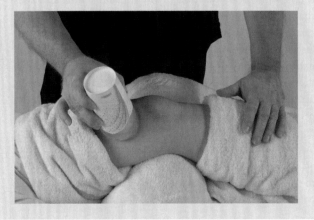

BOX 11-9 **PROCEDURE** Ice Massage Routine (continued)

4. Continue until the area is numb, about 8 to 10 minutes.

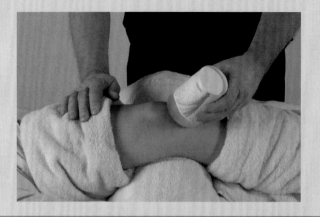

5. Remove ice and dry the area. Tissue will be cold and pink.

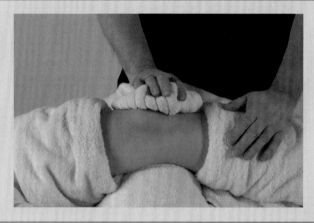

6. Proceed with massage if desired.

Internal Hydrotherapy

Another application of hydrotherapy is the simple and important act of drinking sufficient water. You have an opportunity to educate your clients on the importance of adequate hydration. Drinking water after a massage session can help the body rid itself of cellular and chemical wastes that are mechanically forced into the circulatory system, it can make scar tissue more functional, and it can help prevent fascial adhesion development. Proper hydration of the tissues enhances fluidity of movement and flexibility, whereas dehydration can lead to more tension, restricted movement, muscle soreness, headaches, and fatigue. Dehydration is the primary cause of a "hangover" headache. **Drinking more water may be one of the most important self-care recommendations a therapist makes for the client's treatment plan.**

Water is considered the very core of life on earth and in the human body. Life depends on it. In fact, our bodies can survive for weeks without food, but it is only a matter of days without food and water before our cells dehydrate and our body systems fail, resulting in death. Adult bodies are approximately 60% water (by mass), and our cells and organs require sufficient amounts of water to function properly. The physical body is a complex combination of chemical and biological reactions in which water is the catalyst, transport system, regulator of body temperature, and conduit for transmission of nervous system impulses.

Dehydration is the condition in which there is insufficient water for the physical body to maintain homeostasis. Many minor and major health conditions may result from dehydration, making water the number one nutrient the body requires. Mild dehydration often results in fatigue; headache; general sense of malaise; constipation; and muscle and joint stiffness, pain, and soreness.

No medication in the world can rival the number of beneficial physiological effects of water or is as widely accessible and inexpensive. Water can be used therapeutically as a sedative, antipyretic (reduces body temperature), analgesic, anesthetic, anticonvulsant, and astringent. Depending on its mineral content, water taken internally can have laxative, diuretic, phlegmatic (increases phlegm production), or diaphoretic (induces perspiration) effects. Drinking hot beverages such as hot water or herbal teas will warm the core of the body and stimulate blood flow and healing. Chapter 8, Treatment Plan, discusses internal hydrotherapy and how you can incorporate it into your client's self-care.

Medication and Hydrotherapy

Some pharmaceutical and hydrotherapy interactions should be avoided. Heat therapy should not be applied to any client who is taking medication that promotes vasodilation, including decongestants, migraine headache medications, blood pressure–lowering medications, and attention deficit hyperactivity disorder medications. The increased vasodilation could be dangerous for the client.

Similarly, any client taking medication that causes vasoconstriction such as migraine headache medications with caffeine should not be treated with cold applications that cause further vasoconstriction. Additionally, any nausea, splotchy discoloration on the skin, lightheadedness, dizziness, or headache may suggest that the client's body is having difficulty managing the temperature differential. If any of those signs or symptoms occur, stop the hydrotherapy treatment and wait for the client to return to normal.

Medications that provide pain relief, whether taken internally or applied topically, alter the sensitivity of a person's skin. Hydrotherapy is not contraindicated, but the effects of treatment must be monitored carefully to prevent possible injury.

Some psychiatric medications that affect brain chemistry can compromise the body's ability to regulate a normal temperature. Hydrotherapy is contraindicated if the client's thermal regulation is not functioning normally.

Asian Bodywork Therapy

The goal of this section is to introduce you to the profession of Asian Bodywork Therapy (ABT) and some basic assessment and treatment principles. It covers Yin/Yang theory and the Five Phases along with some basic correspondences. You will be introduced to the primary meridian system and a bioenergetic perspective of the body, along with some basic principles of Chinese medicine. A routine is provided for you to practice, as well as a self-care exercise.

Keep in mind that this section is merely an introduction to an alternate method of hands-on healing, which you may choose to study in depth at another time. As a massage therapist, you may be able to incorporate some of these techniques in your massage therapy sessions; however, full training is required to earn the title "Asian Bodywork Therapist."

The Asian Bodywork Therapy Profession

Asian Bodywork Therapy is the term used to describe all modalities of bodywork that have their basis in Chinese medicine. ABT modalities originated primarily from countries in East and Southeast Asia. Today, these modalities continue to develop in nations around the world. Acupressure, Amma, Chi Nei Tsang, Medical Qigong Therapy, Nuad Bo'Rarn (Thai), Shiatsu, and Tui-na are recognized Asian Bodywork modalities. There are derivatives of these modalities, and other emerging forms, that also fit the criteria.

The American Organization for Bodywork Therapies of Asia (AOBTA) defines ABT as "the treatment of the human body/mind/spirit, including the electromagnetic or energetic field, which surrounds, infuses and brings that body to life, by pressure and/or manipulation."[3]

Asian Bodywork is based in Traditional Chinese Medical assessment and treatment principles, using traditional Asian techniques and treatment strategies to affect and balance the energetic system. The goals of ABT treatment are the promotion, maintenance, and restoration of health. See Box 11-10 for a brief description of some ABT modalities.

Differences between ABT and Massage Therapy

Chinese medicine is a traditional form of healthcare from China with an extensive history, an energetic focus, and natural treatments addressing an individual's life as a whole, and it has a markedly different approach from Western medicine. For example, an identifying feature of ABT is the training and treatment focus on bioenergy and its movement in and around the body. Bioenergy is electric and electromagnetic energy in a living body. The Chinese call it Qi and the Japanese call it Ki. Because of the differences in training, focus, and national certification, ABT is considered its own profession.

In contrast, massage therapy focuses mainly on muscles, connective tissue, the circulatory system, and sometimes the

BOX 11-10
A Brief Description of Some ABT Modalities

- **Acupressure:** A modality in which pressure of varying intensities is applied to acupoints (specific points of energy in the body), generally with the fingers, to meet a therapeutic goal.
- **Amma:** A modality developed in Chinese antiquity that is sometimes considered the "mother" of all massage therapy; a form of skilled-touch therapy that combines deep tissue manipulation with the application of pressure, friction, and touch to specific acupoints, meridians, ligaments, muscles, and joints.
- **Chi Nei Tsang:** A method of internal organ treatment that stimulates or relaxes the internal organs through specific protocols of abdominal work.
- **Medical Qigong Therapy** (also known as external Qigong): This modality affects the Qi surrounding the outside of the body primarily without touch, although some touch may be used.
- **Nuad Bo'Rarn:** Traditional medical bodywork of Thailand that combines yoga poses with bodywork techniques.
- **Shiatsu:** Originally developed 2,000 years ago in Japan, this modality literally translates as "thumb pressure"; it has many forms. See Box 11-11 for a basic Shiatsu routine.
- **Tui-na:** Taught and practiced widely in hospitals in China today, this approach has been in use for over 5,000 years and may be literally translated as "push/pull" or "push/grasp."

lymphatic system. The precise definition of massage therapy is a matter of debate and there is currently no specific scope of practice.

ABT Training and Licensing

ABT entry-level training requirements include a minimum 500-hour curriculum. Included in this training are at least 100 hours of Chinese medical theory and practice, at least 160 hours of techniques of the modality, at least 100 hours of anatomy and physiology, and at least 70 hours of supervised clinical training. Graduation, often coupled with national certification (see National Certification Commission for Acupuncture and Oriental Medicine [NCCAOM] information below), can lead to licensure as an Asian Bodywork Therapist in states that require it.

Legal requirements for ABT and for massage vary from state to state. It has become apparent that all touch therapy is not massage therapy and, in that sense, ABT is not massage therapy. Early massage laws were often written broadly, so that anyone who uses touch in her or his work has to be licensed as a massage therapist. Massage laws generally require training in Swedish massage and/or other Western massage theories and modalities for graduation, national certification, and licensure. They also include a broad legal definition of what massage is. These laws tend to be applied to professions other than massage therapy, including ABT, despite differences in training requirements. There are now some state laws exempting practices that are clearly not massage in the Western legal sense.

Professional Association and National Certification

AOBTA is currently the only nonprofit membership organization representing ABT instructors, practitioners, schools and programs, and students. AOBTA was formed in 1989 through the efforts of dedicated ABT professionals seeking to provide a national organization for an emerging profession. Today, AOBTA represents 1,500 national and international members and offers a quarterly news magazine, monthly email updates, legislative support, continuing education opportunities, and referrals. AOBTA's mission is to promote and protect ABT and its practitioners; support appropriate credentialing; define scope of practice and educational standards; provide resources for training, professional development, and networking; advocate public policy to protect its members; and promote public education about ABT. For more information, see www.aobta.org.

NCCAOM is currently the only entity offering national certification in Asian Bodywork. One can become a Diplomate in Asian Bodywork Therapy (Dipl. ABT [NCCAOM]) by completing all the training and application requirements and passing the exam. For more information, see www.nccaom.org.

Chinese Medicine

This section introduces you to some of the basic principles of Chinese medicine. Chinese medicine has an extensive history and tradition, with energetic principles based in natural phenomena. Included in this section are:

1. Brief history
2. Yin/Yang theory
3. Qi and meridians
4. Acupoints
5. Disease origin and prevention
6. Assessment
7. Five Phase theory

In order to distinguish principles and concepts of Chinese medicine from the familiar words used daily, capitalization is used for the terms. For example, "Heart" is used in Chinese medicine to distinguish from the anatomical heart.

Brief History

Chinese medicine has a long and interesting history, including the discovery of stone acupuncture needles at sites dating back 8,000 years or so. The written history of this discipline is about 3,000 years old. "Oracle bones" (inscribed stone and bone) dating from the Shang dynasty (1766–1122 BCE) are the earliest records of medical information. The *Huangdi neijing,* or "Yellow Emperor's Inner Classic," is considered the first medical text and appears to be a compilation over many years. Dates on this work vary to such an extent (from approximately 3,000 to 2,300 years ago) that it is impossible to determine its true age, although it is certainly at least 2,000 years old. A bronze acupuncture statue was cast in 1027 CE, the earliest known of its kind. Fifteen medical treatises written on silk banners and bamboo slips were discovered in 1973, and date to sometime between 220 BCE and 220 CE.

Early Taoists are given credit for beginning the journey of discovery that has become Chinese medicine. They were interested in longevity and health and experimented with, observed, and experienced all manner of natural phenomena to understand the nature of life and how it could be influenced. These masters passed on their knowledge, and over the centuries as more knowledge has been acquired, the medicine has evolved. The evolution continues today in China and Japan as well as in other parts of the world, including the United States.

Some historians have stated that ABT is the oldest form of healing in the Taoist tradition; acupuncture and Chinese herbal formulae for healing have been in use for centuries. Historically, there are the "Eight Branches of Chinese Medicine" including meditation, diet, exercise, geomancy (the placement of objects; Feng Shui), Chinese astrology, bodywork, herbs, and acupuncture. Additionally, the practice of calligraphy has been, and to some still is, a healing art.

Yin/Yang Theory

The foundation of Chinese medicine is Yin/Yang theory. The terms are used to describe categories of qualities of energy. See Table 11-3 on Yin/Yang correspondences for Yin and Yang qualities.

Yin (YIHN) is the term used to represent the following: the shady side of the hill; the cold, deep darkness of night and wintertime; the feminine principles of nurturing and nourishing; the relentless power of water and stone. Slow, yet continuous, Yin is our grounding and the contracting of consciousness into form.

Table 11-3 Yin/Yang Correspondences

Yin	Yang	Yin	Yang
Cold	Hot	Inferior body	Superior body
Dark	Light	Sunken	Raised
Interior	Exterior	Feminine	Masculine
Deep	Superficial	Heart	Small intestine
Deficiency	Excess	Pericardium[a]	Triple Warmer[a]
Below	Above	Spleen	Stomach
Moon	Sun	Lung	Large intestine
Dense organs	Hollow organs	Kidney	Bladder
Soft, empty areas	Hard, full areas	Liver	Gallbladder
Chronic	Acute	Blood	Qi
Anterior body	Posterior body		

[a]Pericardium and Triple Warmer refer to two Organ Systems from Chinese medicine that do not have anatomical organ correlations in Western anatomy. Pericardium is the Heart Protector and governs circulation. Triple Warmer is the entire trunk of the body separated into three "warmers," the upper warmer being responsible for respiration and circulation; the middle warmer for storage, digestion, and transformation; and the lower warmer for drainage of dregs.

Yang (YAHNG) is the term used to represent the following: the sunny side of the hill, the hot surface of the midday in summertime, the masculine principles of growth and expansion, and the power of the sun. Quick and continuous, Yang is the principle of activity and movement and the realm of the mind and spirit. See Table 11-3 for more correspondences.

Yin and Yang interact continuously with each other, and that interaction brings about all things in the universe. These natural forces are at odds with each other but also cannot exist without each other. This is a fundamental dynamic tension at work in our world, according to centuries of experiences of Taoist masters. They observed natural phenomena at work, shared their perspectives and experiences, experimented, and learned the ways of the energetic principles of life. In fact, this dynamic continues today and is confirmed and quantified by quantum physics theories and modern technologies.

When Yin and Yang are in balanced interaction, there is health and happiness. When Yin and Yang are out of balance with each other, there is dysfunction and disease. The black and white symbol, the Tai Ji (Fig. 11-2), represents the constant ebb and flow of life and the continuous movement between opposing forces, and shows balance through process over time. When Yin is at its strongest, Yang is at its weakest, and vice versa.

Furthermore, Yin/Yang theory teaches us there are certain tenets about how the two interact. They are in mutual creation with each other. They mutually control one another. Yin and Yang can both be subdivided infinitely. They are interdependent and eventually transform into each other. When they are in balance, there is harmony; when they are imbalanced, there is disharmony. The movement from Yang to Yin and Yin to Yang and back again is

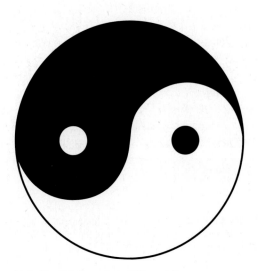

Figure 11-2. The Tai Ji symbol of Yin and Yang.

the great cosmic dance between matter and energy, light and dark, hot and cold.

As humans, we show the interaction of Yin and Yang in many ways. We have active times of our day (and our lives) and restful times. We are happy and laughing; other times we are sad and crying. We have health and we have disease. When we practice Asian Bodywork, or any form of Chinese medicine, we attempt, in part, to facilitate balance in the Yin and Yang aspects of a person. Our goal is the balance of the two, for when there is balance, there is healing, health, and long life.

Qi and Meridians

Qi, pronounced "chee," also spelled **C'hi**, is the Chinese term translated as "Life Force" or "Vital Energy." Qi is one of the **Five Vital Substances** in Chinese medicine—the fundamental substances that make us human and keep us functioning in our bodies. The others are Blood (*xue*), body fluids (*jin-ye*), Essence (*jing*), and spirit or consciousness (*Shen*).

Qi moves through the system continuously and serves four purposes:

1. To warm and protect the body
2. To hold organs and substances in place
3. To be the impetus for movement and to accompany movement
4. To govern smooth, harmonious transformations

A basic premise of Chinese medicine is that Qi moves in pathways called **meridians**, also called channels or pathways, flowing from one area of the body to another much like a highway system carries all manner of goods and people from one place to another. There are many levels of meridians in the body, and they form a three-dimensional matrix for movement of the Five Vital Substances.

Ancient texts say that when Qi and Blood are flowing smoothly and no pathogens are present, there is harmony and health. When Qi is too weak or too strong, or when a pathogen is present, there is a lack of smooth flow and resultant disharmony. Getting regular ABT treatments is a great method for keeping our Qi flowing smoothly and nourishing the body's energetic foundation.

Each meridian in the body is named according to the *zang-fu* (Organ System) to which it is connected. In Chinese medicine, Organ Systems are described according to their function, not their anatomy or structure, although there is an internal meridian trajectory through the associated organ. For example, the Spleen system is responsible, in part, for harmonious transformations of food into Qi. An Organ System also is associated with meridian(s) and acupoints, vital substances, pathogenic influences, and emotions.

The following are the names and abbreviations of the primary meridians and associated Organ Systems (Fig. 11-3 and Table 11-4):

- Lung (Lu)
- Large Intestine (LI)
- Stomach (ST)
- Spleen (Sp)
- Heart (Ht)
- Small Intestine (SI)
- Bladder (BL)
- Kidney (K)
- Pericardium (P)
- Triple Warmer (TW)
- Gallbladder (GB)
- Liver (Liv)

Acupoints

Along the meridian highway are intersections where a change of direction or emphasis can take place and where interaction can occur with other levels. These intersections along the meridians—specifically located points on the body that influence, and are influenced by, body energies—are called **acupoints**, often referred to as acupressure points. Qi tends to pool, or collect, at acupoints, which are often tender upon palpation. If the Qi in an acupoint is excessive, the point will most likely be hard (full) and painful. If the Qi in an acupoint is deficient, the point will most likely be soft (empty) and achy.

Western texts identify acupoints by their meridian name and a number. The meridian name indicates which meridian that point is on, and the number indicates what number point we are using in the direction of Qi flow on that meridian. Lu 1, in the upper chest, is the first point on the Lung channel; Lu 11, on the thumb, is the last.

Each acupoint has its own name, which can also help us remember its actions, but these are not always used in the United States. For example, ST 36 is named *zusanli* and translated as "Leg Three Miles," referring to its action of tonifying (strengthening) Qi and nourishing Blood and Yin. It is said that on long treks on foot, one could stimulate this point when exhausted, then be able to walk three more miles.

Acupoints are worked to activate their actions and are used to stimulate, relax, remove/resolve pathogens, ease

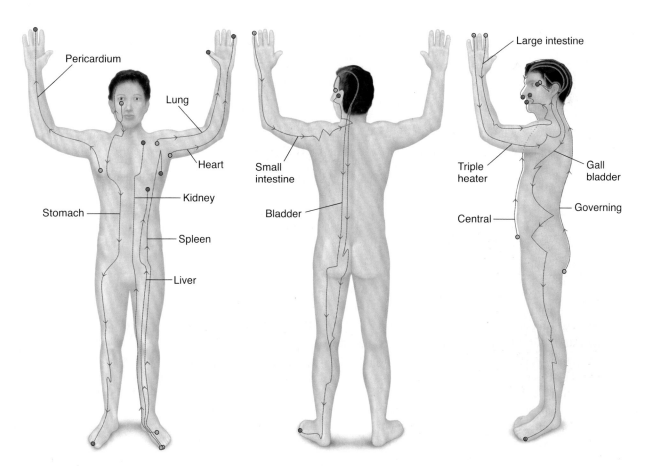

Figure 11-3. Energy meridians.

Table 11-4 Primary Meridian Pathway Descriptions

Meridian	Beginning Point	Pathway	Ending Point
Lung (Lu)	First intercostal space in the lateral chest	Lateral side of the inner arm	Lateral base of the thumbnail
Large Intestine (LI)	Lateral side of the index fingernail	Up the lateral side of the outer arm, across the top of the shoulders and the neck	Outer edge of the nostril
Stomach (ST)	Under the center of the eye in the edge of the orbit	Through the jaw and neck, down the front of the body, lateral edge of the leg, center of the foot	Lateral base of the second toenail
Spleen (Sp)	Medial base of the big toenail	Up the medial aspect of the anterior leg to the outer trunk	On the midaxillary line, in the seventh intercostal space
Heart (Ht)	Center of the axilla	Medial side of the inner arm	Lateral base of the little fingernail
Small Intestine (SI)	Medial base of the little fingernail	Medial side of the outer arm, through the scapula, and up the neck	Temporomandibular joint at the ear flap
Bladder (BL)	The depression between the eyes, on either side of the nose	Over the head and down the back and the back of the legs	Lateral base of the little toenail
Kidney (K)	The depression under the ball of the foot	Up the medial back of the leg, then up either side of the anterior midline	Just under the sternoclavicular joint
Pericardium (P)	1 *cun* lateral to the nipple	Out the center of the inner arm	Lateral base of the middle fingernail
Triple Warmer (TW)	Medial base of the fourth fingernail	Up the outer arm, across the top of the shoulder and around the ear	Outer edge of the eyebrow
Gallbladder (GB)	Outer edge of the eye socket	Zigzags down the lateral aspects of the body	Lateral base of the fourth toenail
Liver (Liv)	Lateral base of the big toenail	Up the inner leg and through the abdomen	In the sixth intercostal space, on the nipple line

pain, and more. They also have specific actions related to the body's vital substances. Acupoints are most often worked in combination to achieve specific results. For instance, working Liv 3 and LI 4 together is a balancing treatment.

Acupoints are highly specific points and must be located exactly according to anatomical landmarks and measurements of body inches. A body inch, called a *cun* (CHUN), is equal to the distance across the thumb knuckle. Each *cun* is measured on each person's body with his or her own thumb knuckle width. One thumb knuckle width is equal to one *cun*.

Disease Origin and Prevention

Although Chinese medicine, like every other form of medicine, cannot treat or cure every disease or condition, it does make great contributions, in part through its health maintenance, early detection, and disease prevention aspects. All branches of Chinese medicine (although astrology and geomancy are not used much today) are used for the healing of disease as well as for health maintenance and disease prevention. Early detection is achieved through assessing imbalances in the bioenergy that may not have yet manifested in the physical.

Unlike Western medicine, Chinese medicine is based in nature and natural processes, and thus the language of its medical model is quite unfamiliar to us. The causes of disease in Chinese medicine are classified as "internal" or "external." The internal causes are the "injurious emotions": anger, excessive joy, worry, sadness, grief, and fear. They can injure the Organ Systems they are associated with if overexpressed or underexpressed (see the section on the Five Phases below). Thus, healthy emotional expression is something that can be very beneficial to one's health.

The external causes are climatic factors: Wind, Heat, Fire, Damp, Dry, Cold, and Summerheat. Sometimes these factors combine, such as Wind-Heat or Damp-Cold; these climatic terms are used to describe the imbalance being assessed and treated. Other causes of disease include wrong treatment, environmental toxins, plagues, unforeseen events, poisons, and parasites.

Regular practice of meditation and *qigong* (or *tai ch'i*) and attention to dietary guidelines are considered fundamental necessities for continued health. Additionally, individuals can prevent disease and maintain their health by regularly visiting a Chinese medicine healthcare practitioner to receive bodywork, herbal formulas, and/or acupuncture treatments. Typically, the practitioner gives the client homework to do, as one goal of this ancient medicine is to help people take responsibility for their own health. This approach is often called "wholistic," meaning that the whole person is treated as one, not as a sum of many parts. As health is a goal but not a destination, so the treatment according to Chinese medicine principles shifts as the person changes. Treatments are designed for each individual, not statistical groups, so the benefits can be measured in individual results.

Early detection of bioenergy imbalances is a skill that is learned over time. There are signs and symptoms that one watches for, and the assessment processes are fairly simple—at least, simple in terms of what format is used; people present with complex conditions! Determining the nature of the imbalance and the appropriate treatment is the art of Chinese medicine. The basic principles are used no matter what modality you practice.

Assessment

In any medical model, there must be a way to gather information, process it, and make a determination for treatment. In this segment, we look at the principles of Chinese medicine assessment including the Four Examinations, the Eight Principles, and the Five Phases. The Four Examinations are for information gathering, whereas the Eight Principles and the Five Phases are the paradigms used to process the information and make a determination of the particular imbalance of an individual.

The Four Examinations

Information is gathered using the Four Examinations. They are as follows:

- Looking
- Listening/smelling
- Asking
- Palpation

Looking includes observing the client's movements, facial characteristics, and overall body type. A practitioner of Chinese medicine also visually inspects several aspects of the tongue, including the size and shape, color, cracks, spots or eruptions, moisture, and the coating. The tongue shows the condition of the interior workings of the body.

Listening refers to assessing all sounds emitted by a client, such as a singing lilt to the voice, shouting, rumbling in the abdomen, wheezing in the lungs, or cracking in the joints. All audible clues are useful. *Smelling* can also be used to assess a client because, despite modern hygiene, smells associated with certain imbalances can be detected in clients. For instance, a burnt smell can indicate Heat, whereas a sweet smell might indicate Dampness.

Asking refers to 10 questions that are usually asked of a client prior to a treatment session. They include questions about preferences for hot or cold, sleep, pain, digestion and elimination, urination, medical history, diet, and family medical history.

Palpation refers to touching acupoints, painful areas, certain areas of the abdomen and back, and checking the pulses. In Chinese medicine, the pulses are taken in three positions on both wrists. There are three depths to each pulse, and 28 pulse qualities to study and learn.

Using the Four Examinations, we can gather the information we require to make a good assessment of the overall condition of the person and determine our treatment strategies. We do that by putting the information into other frameworks that explain what the assessment information means. One of those frameworks is the Eight Principles.

The Eight Principles

The Eight Principles help determine the thermal quality, location, and strength of a client's condition. The parameters are as follows:

- Hot/cold
- Exterior/interior
- Full/empty
- Yang/Yin

If a condition is more "hot," the treatment includes cooling techniques. If a condition is more interior, the treatment strategy will be different than if the condition is more exterior. The "fullness" of a condition tells its strength. Yang

Table 11-5 Five Phase Correspondences

Phase	Organ System	Season	Color	Quality	Climatic Factor	Injurious Emotion
Fire	Heart and Small Intestine; Pericardium and Triple Warmer	Summer	Red	Expanding	Heat/Fire/ Summerheat	Excessive joy
Earth	Spleen and Stomach	Late summer	Yellow	Descending	Dampness	Worry, rumination
Metal	Lung and Large Intestine	Fall	White	Contracting	Dryness	Grief/sadness
Water	Kidney and Bladder	Winter	Navy/black	Resting	Cold	Fear
Wood	Liver and Gallbladder	Spring	Green	Rising	Wind	Anger

and Yin are included as the foundation of them all. Yang is associated with hot, exterior, and full. Yin is associated with cold, interior, and empty (lacking strength).

The Five Phase Theory

Another framework for assessment and treatment is the Five Phase (or Element) theory. The Five Phase theory shows us processes over time, in the sense that a disease process or a healing process can be tracked through the phases by following the natural energetic movement patterns. There are also correspondences associated with each phase that cover nearly every spectrum of existence from foods to existential crises. These correspondences help point us in the direction of a particular phase, whether making an assessment or planning a treatment strategy.

The Five Phases are named according to five energetic forces at work on the earth: Fire, Earth, Metal, Water, and Wood. Fire energy expands and corresponds to the Heart and Small Intestine Organ Systems. Earth energy descends and corresponds to the Spleen and Stomach. Metal energy contracts and corresponds to the Lung and Large Intestine. Water energy is restful and corresponds to the Kidney and Bladder. Wood energy rises and corresponds to Liver and Gallbladder, and then the rising energy expands into Fire again as the cycle continues.

The Pericardium and Triple Warmer are considered part of the Fire phase and are referred to as Supplemental Fire. See Table 11-5 for more correspondences.

The energetic qualities described above move in a cycle of energy creation called the Creation Cycle (Fig. 11-4). This cycle is illustrated by the arrows in the circle on the outer

edge of the symbol. This shows us that each phase fuels the one following it, a cycle of energy creation. Fire burns to ashes to create Earth; Earth compresses to create Metal; Metal becomes Liquid, like Water; and Water nourishes Wood.

The Control Cycle is a built-in balancing system. Fire melts Metal; Metal cuts Wood; Wood penetrates Earth;

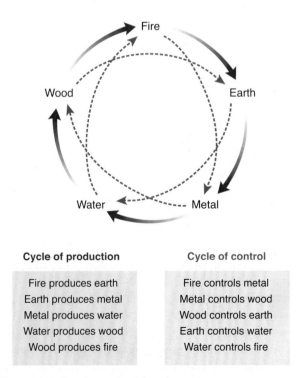

Cycle of production	Cycle of control
Fire produces earth	Fire controls metal
Earth produces metal	Metal controls wood
Metal produces water	Wood controls earth
Water produces wood	Earth controls water
Wood produces fire	Water controls fire

Figure 11-4. Creation cycle of five phases.

Earth dams Water; Water puts out Fire. **When these cycles are moving in the ways they are supposed to, there is health, happiness, and longevity. The key is to keep the energy flowing. When there is imbalance, it can cause a domino effect throughout the system affecting all phases. This imbalance results in disease.**

The Five Phase theory is used to determine the nature of the imbalance as well as treatment strategies. For example, a person who is stuck in a pattern of anger will present with a Wood imbalance. When Qi is stuck, or stagnant, it is called an "excess" (see more in the section Deficiency and Excess Treatment Strategies). We can treat that imbalance by strengthening Metal to help control Wood, dispersing Wood to help move the excess out, and by stimulating Fire to help use the excess as fuel and to move on into the next phase. We effect change by using the appropriate techniques on the corresponding meridians.

Principles of Treatment

One focus for Asian Bodywork practitioners is the facilitation of smooth flow of Qi. The ABT principles of treatment are the same as for any other branch of Chinese medicine: expel/resolve pathogens, tonify deficiency, and disperse excess. In this section, we discuss meridian Qi flow, deficiency and excess treatment strategies, and meridian therapy.

Meridian Qi Flow Directions

In the primary meridian system, there are 12 meridians: 6 Yin and 6 Yang. They are bilateral on the body and are connected in Yin and Yang pairs. The Yin organs are made of dense tissue and serve to create, transform, and nourish: Heart, Pericardium, Spleen, Lung, Kidney, and Liver. The Yang organs are hollow and serve to hold, digest, separate, and eliminate: Small Intestine, Triple Warmer, Stomach, Large Intestine, Bladder, and Gallbladder.

In the bioenergy flow, the Yin meridian Qi flows up from below, whereas the Yang meridian Qi flows down from above. The cosmic energies above and the earthly energies below mix together to create life, and this circulation of energetic opposites continues until we die. The "meridian/energy anatomy" is presented on the body with the arms raised and the palms forward, showing the upward direction of Yin Qi and the downward direction of Yang Qi through the body (see earlier Fig. 11-3).

The Yin channels originate in the feet and flow toward the torso, and from the upper torso, flow to the hands. The Yin meridians are located in the medial and anterior portions of the body.

The Yang channels originate in the hands and flow to the head, and from the head, flow to the feet. The Yang meridians are located in the posterior and lateral portions of the body.

Deficiency and Excess Treatment Strategies

Deficiency and **excess** are terms used to describe conditions of Qi that are considered out of balance. Deficiency means that the system is weak and the pattern is a tiring, draining type of imbalance. When we encounter deficient areas along a meridian, they feel soft, weak, deep, and/or cool to the touch. Long-term deficiency can be quite painful, but short-term deficiency responds well to firm, yet gentle, pressure. The proper treatment for deficiency is to tonify. Tonify means to warm, strengthen, and stimulate. Tonification techniques include clockwise circular motions, which draw the Qi in, and lighter, quicker stimulation. Hot applications may also be used.

Excess means that the system is in full response to an external attack or that the Qi and Blood are stagnant; both present a more robust, feverish type of imbalance. Excessive areas along a meridian feel hard, tight, raised from the surface, and/or warmer to the touch. Excesses are easily irritated by pressure and respond better to a gentle touch. The proper treatment for excess is to disperse. Disperse means to cool, relax, and move out. Dispersing techniques include counterclockwise circular motions, which move the Qi out and away. Pressure is adjusted from lighter and gentler to heavier and deeper as the condition changes and pain eases. Cold applications are also effective.

Meridian Therapy

To practice ABT is to practice "**meridian therapy**." Meridian therapy is the art of working to open and move the joints, release blockages in tissue, balance the Qi moving in the meridians, and stimulate the actions of acupoints as needed. ABT includes the use of range-of-motion techniques for moving the joints, and tonification and dispersal techniques to release blockages and balance the Qi flow. ABT uses direct pressures of varying direction, motion, and intensity to stimulate the actions of acupoints and meridians.

Although meridian therapy uses a wide variety of techniques, its focus is on assessment according to Chinese medicine and/or the individual modality's theory, and the balancing of the Qi movement. To balance the Qi movement in a meridian, one must discover the excesses and deficiencies present. We accomplish this by palpating the meridian, feeling the variations along the pathway, and either tonifying or dispersing as needed.

Begin with light palpation of the meridian and see if you can determine any excesses or deficiencies. Use direct palm pressure and trace the meridian pathway at least three times; try using a gentle, rhythmic series of pressure applications. When you find an excess, you can be sure there is a deficiency somewhere on the channel that is connected to that excess. The fun is in finding it!

Monitor an excess gently and palpate the rest of the meridian with your other hand. When you find the connected deficiency, the excess you are monitoring will respond in some way that is palpable. You can feel the excess "moving" under your fingers each time you touch the connected deficiency. It can feel like a "bumping" under your fingers, or a slight electrical charge, or it may just disappear as soon as you touch the deficiency. It is a fun exploration and treatment process, and clients report wonderful results. See Box 11-11 for a basic ABT routine (Shiatsu routine).

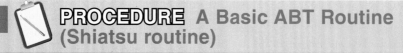

BOX 11-11 **PROCEDURE** A Basic ABT Routine (Shiatsu routine)

Begin with the client in the prone position, on a clean blanket, futon mat, or treatment table. Adjust the suggested body positions below as needed for table or mat.

1. Center yourself and take a few deep breaths. Then focus on the client, and let go of other thoughts.

---

2. Straddle the client, standing on both feet. Place both hands on the client's upper back and shoulder area. After resting there a moment, start a gentle rocking motion that begins in the upper back area and continues all the way to the feet. Do this two or three times to help the client integrate with his or her whole body and loosen up. This is also a great way to quickly gather information of the client's areas of tension.

---

3. Kneel at the client's left side and perform a diagonal stretch to the client's back to help open the BL meridian.
   a. Place your left hand on the client's left scapula and your right hand just below the client's right iliac crest.
   b. Lean forward and apply pressure to move your hands away from each other, and hold for 5 to 10 seconds.
   c. Lean back to relieve the pressure.
   d. Move your left hand to the client's right scapula and your right hand to just below the client's left iliac crest.
   e. Lean forward and apply pressure to move your hands away from each other, and hold for 5 to 10 seconds.
   f. Lean back to relieve the pressure.

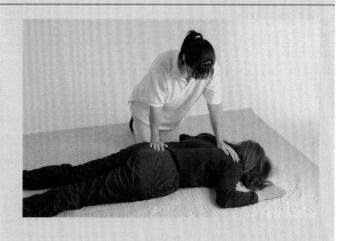

---

4. From that same position, perform a posterior midline stretch to the client's back to open the BL and Governing Vessel (GV; channel that runs up the spine).
   a. Cross your arms, placing your right hand on the upper thoracic spine and your left hand on the sacrum.
   b. Lean forward and apply pressure to separate your hands, and hold for 5 to 10 seconds.
   c. Lean back to relieve the pressure.

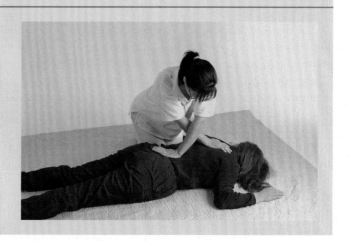

BOX 11-11 **PROCEDURE** A Basic ABT Routine
(Shiatsu routine) (continued)

5. Stand over the client's back, or straddle with one knee down and one up. Apply "cat-walking" technique, leaning in with alternating direct compressions from one hand to another, along the BL meridian from the upper back to the sacrum. Begin with light pressure and proceed deeper as the back warms and loosens and the client allows. Repeat several times.
   a. Place both hands on the upper back on either side of the spine. Rest the heels of your hands close to the spine and let your fingers relax to the sides.
   b. Lean into one hand and then the other, alternating pressure as you make your way down the back.
   c. Continue in this way until you reach the sacrum. Rock back and forth, and gently lean into the sacrum.

6. Apply slow, rhythmic direct compression with both hands simultaneously along the BL meridian, allowing for the client's breath. Again, proceed from the upper back to the sacrum.
   a. Starting at the top of the back, place the heels of your hands on either side of the spine and let your fingers rest along the client's ribs.
   b. Lean forward to apply pressure and hold for 5 seconds.
   c. Lean back to relieve pressure and move your hands 1 to 2 inches down the spine.
   d. Repeat steps b and c until you reach the sacrum, and rock and lean into the sacrum with as much pressure as is comfortable for the client.

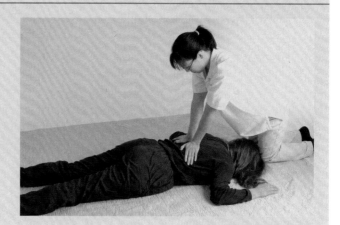

7. Address any particular areas of tension or pain, using meridian therapy.

8. Work the buttocks well; the BL and GB meridians "meet" here. Kneel on the client's side, or stand and use your feet to apply direct pressure to the large muscles.
   a. Using a loose fist or hand, apply alternating pressure to the client's gluteal muscles. Work one side first, then the other.
   b. Standing to the client's side on one foot, use the other foot to lean your body weight into the soft tissue of the buttocks (not on the bones). Adjust the depth and angle of your pressure as needed.
   c. Using both hands, lean into the sacrum and move it slowly in all directions with firm, yet gentle, pressure.

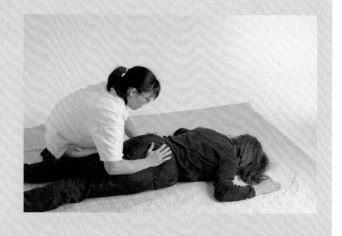

9. Perform range of motion for the left leg; then work the BL meridian with gentle, rhythmic compressions from the ischial tuberosity to the little toe.

10. Work the K meridian in the same manner as above, beginning under the foot and coming up the inside back of the leg.

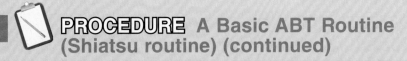

BOX 11-11 📋 **PROCEDURE A Basic ABT Routine (Shiatsu routine) (continued)**

11. "Frog" the leg to the outside: flex the left leg so the foot is above the knee, then raise the entire leg slightly so the left knee comes off the ground. Put your hand under the knee then lean the foot toward the opposite knee. Next, push and slide the left knee up toward the outside of the hip. Work the GB meridian from the piriformis area (GB 30) to the fourth toe.

12. Repeat steps 9 to 11 on the right leg. Ask the client to roll over to a supine position.

13. Perform range of motion for the left leg, then position the leg so the foot is toward the opposite ankle, and support the knee with bolster or your knee. Work the Sp meridian from the big toe to the upper inner leg.

14. Position the leg so the foot is toward the opposite knee, still supporting the knee. Work the Liv channel from the big toe up to the inner leg and thigh.

15. Bring the leg back to a neutral position on the mat or table and work the ST meridian from the upper outer thigh to the 2nd and 3rd toes. Repeat steps 13 to 15 on the right leg.

16. Sit comfortably near the client's right side. Work the abdomen well with direct compressions, following peristalsis (the natural clockwise movement of the digestive and eliminative tracts), in a spiraling pattern toward the lower dan'tien. "Bake" the dan'tien by placing one hand over the lower belly, sliding the other hand under the low back, and generating some penetrating heat between the palms of your hands.

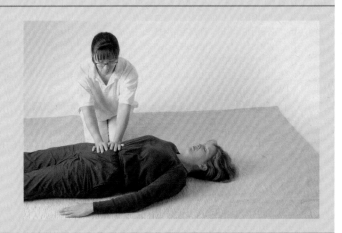

17. With both palms together, lean into the sternum with gentle pressure, making your way up to the sternoclavicular joints. This is more of the K meridian.

18. Take the right arm and perform ROM. Position the arm so the hand is down from the shoulder, the palm up.

19. Work the Lu channel from the upper chest to the thumb.

20. Move the arm so that it is straight out to the side, and work the P meridian from the edge of pectoralis major to the middle finger.

BOX 11-11 **PROCEDURE** A Basic ABT Routine (Shiatsu routine) (continued)

21. Extend the hand and arm up and out from the shoulder, and work the Ht channel from the axilla to the little finger. Place the arm back in a comfortable position.

    Repeat steps 18 to 21 on the left arm.

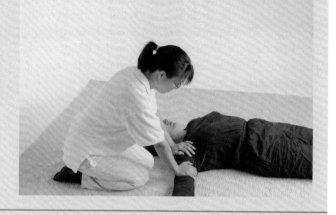

22. Kneel comfortably above the head, and work into the tops of the shoulders with direct pressure. Catwalk on the shoulders and alternate thumb pressure as well. Hold direct pressure on GB 21, halfway between C7 and the top of the humerus, on the edge of the trapezius muscle.

23. Gently work the neck, beginning with gentle exploration of the BL meridian on either side of the cervical vertebrae. Lean into the points on either side of the spine, then plant all your fingers underneath the occipital ridge and apply enough pressure so the chin rises. Hold that for a few seconds.

24. Gently place the head in a comfortable position and work the scalp well using direct pressure and circular motions.

25. Work the face gently, applying direct pressure with fingers together. Begin at the forehead working from the center of the face toward the outside. Work from top to bottom, and end your session with holding one hand under the neck and one hand over the forehead.

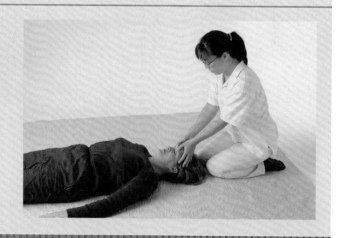

Self-Care

Self-care is a major focus in most ABT trainings. Understanding what Qi is and how it works is not just an intellectual exercise to be applied to clients; taking care of oneself is a fundamental part of Chinese medicine. Qigong, meditation, diet and lifestyle choices, and self-awareness are all integral to a good ABT practice. Acupressure, a bodywork modality in which firm fingertip pressure is applied to acupoints along the energy meridians to regulate the flow of Qi, can also be used for self-care (Table 11-6).

Qigong translates as "Qi work" or "Qi exercise" and refers to a myriad of exercises that have been passed down through Chinese history. These exercises are designed to focus the mind, use the breath, and move the body to achieve harmony and health. There are hundreds of forms of Qigong and innumerable ways to practice it (see Box 11-12). One can find more information through the National Qigong Association and the Association for Traditional Studies, two of the Qigong groups in the United States.

Another very important aspect of self-care is the therapist's body mechanics while doing the work. In ABT practice, especially if working on the floor, therapists use many different body positions, thus the use of proper body mechanics is critical. **One basic thing to remember: *Lean, don't push or press or dig.***

When leaning the body weight, move from the center of gravity (the lower belly) and transfer your weight into the hands. This movement takes the stress off the smaller muscles and joints and uses the body weight effectively. When rising from the floor or when lifting, remember to push into your feet. This way, the leg and hip muscles, larger and designed for more work, do their job properly.

Table 11-6 Acupressure Points for Self-Care

Acupressure Point	Location	Self-Care Applications
LI4 (large intestine 4)	Base of webbing between thumb and index finger	Sinus problems Headaches Constipation Contraindicated during pregnancy!
P6 (pericardium 6)	On forearm, about three finger widths from the crease at the base of the hand, between two tendons	Nausea Anxiety

continues on following page

Table 11-6 Acupressure Points for Self-Care *continued*

Acupressure Point	Location	Self-Care Applications
ST36 (stomach 36)	Front of leg, about four fingers below the kneecap, just lateral to the tibia	Fatigue Depression Lack of grounding Instability
SP6 (spleen 6)	Medial side of tibia, about four fingers above medial malleolus	Irritability Cold and flu Worry Fear Contraindicated during pregnancy!
GB20 (gallbladder 20)	Base of skull, in the hollow on either side of the neck, about 2 to 3 inches apart	Shoulder pain Depression Neck tension Irritability

BOX 11-12 PROCEDURE A Qigong Exercise: Expel the Old

Excellent for practicing between clients, or at the end of the day, whenever you want to calm down, or anytime there are unresolved issues clouding your bodymind (a term used when referring to the total human, the body and mind in connection). This series is designed to move old Qi out and bring fresh, clear, healthy Qi in.

1. Stand with your feet shoulder-width apart, knees relaxed, sacrum slightly tucked, shoulders relaxed, and chin slightly down. Take a deep breath and exhale completely, focusing your mind in your lower dan'tien (lower belly).

2. Put all your weight on your right leg, leaving the left side "empty."

3. Raise both arms over the left side of your body—the empty side. Visualize and connect to the "Qi above" (also called heavenly or cosmic Qi), and inhale as you use your hands to bring this fresh, new Qi through the top of your head and down the left side of your body. Shift your weight slowly as you "fill" your left side with fresh Qi. As you get to the waist, begin slowly exhaling down the left leg, moving any old, stagnant, useless Qi out through the bottom of your foot and replacing it with the fresh Qi. By now, all your weight has shifted to the left side. "Expel the old," letting go of the useless Qi into the ground to be cleansed and recirculated in the earth. Be sure to exhale completely.

4. Next, reach over to the ground below your right leg (now "empty"), and connect to some fresh, clear earthly Qi. Visualize pulling fresh Qi up through the leg, inhaling as you direct the Qi with the hands. The fresh Qi is replacing the old Qi as you inhale and move it through. Shift your body weight again as you "fill" the right side with fresh Qi. As you reach the waist, your weight centered on both legs, bring both hands toward the anterior midline of the body then pull the fresh Qi up through the center of the body toward the esophagus. Open the esophagus as much as you can, then open the throat, directing this fresh Qi through and out the mouth as you exhale. While exhaling, use the hands to expel the old out and *slightly* up from the mouth. Do not push the Qi up over the head, but out of the mouth and slightly up. Make a "haaa" sound as you exhale.

Repeat at least five times. The exercise can be done as often as needed. Regular practice will produce terrific benefits, including balanced stress levels, calm breath and heart, and clear mind.

Ayurvedic Healthcare

Ayurveda is a Sanskrit word derived from two roots: "ayur," meaning science or life, and "veda," meaning knowledge. In Chapter 1, we briefly introduced the ancient Indian scriptural texts called the Vedas. The Ayur Veda, a supplement to one of those scriptures, discusses pharmacology and health and is the basis for the Indian system of health and healing that eventually became known as Ayurveda. This holistic healthcare system addresses a person's physical, sensory, emotional, intellectual, and spiritual well-being. According to the principal Ayurvedic text, Charaka Samhita, health is the result of maintaining a natural state of balance for the individual's body, mind, and spirit on a day-to-day and season-to-season basis (Box 11-13).

The foundation of Ayurveda is built on the five elements of nature: ether, air, fire, water, and earth. Different combinations of these elements create three types of personal natures

BOX 11-13
Ayurvedic Definition of Health

The following definition is from the Charaka Samhita, the principal Ayurvedic text (available at: http://www.ayurvedamedgroup.com/about.html):

"...samadosha samagnicha samadhatu malakriya prasannatmendriyah manah svasya ityaibhiyate..."

Translation: "Balanced qualities, balanced digestion, balanced formation of tissues and organs, and proper release of impurities. Happiness of the senses and the mind, and connection to the higher Self, that is the definition of health."

(doshas), the five senses, and seven body tissues. The energy of all seven body tissues creates Ojas, the energy that connects mind to body. Centered in the heart, Ojas flows throughout the body and helps the body heal effectively. When it is weak, illness can result, leading some to believe Ojas is the fundamental energy of the immune system. The five elements, three doshas, five senses, and seven body tissues are interrelated, and an imbalance in one stimulates change in one or more of the others. Keeping all of these aspects of a person's makeup balanced and functioning naturally and properly allows energy to flow freely, which determines good health.

Ayurveda is consistent with the Traditional Chinese Medicine (TCM) philosophy of maintaining health and well-being. Both identify five elements of nature, both attempt to achieve and maintain a balance of energies, and both recognize energy centers in the body called chakras. Most of all, they are holistic systems of preventive medicine that are instructional and individualized. True Ayurvedic practitioners undergo years of training similar to medical school. It is within their scope of practice to diagnose and prescribe treatments such as diet, herbal teas, medicine, exercise, aromas, massage, color, crystals, and gemstones. Although massage therapists are not Ayurvedic practitioners, it is within a massage therapist's scope of practice to administer massage and educate clients about the Ayurvedic system of healthcare.

Five Elements

Although slightly different from the Five Phases (elements) identified in TCM, the Ayurvedic system also recognizes five elements of nature. These elements are organized in a descending pattern in which the highest element is ether, sometimes called space. Moving downward, the next element is air, then fire, then water, and finally earth. Each element influences different anatomical structures and physiological activities:

- Ether: abdomen, cells, mouth, nostrils, respiratory tract, sound
- Air: movements of cells, intestines, lungs, muscles, touch
- Fire: digestive system, enzyme function, intelligence, metabolism, vision
- Water: blood, digestive enzymes, mucous membranes, plasma, saliva, taste
- Earth: bones, cartilage, hair, muscles, nails, skin, teeth, tendons, smell

As the five elements influence the body's ability to heal, they also define the doshas, or energetic forces, that determine a person's nature or unique combination of these elemental energies.

Doshas

Ayurvedic healthcare focuses on three energetic forces called doshas: vata, pitta, and kapha. Loosely compared to aspects of a person's general nature or disposition, all three doshas are present in everyone (Box 11-14). Each person has a prakruti (also prakriti or prakruthi) state, an individualized balance of doshas like a metabolic blueprint that dictates how that person should live to achieve health and harmony in mind and body. The goal of Ayurvedic healthcare is to preserve and restore the prakruti state, in which the levels of the three doshas are appropriate and balanced for the individual. According to the Ayurvedic philosophy, optimal health is the result of balanced doshas, whereas illness and dysfunction are energetic imbalances that eventually manifest themselves in the body. The imbalanced condition is referred to as the vikruti (also vikriti or vikruthi) state. The doshas interact with biological forces and rhythms of nature such as specific functions of the body and the five basic elements of nature.

Vata is associated with wind, change, and the elements of ether and air, and influences activity and movement. Considered the leading dosha, when vata is out of balance, it tends to force the other doshas out of balance. Someone who is a vata type may be artistic, thoughtful, and imaginative with a weakness for implementing his ideas. Vata imbalances are often manifested as restlessness, anxiety, and exhaustion from mental stress. Regarding human physiology, vata controls muscle movement including heart activity and breathing motions, circulation of blood, the passage of food through the digestive tract, and the transmission of nerve impulses to and from the brain. Excessive vata can result in flatulence (wind); fearfulness (change); and arthritis, constipation, and circulation problems (movement).

Pitta is associated with the sun, influences conversion and transformation, and correlates to the water and fire elements. Pitta types tend to have intense emotions of impatience, anger, and jealousy, but they also demonstrate warm-heartedness and are effective at changing other people's opinions. In the body, pitta affects metabolism, which involves the transformation of energy. Symptoms of excess of pitta may include sensitivity to the sun, including rashes and freckles, diarrhea (water), and premature gray hair or hair loss (transformation).

BOX 11-14
Comparing Doshas to the Ancient Greek "Humours"

Ancient Ayurvedic practitioners who traveled to Greece probably introduced the concept of doshas to the ancient Greeks, who then referred to them as the "humours."

Kapha is related to the elements of water and earth. It is affected by the moon and associated with the principle of cohesion. People who are kapha types are generally sensitive, emotional, methodical, and steady, and dislike change. An imbalance of kapha easily results in weight problems because of a lack of physical activity and the tendency to use food for emotional support. Kapha affects the joints, lymphatics, and mucous membranes. Excessive kapha can result in excessive mucus and fluid retention (water), inactivity or excessive sleep (earth), congestion or sluggish digestion (cohesion).

Energy and Chakras

The Ayurvedic system refers to the life force energy as prana (TCM calls it Qi). Prana animates every aspect of life and must be balanced and flow freely between mind and body to maintain health. Starting as kundalini energy, a powerful form of prana centered at the base of the spine, it flows upward through the body in a spiral fashion, to just above the center of the head. On the way up through the body, prana flows through chakras, which are energy centers along the midline of the body.

The word chakra is Sanskrit for "wheel." These chakras are related to states of consciousness and believed to affect physiology, emotions, and spiritual progression. There are seven major chakras which can be identified by name, number, or anatomical position, and each has a different energetic vibration that correlates to a specific color of the spectrum and a group of emotions. Although the first five chakras are associated with the five natural elements, the last two chakras are more spiritual than earthly and are therefore not associated with the elements. The first five chakras are also located at major nerve plexuses, which are areas rich with the electrical activity of nerve transmission. Figure 11-5 is The Circulation of the Light, a circulatory reservoir of energy in the human body, and illustrates an overlay of Qi meridians and the chakras.

The first chakra is the most inferior, called the root (Muladhara) chakra. It is found at the level of the coccyx, around the perineum. Its energy is represented by the color red and it is associated with the earth element. The root chakra relates to our basic needs of safety and survival as well as our connection to the physical world (grounding). Centered on the coccygeal nerve plexus, the root chakra is physically associated with the spinal column, rectum, legs, bones, feet, and immune system. Symptoms of an

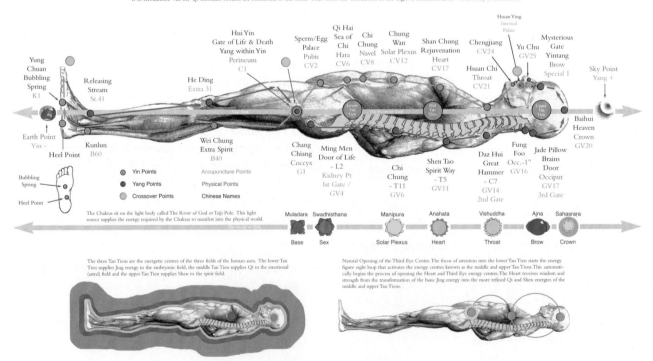

Figure 11-5. The Circulation of the Light, an overlay of Qi meridians, and the chakras. (Reprinted with permission of Kevin Farrow, www. acuenergetics.com.)

Table 11-7 The Chakras

Chakra	Location	Color	Element	Emotional Associations	Superimposed Nerve Plexus	Balanced	Imbalanced
Seventh; Crown; Sahasrara	Just above the center of the head	Violet	None	Spirituality, enlightenment, knowledge	None	Sense of knowledge, wisdom, spiritual connection, creative imagination	Insomnia, restlessness, sensory dysfunctions, negativity
Sixth; Brow; Third eye; Ajna	Between the eyebrows	Indigo	None	Intuition, imagination, power of transcendence, self-reflection	None (superimposes the hypothalamus and pituitary gland)	Sense of clarity, intuition	Neurological disorders, self-absorption, sense of superiority
Fifth; Throat; Vishuddha	Base of the neck	Blue	Ether	Communication, creativity	Cervical plexus	Joy, increased communication	Respiratory problems, frustration, sense of fear
Fourth; Heart; Anahata	Behind center of sternum	Green	Air	Love, wisdom	Cardiac plexus	Love, compassion, sense of calm, relaxation	Mood swings, irregular cardiac activity, sense of panic
Third; Solar plexus; Manipura	Just below the xiphoid process	Yellow	Fire	Will, mental power, happiness	Solar (celiac) plexus	Energy, effectiveness, creativity, spontaneity	Digestive problems, sinus problems, anxiety, mental distraction
Second; Sacral; Pelvic; Svadisthana	Abdomen, near the lumbosacral joint	Orange	Water	Emotional needs, trust, sexuality	Sacral plexus	Sexual fulfillment, optimism, ability to accept change	Muscular problems, sexual dysfunction, self-consciousness
First; Root; Muladhara	Coccyx, perineum	Red	Earth	Safety, survival, grounding	Coccygeal plexus	Sense of security, affection, sensitivity toward others	Chronic fatigue, anemia, low blood pressure, fear, anger

imbalance in this chakra may include chronic fatigue, anemia, low blood pressure, fear, anger, or extreme impulsiveness. A balanced root chakra is manifested as a sense of security, a desire to improve oneself, and feelings of affection and sensitivity toward others.

The second chakra is the sacral or pelvic (Svadisthana) chakra, associated with the element water and the color orange. The energy here relates to emotional needs, trust, and sexuality. The sacral chakra is located in the abdomen, at the level of the lumbosacral joint, overlying the sacral nerve plexus. It is associated with the lower vertebrae, pelvis, hips, reproductive organs, large intestine, appendix, and bladder. An imbalance in this chakra can cause muscle spasms and weakness, sexual dysfunction, defensiveness, or self-consciousness. A balanced sacral chakra can be manifested as sexual fulfillment, optimism, and the ability to accept change.

The solar plexus (Manipura) chakra is third, represented by yellow and the fire element. The energy found here relates to mental power, will, and happiness. Located just below the xiphoid process, at the solar (or celiac) nerve plexus, it is physically associated with the stomach, spleen, pancreas, liver, and gallbladder. An imbalance in this chakra may present as digestive, blood sugar, or skin disorders; sinus or allergy problems; anxiety; or decreased mental focus. A balanced solar plexus chakra can exhibit as energy, effectiveness, creativity, and spontaneity.

Fourth is the heart (Anahata) chakra, associated with air and the color green. It is located at the level of the heart, over the cardiac plexus. The energy found here relates to the emotional power of love and the physical structures of the heart, circulatory system, shoulders, arms, and thorax. Symptoms of an imbalanced heart chakra can include mood swings, increased heart rate, heart palpitations or arrhythmia, or a general sense of panic. A balanced heart chakra is exhibited as love for yourself and others, compassion, and a deep sense of calm and relaxation.

The throat (Vishuddha) chakra is fifth, located at the base of the neck. The energy here is associated with ether, the color blue, and communication and creativity. Located on the cervical nerve plexus, the throat chakra is associated with the cervical vertebrae, jaw, teeth, mouth, and respiratory tract. When an imbalance occurs in this chakra, respiratory and/or bronchial problems, frustration, or a sense of fear can result. A balanced throat chakra can be manifested as a sense of joy, relaxation, and increased communication.

The sixth chakra, called the brow or "third eye" (Ajna) chakra, is centered between the eyebrows, and it is associated with the color indigo. Intuition, imagination, and the power of transcendence and self-reflection are influenced by the brow chakra, as is the brain, pituitary and pineal glands, the eyes, ears, and nose. Although it is not associated with a specific nerve plexus, it is located near the hypothalamus and pituitary gland, both very active areas of the brain. An imbalance in the brow chakra can contribute to neurological disorders, self-absorption, or a sense of superiority. A balanced brow chakra can be revealed as a sense of clarity and intuition.

The crown (Sahasrara) chakra is seventh. Located just above the center of the head, it is associated with the color violet. The energy at the crown chakra relates to spiritual enlightenment, wisdom, and knowledge. Physically, it is associated with the central nervous system and the skin. When the crown chakra is imbalanced, you may experience insomnia, restlessness, sensory dysfunctions, or negativity. A balanced crown chakra can manifest as a sense of knowledge, wisdom, understanding, spiritual connection, and creative imagination (Table 11-7).

When the chakras are open and clear, prana can flow freely from one to the other and health and well-being result. Blocked chakras prevent energy from flowing properly, and without the appropriate prana, anatomical structures and physiological activities suffer, resulting in decreased function or illness. Ayurvedic practitioners are trained to unblock these energy channels to ultimately restore health.

Reflexology

Reflexology is the bodywork modality in which defined points on the feet, hands, or ears are stimulated, resulting in specific reflexive activity of the nervous system. It is also thought that this pressure relieves blocked energy and allows the body to work more efficiently. Evidence suggests that people were applying manual therapy to the feet 5,000 years ago in ancient India. A wall carving in the ancient Egyptian tomb of Ankhmahor, dated about 2350 BCE, shows a person manipulating a patient's

foot, and although many claim that reflexology is being depicted, there is some dispute over the actual subject (see earlier Fig. 1-5). History indicates the use of foot massage in China around 300 BCE, and also in Japan, where it was called sokushinjutsu.

Dr. William Fitzgerald was an ear, nose, and throat surgeon who developed a system of reflexive work called Zone Therapy in 1917. Based on his discovery that pressure on a specific area on the body resulted in a referred anesthetic effect somewhere else, he mapped a pattern of longitudinal zones on the body that had related referral effects. He used pressure points on the tongue, palate, and the back of the pharynx wall to relieve pain, and he discovered that application of pressure on the zones also relieved the underlying cause in most cases. Shelby Riley, MD, worked closely with Dr. Fitzgerald and identified additional horizontal zones across the hands and feet.

In the 1930s, Eunice Ingham, a physical therapist who worked closely with Dr. Riley, refined the familiar modern-day system of foot reflexology. She noticed that congestion and tension in specific points on the foot, called reflex points, corresponded to congestion and tension in specific areas elsewhere on the body. By applying focused pressure to the reflex points, she could create stimulating effects on the body. She integrated all of her findings into the Ingham Method of Reflexology, which improves nerve function and blood supply to normalize body processes and relieve tension.

Reflexology maps and charts are widely available that identify specific reflex points and areas on the hands and feet. They also indicate the body parts that are affected when pressure is applied to those specific reflex points (Fig. 11-6). With sensitive, trained hands, your fingertip pressure on reflex points can relieve stress, pain, and muscular tension; it can restore and maintain homeostasis; and it can encourage healing. Although reflexology techniques can be applied to the hands, ears, or feet, working on the feet is the most common. Learn some of the major reflex points. It is simple to incorporate reflexology into a standard massage session, and many clients are familiar with the technique and request it. Reflexology workshops and certification courses are available worldwide that provide more thorough information and training.

Incorporating Reflexology into a Massage Session

There are three lines you can use as landmarks on the foot to orient you to a person's feet and guide your reflexology work: the diaphragm line, the waist line, and the heel line. Just below the ball of the foot is the diaphragm line. The waist line is an imaginary line from the fifth metatarsal (protrusion on lateral edge of the foot) to the arch.

The point above the heel where the lighter and softer skin becomes the darker, thicker skin of the heel is the heel line (Fig. 11-6A).

The basic foot reflexology techniques include holding, thumb walking, finger walking, and joint movement. Specific passive joint movements of the ankle, metatarsals, and toes are incorporated into reflexology, as are specific deep effleurage strokes (Fig. 11-7). Start and end your reflexology sessions with the back-and-forth technique, ankle rotation, and diaphragm and solar plexus flexing. The back-and-forth technique is a joint movement that does not occur with normal use of the feet, making it particularly beneficial for loosening up the foot at the beginning of a reflexology session. Clockwise and then counterclockwise ankle rotation increases the production of synovial fluid in the ankle joint and also loosens up the fascia in the client's foot. Diaphragm and solar plexus flexing is a tension reliever that should be used at the beginning and end of a reflexology session.

When you apply pressure to a reflex point, use your free hand to apply the holding technique to stabilize the client's foot. You can apply pressure to a reflex point with your thumb or finger, or you can modify the basic pressure technique to cover a larger reflex area by "inchworming" your thumb or finger across the desired area.

More advanced techniques can be learned and used with advanced training and practice. No oil, cream, or lotion is used for reflexology, but you can use powder if the client's feet are damp. Combine techniques into a basic reflexology flow. Box 11-15 describes a basic reflexology procedure.

Indications and Contraindications for Reflexology

Reflexology relieves tension, and stimulates the lymphatic and nervous systems by reflexively affecting different points or zones in the body.

Plantar warts, bunions, and musculoskeletal injuries on the feet are local contraindications for reflexology, as are any areas of numbness and neuromas.

If the client has a foot condition that contraindicates reflexology, you can alternatively use hand or ear reflexology techniques.

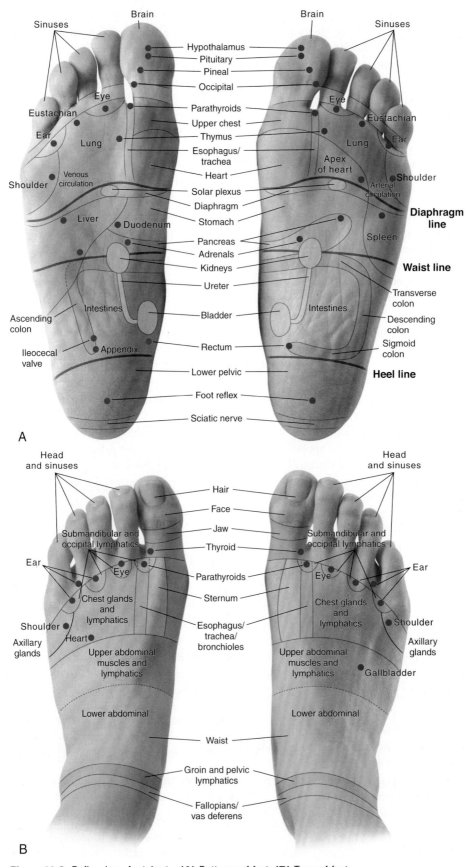

Figure 11-6. Reflexology footcharts. **(A)** Bottoms of feet. **(B)** Tops of feet.

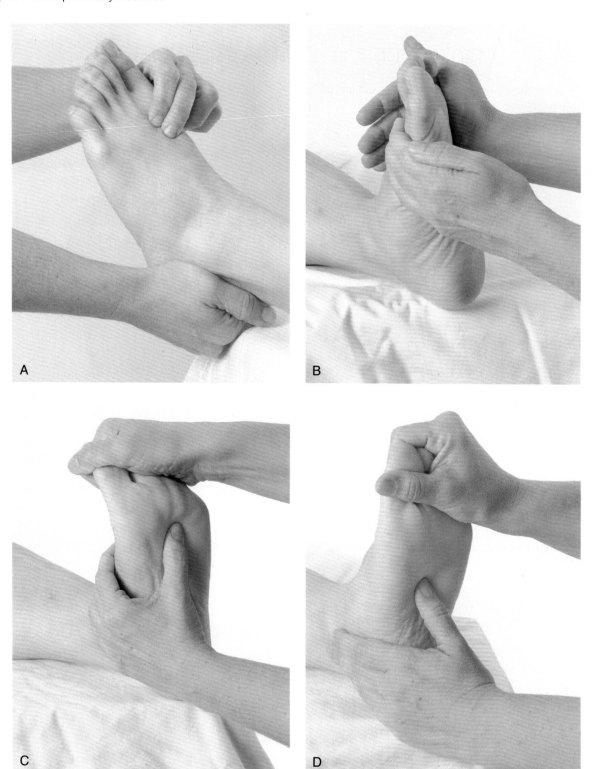

Figure 11-7. Basic reflexology techniques. **(A)** Finger walking—apply pressure with your thumb or index finger and slide it forward in an "inchworm" movement across the client's foot. **(B)** Back-and-forth technique—use one hand to grasp the medial edge of the client's foot and the other hand to grasp the lateral edge. Flex the metatarsals by moving your right hand up and your left hand down, and then switch. **(C)** Diaphragm and solar plexus flexing—apply thumb pressure to the diaphragm and solar plexus reflex point and flex the toes toward you. Then, maintain thumb pressure and extend the toes away from you. **(D)** Holding—place your thumb along the base of the toes and wrap your hand around the toes, resting your fingers on the top of the foot. With your other hand, apply pressure to the desired reflex point.

BOX 11-15 **PROCEDURE** Basic Reflexology Flow

1. Sit at the client's feet, undrape one foot, and find the diaphragm line, waist line, and heel line.

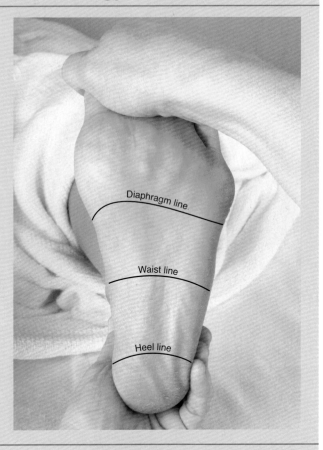

2. Apply back-and-forth movements, ankle rotation, and diaphragm and solar plexus flexing to warm up the client's foot.

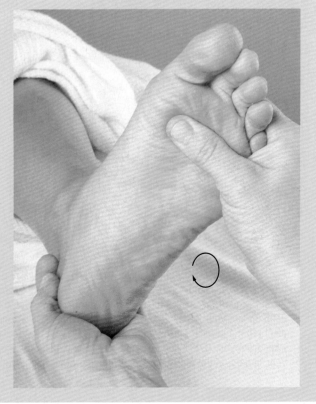

BOX 11-15   **PROCEDURE** Basic Reflexology Flow (continued)

3. Grasp the client's foot with both hands so that the flats of your fingers are on the top of the foot and your thumbs on the soles.

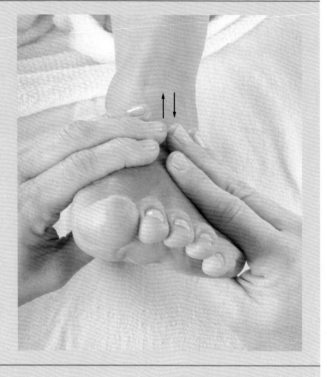

4. Effleurage several times with both hands from the toes to the ankles and from the ankles back to the toes.

5. While holding with one hand, use the other hand to perform thumb or finger walking in the following areas:

   a. The base of all the toes, from the big toe to the little toe

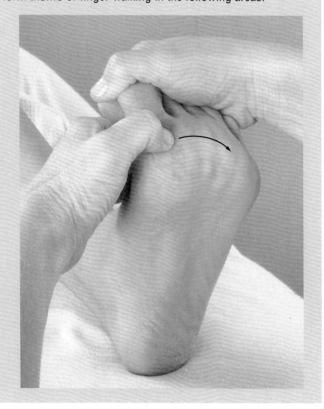

BOX 11-15   **PROCEDURE** Basic Reflexology Flow (continued)

b. Each toe, from the tip to the base, and from the base to tip, from the big toe to the little toe, and back to the big toe

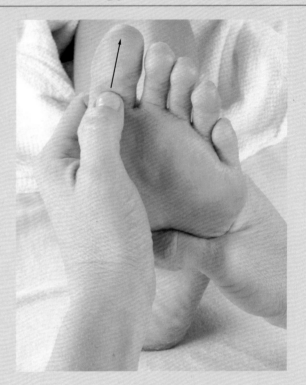

c. The ball of the foot to the base of each toe

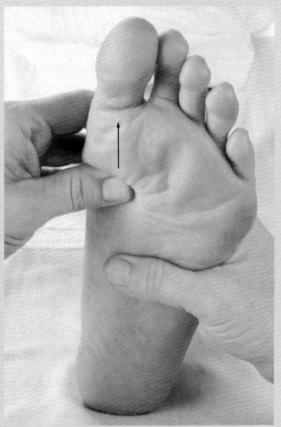

BOX 11-15 PROCEDURE Basic Reflexology Flow (continued)

d. The top of the foot, from the base of each toe and along each metatarsal, from the big toe to the little toe

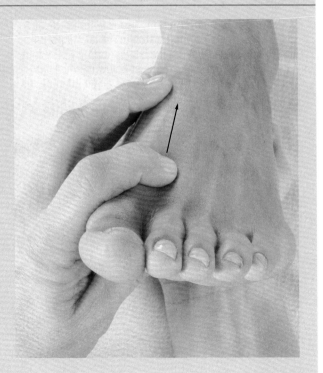

e. From the arch to the lateral portion of the foot, between the waist line and the diaphragm line

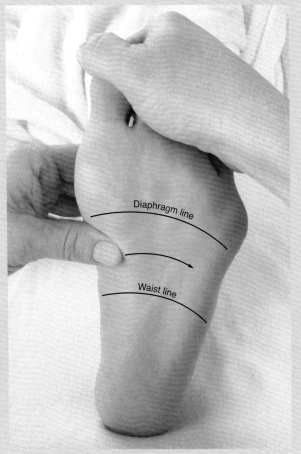

Diaphragm line

Waist line

BOX 11-15 **PROCEDURE** Basic Reflexology Flow (continued)

f. On the left foot, from the heel line to the waist line, moving from the arch to the lateral portion of the foot, then up the lateral portion of the foot. On the right foot, from just below the heel line to the arch of the foot at a 45° angle, then up the lateral portion of the foot.

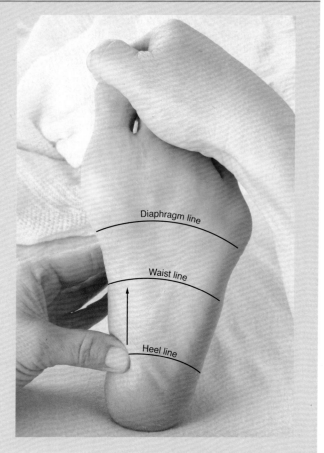

g. The arch of the foot, from the heel line to the big toe

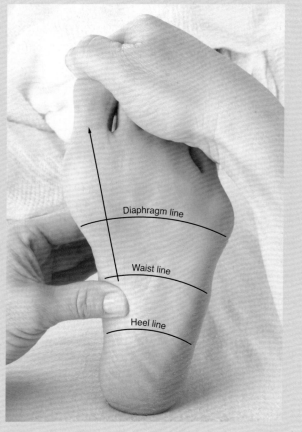

BOX 11-15 **PROCEDURE** Basic Reflexology Flow (continued)

h. From the base of the fifth metatarsal, just below the little toe, down to the heel line

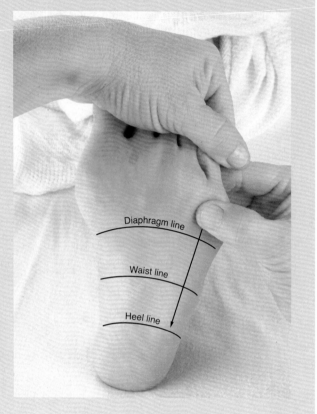

i. Across the heel, just below the heel line

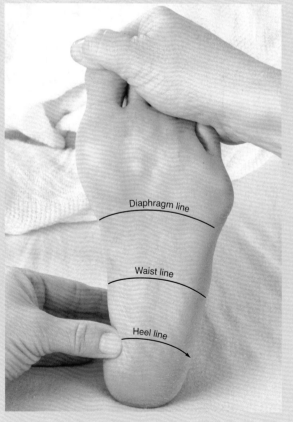

BOX 11-15 **PROCEDURE** Basic Reflexology Flow (continued)

j. Around the lateral malleolus and medial malleolus (ankle protrusions)

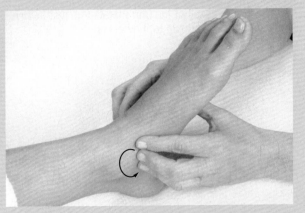

6. Apply back-and-forth movements.

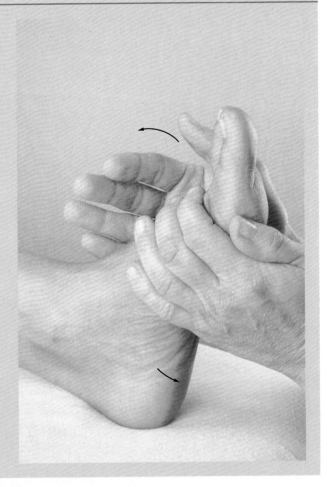

BOX 11-15 PROCEDURE Basic Reflexology Flow (continued)

7. Grasp the foot so that the flats of your fingers are on the top of the foot and your thumbs are on the sole, and effleurage several times with both hands from the toes to the ankles, and from the ankles back to the toes.

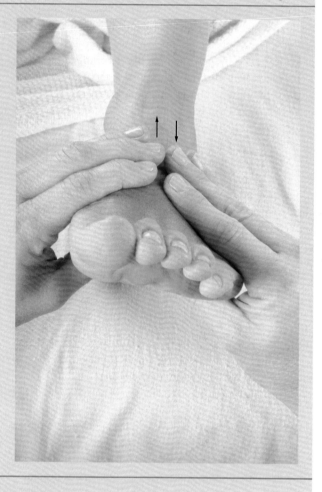

8. Redrape the foot.

9. Expose the other foot and repeat steps 1 to 8.

Adapted with permission from Lidell L, Thomas S, Cook CB, et al. The Book of Massage. New York: Gaia Books Limited/Simon and Schuster, 1984, with permission.

Polarity Therapy

Polarity therapy (PT) is a modality in which very light massage strokes and energy movements are applied on and off the client's body to balance electromagnetic fields, energy nutrition, and develop a higher consciousness. The American Polarity Therapy Association (APTA) defines PT as a comprehensive health system that works with the human energy field (electromagnetic patterns expressed in mental, emotional, and physical experience) and involves energy-based bodywork, diet, exercise, and self-awareness. In PT, health is viewed as a reflection of the condition of the energy field, and therapeutic methods are designed to balance the field for health benefit. PT was developed in the early 1900s by Randolph Stone, DO, DC, ND. He found that electromagnetic fields of the human body are affected by touch, diet, movement, sound, attitudes, experiences, trauma, and environmental factors and suggested that balanced, regular electromagnetic fields allow the body to function properly in a healthy state. When these energy fields are imbalanced or blocked, pain and disease can result. A practical example of this blocked energy is called the "garden hose" effect. When a garden hose is crimped off, some water may trickle through, but most of the water does not flow freely. In the same way, anatomical structures and electrical imbalances can block the flow of energy through the body, preventing the energy from flowing freely.

The energy flows and undulates, projecting outward from a focused center. There are five specific centers of energy in the polarity body called chakras, just as the Ayurvedic centers for energy are called chakras. Each chakra corresponds with the elements of earth, water, fire, air, and ether. According to polarity theory, energy flows in different patterns around the body. The three current patterns are transverse, spiral, and long line. The energy in the transverse pattern spirals upward from the pelvic area to the crown of the head. The energy in the spiral current flows from the belly button area, counterclockwise, over the entire body from the middle of the abdomen to the top of the head. The energy in the long line current flows in parallel streams from the tips of the fingers to the head and from the tips of the toes to the top of the head.

The objective of PT is to adjust and balance the energy flow to create a balanced energy field. The polarity practitioner manipulates the positive and negative currents within the body, and at times, simply "gets out of the way," to facilitate healthy, normal function to all parts of the person's body. As with all bodywork, the therapist is not intending to heal clients, but only to help the body to find its own healthy balance. PT has been used successfully for many conditions, including:

- Easing joint pain
- Easing muscle pain
- Relieving tension
- Reducing headache pain
- Improving circulation
- Enhancing digestion and elimination
- Soothing emotional stress
- Increasing a person's general sense of health and well-being

Alert

Some clients experience profound relaxation following a session of PT, so it is important to disclose to clients some of the normal reactions to polarity: exhaustion, extreme relaxation, lightheadedness, or dizziness.

There is a lot of electrical activity in the body, which also means that there is a lot of energetic activity. For example, nerves and muscles depend on the flow of negatively and positively charged molecules to function. The nature of this electrical activity creates general patterns of energy flow through the body called energy fields. Applying polarity to a client requires you to understand this dual nature (positive and negative) of a person's energy in order to properly manipulate it with your hands. Each part of the body has this duality. In polarity, your hands are considered to each have a charge—the right being positive and the left being negative. The rest of the body carries this dual nature of charge. For example, the top half, the right side, and the back of the body are considered to be positively charged, whereas the lower half, the left side, and the front of the body are negatively charged. Going deeper into the duality, each finger also carries a charge, beginning with the neutral thumb and then alternating from negative to positive such that the index and ring finger have a negative charge, and the middle and the little pinky finger have a positive charge. Completing the electrical circuit by positioning the positive hand on an area of the body with a negative charge ensures that the polarity contact has been made. Further, the fields around one person can alter the fields of another person, which is why PT does not necessarily require touch.

With practice, you can learn to sense the energetic fields surrounding a person's body. Some persons compare the feeling to the repulsion of two magnets, some sense more of a tingling or electrical shock sensation, and others feel vibrations as they approach the fields. Once you can sense energy fields, you can try to manipulate them. Apply your hands directly to the client's body or to the energy fields surrounding the client's body, and focus your energy (using the duality) on your intent to balance the fields. This is a subtle technique that very specifically uses your own energy fields and your conscious intention to redirect the client's energy flow to balance the fields. Because the work is so subtle, you may want to explain the theory and technique to your client before using PT in a massage session. For example, you might use the previously mentioned "garden hose" effect and the concept of the magnets to explain the concepts to your client.

Specific PT techniques are based on principles of energy flow in and around the body, and they can be applied to specific areas of pain. In one technique, you gently place your left hand or left index finger on a client's area of pain, and place your right hand or right middle finger on the area directly across the body from the area of pain, then maintain contact for several seconds until the energy is released. As the energy releases, you may feel heat, tingling, or a pulse that is faster than the cardiac pulse, often called a therapeutic pulse.

This is only an introduction to the basic applications of PT. With advanced training and experience, you can learn how to perform a true PT session that lasts between 60 and 90 minutes and allows clients to remain fully clothed. Registered polarity practitioners learn how to evaluate a person's energetic attributes with palpation, observation, and interviewing skills, and to use various forms of touch and intent to manipulate the energy flow with the intent to enhance their clients' self-healing mechanisms. You should seek more advanced training to apply the principles more appropriately. The APTA standards require a minimum of 675 hours of training to be considered proficient to practice PT. For a list of approved trainings, look at the APTA web site (www.polaritytherapy.org).

CHAPTER SUMMARY

The special techniques discussed in this chapter are only some of the techniques you can incorporate into a massage session. For most massage therapists, they are good techniques to be familiar with and to have available. Most of them can be incorporated into a massage session easily, and clients may request some of these special techniques. Client education and client participation is a big part of healthcare, and these special techniques can serve as good teaching tools to help clients take responsibility for their own health.

Alert

In your clients' best interest, the complementary modalities presented in this chapter should be studied further in depth.

Many therapists continue their education and training to specialize in a particular technique.

CHAPTER EXERCISES

1. Name three indications and three contraindications for:

   a. Cold hydrotherapy applications

   b. Heat hydrotherapy applications

2. Name three physiological effects of:

   a. Cold hydrotherapy applications

   b. Heat hydrotherapy applications

3. Explain the importance of recommending that clients increase their water intake after a massage.

4. What is Asian Bodywork Therapy (ABT)?

5. What is Qi and what are its functions?

6. Describe the starting and ending points for the following energy meridians:

   a. Heart

   b. Lung

   c. Spleen

   d. Liver

   e. Kidney

   f. Small Intestine

   g. Large Intestine

   h. Gallbladder

   i. Governing Vessel

7. List the five elements of Ayurvedic healthcare.

8. Identify and describe the location of each of the seven Ayurvedic chakras.

9. Explain the concept of reflexology.

10. Describe how to apply the specific polarity technique described in this chapter.

REFERENCES

1. Packman H. *Ice Massage: The Ultimate Cryotherapeutic Alternative*. Trafford Publishing, 2006.
2. Ho SS, Coel MN, Kagawa R, et al. The effects of ice on blood flow and bone metabolism in knees. *Am J Sports Med* 1994;22(4):537–540.
3. http://www.aobta.org/about-aobta/about-forms.html, accessed 6.23.12.

SUGGESTED READINGS

Ashton J, Cassel D. *Review for Therapeutic Massage and Bodywork Certification*. Baltimore: Lippincott Williams & Wilkins, 2002.
Brecher P. *Secrets of Energy Work*. New York: Dorling Kindersley Publishing, 2000.
Capellini S. *The Royal Treatment*. New York: Dell Publishing, 1997.
Chaitow L, DeLany JW. *Clinical Application of Neuromuscular Techniques*. Vol 1. London: Churchill Livingstone, 2000.
Chien CH, Tsuei JJ, Lee SC, et al. Effect of emitted bioenergy on biochemical functions of cells. *Am J Chin Med* 1991;19:285–292.
Eisenberg D. *Encounters with Qi: Exploring Chinese Medicine*. New York: WW Norton, 1985.
Fritz S. *Fundamentals of Therapeutic Massage*. 2nd ed. St. Louis: Mosby, 2000.
Gerber, MD. *Vibrational Medicine: The #1 Handbook of Subtle-Energy Therapies*. 3rd ed. Rochester, VT: Bear & Company, 2001.
Gray H, Lewis WH. *Anatomy of the Human Body*. 23rd ed. Philadelphia: Lea & Febiger, 1936.
Henderson J. *What is Polarity Therapy: An Introduction*. American Polarity Association: International Energy Currents, 2005: 9–14.
Henry J. *The Fundamentals of Personal Energy*. St. Paul, MN: Llewellyn Publications, 2004.
Kaptchuk TJ. *The Web That Has No Weaver: Understanding Chinese Medicine*. Chicago: Congdon & Weed, 1983.
Knaster M. Energy Eastern style. *AMTA Massage Ther J* 1998;36:40–46.
Lidell L, Thomas S, Cook CB, et al. *The Book of Massage*. New York: Gaia Books Limited/Simon and Schuster, 1984.
Maxwell-Hudson C. *K.I.S.S. Guide to Massage*. New York: DK Publishing, 2001.
Morningstar S. *Ayurveda: Traditional Indian Healing for Harmony and Health*. New York: Anness Publishing, 1999.
Salvo SG. *Massage Therapy: Principles and Practice*. 2nd ed. St. Louis: Saunders/Elsevier Science, 2003.
Seidler H, Bernhard W, Teschler-Nicola M, et al. Some anthropological aspects of the prehistoric Tyrolean ice man. *Science*. 1992;258:455–457.

Seidman M. *A Guide to Polarity Therapy: The Gentle Art of Hands-On Healing*. Berkeley: North Atlantic Books, 1999.

Warrier G, Verma H, Sullivan K. *Secrets of Ayurveda*. New York: DK Publishing, Inc., 2001.

Werner R. *A Massage Therapist's Guide to Pathology*. Philadelphia: Lippincott Williams & Wilkins, 1998.

Wright J. *Reflexology and Acupressure: Pressure Points for Healing*. Summertown, TN: CRCS Wellness Books/Book Publishing, 2000.

http://healing.about.com/cs/chakras/1/bl_gurmukh_c.htm, accessed 3.17.05.

http://massagetherapy.com/articles/index.php?article_id=767, accessed 4.16.05.

http://massagetherapy.com/articles/index.php?article_id=86, accessed 4.16.05.

http://my.webmd.com/hw/alternative_medicine/tp21271.asp, accessed 2.15.05.

http://naturalhealinginst.com/residential/smt.html, accessed 4.16.05.

http://orientalmedicine.com/acupuncture_faq.htm, accessed 3.5.06.

http://qi-journal.com/TCM.asp?-token.SearchID%EF%80%BDTuinaFAQ, accessed 3.5.06.

http://schools.naturalhealers.com/ntc/?inktomi, accessed 4.12.05.

http://theamt.com/modules.php?name=News&file=article&sid=218, accessed 2.15.05.

http://www.21stcip.com/pages/7bio.html, accessed 3.5.06.

http://www.aaaom.org/HPIRREGULAR%20PERIOD.htm, accessed 3.5.06.

http://www.acupressure.com, accessed 3.5.06.

http://www.acuxo.com/index.asp, accessed 3.5.06.

http://www.aor.org.uk, accessed 3.5.06.

http://www.archaeologiemuseum.it/f01_uk.html, accessed 3.5.06.

http://www.aromytherapy.com/hydro1.htm, accessed 4.16.05.

http://www.asteccse.com/cgi-bin/news.cgi, accessed 4.16.05.

http://www.aworldofacupuncture.com/acupuncture-frequently-asked -questions.htm, accessed 3.5.06.

http://www.ayur.com/about.html, accessed 2.23.05.

http://www.ayurveda.com/online%20resource/ancient_writings.htm, accessed 3.19.05.

http://www.ayurvedamedgroup.com/about.html, accessed 2.23.05.

http://www.balancedlives.net/altmed.htm, accessed 2.18.05.

http://www.bancroftsmt.com/continuing/cont_course.cfm?ID=12&P=6, accessed 4.12.05.

http://www.beyondstress.net/serv04.htm, accessed 4.12.05.

http://www.calmassage.com/spa.htm, accessed 4.11.05.

http://www.chiroweb.com/archives/17/09/34.html, accessed 3.5.06.

http://www.chiroweb.com/archives/17/12/14.html, accessed 3.5.06.

http://www.csha.net/advanced/spa.html, accessed 4.11.05.

http://www.ewcha.com, accessed 4.21.05.

http://www.experienceispa.com, accessed 4.11.05.

http://www.findarticles.com/p/articles/mi_g2603/is_0006 /ai_2603000658, accessed 3.5.06.

http://www.holisticonline.com/hydrotherapy.htm, accessed 3.5.06.

http://www.holisticonline.com/Remedies/Depression/dep_acupressure .htm, accessed 3.5.06.

http://www.howstuffworks.com/question138.htm, accessed 3.5.06.

http://www.internethealthlibrary.com/Therapies/Hydrotherapy.htm#top, accessed 6.22.12.

http://www.kheper.net/topics/chakras/balancing.html, accessed 3.19.05.

http://www.massagemag.com/2005/issue115/history115.htm, accessed 8.6.05.

http://www.massagemag.com/spa/body/mud.html, accessed 4.21.05.

http://www.massagemag.com/spa/treatment/water.html, accessed 8.6.05.

http://www.massagetoday.com/archives/2003/03/20.html, accessed 3.10.06.

http://www.medicalspaassociation.org/vocabulary.htm, accessed 4.11.05.

http://www.mh-hannover.de/aktuelles/projekte/mmm/englishversion /fs_programme/speech/Sharma_V.html, accessed 2.23.05.

http://www.mhvicarsschool.com/summer_school/spatechniques.php, accessed 4.12.05.

http://www.orientalmedicine.com, accessed 3.5.06.

http://www.pdrhealth.com/content/natural_medicine/chapters/201260 .shtml, accessed 4.12.05.

http://www.poconosbest.com/spasheardesign.htm, accessed 4.12.05.

http://www.polaritytherapy.org, accessed 3.5.06.

http://www.qi-energy.com/qigongresearch.htm, accessed 2.23.05.

http://www.qigonginstitute.org, accessed 4.10.05.

http://www.reflexology-research.com/, accessed 3.5.06.

http://www.reflexology-usa.net/facts.htm, accessed 3.5.06.

http://www.sacredcenters.com/chakras.html, accessed 2.18.05.

http://www.secretsofisis.com/noframes/nfhome.html, accessed 4.12.05.

http://www.spacecoastmassage.com/, accessed 4.12.05.

http://www.spafinder.com/Library/glossary_03.jsp, accessed 4.11.05.

http://www.spatherapy.com/education/treatments/thalassotherapy.php, accessed 4.12.05.

http://www.spatrade.com/knowledge/idx/0/085/article, accessed 4.11.05.

http://www.tcminter.net/Artikel/Qigongresearch.html, accessed 2.15.05.

http://www.theenergyconnection.com/energylevels.html#heart, accessed 3.19.05.

http://www.thespaassociation.com/consumer/glossary.htm, accessed 4.11.05.

http://www.thespacenter.com/gscframeset.html, accessed 8.5.05.

http://www.touchamerica.com/Living_Systems_Education/tawork.htm, accessed 4.11.05.

http://www.wholehealthmd.com/refshelf/substances _view/1,1525,705,00.html, accessed 3.5.06.

Special Populations

Objectives

Upon completion of this chapter, the student will be able to:

- Explain the term "special population" as it relates to massage
- Identify at least three different special populations
- Identify at least three benefits of massage for athletes
- Describe how to safely and comfortably position and bolster a pregnant client for massage
- Describe the benefits of massage for infants
- List at least three features of geriatric massage

Key Terms

Athlete: A person who participates in sports on an amateur or professional level.

Chronic illness: Illness that lasts a year or longer, usually limits a patient's physical activity, and may require ongoing medical care and treatment.

Event massage: Administered on the day of the event to help the athlete prepare for and recover from the activity, it includes pre-event, inter-event, and post-event massage.

Hospice: A healthcare approach that caters to the quality of remaining life rather than the quantity of life when a person's life expectancy is limited by a life-threatening illness with no known cure.

Inter-event massage: Performed in between events that occur on the same day and within a given time period, focusing on areas of increased muscular tension that have occurred as a direct result of participation in the activity.

Maintenance massage: Performed in between sporting events to maintain flexibility and ensure that muscles are relaxed and lengthened to prevent injuries from occurring during training.

Post-event massage: Performed within 2 hours of the athletic performance, it focuses on circulatory enhancement to aid in recovery from the activity as well as decrease muscle and connective tissue tension.

Pre-event massage: Performed just before the client participates in an athletic event, it focuses on circulatory enhancement and warming up the tissues.

Restorative massage: Performed 6 to 72 hours after the athletic performance, it is intended to increase circulation and restore the normal resting length of muscles; also called curative massage and post-recovery massage.

Special populations: Segments of the population whose massage requires special considerations.

Treatment massage: Intended to facilitate the healing process when an injury has occurred or when chronic strain has diminished the athlete's performance.

Special populations are segments of the population whose massage requires special positioning, physical assistance, or a therapist who understands and can manage unique physiological characteristics. Various massage routines have been developed for some of these special populations, but a standard routine can significantly limit the benefit to the client. Although standard routines do not allow the therapist to read and address the individual client's tissues, they can serve as a good foundation for the massage. A routine may include an efficient flow for the massage or a set of basic strokes that are appropriate for the particular physiological needs of the client. A quality therapist can specialize and alter the routine to better accommodate each client. To be fully qualified to work with clients who have specific physiological needs, you should seek additional advanced training for the particular population you are interested in treating. The special circumstances and special populations discussed in this chapter include:

- Athletes
- Pregnant women
- Infants
- Geriatric clients
- Chronically ill clients
- Disabled clients

Athletes

Athletes participate in sports at levels ranging from casual to amateur to competitive to professional. A casual athlete, sometimes called the "weekend warrior," may not need massage as often as a competitive athlete. As a general rule, the weekend warrior exercises up to three times a week, whereas the competitive athlete typically works out five or more days a week. Because athletes often train in only one sport, they are prone to muscular tension and strain from repetitive overuse. One of the best ways for athletes to avoid muscular pain and discomfort is to incorporate massage into their routine. Sports massage is the general term that refers to massage for athletes, and it uses the basic massage strokes and therapeutic techniques. **The distinguishing factor of sports massage is that the therapist should know which muscles and motions athletes use most often in a particular sport (Box 12-1).** For example, the muscles actively used for running or jogging are the leg muscles. The massage therapist might focus on a runner's psoas major, hamstrings, quadriceps femoris group, tensor fascia latae, gastrocnemius, soleus, peroneus group, and anterior and posterior tibialis. The upper body counterbalances the leg movements of running with core strength and an arm swing, so it is important to also treat the postural muscles and the muscles responsible for shoulder flexion and extension. Particularly important to running is a normal gait pattern, because if a runner deviates from an even, fluid gait pattern, compensation patterns will result. This process of determining which muscles and motions are most often used is also helpful in nonathletes. Specifically, it will help you understand which muscles endure repetitive motion and tension, it will help you conceptualize your client's compensation patterns in everyday activities, and it will thus help you determine appropriate treatment goals and an effective treatment plan.

Massage is gaining popularity in all segments of the population, but athletes tend to embrace the importance of massage for flexibility, enhanced recovery from muscle fatigue and injury, and improved performance. Massage has been widely used in several amateur and professional sports

---

BOX 12-1

Major Muscles Involved in Some Common Sports

- Basketball: gastrocnemius, anterior tibialis, quadriceps femoris, hamstrings, gluteal muscles
- Bicycling: neck extensors, trapezius, erector spinae, gastrocnemius, quadriceps femoris, hamstrings, gluteal muscles
- Bowling: finger flexors, wrist flexors, wrist extensors, anterior serratus, pectoralis major, anterior deltoids, triceps brachii
- Downhill skiing: quadriceps femoris, anterior tibialis, toe flexors, plantaris, peroneus group, adductor group, erector spinae, trapezius
- Golf: levator scapulae, triceps brachii, trapezius, infraspinatus, supraspinatus, rhomboids, quadratus lumborum
- Racquet sports: finger flexors, wrist flexors, triceps brachii, deltoids, subscapularis, trapezius, infraspinatus, pectoralis major, quadriceps femoris, gluteal muscles, hamstrings
- Rowing: most major muscle groups
- Running: anterior tibialis, psoas major, quadriceps femoris, hamstrings, gluteal muscles, gastrocnemius
- Swimming: (depends on the stroke, but these are some of the primary muscles) infraspinatus, supraspinatus, subscapularis, teres minor, deltoids, pectoralis major, gluteal muscles, trapezius, latissimus dorsi, triceps brachii
- Volleyball: most major muscle groups

for years and has been a part of the official Olympic medical team since the 1996 summer games in Atlanta, Georgia. Massage can provide many benefits to athletes:

- Reduce muscle pain
- Relieve acute and delayed onset muscle soreness
- Relieve muscle tension and spasms
- Enhance generally flexibility and range of motion (ROM)
- Reduce recovery period
- Enhance proprioception and body awareness for coordination
- Restore normal resting length to hypertonic muscles
- Break up fascial restrictions
- Improve circulation of blood and lymph
- Enhance the health of muscle tissue

The many different applications of massage for athletes include event massage, restorative massage, maintenance massage, and treatment massage. **Event massage** is administered on the day of the event to help the athlete prepare for and recover from the activity. **Restorative massage** is a more therapeutic massage, which focuses specifically on circulatory enhancement and restoring the resting length to muscles involved in the athletic performance. **Maintenance massage** is performed in between sporting events to maintain flexibility and ensure that muscles are relaxed and lengthened to prevent injuries from occurring during training. **Treatment massage** is intended to facilitate the healing process when an injury has occurred or when chronic strain has diminished the athlete's performance. In order to perform restorative, maintenance, and treatment massage for athletes, the therapist must understand the relevant anatomy, physiology, and mechanisms of healing and injury repair as well as be experienced with ROM and connective tissue manipulation techniques. In order to provide sports massage or therapeutic massage to athletes, you should continue your education in this specialty via the many workshops that are available so you can learn more about the general characteristics and treatments of a variety of common sports injuries. This will enable you to work with athletes both individually and with their healthcare and performance team.

Event Sports Massage

Event sports massage, which includes pre-event, post-event, and inter-event sports massage, specifically addresses athletes who are preparing for and recovering from the physical exertion associated with a specific athletic performance. As such, it is performed at the site of and on the day of the

sporting event. Event sports massage is generally a fast-paced application and most often involves a basic set of strokes and flow. Depending on whether it is performed with or without lubricant, the combinations of strokes will vary. Without lubricant, your flow of strokes may follow a sequence such as:

- Compression
- Pétrissage
- Friction
- In pre-event sports massage, end with tapotement

With lubricant, your flow of strokes may follow a sequence such as:

- Effleurage
- Pétrissage
- Stretching
- In pre-event work, end with tapotement
- In post-event work, end with effleurage

When creating good event sports massage flows, you should follow the general guidelines of working from general to specific and superficial to deep.

Event sports massage involves touching many bodies in a short time and can be overstimulating and overwhelming, so it is important for you to maintain an emotional and energetic barrier for yourself. **If you plan to be at an event for several hours or all day, during which you will be doing event massage, you must continually be aware of and maintain your own energy level.** Be sure to schedule breaks to periodically rest and keep yourself grounded. Sometimes food and drinks are provided for you, but not always. Come prepared with food and drink, and schedule breaks at least once an hour to take a walk or use the restroom.

Pre-event Massage

Pre-event massage is performed before the client participates in an athletic event. It is most beneficial when performed about 2 hours before the actual event; however, because the effects of pre-event massage can last for a day or two, some athletes may still benefit from massage up to 2 days before the event. The focus of the pre-event massage is not to replace, but rather enhance, the athlete's warm-up routine. (See Box 12-2 for pre-event sports massage features.) More specifically, pre-event massage is intended to:

- Increase circulation to the primary large muscles that will be used in the event
- Increase the temperature of the muscles
- Soften the connective tissues

BOX 12-2

Pre-event Massage to Increase Circulation and Warm the Tissues

- Also applied to reduce muscular tension and increase flexibility and ROM
- Can reduce anxiety and heighten the athlete's sense of well-being and ability to concentrate
- Usually onsite
- Performed 2 days to 10 minutes before the event
- Clients are usually wearing athletic apparel or warm-up suits
- 15 to 20 minutes or less of brisk treatment
- Use light, nonspecific rhythmic compression; kneading; superficial friction; tapotement; vibration; and stretching and joint movements
- Focus on the primary muscles involved in the event
- Little or no draping
- No lubricant
- No changes are made to the length of muscles
- No comments are made regarding client's tissues unless you suspect an injury, at which point you refer the client to the medical tent
- The techniques should not be deep or painful

No significant changes are made to the length of the muscles or fascia during pre-event massage, because the client's kinesthetic awareness could be altered.

- Decrease muscle tension
- Enhance ROM
- Increase general kinesthetic awareness
- Reduce general anxiety

Pre-event massage is often based on a routine in which clients typically lie on a table for a minimum of 15 to 20 minutes, during which you have access to most of the body. Psychologically, pre-event massage benefits athletes by reducing anxiety and heightening their sense of well-being and ability to concentrate. Because this massage is so brief, try to focus on the muscles that the athlete will use during the upcoming event as well as any muscles that might be held in passive contraction for extended periods.

The session should be light and nonspecific. The strokes used most often include rhythmic compression, kneading, superficial friction, tapotement, vibration, and stretching and joint movements to increase flexibility. They are applied briskly, slightly faster than 1 compression stroke per second, and are intended to enhance circulation and energize the

client (Box 12-3). Use joint movements to stimulate synovial fluid production for lubrication and shock absorption at the joints.

Alert

Do not use joint movements to extend the ROMs or change the shape or position of soft tissues.

In other words, if a client has been training for a 10-km run with a tight right psoas major muscle for 2 weeks, her body may have developed some compensation patterns that alter her posture and muscular coordination. The psoas major muscle is responsible for initiating a stride, slightly drawing the femur forward with hip flexion. If you were to lengthen the psoas and stretch the surrounding fascia immediately before the run, the athlete's body would be unfamiliar with the new length of the psoas muscle and the new body position. As a result, old patterns of coordination and kinesthetic awareness could cause the athlete to trip or otherwise negatively affect the performance.

Before an event, the athlete's mental state is often focused and possibly anxious. Athletes may be extra sensitive to comments regarding their physical condition. You can encourage the athlete to perform well but should not make any comments regarding an athlete's muscles or physical condition during a pre-event massage. For instance, you might notice that your client's left hamstrings are a bit tighter than the right hamstrings or that the ROM of the right shoulder is restricted. Instead of sharing that information before the event, keep that kind of information to yourself. Such thoughts can easily have a psychosomatic effect on a client. Because the athlete's mental state is so closely related to the physical state, negative thoughts can create a real physiological condition. As with a self-fulfilling prophecy, athletes who assume they cannot perform well may not try to perform well, believing that they are not capable. Then, when their performance is not successful, they have a "reasonable" explanation. If you notice a possible injury, however, you should suggest that the client visit the medical tent before the event.

Inter-event Massage

Inter-event massage is performed in between events that occur on the same day and within a given time period, for example, at half-time or between heats at an event. This type of event sports massage typically lasts no more than 10 minutes and focuses on any areas of increased muscular tension that have occurred as a direct result of participation in the activity. Often, the athlete will direct you to their specific areas of concern, but you can also gather information while working with the athlete directly and by being familiar with the muscles that are involved in their particular sport.

BOX 12-3 **PROCEDURE** Pre-event Massage Routine for a Long-Distance Runner

---

Client in the prone position

1. Compression: 4 strokes that move distally along the client's left arm

---

2. Pétrissage: approximately 6 seconds to the left trapezius, levator scapula, and posterior deltoid

---

3. Tapotement: approximately 6 seconds of hacking to the left upper back

---

4. Brisk effleurage: 2 strokes to brush down the left back

---

5. Compression:
   a. 6 strokes to the left gluteals
   b. 4 strokes that move inferiorly, to the left iliotibial band
   c. 4 strokes that move inferiorly, to the lateral side of the left hamstrings
   d. 4 strokes that move inferiorly, to the center of the left hamstrings
   e. 4 strokes that move inferiorly, to the medial side of the left hamstrings

---

6. Pétrissage: approximately 8 seconds to the left thigh

---

7. Tapotement: approximately 8 seconds of hacking to the left gluteals and thigh

---

8. Compression:
   a. 3 strokes that move inferiorly, to the lateral side of the left calf
   b. 3 strokes that move inferiorly, to the lateral side of the left gastrocnemius
   c. 3 strokes that move inferiorly, to the medial side of the left gastrocnemius

---

9. Pétrissage: approximately 8 seconds to the left calf

---

10. Brisk effleurage: 2 strokes to brush down the left leg

---

11. Repeat steps 1 to 10 for the client's right side

Client turns over to the supine position

12. Compression:
    a. 3 strokes that move inferiorly, to the lateral side of the left quadriceps femoris
    b. 3 strokes that move inferiorly, to the center of the left quadriceps femoris
    c. 3 strokes that move inferiorly, to the medial side of the left quadriceps femoris

---

13. Pétrissage: approximately 8 seconds to the left thigh

---

14. Compression:
    a. 4 strokes that move inferiorly, to the left anterior tibialis
    b. 4 strokes that move inferiorly, to the left peroneus group

---

15. Joint movement:
    a. Passive left knee and hip flexion
    b. Passive left ankle rotation

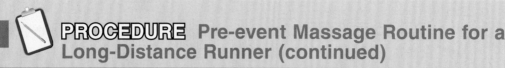

BOX 12-3 **PROCEDURE** Pre-event Massage Routine for a Long-Distance Runner (continued)

16. Brisk effleurage: 2 strokes to brush down the left leg

17. Repeat steps 12 to 16 for the client's right leg

18. Brisk effleurage:
    a. 1 stroke, simultaneously with both hands, to brush down both of the client's arms
    b. 2 strokes, simultaneously with both hands, to brush down both of the client's legs

---

Alert

Be sure your focus is on improving the athlete's recovery between events and do not massage tissues to the point that the athlete is too relaxed to compete.

Post-event Massage

Post-event massage is most optimally performed within 2 hours of the athletic performance and focuses on circulatory enhancement to aid in recovery from the activity as well as decrease muscle and connective tissue tension. (Box 12-4 lists some of the features of post-event massage.) Athletes should cool down and, if possible, put on dry clothes if they are receiving treatment immediately after their event. Post-event massage generally focuses on the larger muscle groups specific to the sport, and the purpose of post-event massage is to:

- Encourage circulation in and around the muscles
- Reduce muscular tension
- Increase circulation
- Minimize potential delayed onset muscle soreness
- Restore flexibility
- If necessary, relieve muscle cramps

Immediately following performance, the athlete typically cools down and stretches. Often, the athlete's musculature is suffering oxygen debt. One of the greatest benefits of massage is increased local circulation, which delivers oxygen to the tissues and reduces the metabolic buildup in the muscles. Metabolic byproducts are chemicals that build up in the muscle tissue and make the athlete feel sore and achy for the next few days. The stiffness and sore muscles, which often discourage people from exercise, can be prevented with massage.

Post-event massage usually lasts 15 to 20 minutes. The session focuses on the muscles used during the athlete's event and is slower paced, providing relaxation and general relief from exhaustion. Effleurage is the primary stroke used in post-event massage, mostly applied toward the heart. Lubricant increases the comfort of effleurage strokes and enhances the slip to alleviate some of the pressure. Avoid deep strokes because they can damage the fatigued tissues. Gentle compression and joint movements are commonly included in post-event massage routines.

BOX 12-4

Post-event Massage to Increase Circulation

- Applied to reduce muscular tension, congestion, and potential muscle soreness; restore flexibility; and, if necessary, relieve muscle cramps
- Usually onsite
- Performed within 6 hours after the event
- Clients are usually wearing athletic apparel or warm-up suits, or, if possible, dry clothes
- 15 to 20 minutes or less, moderately paced treatment
- Use effleurage, gentle compression, stretching, gentle joint movements, and fulling and lifting
- Focus on the major muscles involved in the athletic event
- Use lubricant
- Little or no draping
- No deep strokes

Alert

Open skin is an invitation for infection, and intact blisters can easily break open, so massage should be avoided over broken and unbroken blisters.

To avoid causing a muscle cramp during an athlete's post-event massage, be sure the pace of your application is slow. Massage strokes applied too rapidly may actually cause cramping to occur. Very gentle stretching and joint movement may also be applied to relax tense muscles and encourage circulation.

Some variations of the basic massage strokes that are commonly used in post-event massage include fulling and lifting. These two-handed strokes travel across the muscle fibers instead of along the length of the fibers. Fulling, also called broadening, spreads the muscle fibers out and away from each other. To perform fulling on the quadriceps femoris, bring your hands together and rest the heels or palms of your hands on the quadriceps femoris. Effleurage with both hands simultaneously so that one hand slides to the medial thigh and the other hand slides to the lateral thigh. Lifting is essentially the opposite of fulling, basically picking up the muscle and pulling it away from the underlying bone. Using the quadriceps femoris as an example, you start with one palm on the lateral side of the thigh and the other palm on the medial side of the thigh. Simultaneously slide both hands toward the front of the thigh, compressing and lifting the quadriceps femoris up and away from the femur. Together, fulling and lifting are similar to a pétrissage stroke. As with all strokes, pay attention to your body mechanics and make sure your wrist position does not put excessive pressure on the structures running through the carpal tunnel (Box 12-5).

Equipment for Event Sports Massage

As previously stated, event sports massage is performed onsite at the athletic event, either indoors or outdoors. For outdoor venues, you need to consider temperature and weather, which could be cold, windy, rainy, hot and humid, or unusually dry. Dress appropriately with layers of clothing that you can add or remove to stay comfortable. Consider shelter to stay out of the bright sunlight or the rain. Large corporate and/or well-organized events may provide a tent for you, but it is best to find out before you arrive. The larger the event, the more activity there is around you. Athletes and their supportive family members and friends, event organizers, vendors, music, loudspeakers, starting pistols, and roaring crowds are some of the aspects of a sports massage environment. Massage therapists typically bring their own tables, but because clients often wear their athletic apparel or warm-up suits during the massage, linens are generally not used. Instead, you need to bring spray or wipes to properly disinfect your equipment before and between athletes, as well as a trash container to properly dispose of waste. Some therapists bring sheets and/or towels to drape their equipment or the athletes. Towels of various sizes are especially

versatile—you can use towels for bolstering, to absorb sweat or spills, to cover clients for warmth, and to cover your equipment.

Contraindications for Event Sports Massage

As with any massage application, it is important to know when massage is indicated and even more important to recognize when it is contraindicated. The general indications and contraindications for massage apply to event sports massage. Typical contraindications you might encounter in event sports massage are:

- Blisters
- Open cuts and/or wounds
- Sprains
- Strains
- Dehydration
- Severely compromised core body temperature

Follow the rule of "When in doubt, don't," and make sure to familiarize yourself with the locations of medical tents or healthcare professionals at the sporting events in case you need to send an athlete for first aid or to be evaluated for a health condition. You could be faced with first aid situations in the post-event massage setting; however, it is important to remember to stay within the massage therapy scope of practice. Typically, there are healthcare professionals available at sporting events to handle health conditions such as shortness of breath, dehydration, hyperthermia, hypothermia, ligament sprains, cuts, or scrapes.

Restorative Massage

Restorative massage, also called curative massage and post-recovery massage, takes place 6 to 72 hours after the athletic performance. The purpose of restorative massage is to increase circulation and restore the normal resting length of muscles. During an athletic event, some muscles contract repeatedly, usually with a lot of force. After the event, the muscles that have been contracting can easily develop a shorter resting length unless they are lengthened and their antagonistic muscles are activated. Restorative massage is the perfect opportunity to lengthen the muscles that were particularly active during the event and to stretch the fascia that surrounds those muscles. (See Box 12-6 for restorative massage features.)

Restorative massage typically takes place in your standard massage treatment room because clients are not usually at the event 6 to 72 hours after their performance. It is generally safe to use all of the basic massage strokes, ROMs,

BOX 12-5   **PROCEDURE** Post-event Massage Routine for a
Long-Distance Runner

Client is in the supine position
Right leg

1. Distal compression strokes to the quadriceps femoris

2. Proximal effleurage strokes to thigh

3. Fulling strokes to thigh

4. Lifting strokes to thigh

5. Distal compression strokes to the anterior tibialis

6. Proximal effleurage strokes to anterolateral lower leg

7. Passive joint movement to knee, hip, and ankle

8. Brisk effleurage strokes to brush down the leg

Left leg
• Repeat supine steps 1 to 8.

Client turns over to the prone position
Right leg

9. Compression strokes to the gluteal muscles

10. Distal compression strokes to the hamstrings

11. Proximal effleurage strokes to thigh

12. Fulling strokes to thigh

13. Lifting strokes to thigh

14. Distal compression strokes to the gastrocnemius

15. Proximal effleurage strokes to calf

16. Brisk effleurage strokes to brush down the leg

Left leg
• Repeat prone steps 9 to 16.

BOX 12-5   **PROCEDURE** Post-event Massage Routine for a Long-Distance Runner (continued)

Back

17. Effleurage strokes across the low back

18. Effleurage strokes from the left iliac crest to the left shoulder

19. Effleurage strokes from the left shoulder to the occipital ridge (walk to the client's right side)

20. Effleurage strokes from the right iliac crest to the right shoulder

21. Effleurage strokes from the right shoulder to the occipital ridge

22. Brisk effleurage strokes to brush down the back

Alert

Sometimes athletes experience muscle cramps after intense physical exertion in their event.

BOX 12-6

Restorative Massage to Increase Circulation and Restore Normal Resting Length to the Muscles

- Usually in your treatment room
- Performed 6 to 72 hours after the event
- Clients are usually undressed and modestly draped
- 30- to 60-minute treatment
- Use effleurage, pétrissage, compression, ROM, PNF techniques, and stretches
- Focus on the major muscles used in the athletic event
- Use lubricant

Alert

Localized areas of inflammation are contraindications for massage.

---

and therapeutic applications unless the athlete has an injury. Proprioceptive neuromuscular facilitation (PNF) techniques are especially effective during post-event massage to restore normal resting length to muscles. Remember to stretch the fascia in and around the muscles that are lengthened, and hold the stretch to allow a tendon reflex to further relax the muscle.

Maintenance Massage

Maintenance massage is for the ongoing and regular treatment of muscle tension and soreness due to chronic repetitive stress from an athlete's particular sport. It is generally a 30- to 90-minute session in which you focus specifically on body areas or perform a full-body massage, depending on the needs of the athlete at the time of the session. The therapeutic techniques are anatomically directed to the muscles, musculotendinous junctions, fascia, and ligaments in order to address the myofascial and neuromuscular systems of the body. The focus of maintenance massage follows the general application of working from general to specific, then superficial to deep, and according to the needs of your client.

When determining the specific needs of your client as an athlete, you must first consider whether the activity is lower or upper body dominant or a combination of both. For example, consider cycling, which is a lower body–dominant sport with some upper body stress points. In a 60-minute maintenance massage session, you would warm the tissues with basic massage strokes, devote approximately half the massage to the lower body muscles and spend the rest of the session addressing the back, neck, and chest areas as they are also used when cycling.

Treatment Massage

When clients come to you as a result of soft tissue trauma, repetitive overuse, or muscle strain, ask about their physical activity patterns and goals, and perform both general and specific assessments to determine their stage of healing, pain, and compensation patterns. Different kinds of pain have different causes and thus require different treatment. Treatment massage can be integral to the athlete's overall treatment plan and by using massage to address soft tissue trauma, the goals of treatment massage are to:

- Decrease pain
- Decrease swelling
- Restore ROM
- Restore normal function

The application of treatment massage combines specific massage techniques to enhance soft tissue healing and enable the athlete to return to his or her normal level of activity. **It is important to understand what other treatments the athlete is receiving in his or her recovery in order not to overtreat the client's soft tissue and potentially diminish healing by creating more injury.** Additionally, if the athlete is using anti-inflammatory or pain medication as part of his or her treatment, be sure to adjust your techniques for his or her diminished awareness of the depth and intensity of the application of treatment techniques.

During and immediately following the physical activity, muscles may burn and feel fatigued as a result of oxygen debt. The pain subsides after exercise stops and the oxygen debt is repaid, which usually occurs within minutes. The pain and discomfort resulting from the buildup of metabolic muscle waste and shortened muscles may worsen over 2 to 3 days before it gets better, but the soreness usually only lasts a few days. When muscle tissue is torn, the healing mechanism is initiated, and inflammation results.

Depending on the client's health and the severity of the injury, healing can occur within several weeks or it can take up to a year or more. Clients who exercise regularly but are trying a new sport will heal differently and probably much quicker than someone who has been inactive for years and has started a strenuous exercise program. The pain cycle will aggravate the healing process, and clients who have been caught in a pain cycle for more than a month will benefit greatly from therapeutic massage. The more you understand your clients' physical activity, the better you can address their soft tissue complaints.

Discuss the healing mechanism and the effects of restricted fascia. Athletes frequently repetitively overuse and stress their muscles, which causes them to suffer the resulting soreness, stiffness, ROM limitations, muscle fatigue, and generalized body pain.

When an athlete is in the acute stage of injury, the goal is to control and stabilize the injured area. Treatment massage includes rest, ice, compression, and elevation at the local area of concern, as well as lymphatic massage techniques incorporated into the full-body massage to initiate and enhance the healing process. The rest prevents further injury, the ice provides pain relief and reduces circulation to the area, compression prevents lymph from accumulating, and elevation encourages lymph to drain away from the injured area. Once the ice is removed, the body floods the area with oxygenated blood to encourage healing, and the cellular and chemical wastes are removed. Lymphatic techniques to reduce edema are covered in detail in Chapter 10.

In the subacute phase of healing, the treatment goal is to enhance and improve healing. In this phase, connective tissue begins to form, edema and pain are diminishing, and ROM and muscle function is beginning to be restored. You should continue applications of ice and lymphatic techniques to enhance healing. Once edema has decreased, you may apply friction techniques to influence the functional formation of scar tissue to restore mobility with minimal restriction. **It is important to note that ice should be applied before lymphatic techniques because ice and cold temperatures diminish lymphatic flow.** In the maturation phase, or phase III, of healing, the treatment goals are to create functional adhesions and/or scars, improve flexibility, and restore function to the area of injury. Treatment massage during phase III includes a combination of gentle movements of the injured area in addition to lymphatic, myofascial, and neuromuscular techniques to reduce swelling, enhance connective tissue mobility and flexibility, and reduce muscle tension. It is also important to assess and treat any compensation patterns that may have formed as a result of the injury so that the likelihood of the injury reoccurring will be reduced. Most athletes are seriously interested in healing and will be grateful for information that helps them heal faster and more functionally.

Common Athletic Injuries

There are some common athletic injuries that you will likely encounter in treating amateur and competitive athletes. These injuries include but are not limited to:

- Acute or chronic muscle strains
- Acute or chronic ligament sprains
- Acute or chronic bursitis
- Hip or shoulder pointers (a collision at or fall onto a bony prominence such as the iliac crest, greater trochanter, or acromion-deltoid area that usually develops a hematoma)
- Charley horse (a contusion of the quadriceps that results in a muscle spasm and sometimes a hematoma)
- Neurovascular compression or tension syndromes

See Chapter 5 for more specific information on the indications and contraindications for massage in some of these conditions.

Cramping and Thermoregulatory Conditions

Because this might occur as a result of participating in exercise or an athletic event, you should be aware of what causes muscle cramping and how to alleviate it. Cramping is a forceful, painful, involuntary contraction of the muscle fibers that may be caused by trauma, overload, fluid loss, electrolyte imbalance, or excessive temperatures. You can alleviate cramping via ice massage, which decreases nerve impulses and muscle spindle cell activity, or you can use reciprocal inhibition, direct manipulation, or compression.

Athletes may also experience thermoregulatory conditions such as hypothermia (core body temperature that drops below the normal range), heat cramps, heat exhaustion, or heat stroke. Any time athletes complain of feeling excessively hot or cold, you notice that their tissues are abnormally hot or cold, or they feel faint, disoriented, or dizzy, you should refer them immediately to the emergency medical technicians or medical tent for treatment.

Self-Care for the Athlete

During athletic activity, muscles contract repeatedly and can easily establish a shorter resting length once the activity stops. Lengthening and stretching muscles immediately after exercise is a very effective and beneficial technique clients can use for self-help. For example, to lengthen and stretch their gastrocnemius muscles, they can use a post-isometric relaxation technique on their own:

1. Stand on the balls of the feet on the edge of a step or raised platform.
2. Let the heels slowly drop down to extend the gastrocnemius muscles to the end feel.
3. Rise up on the toes just a bit to contract the gastrocnemius muscles slightly.
4. Hold the position for a minimum of 7 to 10 seconds.
5. Slowly relax the gastrocnemius muscles and let the heels drop down, extending the gastrocnemius to the end feel.
6. Hold the position for a minimum of 7 to 10 seconds and wait for a tendon reflex to relax and lengthen the gastrocnemius muscles further.

Additionally, you may recommend yoga poses, Pilates, and other forms of stretching and strengthening to the athlete for his or her return to an optimal level of activity and for ongoing maintenance of soft tissue flexibility. It is your job to help clients help themselves. The combination of education, self-help activities, and massage treatment can be highly effective if your clients are willing to participate in their healthcare. In order to do this, it is wise to have some references on stretching, yoga, and Pilates in your office.

Pregnant Women

There is some controversy regarding pregnancy and massage. Some suggest that women should not receive any massage at all during the first 3 months of pregnancy. However, others suggest that very light massage is appropriate and beneficial during the first 3 months. Many people specifically avoid massaging women with a history or risk of miscarriage. Some recommend against the prone position at any point during the pregnancy, and others consider a bolstered prone position safe. Generally, healthy women with a low-risk pregnancy can receive the benefits of massage throughout their pregnancy, during labor, and through the postpartum period. Ask your pregnant clients to discuss the benefits of or contraindications to massage with their obstetricians before you agree to treat them.

The physical condition of pregnant women involves some important considerations and contraindications for massage. A pregnant body undergoes many changes that create stress, pain, and discomfort. Stress can complicate the pregnancy and delivery in numerous ways. Massage can provide relief from many of these symptoms, as long as it is applied carefully and knowledgeably.

First Trimester

The first trimester includes the first 3 months of pregnancy. Some women are unaware of their pregnancy for the first month or two. Once they are aware of their pregnancy, some women will openly inform you of it, but others keep their pregnancies private for some time. It is nearly impossible to be aware of every pregnancy during the first trimester, even if you ask every female client before every massage whether she is pregnant. After fertilization, the embryo floats free in the uterus until it embeds itself in the uterine lining, which occurs within about 7 days. The embryo undergoes the important developmental stages of becoming a fetus during the first trimester. Considering the possibility that there is an undisclosed pregnancy, yet knowing that the first trimester is a critical time for the developing fetus, you can see why massage during the first trimester is so controversial.

Physically, the client may experience nausea, vomiting, taste and smell sensitivities, exhaustion, constipation, and mood swings, but her shape and size will be relatively unchanged. Assuming you are aware of your client's pregnancy, you must be sensitive to her emotions and her physical condition and especially attentive to her comfort.

Positioning for the First Trimester

Although some persons recommend against the prone position during the first trimester, in reality, many women sleep in the prone position without being completely aware of it, and obstetricians do not typically recommend against the prone position during the first trimester. If you practice client-centered massage and pay attention to both verbal and nonverbal cues, you will know whether your client is comfortable or not and make appropriate adjustments to technique or client positioning.

Second Trimester

The client may start "showing" during the second trimester, and she may feel the fetus moving. The mother's body has to make some physical changes to accommodate the size of the baby. Her ribs may start spreading apart, and her organs may get pushed aside. Connective tissues are stretched, sometimes past their limits. Stretch marks, shortness of breath, varicose veins, hemorrhoids, heartburn, frequent urination, and backaches are common symptoms that result from the physical changes of the second trimester. The lymph circulation is also affected. As the fetus gets larger, it puts pressure on the larger lymphatic vessels in the abdominal and pelvic cavities. The lymphatic vessels rely on gravity and skeletal movement to create lymphatic flow, and when the flow is restricted so close to the lymphatic ducts, lymph can accumulate in the tissues. This undrained lymph creates swelling, or edema (eh-DEE-mah), which is common during pregnancy, particularly in the areas that are least assisted by gravity, such as the ankles.

Unusual levels of hormones are produced during normal pregnancy, which affect a pregnant woman's emotions, body temperature, and ligaments. Because her body temperature may run a little higher than normal, fresh air or a breeze may help keep her comfortable. In the second trimester, the woman's body will start to manufacture relaxin, a hormone that changes the collagen composition, allowing the pubic symphysis to loosen and expand the pelvis for delivery of the baby. Unfortunately, relaxin affects ligaments as well. Be extra careful with joint movements because the ligaments will not stop the ROM that normally occurs.

Positioning for the Second Trimester

The size of the client and the size of the fetus create a need for special positioning and bolstering. Because a pregnant woman's breasts often become sensitive and because her abdomen may protrude during the second trimester, the prone position may not be favorable. Pregnant women who prefer the prone position for massage can be sufficiently bolstered to minimize pressure on the breasts and uterus, but the easiest and safest way to position clients during the second trimester is in a seated or side-lying position. The supine position may be appropriate for the early part of the second trimester, but the fetus puts pressure on the aorta and lymph vessels, which restricts the delivery of oxygenated blood and lymph. Large or multiple fetuses put excessive pressure on the abdominal aorta when the mother is in the supine position, a condition sometimes called supine hypotension. With large and multiple fetuses and toward the later part of the second trimester, a woman's time spent in the supine position should be limited to 10 to 15 minutes. As a safer alternative, the client can be placed in a semireclined position.

Special massage tables have been designed for pregnant women that provide holes for an extended belly and for enlarged breasts. These tables allow pregnant women to lie prone, which otherwise can be uncomfortable and nearly impossible as the pregnancy progresses. As part of the controversy over the prone position, these pregnancy tables are considered ridiculous and worthless by some. In practical terms, these tables are more expensive than standard massage tables; given the conflicting opinions, the side-lying position is a simpler alternative for clients in their second trimester of pregnancy.

Third Trimester

During the final few months of pregnancy, the fetus grows considerably. The maternal conditions and symptoms of the second trimester continue and often are more pronounced. Edema can be a significant problem during the third trimester, particularly in the lower legs and feet, but also in the forearms and hands. Massage is especially effective at encouraging lymphatic flow. The size of the baby or unusual positioning of organs can also compress nerves and cause symptoms such as numbness, fatigue, tingling, a feeling of pins and needles, and sometimes pain. Compression on the brachial plexus can cause symptoms in the shoulders, arms, hands, or all three. Pressure on the tibial nerve can create similar symptoms in the feet or ankles.

Other common symptoms that can develop during the last trimester include muscular cramps, incontinence, sacroiliac joint pain, pelvic discomfort, indigestion, frequent urination, stress and worry, and sleeplessness. Massage can provide some relief to these symptoms, but it cannot eliminate them.

Positioning for the Third Trimester

Due to the size of the baby in the final trimester, the mother should be placed in the supine position for a maximum of 10 to 15 minutes. A slightly modified supine position, in which the woman's head, shoulders, and upper back are elevated with bolsters, can be used for a longer period, but the side-lying position is easiest and usually the most comfortable. Even in the side-lying position, the woman should be well bolstered for comfort.

Considerations for Pregnancy (Prenatal) Massage

Pregnant women can be massaged in a side-lying position with proper bolstering for most of their pregnancy. (See earlier Fig. 9-2 for bolstering prenatal clients in the side-lying position.) During all stages of pregnancy, watch for the client feeling faint during the massage session. If this occurs, change the client's position; the therapist must pay close attention to the client's level of consciousness. Of course, this holds true for any client, pregnant or not, but there is a greater chance that woman whose baby is putting excessive pressure on her aorta will feel faint. There are some contraindications for massaging pregnant women. Massage can interfere with the body's processes, aggravate conditions created by pregnancy, endanger anatomical structures, or encourage labor:

- Joints—because of the activity of relaxin, be cautious with any ROM to prevent injury
- Abdomen—light abdominal massage is acceptable, but deep work can traumatize the uterus or fetus and should be avoided
- Connective tissue—the activity of relaxin can affect the fascia, so myofascial manipulation and connective tissue work should be avoided to prevent injury
- Varicose veins—caused by collapsed valves in the veins and resulting in blood collecting at the most distal functional valve, they are to be avoided at all times to prevent further injury to a faulty vein
- Acupressure points—a few are known to encourage uterine or cervical activity and should be avoided during pregnancy (see earlier Table 11-6, for maps of acupressure points)
  - Spleen 6—on the medial side of the tibia, approximately 3 to 5 inches from the medial malleolus
  - Large Intestine 4—in the web between the thumb and index finger, at the base of the crease created when adducting those two metacarpals
  - Gallbladder 21—directly lateral of C7, midway between C7 and the acromion process
- Essential oils—a number of essential oils (not necessarily the raw ingredients from which they originate) could be harmful to a pregnancy, including:
  - Angelica
  - Basil
  - Chamomile
  - Clary sage
  - Fennel
  - Jasmine
  - Juniper
  - Peppermint
  - Wintergreen

Massage is appropriate for most pregnant women and can be very beneficial. The same techniques used in a regular massage session can be used in a prenatal massage, but you must be aware of the client's special needs. Massage therapists should take additional training to specialize in pre-natal massage.

Postpartum Massage

Having a baby is a physically, emotionally, and spiritually life-changing event. Labor and delivery can be both exciting and exhausting for new mothers who now must attend to their new baby or babies. There can also be changes in the dynamics of relationships with her partner, other children, family members, and friends. Postpartum mothers often experience exhaustion along with muscular tension and sore-ness in the neck, shoulders, arms, and upper back from deliv-ering the baby and learning to breast-feed. Cesarean section (C-section) deliveries can result in a lot of back pain and dis-comfort because of the extended recovery from surgery and the prolonged inactivity. This tension may also increase when she starts moving around and hunches over to compensate for the abdominal pain associated with the surgery.

Use the basic massage strokes and lymphatic drainage techniques to facilitate relaxation, increase circulation to flush out chemical and cellular waste, and reduce edema. The side-lying position may be most comfortable for a new mother for up to 3 days postpartum, but the prone and supine positions are acceptable. Be sure to bolster your client so she is comfortable while receiving massage. Your focus should be on nurturing and supporting the mother during this time.

Although postpartum massage is beneficial for many reasons, you should be aware that there are risks for deep venous thrombosis or blood clots for up to 6 weeks postpartum and no massage should be applied to the medial side of the legs.

There is occasionally pain and soreness at and around the site where an epidural anesthetic was administered. Massage is indicated around, but not on, the site to relieve the pain and soreness. Consult with her physician if there have been complications with birth and prior to using any abdominal techniques on a mother who had a C-section delivery.

Infants

The benefits of massage are not limited to adults. **Increased circulation, more effective digestion, reduced stress, and deeper and more regular sleep patterns are some benefits that are as good for babies as they are for adults.** Premature infants who receive massage have shown increased weight gain, reduced stress, and better developmental progress. Dr. Tiffany Field has scientifically studied the effects of mas-sage on groups of infants in various stages of health or dysfunction. Babies born prematurely or with drug addic-tions, AIDS, breathing disorders, or diabetic conditions have all shown improved health after receiving regular massage while still hospitalized. Additionally, their improved health decreases the amount of medical intervention needed and reduces their hospital costs.

Massage can provide physical benefits to the baby as well as strengthen the bond between the baby and the per-son giving the massage (Fig. 12-1). Touch is a form of com-munication, and a new baby understands touch more than words. In fact, touch may be as important as food to babies, so the more they are touched with a caring, loving intent, the healthier they are. Ask the baby's parent or parents to be present while you massage their baby, for both professional courtesy and legal protection. While they observe, you can describe some of the different strokes you use, explain the

physiological benefits of the strokes, and encourage the parents to massage their baby on a regular basis, even daily. Incorporating massage into the bedtime or bath routine is often easiest, but massage will provide quality time for the infant and parent whether it is used daily or weekly, regu-larly or not. There are infant massage videos, books, and classes available for parents who are interested.

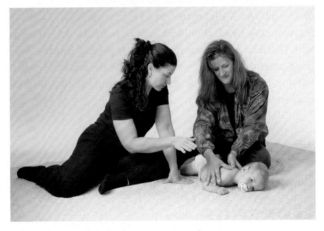

Figure 12-1. Massage therapist teaching a parent how to perform infant massage.

Infant Massage

Therapists wishing to specialize in infant massage should receive additional training to learn techniques and flow. Keep in mind that to some degree, babies control the massage. The infant massage typically lasts only 15 minutes or so, but the duration is often determined by the baby's patience or willingness to accept the massage. An infant may dislike being touched in certain areas, may dislike particular strokes, or may dislike certain positions. Stay focused on the baby's comfort and change the massage as the baby expresses likes or dislikes.

During the massage, the baby may or may not wear a diaper. You may use a dry lubricant, such as cornstarch, or one of the many lotions and creams available for infant massage. Natural oils are better than synthetic or petroleum-based products, and vegetable or nut oils are preferable to mineral or animal-derived oils. Synthetic, mineral, and animal-based products are more likely to clog the baby's pores and irritate the skin.

Effleurage, pétrissage, and tapotement can be used cautiously on infants. Some variations of these strokes have been specially developed for infant massage. One technique, called "milking," is commonly used. You hold the baby's hand or foot with one hand and form a sort of ring around the baby's limb with your other hand, gently squeezing the limb while sliding your hand toward the baby's body. It is like a long effleurage stroke of the entire limb. Another variation, wringing, is similar to milking, but has an added twisting action as the stroke moves proximally. Milking and wringing encourage both lymphatic and venous flow, they warm the tissues, and they are soothing strokes.

The baby can be positioned supine first, which allows you to see the baby's facial expressions and lets the baby fix his or her gaze on the person massaging. This positioning helps the baby trust the therapist and become familiar with the process. The strokes mentioned above may be used while the baby is supine. The baby's arms, legs, feet, face, and abdomen can all be massaged in this position. When massaging the abdomen, follow a clockwise pattern for abdominal massage as discussed in Chapter 9. As the baby is supine with you at the baby's feet, looking at the baby's face, move your hands clockwise on the baby's abdomen. Clockwise effleurage strokes encourage peristaltic activity, which moves the contents of the intestines in the same direction.

You can attempt to put the baby in the prone position after the supine position for access to the baby's back, neck, scalp, legs, and arms. Wringing and milking might stress the baby's joints while prone, so limit your strokes to effleurage, pétrissage, and tapotement of the baby's back and gluteal muscles in this position.

Return the baby to the supine position to complete the massage so that you can communicate to the baby that the massage is finished.

It should be common sense to use minimal pressure in infant massage. Being relaxed and patient will help the massage flow smoothly. Babies are very sensitive to emotions and will respond negatively if you are nervous or emotional. If the baby is not enjoying the experience or seems to be in pain, it may be best to stop the massage, comfort the baby, and try massage again at another time.

Geriatric Clients

The geriatric population continues to grow as our life expectancy increases. Massage for geriatric clients is a specialty that provides them with both physical and mental benefits. Many health problems are associated with aging that range from mild discomfort to significant disease processes. Compounding existing problems, most geriatric persons are not very physically active, which diminishes the circulation of blood and lymph. Without sufficient oxygen, cells suffer and eventually die.

Geriatric Massage

Many people over the age of 65 lead perfectly healthy, active lifestyles and can benefit from massage, but others have special needs. The condition of the client's tissues will determine the strokes and techniques used, but most of the work is accomplished with light, gentle effleurage strokes and passive ROM (Box 12-7). For geriatric clients who are in very good health, are active in sports and other activities, and have healthy tissues, the massage can include faster, deeper, and more stimulating kinds of techniques.

All of the client's body systems are affected by increased circulation and the movements of the massage. The body needs some time to readjust and recover, so the session should be shorter than usual to avoid overwhelming the client's body. Massage for geriatric clients is typically 30 minutes instead of 60 minutes. Given by a therapist with proper training, geriatric massage can provide the following benefits:

- Increased circulation of blood
- Increased circulation of lymph
- Pain relief

BOX 12-7
Geriatric Massage Features

- Clients may require physical assistance.
- Sessions usually last 30 minutes.
- Primarily gentle, more superficial strokes; use of deeper work depends on the client's health and condition of the soft tissues.
- Almost always incorporates ROM techniques, active or passive, unless client has osteoporosis, recent fracture, or surgery.
- Use gentle massage strokes on hands and feet.

- Reduced stress and anxiety
- Improved joint ROM
- Personal attention and feelings of reassurance, which lead to a healthier disposition
- Improved sleep patterns
- Possible reduction of symptoms of Alzheimer's disease

The increased circulation of blood and lymph helps deliver oxygen and other nutrients to the cells of the body and remove cellular debris. As a result, healing processes are more efficient. Bedsores and other circulatory problems can be prevented by maintaining sufficient circulation.

Some senior clients are less modest and may attempt to undress while you are still in the treatment room. You may need to explain that the client should undress after you step out of the room. Occasionally, a client is unable to undress independently and requires assistance. Some senior clients, like persons of any age, prefer to remain clothed for the entire massage. Keep a wide, firm step stool nearby to help clients get on and off the table and be prepared to help clients turn from the supine to the prone position, or vice versa. Some clients are reserved and may be shy about asking for help, so it is better to offer assistance and not wait for the client to ask for it.

Receiving human touch along with someone's undivided attention for 30 minutes or more is a luxury many geriatric clients may not have experienced for some time. Many have lost their spouses and feel lonely or depressed, confused, or anxious. Your presence and the massage combine to leave the geriatric client usually in a more positive mental state that facilitates health and well-being. Your use of either active or passive ROM techniques for the synovial joints promotes the production of synovial fluid. The lubricating function of the fluid then improves ROM.

Massage Environment for Geriatric Clients

Your geriatric clients may come to your office, but it is more convenient for those with special needs if you go to them. You can take your table and all of your supplies to their home, a nursing home, or an assisted living arrangement, just like any other outcall. Before you transport your table, ask about the special needs of your geriatric clients to find out if they are bedridden or unable to use your table. Clients who cannot get on the massage table are still able to enjoy the benefits of massage, but you have to adapt your massage to their needs. You can massage bedridden clients in their beds, despite the awkward body mechanics. Often, bedridden clients cannot withstand a lot of pressure or a lot of movement. If they can get out of bed and sit in a chair, you can also offer them a massage in a wheelchair or household chair.

Considerations for Geriatric Clients

The aging process affects all parts of an organism. As we get older and less physically active, it becomes more difficult to reach our feet to take care of them. Geriatric clients commonly have feet that are in poor condition. Despite the shape and condition of their feet, massage and joint movement is very beneficial for their feet. Another common effect of aging is memory loss. Call or contact your geriatric clients that morning to remind them of their appointment. Depending on the extent of their memory loss, you might want to contact them even an hour before the appointment. At the same time, if a geriatric client misses an appointment, do not get frustrated or offended. You can talk to the nursing home administrators or family members to find out if there is an activities director or someone else who can help your clients make it to their appointments.

There are special conditions in the geriatric population that are contraindications for massage:

- Bedsores
- Arthritic joints
- Varicose veins
- Recent surgery
- Blood clots or history of blood clots
- Blood thinners

As with each special population, specialized training is available for geriatric massage. Every massage therapy student should experience geriatric massage. In many cases, students who did not expect to enjoy the work end up loving it.

Chronically Ill Patients

A **chronic illness** is one that lasts a year or longer, usually limits the patient's physical activity, and may require ongoing medical care and treatment. Some chronic illnesses you may recognize include:

- Alzheimer's disease
- Arthritis
- Asthma
- Cancer
- Diabetes
- Epilepsy
- Glaucoma
- Heart disease
- Hepatitis
- HIV
- Lupus
- Multiple sclerosis
- Parkinson's disease

Each of the above chronic illnesses has its own symptoms, but many chronically ill patients are commonly burdened with high medical costs, difficulty holding a job, family stress, and depression. Massage can offer relief from some of the associated physical and emotional stress and tension, but you must understand the anatomy and physiology of the illness before you incorporate massage into the client's treatment. Communicate with the client's other healthcare professionals and try to establish a team approach that includes the client's input. Ruth Werner's book, *A Massage Therapist's Guide to Pathology,* is an excellent and comprehensive resource that includes a number of illnesses, their causes, treatments, and the indications and contraindications for massage.

Hospice Massage

Sometimes, diseases and illnesses cannot be cured with current medical treatment. When a person's life expectancy is limited because of a life-threatening illness and there is no known cure, **hospice** (HAHSS-pihss) care caters to the quality of remaining life rather than the quantity of life. It addresses all of the symptoms of the disease and provides emotional, spiritual, and practical support to the patient as well as the friends and family members. Massage therapy is frequently included in hospice care to make patients more comfortable and reduce stress. It can also be helpful for the caretakers to ensure that their loved one is receiving caring touch when a cure is unavailable. Typically, relaxing techniques such as light effleurage, connecting strokes, and simple resting strokes may be used in this type of massage. As with most special populations, you can discuss the person's condition with the healthcare professionals to incorporate massage into the treatment plan safely.

Disabled Clients

Many persons with disabilities receive massage, including those with visual and hearing impairments, paralysis, amputation, and psychological issues. The massage itself is not so different, but your approach to caring for these clients requires that you understand their conditions and make special accommodations to ensure their safety and comfort.

Visually or Hearing Impaired

Visually or hearing impaired clients need some special assistance, but the actual massage is minimally affected by these disabilities. These clients may need an auditory or visual signal to let them know it is time to turn over during the massage, but the strokes and flow are the same as in a typical session. If the client has a companion dog that must stay in the treatment room, the dog can either lie in a corner of the room, out of the way, or under the table. These companion dogs are at work, so do not expect them to be playful and do not distract the dogs by trying to play with them.

Physical Disabilities

With proper training and experience, massage therapists can specialize in massage for the physically disabled. For some massage therapists, working with the physically disabled is uncomfortable at first, but massage students are encouraged to experience the challenges and rewards of working with this special population.

Using crutches requires excessive use of the triceps brachii muscles, puts the wrists in an unnatural position, and can compress the structures running through the carpal tunnel. Manual wheelchairs also require a lot work from the arm muscles, particularly the latissimus dorsi, triceps, pectoralis, and coracobrachialis. You may need to alter your body mechanics to accommodate a client in a wheelchair or bed, but the correct principles of body mechanics are basically the same. In fact, massage is especially beneficial for clients who are bedridden and wheelchair bound.

If you think about the joint movements involved in your client's physical limitations or compensation patterns, you can use the special muscle chart in Chapter 4 to determine which muscles to evaluate and treat. (Earlier Table 10-1 can also help you determine antagonistic muscles to assess or to use in PNF techniques.)

The flow of massage need not change if the client can lie on the massage table. If, however, the client must remain in a wheelchair or bed, a massage can still be given. The flow must change, and it may take a longer time to address the entire body. Shorten the session for a new client because the body needs to reestablish a balance following the soft tissue manipulation and circulatory enhancement. This can be an exhausting experience for anyone, but even more so for a client whose nervous and muscular systems are not functioning normally.

Paralysis

Paralysis is accompanied by a loss of sensation, the effects of which are important for the massage therapist to understand. Since the client cannot sense pain, be especially careful to avoid injuring the tissues. To ensure the safety of the tissues, use enough bolstering to support the client's body. Position the client's muscles in passive contraction before working on them, to provide the softest, most relaxed position of the muscles. Strokes used for a person with paralysis are the same as those in a "regular" massage but must be gentler and more sensitive. Strokes have more therapeutic benefit for a paralyzed client if they are directed toward the heart to increase venous and lymphatic flow. ROM techniques are very beneficial but must be done with extreme care for a paralyzed client. The person's tissues are probably stuck together and shortened, significantly limiting the ROM. You must understand that, because of this hypertonicity, the movements may be barely perceptible, and therefore you must pay close attention to feel the limits of the tissues.

The circulation of a paralyzed client and anyone bedridden or confined to a wheelchair is usually greatly compromised. Without muscular activity, small blood vessels do not receive normal amounts of blood flow, and the extremities can easily become ischemic. Likewise, the lymph, which does not have a pumping force behind it, does not flow well. Massage acts as an external pump that increases blood and lymph flow. Be extremely careful with clients who are paralyzed, bedridden, or significantly inactive. Their muscles are probably atrophied, their fascia severely restricted and bound down, and their joints very stiff; movement of any kind can hurt. Discuss their condition with their caretakers and/or physician to understand as much as you can about the client's health. Moving these clients into a chair or onto a table might not be appropriate, even if the client or the caretakers think it is. Use your best judgment, with a client-centered focus, and give your disabled clients a massage in the safest and most beneficial place.

Amputation

In the process of amputation, the surgical removal of part of a limb, nerves are severed. Many amputees, or persons who have undergone amputation, suffer a phenomenon called phantom pain, which is the sensation of pain in the missing limb. The point where the limb was amputated, called the stump, is often very sensitive to pain. In addition to coping with the emotional hardship of losing the limb, amputees must deal with the physical pain caused by faulty nerve signals. Massaging the stump can help quiet the pain, but you must go slowly and carefully, paying close attention to the client's tolerance.

The posture of an amputee is significantly affected, because the entire balance of the body is permanently offset. Whether the amputation occurs at an arm or leg, necessary compensation patterns develop to establish a posture that allows the amputee to balance and function normally. Address the muscular aches and pains, but use a knowledgeable approach when applying therapeutic techniques to ensure that you are not disturbing the necessary postural compensation patterns.

Psychological Issues

Treating mental impairment and emotional and psychological disturbances is not within the scope of practice for wellness or therapeutic massage. However, it is within the scope of practice to provide massage to clients who suffer from emotional and psychological issues. Transference and countertransference can easily develop in relationships with clients who have psychological diagnoses, so you need to recognize and avoid these situations. Transference is the client's dependence on you for friendship or companionship in addition to therapeutic treatment, and countertransference is your tendency to react emotionally when clients do not behave or respond to you or your treatment as you had expected. Offer clients your massage, education, and recommendations for self-care. Expect prompt payment, professional respect, and cooperation with your policies and business practices. Establish and maintain a professional client–therapist relationship to avoid complications and potential problems.

If you suspect that a client has a psychological impairment, emotional instability, or mental disturbance, you can neither diagnose nor treat it. You can gently refer clients to an appropriate healthcare professional, but you cannot force them to make or attend an appointment. **If you suspect that a client is being abused or that a client's life is in danger for any reason, you may have a legal responsibility to report it to the local authorities.** Be sure you check with your local government's child welfare, family services, or social services department to determine your legal responsibilities as a massage therapist.

Clients with psychological issues may respond to massage with defense mechanisms such as extreme laughter, sadness, introversion, or extroversion. They may have an emotional release, which is similar to a flashback of an emotional experience. Do not encourage clients to have emotional releases, but do not suppress them when they occur. You are not allowed to treat the emotional disturbance, but you can offer support, understanding, and patience to clients who experience an emotional release. There are advanced courses that teach massage therapists how to best handle and facilitate these emotional releases. The intent is to relieve the fascial restrictions that affect the soft tissues of the body.

You must respect the coping mechanisms and behaviors of persons who have suffered abuse, be it physical or psychological. For example, they may want to leave all of their clothes on, they may ask for additional draping despite the room temperature, and they may be uncomfortable in certain client positions. You may or may not be informed of a client's abuse history, but by paying attention to nonverbal communication and using a client-centered approach, you can offer a safe massage to all clients.

Chemical imbalances such as depression, anxiety, and bipolar disorder can usually be treated medically, but persons with chemical imbalances commonly avoid their medications. If you notice that a client who is supposed to be taking medication is behaving inconsistently, carefully and cautiously inquire about the medication. You could casually ask the client about medication during the assessment process or as you set the next appointment by saying something like, "How are things going, anyway? . . . Medications ok? . . . Sleeping ok? . . . Is anything new or interesting going on?" If they admit that they are not taking their medication, you could gently suggest they talk to their doctor about the medication or dosage to see if there might be a better alternative. If they are not willing to tell you about their use of medication, you cannot force the issue unless you suspect that they are endangering their life or someone else's.

CHAPTER SUMMARY

The benefits of massage are available to anyone, male or female, young or old, pregnant, athletic, sedentary, healthy, ill, or physically or psychologically disabled. The special needs of each population may require that you modify the massage in one way or another, but those needs should not prevent anyone from receiving the benefits of massage. Learn about the physical and psychological needs of those in these special populations and the contraindications for massage, cooperate with the other members of the client's healthcare team, and be careful to stay within the clients' tolerances. Students are encouraged to work with as many special populations as possible to learn about differences and face the challenges. Massaging members of these populations can be a very rewarding experience.

CHAPTER EXERCISES

1. Compare and contrast pre-event massage, post-event massage, and restorative massage. Include details of timing, duration of the massage, strokes used or techniques to avoid, purpose, location, and equipment.

2. Find at least three different volunteers on whom to practice a pre-event massage routine. Ask them to identify a sport that they participate in so you can tailor their pre-event massage to the muscles involved in that sport. Remember to incorporate grounding and centering techniques.

3. Use the same three volunteers from exercise 2 and practice an appropriate post-event massage routine

on each of them. Include grounding and centering for each massage.

4. List at least five contraindications of massage for pregnant women.

5. Describe an important contraindication for post-partum massage.

6. List at least three benefits of massage for infants.

7. Describe some of the features of geriatric massage, including at least four contraindications, four benefits, and special considerations for the physical condition or mental capacity of geriatric persons.

8. Describe how you can communicate with visually impaired clients during a massage session to ensure their safety and comfort.

9. Go to the Touch Research Institute web site, www.miami.edu/touch-research.com, and find at least two research articles. Summarize at least two studies that are interesting to you.

10. Research hospice organizations in your area and list at least five different services they offer for patients as well as services they offer the friends and families of persons whose life expectancy is limited.

SUGGESTED READING

American Massage Therapy Association Sports Massage Tool Kit. Evanston, IL: American Massage Therapy Association, 2003.

Anderson MK. *Fundamentals of Sports Injury Management.* 2nd ed. Baltimore: Lippincott Williams & Wilkins, 2003.

Archer P. *Therapeutic Massage in Athletics.* Baltimore: Lippincott Williams & Wilkins, 2007.

Ashton J, Cassel D. *Review for Therapeutic Massage and Bodywork Certification.* Baltimore: Lippincott Williams & Wilkins, 2002.

Cady SH, Jones GE. Massage therapy as a workplace intervention for reduction of stress. *Percept Mot Skills* 1997;84(1):157–158.

Chaitow L, DeLany JW. *Clinical Application of Neuromuscular Techniques.* Vol 1. London: Churchill Livingstone, 2000.

Field T, Ironson G, Safari F, et al. Massage therapy reduces anxiety and enhances EEG pattern of alertness and math computations. *Int J Neurosci* 1996;86:197–205.

Field T, Quintino O, Henteleff T, et al. Job stress reduction therapies. *Alter Ther Health Med* 1997;3(4):54–56.

Johnson J. *The Healing Art of Sports Massage.* Emmaus, PA: Rodale Press, 1995.

Osborne-Sheets C. *Pre- and Perinatal Massage Therapy: A Comprehensive Practitioners' Guide to Pregnancy, Labor and Postpartum.* San Diego, CA: Body Therapy Associates, 1998.

Rattray F, Ludwig L. *Clinical Massage Therapy: Understanding, Assessing and Treating over 70 Conditions.* Toronto, Ontario: Talus Incorporated, 2000.

Stephens R. *Therapeutic Chair Massage.* Baltimore: Lippincott Williams & Wilkins, 2006.

Werner R. *A Massage Therapist's Guide to Pathology.* 3rd ed. Baltimore: Lippincott Williams & Wilkins, 2005.

http://www.americanhospice.org, accessed 3.5.06.

http://www.amtamassage.org/about/terms.html, accessed 3.5.06.

http://www.applesforhealth.com/AlternativeMedicine/agrowkn3.html, accessed 3.5.06.

http://www.childbirthsolutions.com/articles/birth/acupressure/index.php, accessed 3.5.06.

http://www.daybreak-massage.com/massage-day-break-about-us.htm, accessed 3.5.06.

http://www.disabilitymuseum.org/lib/docs/954.htm, accessed 3.5.06.

http://www.essentialoils.co.za/pregnancy.htm, accessed 3.5.06.

http://www.findarticles.com/cf_dls/g2603/0003/2603000386/p1/article.jhtml, accessed 3.5.06.

http://www.findarticles.com/cf_dls/g2603/0004/2603000452/p1/article.jhtml?term_infantmassage, accessed 3.5.06.

http://www.hospicefoundation.org, accessed 3.5.06.

http://www.hospicenet.org, accessed 3.5.06.

http://www.montaine.com.au/corporate.htm, accessed 3.5.06.

http://www.pslgroup.com/dg/42772.htm, accessed 3.5.06.

Professional Massage Practice

Objectives

Upon completion of this chapter, the student will be able to:

- Properly set the height of the massage table
- Describe the purpose of standard precautions
- Demonstrate the proper handwashing procedure
- Name at least five policies or rules to include on the policies and procedures form
- Name at least three different kinds of advisors a massage therapist should consult when starting a massage practice
- Design a business card that includes appropriate information

Key Terms

Artificial respiration (also called artificial resuscitation, mouth-to-mouth respiration, and rescue breathing): A mechanical or manual technique of forcing air into a person's lungs if he/she is not breathing but has a pulse.

Cardiopulmonary resuscitation (CPR): A combination of artificial respiration and chest compressions that restores circulation for a person who is not breathing and has no pulse.

Corporation: A business arrangement that has one or more owners who are legally separate from the business.

Networking: The practice of establishing mutually beneficial professional relationships with other persons in a business or networking group.

Partnership: A company in which two or more persons share ownership and personal liability for all business transactions.

Sole proprietorship: A business arrangement in which one person owns the business and is personally liable for all business transactions.

Standard precautions: Specific procedures that maintain a hygienic and sanitary practice and reduce the risk for germ transmission.

Now that you have a foundational understanding of massage therapy, it is time to learn how to put it all together to build a successful practice. The first consideration is equipment and supplies. A basic massage session utilizes properly assembled, dependable equipment in a safe and sanitary environment. Most massage equipment is designed to keep the client comfortable, but it also influences the massage you give by determining how much access you have to the client's body. The massage table is the primary piece of equipment, but there are a variety of other pieces of equipment and accessories that you may consider using, including massage chairs, massage mats, and body cushions. Massage tools and gadgets can reduce the stress on your joints and reduce the amount of physical work required to do massage for a living. Some of the supplies you will need are so important for the comfort and safety of the client that they may be considered pieces of equipment. These include lubricants, sheets and other draping supplies (towels and blankets), a collection of massage music, a sound system, treatment room furnishings, disinfectants, and safety-related items.

Sanitation and safety are critical components of a successful massage business. The health and well-being of the client are the primary goals for massage therapy, so every therapist should know how to maintain a healthy, hygienic practice with specific methods called standard precautions and transmission-based precautions. It is also important to be aware of safety issues that may present legal liabilities, fire codes and regulations, and how to handle medical emergencies.

As a massage therapist, you can understand and be skillful in massage techniques, anatomy and physiology, and documentation, but without being familiar with the basics of professionalism, how to run a business, and how to be a valued and healthy employee, your massage career may be limited. This chapter introduces the components of building a business, including the financial aspects, marketing and promotion, networking, long-term business development, and self-care. Developing and maintaining a self-care plan is critical to maintaining a long-term practice. Therapists often burn out of the profession because they neglect their own health and well-being. Coupling a professional massage business with a devotion to an effective self-care plan will help you become and remain successful.

Equipment

The equipment and supplies you need to practice massage are available in a huge range of prices, sizes, types of construction, appearance, durability, and maintenance requirements. New equipment is readily available in specialty stores, in catalogs and magazines, and through online suppliers. Discontinued models and colors or demonstration models can sometimes be found at a discount.

Used equipment is available and much less expensive, but you need to know its history: where it has been, how old it is, how long it was used, any substances or odors it was exposed to, if it has been damaged or repaired, and how it has been maintained. Without knowing the equipment's history, its reliability is questionable. Some sources for used and more reliable equipment are massage schools and massage therapists. Students who were unable to complete their massage education may be interested in selling their gently used equipment. Practicing therapists may know people who were unable to maintain a massage business and need to sell their used equipment.

Another alternative to purchasing new equipment is to borrow it. Recent graduates interested in helping new students may be interested in sharing their tables for a short time. Even better, some massage schools offer equipment rental to their students. Learning massage requires hands-on practice to develop good techniques, so whether you buy a new table, buy a used one, or borrow one, make sure you have one.

Equipment Specifications

The process of choosing your equipment can be challenging, especially because of the many options available. Once you start looking at the brochures and advertisements, you will discover the seemingly endless choices. Massage suppliers feature equipment with a range of prices, comfort levels, strength and stability specifications, and warranties. Sifting through all the numbers and tests and comparing specifications can make it difficult to know what to look for.

Price

To build a successful practice, you have to give clients an experience that invites them back. Clients form impressions about you and your massage practice on the basis of many factors, from your massage room and equipment to the actual massage. With this in mind, think of the equipment you purchase as an investment in your professional image and the success of your practice.

Comfort

Focusing on client-centered care that delivers a comforting massage session will encourage clients to come back. Just the right amount of padding on your table and face rest (face cradle) as well as quality construction will influence your client's experience. Imagine yourself climbing onto a table that squeaks, has minimal padding and a stiff plastic covering, and then imagine how different it would seem to climb onto a table of solid construction with generous foam padding and ultrasoft covering. When determining which equipment to purchase, ask yourself whether the equipment will enhance the comfort and relaxation of your client or detract from it.

Strength and Stability

Strength and stability in a table come from quality construction in which each component reinforces the other components of the table. Your equipment holds your clients and allows them to relax, so its stability and structural integrity are very important. Underwriters Laboratories (UL) listing and static and dynamic load capacities specify the strength and stability of a table.

Underwriters Laboratories Inc. is an independent, nongovernmental, not-for-profit company that objectively tests products for safety. Products that pass their tests receive the UL listing and products that do not pass do not get the listing. The results are vague and not necessarily helpful in deciding what to buy. Basically, massage equipment with the UL listing has been tested and determined to be safe if used properly.

Equipment companies boast static loading capacities of 3,000 pounds or more and show photos of a truck, a pyramid of people, or a pile of barbell weights on a massage table. Static loading simply tests how much weight a table can withstand as long as the weight is evenly distributed and not moving. The images are impressive, to say the least, but are generally not useful when determining the working strength and stability of your table. Essentially, tables that can carry static loads of 2,000 pounds or more have a strong structure that is dependable.

Dynamic loading measures the weight that can be loaded unevenly on the table. Some companies refer to this measurement as the table's working weight. It tests the amount of weight that can be set on one end of the table or on the center of a hinged table. Testing the dynamic load, or working weight, best replicates how you and your clients will use your table, making it the most helpful statistic to check. The dynamic loading capacities of good-quality massage tables will be about 450 pounds or more.

Warranty

Most reputable equipment companies offer product warranties that may be a bit confusing, often with different durations and transferability. For instance, a massage table made by a respectable company may have a 5-year warranty on the padding and a 3-year warranty on the vinyl covering, all of which is transferable if the table is sold. Another table made by the same company may have a nontransferable guarantee of only 2 years on the padding and vinyl. The specifics of these guarantees are not as critical as the company's willingness to stand behind the products and replace or repair anything that they designed or made poorly. A company that guarantees its workmanship likely makes a good-quality product that should stand the test of time as long as you use it properly. All of the guarantees exclude any damage that occurs to the tables due to accident, neglect, or improper use.

Tables

For most massage therapists, the primary piece of equipment is a massage table. It provides a flat surface that allows clients to lie down during the massage in a position that gives you access to their whole body. Almost all tables have a padded rectangular top with a washable covering that is supported by a stabilized wooden framework. Some massage tables are made with an aluminum framework, and although they are not as popular, they withstand exposure to water much better than tables with a wooden framework. There are also electric-lift, stationary massage tables, whose height you can adjust by a foot pedal; however, these can be very expensive, so they might not be an option for a beginning practitioner. Generally, massage tables are categorized as portable or stationary because the purpose and design of the two are so different. The wide variety of massage table sizes, features, and prices is mostly a function of the tabletop and the support structure.

Tabletop

The most common shape of massage tabletops is a rectangle, but there are also rectangles with rounded corners, contoured shapes, ovals, and a relatively new option of a breast recess. Table widths range from 22 to 33 inches, and lengths run between 65 and 78 inches. The most common tabletops are about 28 to 30 inches wide and 72 to 73 inches long. Some tables are designed for special applications such as Feldenkrais techniques, prenatal or pregnancy tables, or have an easy access end panel for several different techniques (Fig. 13-1).

A wider top provides a larger and more comfortable base that increases client comfort and security, but there are some disadvantages of a wide table. Accessing the center of the clients' bodies requires a longer reach, which is especially

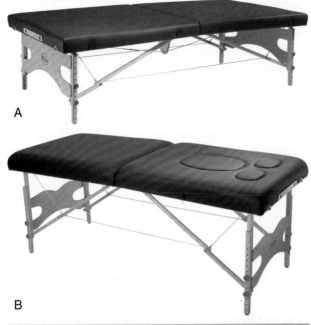

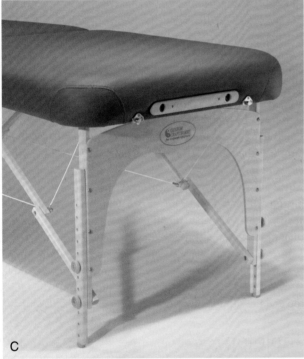

Figure 13-1. Specialty tables. (A) Feldenkrais. (B) Pregnancy. (C) Easy access panel. (Photos courtesy of Customcraftworks.)

problematic for shorter therapists. The wider the table, the heavier it is and the more awkward it is to transport. It may also require deeper pocket sheets to cover the table.

There is a breast recess option for the tabletop that can help therapists provide a more comfortable option for larger-chested clients (Fig. 13-2). Traditionally, the tabletop of a massage table is flat, which compresses the clients' breasts and elevates their torsos. This position rolls the shoulders forward and moves the scapulae laterally, pulling

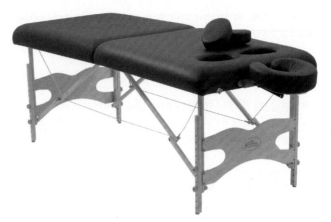

Figure 13-2. Breast recess table. (Photo courtesy of Customcraftworks.)

and lengthening the muscles that are medial to the scapulae. Instead of being soft and pliable, these muscles get stretched out like a tight rubber band, becoming taut and more challenging to massage. A table with breast recesses maintains a more natural position for the scapulae and can minimize the tightness that accompanies soft tissues surrounding the shoulders. It makes these regions more pliable and gives you deeper access to the muscles and tendons with less effort.

The tabletop is padded for comfort. The padding is usually made of foam or multiple layers of different kinds of foam. Padding is usually between 2 and 3 inches thick, and although thicker and firmer padding is more comfortable for clients, it tends to be heavier and bulkier. If you plan on carrying your table a lot, you may want to consider a 2-inch layer of padding instead of 3 inches (Fig. 13-3). Natural fibers such as cotton and wool are also available as padding material, but they are usually a separate layer that can be placed on top of the finished table.

Over the foam, the entire tabletop is covered by a durable, leatherlike, vinyl fabric that can withstand regular cleaning with disinfectant. The covering is available in a wide range of colors, giving you an opportunity to individualize your practice and express your personality. Dirt and stains are more noticeable on the lighter colors, but clients usually only see the sheets or towels on top of your table instead of any stains or the color of the table.

Some table coverings are buttery soft and supple to the touch. They are more expensive than the standard vinyl,

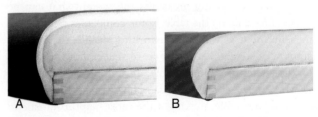

Figure 13-3. Foam padding. (A) Three layer. (B) One layer. (Photos courtesy of EarthLite.)

implying that they are better or more comfortable. These soft coverings tend to be less durable than the standard vinyl and are more susceptible to scratches and tears. The standard vinyl is a more practical option for tables that are moved around a lot or that receive a lot of use.

Table Support

Massage tabletops are supported by four wooden or metal legs or a single metal pedestal. Tables are occasionally constructed with a fixed height, but most tables can be adjusted to different heights, providing the following benefits:

- Different therapists of different heights can use the same table.
- Clients of different sizes and thicknesses can be positioned at the same working height.
- Variable table height accommodates multiple body-work techniques.

Manually adjustable tables are the most common with massage therapists due to their affordability and portability. The legs are constructed of two pieces of wood or metal that can be bolted together in different positions to create different lengths. As clients get on and off the table and as the table is moved or cleaned, the table experiences torque, or twisting forces, and uneven weight distribution. These mechanical forces can wiggle the bolts loose, making the table leg weak and wobbly. **The table leg bolts must be checked for tightness on a regular basis to maintain the table's stability.**

A guideline for checking leg bolts is every 5 to 10 clients or each time the table is moved. An unstable massage table can flex, shift, and squeak during the massage. The movement and noises can distract clients into thinking the table might collapse, which obviously does not promote a feeling of comfort and safety. The stability of the table is reinforced with bracing to keep the table from collapsing. There are usually wooden dowels and/or plastic-coated wire cables that attach the legs to the tabletop. Between the two legs at either end of the table, wooden panels or cross braces of different shapes and sizes provide additional stabilization.

Electric-lift or hydraulic massage tables are designed to allow you to raise and lower the table, making height adjustment quick and easy. The trade-off for this easy adjustability is a higher price and the fact that their placement is fairly permanent. They are supported by a central hydraulic pedestal instead of four legs at the corners of the table. The ease of adjustment allows you to customize your techniques according to the client's size and ability to maneuver on the table. For elderly clients or clients who do not move well or who have difficulties with balance, the hydraulic tables enable you to lower the table for them to get on the table,

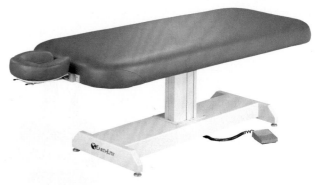

Figure 13-4. Electric-lift table. (Photo courtesy of EarthLite.)

raise the table to perform the massage, and then lower the table again for them to get off the table. The hydraulic lifts also allow you to adjust the table, and subsequently your technique, to the person on the table. For example, you can easily lower the table if a client has a larger frame or raise it if a client has a smaller frame, allowing you to protect your body and hands with proper alignment and body mechanics. This ease of adjustment may contribute to the longevity of your career. These hydraulic lift tables may qualify for a tax credit for American Disabilities Act. Check with your accountant and the table manufacturer to see if you qualify for this credit (Fig. 13-4).

Proper Table Height

You need to set your table at the proper height to use it efficiently. Most tables can be adjusted to heights between 24 and 34 inches, but special Shiatsu tables, mat tables, and Feldenkrais tables can be set as low as 17 inches. For general relaxation massage, if you are standing next to the table with your arms relaxed at your sides, the top of the table should be about even with the middle of your index finger or the middle of your thigh. This is a general guideline for setting your table height, but experience may lead you to a different, more comfortable setting (Fig. 13-5).

Make sure your table legs are all set at the same heights. If you need to adjust the height of the legs by yourself, make adjustments carefully and make sure no one puts any weight on the table while you are changing the lengths of the legs. Massage school tables are typically used by multiple students of different heights and are adjusted daily. It is likely you have adjusted the table you use in class. **Make sure all four legs are adjusted to the same setting and the bolts are all secured before a client or anyone gets on the table.**

Stationary Tables

Now we explore the different purposes and designs of stationary and portable tables. Stationary massage tables are

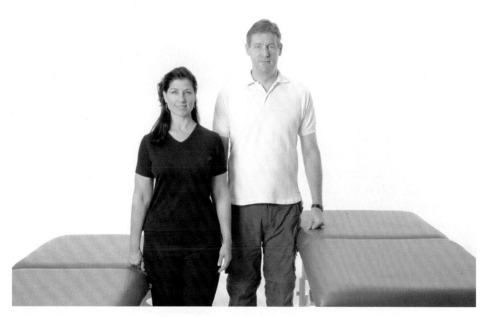

Figure 13-5. Proper table height.

intended to stay in one place for long periods. They are designed and constructed as solid, stable, permanent pieces of equipment that are very sturdy and heavy (Fig. 13-6). The benefits of a stationary table are also its disadvantages, depending on the table's purpose and your needs. In a treatment room, the stationary table remains in place and everyone and everything must work around it. The permanence gives some people a sense of familiarity and comfort, but for those who need to take their table to different places, a stationary table is impractical.

Portable Tables

If you plan on taking your table to different locations such as sporting events, outcall appointments, or your home, you need a portable table. Portable massage tables are designed and built for transport with minimal trouble, so their construction is very different from the stationary

ones (Fig. 13-7). They have four collapsible legs and a top that can be folded in half via a hinge that is secured to both halves. The hinge is a structural weak spot, so a hinge that spans the width of the table provides more stability than a couple of small hinges placed along the fold. There are usually two clasps at the end of the table to keep it locked in the folded position for safe transport.

The portability of the table is relative. Even folded up, these tables are still awkward to carry around because of their size, shape, and weight. The lightest table, which is about 22 pounds, is still unwieldy. The folded table may or may not fit in the trunk or backseat of your car, so you should try to fit different-sized tables into your car before buying a table.

There are equipment accessories that make carrying your table a lot easier (Fig. 13-8). Carrying cases are available and highly recommended. They have a shoulder strap and handle that make it easier to carry the table, and their rugged fabric protects tables from bumps, scratches, and tears. Another option, which you can use with or without a

Figure 13-6. Stationary table. (Photo courtesy of EarthLite.)

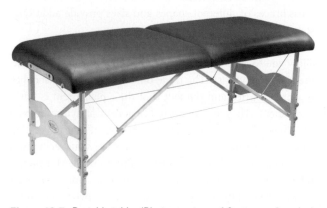

Figure 13-7. Portable table. (Photo courtesy of Customcraftworks.)

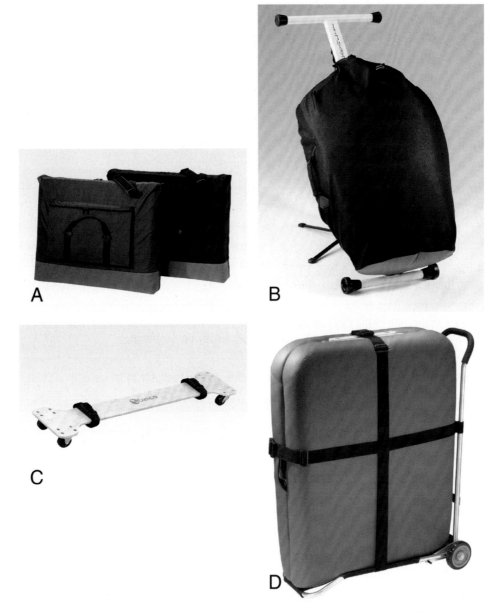

Figure 13-8. Massage accessories. **(A)** Massage table bag. **(B)** Massage chair bag. **(C)** Massage table skate. **(D)** Massage table cart. (Photos A–C, courtesy of EarthLite; D, courtesy of Customcraftworks.)

carrying case, is a set of wheels. You can put your table on a luggage dolly, massage table skate, or massage table cart to roll it around instead of carrying it. Using both the carrying case and a set of wheels greatly reduces the stress and strain on your body.

Portable Table Set-up and Takedown

Setting up a portable massage table is not complicated, but it does take some practice. See Box 13-1 for the portable table set-up procedure. Again, if you have to stand the table up by yourself, avoid any torque or twisting motion by pulling on the handles evenly. Better yet, ask someone to help you pick

up the table. Each of you can grab an end of the table with both hands, carefully rotate it until it is upright, and gently set it down.

The breakdown procedure is just the opposite of set-up. Carefully place the table on its side, on the little rubber feet, fold up the legs and top, making sure the cables or dowels are stored in their appropriate places, and then lock the clasps. Check with your massage equipment manufacturer for specific directions and procedures for setting up your table, adjusting your table, and putting your table away.

Once you have practiced table set-up and breakdown as well as transporting a table in and out of buildings and cars, you may find that you like it or that it is too much trouble.

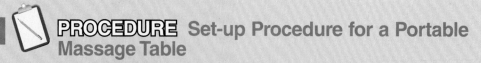

BOX 13-1 **PROCEDURE** Set-up Procedure for a Portable Massage Table

1. First, gently set the table on its edge, on the little rubber feet.

2. Unlock the clasps and open the table up slightly.

3. Flip the clasps closed to keep them from sticking out and poking someone.

4. Continue to open up the table, unfolding the legs and the top.

5. Adjust the cable system or wooden crosspieces and open the table completely while it is on its side.

6. Stand between the legs of the table, facing the center hinge.

7. Hold the handles on the side of the table (or grab the edge of the table with your hands, one hand for each half of the tabletop) and slowly walk backward while pulling down gently on the handles.

8. Let the legs that are closest to the ground stay in place while you tip the table to an upright position.

You may decide that you do not want a massage table of any kind or that you want to add variety to your practice with other equipment. Some equipment options include massage chairs and massage mats.

Face Cradles

The most awkward part of lying face down is the head placement. Generally, clients are most comfortable when the neck is in a neutral position (no neck rotation, lateral flexion, excessive extension, excessive flexion, projection, or retraction). The face cradle allows clients to keep a neutral neck and still breathe through their nose and mouth. Some clients are uncomfortable with face cradles, despite the neutral neck position. They may feel confined, there may be too much pressure on their sinuses, or they may have difficulty breathing through the hole. Most people, however, prefer using a face cradle.

Sometimes called a face rest, headrest, or head support, this horseshoe-shaped support is padded and covered like a massage table (Fig. 13-9). The covered padding is usually attached to a wooden support base with Velcro, so you can remove the padded part and use it as a neck bolster in the supine position. The Velcro also makes it possible for you to adjust the position of the padding closer to or farther from the table, essentially extending the length of your table or

using it as a neck bolster, which works especially well for the side-lying position.

Fixed face cradles attach to the end of the table, and their padded surface is level with the padded tabletop. They eliminate neck rotation and lateral flexion, but the size or posture of your clients may force their necks into flexion, extension, projection, or retraction.

Adjustable face cradles also attach to the end of the table; however, they can be adjusted to accommodate differences in clients as well as provide greater access to the neck area. Most adjustable face cradles offer tilt adjustment that uses a pivot mechanism to raise or lower the forehead. Some adjustable face cradles also offer height adjustment that uses a telescoping mechanism to raise and lower the face cradle while keeping its surface horizontal. This is especially beneficial for persons with a large frame or a large chest. The prices vary with construction and gradually increase with additional adjustable options.

Table Extensions

Table extensions are not used as much as some of the other accessories, but they offer clients additional support and comfort. They are especially beneficial for clients who are tall or wide or whose arms rest in an abducted position. Table extensions such as footrests and ankle rests attach to the end of the table to increase its length. Arm shelves hang

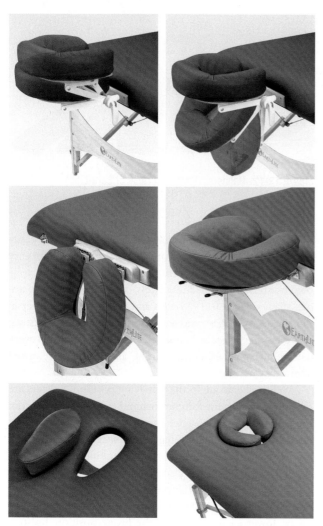

Figure 13-9. Face cradle assortment. (Photos courtesy of EarthLite.)

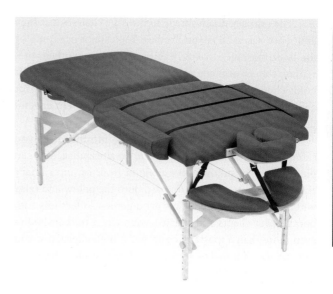

Figure 13-10. Table with arm shelves and armrests. (Photo courtesy of EarthLite.)

give chair massages at public venues, health fairs, conference halls, and business offices. Chair massage is an excellent marketing and promotion tool for your business because you can demonstrate massage therapy in public, out in the open, to large numbers of people.

beneath the face cradle to give clients a place to rest their arms while in the prone position. Armrests attach to the sides of the table, adding extra width that allows clients to rest their arms comfortably at their sides (Fig. 13-10).

Massage Chairs

Massage chairs are designed to support fully clothed clients in a seated position, leaning forward and relaxed. They have a padded seat that tilts forward; padded platforms for the client's shins, chest, and arms; and a padded face cradle (Fig. 13-11). Different designs and construction are available, and their weight varies accordingly. Like massage tables, the size and shape are more troublesome than the weight.

The main benefit to using a massage chair is that they can be used almost anywhere. They are portable and take up less floor space than massage tables. Since clients remain fully clothed, privacy is not an issue. As a result, you can

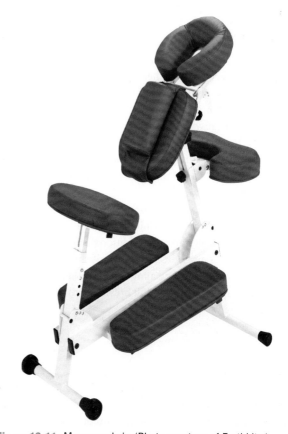

Figure 13-11. Massage chair. (Photo courtesy of EarthLite.)

The primary disadvantage to massage chairs is that they limit your access to clients' bodies. You cannot use some of the basic massage strokes because clients are clothed, preventing skin-to-skin contact. Because the design of the chair holds clients in a fairly confined position, it restricts your ability to manipulate their bodies and move them around during the massage.

When clients have trouble getting into the chair, you can offer your assistance or provide an alternative. You can put a pillow or pillows on a table in front of an ordinary chair, and clients can lean forward onto the pillow and relax without being confined. This arrangement offers less support to your clients and restricts your access to their bodies even more than a massage chair, but it is an alternative you can consider if it makes your clients more comfortable.

Massage Mats

Rather than using a massage table or chair, you can also use a massage mat or Shiatsu mat as your primary piece of equipment. These padded mats are placed on the floor and provide a supportive, comfortable surface for your clients to lie on. They come in a variety of prices and styles, ranging from those with organic cotton padding and coverings to those that resemble the tops of massage tables. The construction and materials of massage mats determine their ability to be rolled up or folded for storage and transport.

A variation of the massage mat is a set of specially shaped cushions called body cushions, body support systems, or body positioning cushions. By placing them on a large, flat surface such as the floor or a table, you can use these cushion systems as a lightweight alternative to massage tables in almost any home or office. They offer a less expensive alternative, but some drawbacks accompany their versatility. It may not be possible to properly disinfect the table or floor that supports the cushions, clients may find them unpleasant to lie on, and you may have difficulty accessing a client's body.

Depending on which support pieces you use, and in what combination, these cushion systems can also be used on top of a massage table for additional support and comfort. They reduce pressure on joints, tilt the pelvis forward to relax the lower back, and allow clients to keep their necks neutral (facing forward) and still breathe comfortably in the prone position.

Bolsters

A bolster is a pillow-like cushion that offers additional support for client positioning. Massage equipment manufacturers sell vinyl-covered bolsters in a variety of sizes and shapes

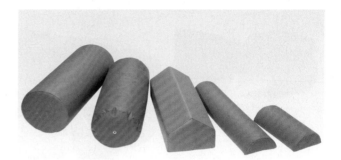

Figure 13-12. Bolsters. (Photo courtesy of EarthLite.)

(Fig. 13-12). They are convenient because they can be easily disinfected, are durable, and are slippery, making them easy to position and remove. Another option is to make your own bolsters with rolled-up towels, pillows, or foam of various shapes (Fig. 13-13). Towels and pillows are more versatile, more convenient, and less expensive than retail bolsters; however, they must be laundered and disinfected after every use or have a covering that can be disinfected or removed after every massage.

When clients are in the side-lying position, bolsters are especially important for comfort and necessary support in the following places: under the neck and head to prevent neck strain, under the top leg that is flexed forward, under the top arm that is flexed forward, and along the client's back. Supine clients can also benefit from properly placed bolsters at the cervical curve of the neck and the head, under the knees, or under the entire lower leg, including the knees, lower legs, and feet. In the prone position, bolsters are typically used under the ankles, under the pelvis, and under the chest, just below the sternal notch.

Massage Tools

When you give several massages on a daily basis, your body will, at some point, develop aches and pains. You may want to try using some of the many tools and gadgets available in

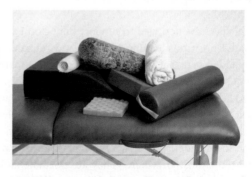

Figure 13-13. Homemade bolsters: pillows, rolled-up towels, and foam.

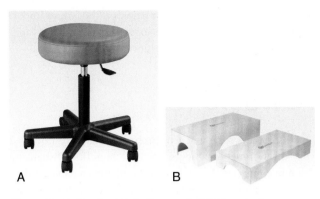

Figure 13-14. Stools. **(A)** Rolling stool. **(B)** Step stools. (Photos courtesy of EarthLite.)

retail stores that can minimize the physical stress of giving a massage. While many of these tools are marketed toward people who are not massage therapists, you can also find professional tools advertised in the massage trade journals and magazines and at trade shows.

Instead of using your own thumb or finger to deliver the pressure, which puts undue stress on your joints, you can hold tools in the proper position in your hand and simply lean on them to deliver the pressure. There are electric massage machines that thump and vibrate, which are good for clients with very restricted tissues. Sometimes, when such clients get on the table, it can take 20 minutes or more to soften the tissues enough to work through the layers. Instead of using your own physical work to soften and warm those restricted tissues, you can use the machine to do that work. These tools can also be recommended to clients to use for self-care, as long as you remember to specify durations and frequencies for using them.

Standing requires more work than sitting, so you can save a little energy by doing some of your work while you sit down. Ordinary chairs are adequate, but rolling chairs or rolling stools are preferred because they let you keep your hands on your clients while you roll the chair to a new position. Step stools are handy for clients who need help getting on and off your table (Fig. 13-14).

Lubricants

Lubricants are products used to reduce friction between your skin and the client's skin and increase the comfort of the massage strokes (Fig. 13-15). Most people think of lubricants as wet substances such as oils, lotions, creams, and gels; however, you can also use dry powders as massage lubricants. Experiment with a variety of products to get an idea of:

- How much slip they provide
- How long they stay slippery on the skin before they dry out
- How much you need to use for the amount of slip you want

- How easily they can be dispensed during a massage
- Cost

Lubricants can be expensive, so rather than purchase different types, try to find free samples. Some lubricant suppliers market their products to massage schools and massage students by giving out trial-sized samples. These suppliers usually have online stores or phone numbers you can use to request samples. Retail stores occasionally offer samples of massage lubricants, but one of the simplest ways to get different kinds of lubricants is to share and trade with other massage therapists.

The lubricants you use will contribute to the environment of your massage practice by influencing the strokes and techniques you use. The information here is to help you familiarize yourself with lubricants. Lubricants that are slipperier deliver a very smooth and comfortable massage stroke, but they can leave the client feeling greasy or oily after the massage. On the other hand, lubricants that are less slippery allow you to manipulate the client's body parts without dropping them and use deeper pressure without slipping, but clients may feel their skin getting dragged or pulled during the massage strokes. With practice, you will be able to determine just the right amount of lubricant to use with the technique you are applying.

Scented lubricants are widely available and can strongly affect the atmosphere and environment. You can create your own aromatherapy oils by adding plant and flower

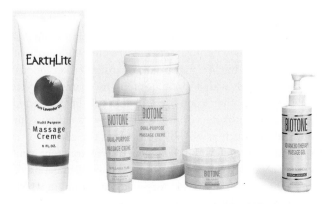

Figure 13-15. Lubricants. (Photos courtesy of EarthLite.)

essences to unscented carrier oils. Without being aware of it, you may be overwhelming clients with fragrances on your body, in your hair, in the air, on the carpet, in the laundry, in the bathroom, and in candles. Too many fragrances can cause the nervous system to "ignore" the sensory input and not respond to it. Basically, if you use a lot of scented products, you could actually decrease the effect of any one fragrance or essential oil by overstimulating the client's nervous system.

Oils

Oil spreads easily, and a little goes a long way. You can use oil for clients who have a lot of body hair because it is slippery and helps you slide over the body hair rather than pull it. The client is not likely to tell you when body hair is pulled during a massage, so it is up to you to use oil as your lubricant or use sufficient amounts of other lubricants. The disadvantages to using oil: it spills easily, it tends to stain sheets and clothing, and it is difficult to clean out of carpet.

Oils can degrade with heat, sunlight, and air, so they must be stored in a cool, dark place in an airtight container. A flip-top or pump bottle that holds just a small amount of oil is best to use in the treatment room because it allows you to store most of your oil properly and minimizes the amount of oil you can spill during a massage. Oils made from natural sources, such as fruits, vegetables, and nuts, are preferable because they are gentle on the skin and are not associated with the health risks of mineral and animal-based products. Prolonged, repeated exposure to mineral oil can irritate the skin and mucous membranes and increases the risk for cancer.[1] **Some persons have sensitivities to nut oils, so be sure to ask clients if they have any skin allergies.**

Lotions, Creams, Gels

Lotions, creams, and gels are wet lubricants that are alternatives to oils. Although laundry is not the determining factor for lubricant choice, the water-based products are easier to wash out of sheets and clothing. Dispensing wet lubricants with pumps and flip-top bottles is an easy, one-handed operation unless you use the thicker creams, in which case it is better to use a small disposable dish or cup that holds just enough cream for one massage. The benefit to using thick lubricants is that they cannot be spilled, which is helpful when you are learning how to do massage because you can focus on technique instead of your lubricant. Check the ingredient lists for several different lubricants and notice how they vary. Lanolin is an animal-based product blended into a number of lotions and creams, depending on the

manufacturer. It can cause skin irritation, but more importantly, it can contain cancer-causing pesticides, making lanolin a controversial ingredient in lubricants.[2]

Powders

Dry lubricants such as cornstarch and chalk are not used very often; however, they have some benefits. Dispensing dry lubricants is tricky to do without making a cloud of dust that can irritate the client's and/or your respiratory system, but the advantages are worth considering. Powders work particularly well when you use both gliding strokes and deep compressive strokes in one massage, because they let you slide across the skin yet still apply deep pressure without slipping. Clients who need to return to work after their massage will not want to feel greasy or sticky afterward. To avoid that altogether, you can use dry lubricants.

Cornstarch is a plant product that is safe to use because it does not have any toxic effects. Chalk is available as a powder with negligible health risks, but because it is a mineral product, it can irritate the skin.[3] Talcum powder is not recommended because talc is a mineral product that often contains asbestos-like structures associated with cancer risks and respiratory illness.[4]

Lubricant Storage

To protect your lubricants from contamination, there are some sanitary practices you should follow. Basically, the lubricant should be isolated so that it only comes in contact with skin when it is dispensed into your hands for immediate use on a client. Isolate your lubricant by using two different containers: a small dispenser and a larger storage container. In your treatment room, keep the lubricant in a small container that does not contact the client's skin such as a pump dispenser, flip-top bottle, or squeezable tube. The larger supply of lubricant can be kept in a big container either in or outside the treatment room, as long as it is kept at room temperature and kept out of direct sunlight. When your smaller dispenser runs low on lubricant, you can refill it from the large supply container. Oils and thin lotions can be poured directly into your dispenser with minimal risk of contamination, but you may need to transfer thicker lotions, creams, and gels with a spoon or pump mechanism. If you use a spoon or other scoop-like tool, it should be disinfected before being introduced into your supply. Isolating your lubricant as much as possible minimizes the chance of it being contaminated with germs from the environment, you, or your clients. The biggest problem with contamination of your lubricant is the risk for cross-contamination, in which germs are passed from person to person via the lubricant.

Application of Lubricants

It takes practice to learn to use lubricants effectively and efficiently. First, lubricants should always be dispensed into your own hands instead of being applied directly to the client's skin. Although the recommended amount of lubricant to use varies, depending on the type of lubricant, your school, the instructor, the area of the body receiving the lubricant, the techniques you use, and the condition of the client's skin, there are sometimes directions for use on the product label. Generally, you will use more lubricant for wellness massage than for therapeutic massage because there are several therapeutic techniques that require minimal slip on the skin or require you to hold and move your client's body securely.

Because it is easier to add more lubricant than remove it, it is more practical to start out with a small amount. **Less is more when it comes to the amount of lubricant you use.** A series of steps for dispensing and applying the lubricant is outlined below. (Note: the specific directions for the left and right hands are for right-handed persons; if you are left handed, use the opposite hands as specified in the directions.)

1. Leave your left hand on the client's skin while you dispense about a penny- or nickel-sized amount of lubricant.
    a. If you are using a pump dispenser, use your right hand to push the pump once and catch the lubricant.
    b. If you are using a squirt bottle or squeezable tube, use your right hand to pick up the bottle and squirt lubricant into the palm of your left hand.
    c. If you are using an open cup or dish, use one or two fingers from your right hand to scoop out some lubricant and smear it onto your left palm.
    d. If you are using a powder, use your right hand to lift the container and carefully shake or pour a thin layer of powder into your left palm.

2. Rub your palms together to spread the lubricant evenly on both hands and warm it up a little.
3. Gently apply the lubricant to your client's skin.
4. If you feel your strokes pulling on the client's skin or body hair, you can try using more lubricant.

Lubricants are usually spread thinly and evenly in a slow, sweeping motion using both hands. The objective is to dispense enough lubricant to cover the whole area you will be immediately working on so you will not need multiple applications of lubricant to one area. The massage will flow more smoothly and you will be less distracted if you use enough lubricant on the first application.

Initial touch has a stimulating effect on the body, whereas sustained touch has a more relaxing effect. For this reason, you should minimize the number of times you break contact with the client's skin during the massage, even when you need more lubricant.

Occasionally, you will find that your lubricant dispenser is out of reach when you need it. This is an awkward situation for the beginning student who wants to maintain contact but needs to retrieve the lubricant dispenser. When this happens, you have some options:

- You can break contact briefly to retrieve the dispenser.
- You can slowly "walk" your hands along the client's body to retrieve the dispenser.
- You can slowly and gently slide your contact hand along the client's body to retrieve the dispenser.

You can avoid this situation altogether by having several containers of lubricant placed in strategic places around the room or by keeping your lubricant dispenser in a holster that straps to your waist. Lubricant holsters keep you from dropping your lubricant or leaving it out of reach. Massage supply companies offer holsters for containers of different sizes and shapes. Before you buy one, try using one for a few massages, if possible. Although these holsters sound very helpful, some therapists do not like to use them.

Hygiene and Sanitation

A successful therapist understands and practices good personal hygiene, standard precautions, and, if necessary, transmission-based precautions and sanitation procedures. **Standard precautions**, which are specific procedures that maintain a hygienic and sanitary practice, reduce the risk for germ transmission. This section focuses on understanding the methods necessary for preventing disease transmission and minimizing the risks for allergic responses. Some of the massage laws and regulations (see www.massagetherapy.com) include guidelines for sanitation and safety, but at the time of publication, national regulations for massage have yet to be standardized.

Your client-centered focus requires that you do everything you can to keep your clients healthy and safe. In addition to following the guidelines for sanitation and safety, you need to know about diseases and how they are transmitted before understanding how to prevent the spread of diseases.

Disease

A disease is an abnormal condition of the appearance, structure, or function of an organism or its parts. There are two categories of disease: noninfectious and infectious.

Noninfectious Disease

A noninfectious disease is caused by internal and external factors that cannot be transmitted with any kind of contact.

Noninfectious diseases cause symptoms and can be generally separated into the following nonexclusive categories (Table 13-1):

- Cancer
- Degenerative
- Environmental
- Genetic
- Metabolic
- Neurologic–psychiatric
- Nutritional

Generally, massage therapists cannot protect clients from noninfectious diseases; however, massage therapists may help clients manage noninfectious diseases. **Take special precautions for the client who has environmental allergies and sensitivities to chemicals, pets, pollen, and materials.**

Table 13-1 Categories of Noninfectious Disease

Noninfectious Disease	Description	Examples
Cancer	Cells replicate and grow at abnormally high rates	Breast cancer Leukemia Skin cancer Lymphoma
Degenerative	Part of the organism is deteriorating	Alzheimer's disease Multiple sclerosis Osteoarthritis Osteoporosis Autoimmune diseases such as AIDS and lupus erythematosus
Environmental	Chemicals, particles, and radiation from the environment cause symptoms	Allergies Lead poisoning Asbestosis
Genetic	The genetic coding in the DNA is abnormal	Cystic fibrosis Down syndrome Hemophilia
Metabolic	The cells or tissues function abnormally	Diabetes Cardiovascular disease Hypoglycemia
Neurologic–psychiatric	A complex interaction of brain chemicals and psychological disorders	Depression Addiction Seasonal affective disorder
Nutrition	Deficiency of nutrients acquired through diet	Iron deficiency anemia Scurvy

During the initial intake, inquire about client's allergies and sensitivities and make sure that the offending allergens or products are not present in your practice. Some allergies are life threatening; if you know a client is allergic to something in your practice, you have a responsibility to share that information with him or her and offer a referral to another qualified therapist. Sensitivities are generally not as critical as allergies, but you should still make your clients aware of anything in your practice that could trigger an immune reaction. Let those clients decide whether they want to continue with treatment or need a referral to another therapist. As a massage therapist, it is important to know that specific nutritional recommendations are not within your scope of practice, but you can educate clients about nutritional deficiencies and refer them to the appropriate healthcare practitioner. One way to educate clients is to have nutritional reference books and/or articles so you may look up particular questions, show the client, or give them a copy of the information to take home.

Infectious Disease

Infectious diseases are more critical to understand because they can be transmitted by contact with germs. A germ is a common term for a pathogen, or pathogenic microorganism, which is a microscopic organism that can cause disease in other organisms. There are thousands of different kinds of microorganisms, which come in the forms of algae, bacteria, fungi, protozoa, and viruses, but only a small percentage of them are pathogens. In fact, there are normally millions of microorganisms in and on our bodies that are nonpathogenic and beneficial to us. For a pathogen to be transmitted, it must be acquired by an organism in one of three ways:

- Contact transmission
  - Direct contact—a host organism physically transfers a pathogen to another person via touching, kissing, or sexual intercourse
  - Indirect contact—a host organism leaves a pathogen on a fomite, or inanimate object such as a doorknob, table, or chair, and the pathogen is transferred to someone else who touches that fomite
  - Droplets—a host organism forcefully expels mucus by spitting, sneezing, or coughing on another person, and a pathogen in the mucus is transferred to another person
- Vehicle transmission
  - Air—pathogens are either suspended in a mist of very fine mucous droplets or have become airborne as a result of evaporation of a mucous droplet, and they are transferred to someone who contacts them in the air
  - Food—pathogens residing in food are transferred to persons who eat the contaminated food
  - Liquid—pathogens residing in water or other liquids are transferred to persons who drink the contaminated liquid
- Vector transmission
  - Mosquitoes
  - Flies
  - Rats

Healthy immune systems normally inactivate or destroy acquired pathogens, but when the immune system does not do its job, pathogens can establish themselves, multiply, and cause disease in the host organism. You cannot know how effective your client's immune system is or who might be carrying pathogens. **Do your best to keep everyone healthy with procedures that prevent any existing pathogens from being transmitted.** To achieve this, use the information in the remainder of the chapter to guide you.

Hepatitis and Human Immunodeficiency Virus

Of the numerous pathogens you may encounter, two in particular have become the focus of public health: hepatitis and human immunodeficiency virus (HIV). Public awareness has been raised for these viruses because of their modes of transmission and the symptoms of their associated illnesses.

Although hepatitis is directly translated as "an inflammation of the liver," it is a condition usually caused by a virus (hepatitis A to G, with A, B, and C being most common) that can wreak havoc on a person's health. Hepatitis A is a short, acute infection transmitted via the fecal–oral route, via contaminated food or water. Symptoms of hepatitis include headache, nausea, vomiting, abdominal pain, jaundice, diarrhea, and fatigue that generally last up to 6 months. For example, if John is infected with hepatitis A and does not properly wash his hands after using the toilet, he can transfer the virus from his hands to anything he touches, such as a doorknob, chair, cash, phone, or water cooler. Anyone who touches those surfaces can then pick up the virus, and the next time they touch their mouth or eat food, the virus can enter and potentially infect that person. Proper handwashing can significantly decrease the spread of hepatitis A. Hepatitis B virus is transmitted via bodily fluids such as blood, semen, vaginal fluid, and sometimes saliva. A person typically recovers with immunity and no serious issues; however, 5% of those infected with hepatitis B suffer long-term chronic infections and are carriers of the disease. Massage that enhances circulation is contraindicated in the acute phase of hepatitis B but is fine for those who recover with no symptoms. Hepatitis C is a bloodborne infection that causes mild fever, nausea, weakness, and sometimes jaundice that often do not appear for years after the person contracted the infection. It is transmitted via blood transfusion, shared needles, or tattoo or body piercing instruments. Circulatory massage in the acute phase of hepatitis C is contraindicated. Treatment for each type of hepatitis differs, depending on which virus is involved and the length the infection. For example, hepatitis A usually resolves itself in time, but hepatitis B and C require intensive medical treatment, often involving one or more medications. **If a client currently has or has had any form of hepatitis, you should check with his or her primary healthcare professional before proceeding with massage.** You should also follow the standard precautions found in this chapter.

HIV attacks specific cells of the immune system, compromising the body's ability to fight pathogens. The progression of the virus occurs in five phases. It is in the first phase, in which the virus is activated but no symptoms are present, that a person is most contagious. This phase lasts for an average of 3 weeks to 6 months but can last for up to a year. HIV is spread through the exchange of intimate fluids including blood, semen, vaginal secretions, and breast milk. To date, there is no data showing that HIV is concentrated enough in body fluids such as saliva, sweat, or tears to transmit the disease. Neither has it been proven that HIV can spread through casual contact. In the second phase, usually lasting 2 weeks, the early flu-like symptoms of HIV emerge—fever, weight loss, headache, fatigue, and enlarged lymph nodes. During phase three, the symptoms disappear and the virus duplicates itself, generally over a period of 1 to 15 years, depending on the general health of the person infected. Medical treatment is most helpful during this phase to help prolong the life expectancy of a person with HIV. Phases four and five occur when the virus reaches the advanced stages of HIV infection, which is called acquired immunodeficiency syndrome (AIDS). According to the Centers for Disease Control and Prevention (CDC), AIDS is diagnosed when a person's helper T-cell count drops below 200. Due to the body's inability to fight pathogens, a person with AIDS often suffers the symptoms of opportunistic illnesses such as:

- Pneumocystis carinii pneumonia: infection of the lungs
- Kaposi's sarcoma: type of skin cancer
- Non-Hodgkin's lymphoma: type of cancer that affects the lymph nodes
- Cytomegalovirus: type of herpes virus

A person is often unaware that he or she is infected with the HIV virus, so someone who comes in contact with body fluids, such as in intimate contact, shared needles, contaminated blood via transfusion, or breast milk can potentially be infected. Massage is contraindicated in phase two, when flu-like symptoms are present, and in phases four and five, when circulatory massage may further compromise the immune system. Massage is indicated in phase three when the client is asymptomatic. Before performing any massage treatment, it is best to consult the client's primary healthcare professional regarding massage to develop a complementary treatment plan.

Preventing Transmission of Pathogens

Most likely, you will not know if you or your clients are harboring harmful pathogens; therefore, it is wise for you to assume that pathogens are present and use the appropriate procedures to keep them from being transmitted via direct contact, indirect contact, and vehicles such as air, food, and liquids. In 1987, the CDC created an overall approach to infection control called universal precautions to prevent the spread of bloodborne pathogens such as hepatitis B and HIV. The CDC updated its infection control protocols in 1996 and again in 2007 in which it outlines a set of standard precautions and transmission-based precautions to prevent the spread of pathogens that reside in *all* body secretions—blood, semen, vaginal secretions, tears, saliva, nasal secretions, urine, feces, and vomitus. These precautions are the practical applications of universal precautions. **Because massage therapists are exposed to pathogens from all body secretions instead of just bloodborne ones, it is critical for you to follow standard precautions and be aware of transmission-based precautions in your massage practice.**

Standard precautions include:

- Proper hand hygiene
- Barrier techniques
- Proper cleaning and sanitizing procedures
- Proper disposal techniques

Transmission-based precautions are in addition to standard precautions and include

- Contact precautions—environmental preventions such as personal protective equipment (PPE) (gowns, masks, gloves) as well as disinfection of the environment
- Droplet precautions—protecting against respiratory or mucous membrane secretions via PPE
- Airborne precautions—protecting against pathogens that travel over long distances such as measles, chickenpox, or tuberculosis (TB), which requires isolation

in a hospital setting. In massage, these conditions are contraindicated and massage sessions should be postponed until the client has recovered.

In addition to the standard precautions and transmission-based precautions that are intended to prevent pathogen transmission by direct contact, by indirect contact, and through the air, you will also need to use some common sense to keep your clients safe from germs. If you know you are infected with a pathogen such as the influenza virus (the flu) or streptococcus bacteria (strep throat) or any other contagious condition, inform your clients and either postpone their appointment/s or refer them to another massage therapist until you recover and are no longer contagious. Additionally, avoid offering clients food or drinks that are not individually wrapped and sealed or that are not dispensed from sterile containers. For example, homemade baked goods or a cup of hot tea may seem like a nice treat to offer clients, but you cannot be sure that they do not contain harmful pathogens that could cause illness. It is acceptable to offer individually wrapped mints, snacks, or tea bags. You can safely offer clean, disposable cups and water from a cooler that holds 5-gallon bottles that are sealed when you purchase them. Knowing the mechanisms for pathogen transmission will help you minimize the pathogenic risks to your clients. For a more advanced text on massage-specific disease prevention, you can refer to *Massage for the Hospital Patient and Medically Frail Client* by Gail MacDonald (Lippincott Williams & Wilkins, 2005).

Hand Hygiene

The CDC has shown that when hand hygiene procedures are followed, the spread of pathogens is reduced. Further, it is important to keep your fingernails short and avoid wearing artificial fingernails. The CDC makes no specific recommendations regarding jewelry; however, because it may scratch or be uncomfortable to clients and lubricant can accumulate in the jewelry and potentially harbor pathogens, it is wise for you to remove jewelry from your hands during massage. Make sure your hands are kept moisturized with lotions or creams to prevent them from cracking and increasing the risk of pathogen transmission. Above all, wash your hands properly. **The CDC has determined that handwashing is the single most important procedure for the prevention of infection.** Thoroughly wash your hands immediately before and immediately after massaging your clients, immediately after contacting any bodily fluids, and immediately after taking off protective gloves. You can use traditional soap and water, antimicrobial soap and water, or alcohol-based hand rubs. It is safer to use pump dispensers for soap because soap can harbor some pathogens. Box 13-2 illustrates proper handwashing technique.

In addition to washing with soap and water, the CDC has determined that healthcare workers can also use alcohol-based hand rubs as a suitable alternative. These rubs significantly reduce the pathogens on your skin very quickly, and they are not as likely to cause skin irritation with repeated use. Before and after massaging each client, you can apply the alcohol-based hand rub (as directed on the product) to the palm of your hand, rub your hands together to cover all of your hands and fingers, and continue rubbing until your hands are dry. Antimicrobial disposable wipes are not as effective as handwashing or alcohol-based rubs and should not be used in their place.

Barrier Techniques

On the rare occasions when a client leaves bodily fluids on your massage table or anywhere else in your practice, you need to know how to safely use barrier techniques. There are numerous protective physical barriers defined by the CDC as PPE, such as latex gloves, gowns, aprons, masks, or protective eyewear that can reduce the risk of acquiring pathogens on your skin or mucous membranes any time you contact blood or bodily fluids (Fig. 13-16).

You should wear latex gloves if you have to touch any bodily fluids except sweat, any surfaces that have bodily fluids on them, your clients' mucous membranes, and clients' skin that is not intact (has a cut or open wound). Remove gloves and properly dispose of them into a closed container after contact with each patient or contaminated surface. You could accidentally be contaminated by small defects in the gloves or while you are removing the gloves, so you *must* wash your hands and other exposed skin surfaces immediately after removing the gloves. Using gloves does not eliminate the need for hand hygiene, and the use of hand hygiene does not eliminate the need for gloves.

You may find it challenging to work with gloves on. They reduce the sensitivity of your hands, and you and/or your client may be allergic to latex. If you or your clients have latex sensitivities or latex allergies, there are substitutes you can use. Vinyl gloves are similar in cost to latex, but because they are not as durable, avoid wearing them for longer than 30 minutes. Gloves made of nitrile, neoprene, and thermoplastic elastomers are suitable alternatives whose durability and strength equal or exceed those of latex. **Before you use gloves in sessions, be sure to ask your clients if they have allergies to latex.**

Aseptic Techniques

Asepsis is the process of removing pathogens or protecting from infection. Using aseptic techniques will help keep you,

BOX 13-2 **PROCEDURE** Proper Handwashing Technique

1. Remove rings, watch, and bracelets and push sleeves up to the elbows. Stand close to the sink, but do not allow your clothing to touch it.

2. Turn on the water and adjust the temperature to warm (water that is too hot or cold can cause skin to crack or chap, increasing the risk of infection). Wet your hands and wrists under warm running water, apply liquid soap, and work the soap into a lather by rubbing your palms together.

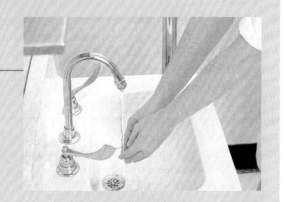

3. Scrub the palm of one hand and wrist with the fingertips of the other hand to work the soap under the nails of that hand; then reverse the procedure and scrub the other hand and wrist. This step should take at least 30 seconds.

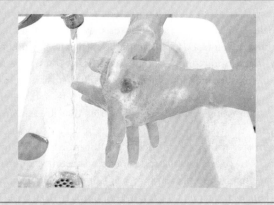

4. With fingers pointing downward, and hands lower than the elbows and wrists, rinse hands and wrists thoroughly under running warm water. Do not touch the sink or you will have to repeat the entire process.

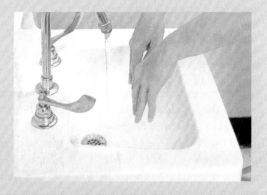

5. Dry hands and wrists thoroughly with a paper towel. Discard the paper towel in the waste can when finished. Use another paper towel to turn off the faucet, and discard that paper towel.

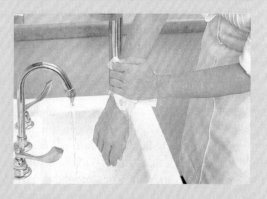

Figure 13-16. Using latex gloves as a protective barrier during massage.

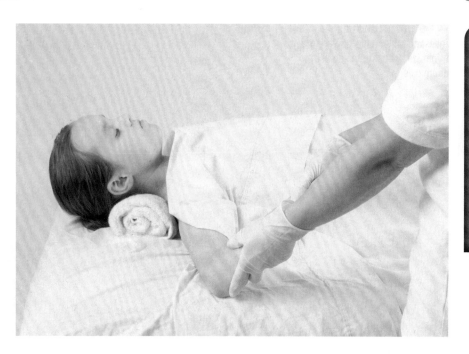

the massage therapist, and your clients from transmitting infectious agents. There are three aseptic techniques that can be used to minimize infectious agents: antiseptics, disinfectants, and sterilization. Antiseptics, such as hand soap, rubbing alcohol, and hydrogen peroxide, are safe to use on your skin and minimize (but do not totally destroy) germs and bacteria. Disinfectants are strong solutions that are very effective in destroying bacteria and germs on equipment and surfaces. They are generally too strong to apply with your bare hands, so gloves are recommended. Bleach, phenolic solution or spray, and quaternary ammonium compounds (quats) are examples of disinfectants. Finally, sterilization techniques such as baking, boiling, or steaming surfaces and/or tools use high heat for a period of time to kill germs and bacteria. Massage therapists can generally maintain asepsis if they use handwashing and/or hand sanitizers before and after massages along with disinfectants to keep massage equipment and other surfaces free of germs and bacteria.

Cleaning and Sanitizing Procedures

Keep your massage room and office or home space clean and clear of debris, pests, trash, spills, or any other potential hazards. Clean and disinfect toilets, sinks, and other surfaces that are touched frequently: doorknobs, light switches, faucet handles, water dispenser handles, lotion/oil dispensers, telephone, chairs, and desktops. The surfaces that need to be cleaned when they appear dusty or dirty include the walls, blinds, and window treatments.

It is critical to clean your equipment. **The massage table, face cradle, vinyl-covered bolsters, table extensions, stools, and linens must be properly disinfected after every client.**

Even if you use disposable linens and face cradle covers, your equipment needs to be disinfected after every use (Fig. 13-17). Antimicrobial and antibacterial products are not strong enough to eliminate most pathogens, so make sure the solution you purchase is labeled a disinfectant. Sodium hypochlorite is an Environmental Protection Agency (EPA)-approved disinfectant and is commonly available as household bleach (which is usually 5.25% sodium hypochlorite). You can mix household bleach and water in different concentrations, depending on the strength disinfectant you need. Household bleach is the least expensive, most readily available solution with which to make an appropriate disinfectant. The disadvantage to using bleach is that it degrades quickly, and it is a harsh, caustic, corrosive chemical. Bleach solutions must be mixed daily to guarantee their ability to disinfect, and the solutions must be mixed carefully in a ventilated room. Phenolic disinfectant spray such as Lysol is readily available, easy to use, and EPA-approved, but aerosol products are discouraged by the CDC. The surfaces that need disinfection and the pathogens that need to be eliminated determine the steps required to prevent pathogen transmission. There are three generally recognized levels of infection control: high, intermediate, and low. Below is a list of the infection control levels and appropriate disinfection procedures you can use:

1. **High-level** exposures include spills of bodily fluids.

    a. Put on latex or other acceptable barrier gloves.

    b. Absorb the spill with disposable towels.

Figure 13-17. Sanitizing the massage table using gloves to minimize exposure of the skin to chemicals.

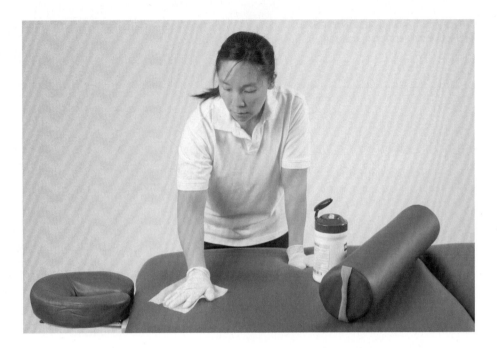

c. Apply disinfectant to the area and let it sit for 20 minutes—sodium hypochlorite (household bleach) diluted 1:50, or about 2 tablespoons per quart of water (this is a strong and corrosive mixture, so be careful with it).

d. Absorb the disinfectant solution with disposable towels.

e. Dispose of all articles with bodily fluids and used disinfectant, including gloves, in plastic bags, and seal the bags.

f. Wash hands.

g. Allow the area to dry completely.

2. **Intermediate-level** exposures include smooth, hard surfaces that come in contact with mucous membranes or broken skin.

   a. Apply enough disinfectant (identified as EPA-approved tuberculocides) to wet the entire surface and let it sit on the surface for about 10 minutes:

      i. 70% to 90% ethyl alcohol or isopropyl alcohol

      ii. Phenolic disinfectant (Lysol or equivalent), per label instructions

      iii. Sodium hypochlorite (household bleach) diluted 1:50, or about 2 tablespoons per quart of water (this is a strong and corrosive mixture, so be careful with it)

   b. Absorb the disinfectant solution with disposable towels.

   c. Dispose of towels in trash receptacle.

   d. Wash hands.

3. **Low-level** exposures include smooth, hard surfaces touched by intact skin.

   a. Apply enough disinfectant (labeled as EPA-approved hospital disinfectants) to wet the entire surface and let it sit on the surface for about 10 minutes:

      i. 70% to 90% ethyl alcohol or isopropyl alcohol

      ii. Phenolic disinfectant (Lysol or equivalent), per label instructions

      iii. Sodium hypochlorite (household bleach) diluted 1:500, or about 2 teaspoons per gallon of water

   b. Absorb the disinfectant solution with disposable towels.

   c. Dispose of used towels in trash receptacle.

Linens and Laundry

The CDC has found that although soiled linens are a source of pathogens, there is negligible risk of transmission. It recommends hygienic and common sense processing and storage of linens. All of your linens, including your sheets, towels, pillowcases, and blankets, require infection control and must be laundered after every use. Soiled sheets should be handled as little as possible and stored in a closed receptacle such as a hamper. Unless there are bodily fluids on the linens, they can be laundered in hot water at 160°F for 25 minutes with regular detergent or at a lower temperature with a disinfectant such as bleach. Dry your linens completely in a dryer instead of outside in fresh air.

If your linens are contaminated with bodily fluids, you need to handle them carefully. Wear gloves made of latex (or other material if you or your client has allergies to latex), carefully place contaminated linens in plastic bags, seal the bags, and label the bags as contaminated laundry. Use ¾ cup of household bleach per wash load of contaminated laundry, and dry your linens completely in a dryer.

Clean sheets should be stored in a way that ensures and maintains their cleanliness. Keep them off the floor, away from food or drinks, and apart from used linens. For more detailed procedures and updates on sanitation and standard precautions, you can refer to the CDC at www.cdc.org or the American Red Cross at www.redcross.org.

Safety

A clean and safe practice minimizes the risk of getting sick and getting hurt, both for you and your clients. The safety of your practice depends on sanitation as well as regular maintenance of all aspects of the business—parking lot, walkways, stairways, doors, windows, floors, furniture, electricity, and fire safety. Fire codes are government regulations for fire safety at a place of business, which deal with evacuation plans, smoke detectors, fire extinguishers, and electrical cords and outlets. Additionally, insurance coverage protects you against the legal and financial ramifications for any injuries your clients sustain on your premises.

Basic first aid training and cardiopulmonary resuscitation (CPR) certification are required for many massage therapists and highly recommended for all. Although this text is not an adequate training tool for these skills, some of the first aid and CPR skills taught by the American Red Cross and the American Heart Association are presented to give you an idea of what they teach. In addition to the primary assessment of a person in an emergency situation, first aid for choking and hot and cold weather–related conditions are included.

Every therapist should have a first aid kit on the premises. A first aid kit should minimally contain the following (see www.redcross.org for more information on classes and kits):

- Scissors
- Latex-free gloves
- Antiseptic wipes
- Gauze pads and roll
- Compresses
- Adhesive tape
- Adhesive bandages
- Antibiotic ointment
- Aspirin
- Hand sanitizer
- Hydrocortisone packets
- One-time-use thermometer
- One CPR one-way valve face shield, latex-free

Fire Safety

Fire safety is an important aspect of your practice. Check with your local fire department for specific details regarding the use of:

- Candles
- Smoke detectors—placement and regular testing
- Evacuation plans
- Fire drills
- Fire extinguishers—instructions, approved types, inspections
- Electricity—fixtures, outlets
- Stairways, walkways, doors, locks
- Fire hazards

You can also look up the US Fire Administration (http://www.usfa.fema.gov/safety) for more information on fire safety.

Primary Assessment in an Emergency Situation

An emergency situation is when someone's illness or injury requires immediate care to prevent the person from dying or being permanently disabled. There is a series of steps that determine what is wrong and what needs to be done:

1. Check the person for consciousness by pinching them and loudly asking, "Are you okay?"

2. If there is no response, assume the person is unconscious and needs help.

3. Shout, "Help!" or look at a specific person and firmly instruct them, "Dial 911!"

4. Evaluate the condition of the person using the primary assessment tools for an emergency situation that are sometimes called the ABCs:

   i. **A**irway—Tilt the person's head back and lift the chin to make sure the mouth and throat are clear of any obstructions, including the tongue. If necessary, turn the person's head to the side and perform a finger sweep to clear the mouth.

   ii. **B**reathing—Lean over the person with your ear near the person's mouth and nose to detect breathing by watching for the rise and fall of the chest, feeling air on your cheek, and hearing breath sounds. Air movement and chest movement are both required for breathing to occur. If the person is not breathing, begin artificial respiration as you were trained.

iii. **Circulation**—Determine if the person has a radial or carotid pulse. If there is no pulse, CPR must be performed immediately by a trained person. If the person is bleeding, use appropriate care for wounds and bleeding.

These assessment ABCs help you identify and correct life-threatening problems that can be dealt with before emergency medical personnel arrive. They also help you communicate the status of the victim to the emergency personnel.

Artificial Respiration

When initial assessment ABCs have determined that a person is not breathing but has a pulse, artificial respiration (also called artificial resuscitation, mouth-to-mouth respiration, and rescue breathing) is a technique that manually or mechanically forces air into a person's lungs to deliver oxygen to the person's bloodstream. **Only a person who has received supervised training and certification in first aid and CPR should administer artificial respiration.**

There are several different techniques for administering artificial respiration, but the general steps are as follows:

1. With the victim in the prone position, lift the chin with one hand, protracting the lower jaw, and use the other hand to tilt the forehead back.
2. Using the hand holding the forehead back, pinch the victim's nose closed.
3. Seal your mouth tightly over the victim's mouth.
4. Attempt to blow 2 full breaths (1 to 1.5 seconds each) into the victim.
5. If air does not enter, repeat the chin lift, head tilt, finger sweep and possibly abdominal thrusts, and try again. If air enters, give 2 full rescue breaths.
6. Check for a carotid pulse.
   a. If there is a pulse, give 1 full rescue breath every 5 seconds followed by a check for a carotid pulse. Continue until emergency medical personnel arrive or you are relieved by a trained person.
   b. If there is no pulse, begin CPR.

Cardiopulmonary Resuscitation

When a person is unconscious, not breathing, and has no pulse, cardiopulmonary resuscitation (CPR), a combination of artificial respiration and chest compressions, can be applied to him or her as an emergency attempt to restore circulation. These chest compressions must be learned in a supervised environment and only certified individuals should perform them in an emergency. The general steps for CPR for an adult are

1. Once you have successfully delivered 2 rescue breaths and found no pulse, you start a series of 30 chest compressions with the person on a firm, flat surface, if possible. These thrusting compressions are performed at a rhythmic rate of at least 100 per minute, compressing the chest by 2 inches.
2. After 30 compressions, deliver 2 rescue breaths by tilting the head and lifting the chin up, pinching the nose shut and making a complete seal over the person's mouth.
3. Repeat the pattern of "30 and 2" for four cycles.
4. Recheck for ABCs, and continue the "30 and 2" for four more cycles. Repeat this series of rechecking and four cycles until emergency medical personnel arrive or you are relieved by someone else trained in CPR.

Choking

When someone is choking, a foreign object is caught in the airway and obstructing the flow of air. If the person is conscious, there may be a partial or complete obstruction. In a partial airway obstruction, a limited amount of air will be able to pass the object to get into the lungs and the victim will be able to speak, cough, or breathe. Encourage the person to continue coughing. If the small amount of air passing through the airway is not enough, the skin may start to turn bluish and coughing may become weak with a high-pitched wheezing sound, which means the person needs immediate help before he or she loses consciousness. When someone's airway is completely obstructed, no air can pass the foreign object, so they are unable to talk, whisper, or cough. This person needs immediate attention or he or she will lose consciousness. Someone with a completely obstructed airway often makes the universal sign for choking, where both hands grab at the throat while the person's mouth is open. In this case, you should properly perform subdiaphragmatic abdominal thrusts (formerly called the Heimlich maneuver) until the obstruction is expelled or until the person becomes unconscious and emergency medical personnel arrive. For obese or pregnant victims, use chest thrusts instead of abdominal thrusts.

If the person becomes unconscious due to a partial or complete airway obstruction, you will need to perform more advanced first aid. The general steps are outlined below, but you must be properly trained by an organization such as the American Red Cross (www.redcross.org):

1. Yell for help or for someone to call 911.
2. Place the person in a supine position.

3. Lift the person's tongue and jaw with one hand and use your other hand to perform a finger sweep in an attempt to clear the obstruction from the airway.

4. Open the victim's airway using the head-tilt and chin-lift and attempt to give 2 rescue breaths.

5. Straddle the victim and give 6 to 10 abdominal thrusts with the palms of your hands.

6. Repeat the finger sweep, opening the airway, attempting rescue breathing, and performing abdominal thrusts until:

    a. The object is expelled, in which case you use the assessment ABCs

    b. Victim regains consciousness

    c. Emergency medical personnel (or a properly trained person) relieves you

Weather-Related Conditions

When the body is exposed to environmental conditions for long periods of time, there are a number of homeostatic mechanisms that keep the body functioning properly: body temperature must be kept within a safe range, blood volume must be maintained, and salt concentrations must be held at the right levels. At sporting events and other outdoor activities, clients who have been exposed to the weather for extended periods of time sometimes have difficulty coping with the elements. As part of your client-centered practice, you should recognize the signs and symptoms of weather-related or temperature-related conditions.

Heat-Related Conditions

The process of sweating is one of the natural mechanisms our body uses to cool itself down. There are some situations, however, when sweating cannot keep the body temperature within the safe range. Heat cramps, heat exhaustion, and heat stroke are conditions (from mildest to most severe) brought about by prolonged exposure to hot temperatures. Dehydration is a complication of exposure to high temperatures that results from the body's attempt to cool itself by sweating. Symptoms of dehydration include a dry or sticky mouth, dizziness, muscle cramps, fatigue, and headaches.

Heat cramps are painful, involuntary muscle spasms that usually result when a person sweats a lot during strenuous physical activity (often in hot weather) and does not drink enough fluids. The cramps are a direct function of salt concentration imbalances in the muscle tissue, and as a result, sports drinks and other fluids with salts and sugars (fruit juice or the like) are better than plain water as

treatments for heat cramps. These cramps, which often occur in the legs, abdomen, back, and arms, do not usually last more than an hour. If they do, the person should seek medical attention. Heat cramps are some of the first symptoms of heat exhaustion, so it is important to stop physical activity, sit quietly in a cool place, and drink fluids. Because heat cramps are some of the first symptoms of heat exhaustion, it is important that the person not return to their previous activity for at least a few hours.

Heat exhaustion is more severe than heat cramps. Sometimes the symptoms begin several days after strenuous physical activity or prolonged exposure to hot weather, but other times the symptoms begin suddenly after heavy exercise, excessive heat, and insufficient fluid intake. A person suffering from heat exhaustion may appear ashen or pale; feel faint or dizzy; and have a rapid, weak pulse, with rapid, shallow breaths. It is important to cool down a person with heat exhaustion using a cool shower or bath, air conditioning, or shade if nothing else is available. Get them to drink cool (not iced) fluids with electrolytes, if possible, loosen their clothing, lay them down, and elevate their feet. If the condition does not improve in an hour, or the person develops a fever of 103°F, shows signs of confusion, or has seizures, it is critical that you seek medical attention before the person suffers heat stroke.

Heat stroke is the most serious of all heat-related conditions. The body loses its ability to regulate temperature, the sweating mechanism fails, and the rapidly rising body temperature can exceed 104°F in just minutes. Signs of heat stroke include:

- No sweating
- Red, hot skin
- Fever
- Rapid pulse
- Rapid and shallow breathing
- Irritability
- Confusion
- Dizziness
- Fainting
- Unconsciousness

Immediately call for emergency medical assistance, and while you are waiting, do what you can to cool the person's body: administer cool fluids, move the person to a shady area or air conditioning, fan the person, and loosen the person's clothing.

Cold-Related Conditions

Cold temperatures can also stress the body's ability to maintain homeostasis. Dehydration, hypothermia, and frostbite are conditions that can result from exposure to cold temperatures.

Dehydration is a common condition that occurs in cold weather. People generally associate sweating with hot weather, and unfortunately tend to forget about dehydration during cold weather. The simple act of breathing cold, dry air depletes our bodies of water with every exhalation. Physical activities such as shoveling, sledding, skiing, or skating cause us to sweat, increasing fluid loss even more. Just as in hot weather, it is important to increase fluid intake during cold weather to avoid dehydration.

Prolonged exposure to cold temperatures causes the body to lose heat faster than it can be generated. Hypothermia is the condition in which core body temperature drops below 95°F, which is too low to maintain proper metabolism. The nervous system cannot function effectively, which, in turn, influences all body systems. Signs of hypothermia include shivering, drowsiness, slurred speech, confusion, pale skin, and poor muscle coordination. If you think someone might be suffering from hypothermia, get immediate medical assistance and try to warm the person's body: move the person to a warmer place; administer warm (nonalcoholic) beverages if the person is conscious; remove any wet clothing; and wrap the person in dry, warm blankets or clothing. If the victim is unconscious, use the primary assessment ABCs and administer CPR as necessary until medical personnel arrive.

Frostbite is a condition in which parts of the body have been exposed to very cold temperatures long enough that the skin and underlying tissues freeze. Circulation ceases, resulting in numb, pale grayish-yellow skin that has a hard, cold, and waxy feel. Someone suffering from frostbite may also be suffering from hypothermia, which is a more serious condition that requires emergency medical attention. As long as there are no signs of hypothermia, frostbite can be treated as follows: get the victim to a warm environment and submerge the affected body part in warm (not hot) water, or use your own body heat to hold (not rub) the frostbitten area. Do not walk on or attempt to use frostbitten body parts, do not rub or massage them, and do not use any kind of heating pads or other sources of heat to warm the affected parts; all of these techniques can damage the tissues.

Becoming a Professional Massage Therapist

By now, you have undoubtedly spent a significant amount of time studying, practicing, and learning about the fundamental components of massage therapy. It is likely that beyond your learning these fundamentals, your life has been affected and changed. Beyond this learning, you most likely have greater personal and body awareness along with the basic skills to facilitate healing in the people you touch through massage therapy. This final section addresses how to translate what you have learned into becoming a successful, professional massage therapist. We present professional concepts, employment options, business start-up concepts, finances, marketing and promotion, networking, long-term business development and, last but not least, self-care.

Professional Concepts

Although there is no specific, iron-clad recipe for success, there are components that promote longevity in the massage therapy profession, including self-awareness and confidence, clear boundaries, continued learning, support from others, and perseverance.

Self-Awareness and Confidence

Once you have been through massage therapy training and received a significant amount of massage and/or bodywork, it is likely that you have a heightened self-awareness. The very essence of giving and receiving touch and energy creates a multidimensional effect on both the giver and the receiver that will result in varying experiences on a continuum from minimal to life changing. It is important to maintain this awareness, perhaps new or expanded, of the powerful physical, psychological, emotional, and spiritual effects of massage therapy. It is important to sustain this self-awareness as you begin working with your own clients in your massage practice. Additionally, it is important for this awareness to be coupled with the certain level of maturity and responsibility that it takes to facilitate healing in a client. Success often depends on the confidence you and your clients have in your ability to facilitate a comforting and stimulating response in them. In general, there are many ways to create confidence; however, specific to massage therapy are clear boundaries, maintaining a client-centered focus, and continued learning.

Clear Boundaries

Creating and maintaining clear boundaries is the first way to build confidence. Any time you give and receive touch, it is important for you, as the professional, to have and maintain clear boundaries around the parameters of the session. For review on this topic, see the sections in Chapter 2 on Ethics and Professionalism. As you continue to practice, it is important to continue your education on this topic. You can do this by reading articles and books on ethics and professional re-lationships and/or taking continuing education (CE) hours in ethics, boundaries, and/or professional relationships (see Suggested Readings and web sites at the end of this chapter).

Continued Learning

As you near the end of what has most likely been a rich and rewarding learning experience, it may be challenging to under-stand the value of continuing to learn more about any com-ponent of massage therapy—be it more anatomy and physiol-ogy, refining your technique(s) or learning new ones, or any other related topic. However, continual learning will help you keep your passion for health and healing through massage alive as well as offer the opportunity for you to connect with other professional massage therapists. If you voluntarily de-cide to or are required by law to obtain National Certification in Therapeutic Massage and Bodywork (NCTMB), you will have to take a certain amount of continuing education hours, commonly known as CEs. If this applies to you in your lo-cale, be sure to check the National Certification Board web site (www.ncbtmb.com) for updates on the requirements for maintaining certification. You may also be required to have CEs for your local or state regulation. Your school program should provide you with this information; however, you are ul-timately responsible, so be sure to check with the appropriate agency in your area to ensure you are in compliance.

More than desire or requirement to learn, you will most probably experience a natural curiosity to learn more as you treat clients with different conditions and/or states of soft tissue health. You may also find that you are inter-ested in learning more about a particular part of the body in which you have experienced injury, discomfort, and/or pain. For example, if you have chronic discomfort in your lower back, you might find yourself drawn to learning more assessment and/or techniques for this area. No matter how you come to the decision to take CEs, you and your clients will undoubtedly benefit from it.

Support from Others

If you are like most massage students, you have not only re-ceived a basic education in massage therapy, you have come together with your classmates in a way that is different from most group experiences. When you move from the cocoon of massage school where you learn a lot of information and receive support to becoming a professional massage therapist practicing on your own or in a massage setting, it is wise to seek continued support. Hopefully, you have the personal support of family and friends as your foundation. Professionally, it will be helpful for you to network with other massage therapists and/or seek out one or more men-tors. Your success may be directly related to the amount of support you seek and receive. Having the support of other massage professionals and/or a mentor offers you a chance

to discuss a variety of situations and challenges that may occur with clients or with your business situation. It will also help renew your passion for massage therapy and help you feel connected to others within the profession. You can network and/or find mentors in several ways:

- Have regular meetings with a few classmates and/or local massage therapists
- Join a professional association such as the American Massage Therapy Association (AMTA) or Associated Bodywork and Massage Professionals (ABMP)
- Attend local and national massage, bodywork, and/or spa meetings and conferences
- Join a business networking group
- Attend CE workshops
- Meet regularly with a person who is willing to be your mentor—someone with whom you can process challenges and opportunities (this can be a seasoned massage therapist, a friend, or someone who is in another helping/service profession)

Most of all, you need to be supportive of yourself by doing what it takes for you to maintain the balance and self-care it takes to spend your valuable energy on your clients in order to facilitate their health and healing (see later section on self-care)

Perseverance

Although you may have started massage school for a myriad of reasons, it can be challenging to make the transition from massage student to professional massage therapist. In fact, you should expect it to be challenging. You should expect to face obstacles. You need to keep practicing massage until you find your own rhythm of how you want to practice massage therapy, which may include but is not limited to:

- Building up endurance and stamina
- Where you want to work—self-employed or employee or a combination of both
- What kind of techniques you offer
- What kind of clients you like to work with
- How many massages you would like to give in a day
- How much money you need to earn to make a living
- Determine how to maintain a self-care plan and balance within yourself so you can give as many ses-sions as you want and need to earn a living

This is just a beginning to your own personal list of what it will take to find your own rhythm. If you are willing to persevere through all of the day-to-day realities of becoming and being a professional massage therapist, you will be able to fully participate in a profession that is filled with people who often passionately care about the health and well-being of others. **It is important for your success that you do not waste your time, energy, and talent for facilitating healing by not caring enough about the components of what it takes to become, and ultimately be, a professional massage therapist.**

Employment and Business Options

There are a few options to consider when entering the professional practice of massage therapy, each with its own distinct advantages and disadvantages: self-employment, partnerships, corporations, and working as an employee. Some therapists prefer working part-time in more than one employment structure, enjoying the benefits of the different systems. Some therapists prefer the security of keeping a current job with a stable paycheck while they start their massage business as a part-time commitment. When considering the different business structures, think about the following:

- Your vision for the size or nature of the business
- The level of control you want
- The amount of structure you are willing to manage
- Your vulnerability to lawsuits
- The tax implications of the different business structures
- Your expected profit (or loss)

Because this chapter presents very basic information, it is highly recommended that you consult with one or more advisors before deciding how to practice: a financial advisor, an attorney, a certified public accountant (CPA), a public accountant, or an Internal Revenue Service (IRS)-approved enrolled agent. Because there are good and bad advisors, ask friends and family members for referrals and make sure the advisor specializes in small business.

The Small Business Administration (SBA) is an excellent source of help and guidance for people who are looking at starting a small business (www.sba.gov). This federal government office offers help with technical, financial, tax, and legal matters and can assist you with contracts and regulations. In an effort to promote small businesses, the SBA offers financial loans, with special support for women, minorities, Native Americans, youth, and veterans, among others. The SBA has a volunteer service corps of retired executives (www.score.org) that offer resources that are very useful as you begin your business. These mentors are a good source of business counseling information, they have experience, and they are interested in being helpful. You can also consult the IRS web site (www.irs.gov) for additional tax information.

Regardless of how you practice massage, you should join a professional massage therapy association such as the AMTA or the ABMP. Look into national certification through the National Certification Board for Therapeutic Massage and Bodywork (NCBTMB), which is an organization that makes an effort at standardizing the massage profession. To become a certified member, you must meet and maintain certain requirements and pass an objective test. National certification is required by law in some states to obtain a license to practice. In most states, the Federation of State Massage Therapy Boards (FSMTB) Massage and Bodywork Licensing Exam is also accepted to obtain a license to practice. Professional organizations, such as the AMTA, ABMP, NCBTMB, and FSMTB, work for and on behalf of the massage industry, learning about and improving the profession. The AMTA and ABMP provide insurance, numerous resources, and professional massage therapy journals that keep you informed about trends and changes in the industry, techniques, and workshops for enhancing your education.

Self-Employment

Self-employment is a business arrangement in which you work for yourself, either in a sole proprietorship or as an independent contractor. These simpler ways to begin a business may be regulated by state, county, or city governments. Your local SBA office, city hall, department of planning or zoning, city/county office, or Secretary of State's office can help you determine and follow the appropriate regulations for business licenses, DBA (doing business as) permits, local fire and safety codes, local regulations, and appropriate property insurance. **To avoid a tax penalty by the IRS, persons who are self-employed make quarterly estimated tax payments on April 15, June 15, September 15, and January 15 in accordance with tax guidelines and regulations.** Generally, set aside 20% to 30% of your total income each week to cover these quarterly tax liabilities, and consult the SBA or a tax advisor such as a CPA for more specific guidelines. You might otherwise easily spend all the money received from clients, especially if you are used to receiving a paycheck with taxes already taken out and paid by the employer.

Sole Proprietorship

A sole proprietorship is a business owned by one person who is personally liable for all of the business transactions (Box 13-3). It is relatively easy to set up, the owner has complete control over the business, and the owner receives all the income. As the owner, you determine the business parameters such as hours of operation, fee schedule, services offered, and rules. All income and expenses, hiring, firing, taxes, banking, marketing, establishment of utilities, legal compliance, and insurance are managed by the therapist/owner or may be hired out to someone else who takes care of these important details.

Sole Proprietorship Pros and Cons

+ It is simple to organize.
+ The owner has complete control over the business.
+ The owner receives all of the income.

− The owner has unlimited liability.
− Benefits are not business deductions.

Some of the tax forms you will need:

- Form 1040: Individual income tax
- Form 1040ES: Estimated tax for individuals
- Form 4562: Depreciation/amortization
- Form 8829: Expenses for business use of your home
- Schedule C: Profit/loss
- Schedule SE: Self-employment tax

The drawbacks of being the sole proprietor are that you are personally liable for all of the business and your benefits are not business deductions. Being responsible for your schedule, vacation, pay rate, retirement benefits, taxes, and insurance can be challenging, but the pride of ownership can be a greater source of fulfillment.

Independent Contractor

Being an independent contractor provides many of the benefits of self-employment without the large responsibility of running a business. Typically, an independent contractor rents space in a business such as a spa, massage clinic, physician's office, salon, or fitness center, and signs a contractual agreement with the business owner or the person who is contracting the massage services. The therapist is responsible for appointments, fee schedule, and other business parameters and assumes liability according to the specifications in the contract. Before signing a contract as a contractor, communicate and put in writing all of your needs and expectations clearly to the owner or manager of the business regarding:

- Space
- Lighting
- Electrical outlet requirements
- Safety
- Accessibility to the building and treatment room
- Accessibility to a restroom and sink
- Housekeeping responsibilities
- Maximum number of massages performed on any given day
- Security

Partnerships and Corporations

The other two forms of business ownership, partnerships and corporations, are more complicated to set up than sole proprietorships. Setting up one of these business entities requires more paperwork and they are more complicated to maintain, but in some situations these arrangements can be more beneficial for the therapist. Generally speaking, however, the benefits do not outweigh the costs and the complexity of maintaining one of these entities unless your massage practice's federal taxable income is at least $15,000. **Although not legally required, it is highly advisable to seek the assistance of a tax advisor such as a CPA.**

A partnership is a company in which two or more persons not only share ownership and all of the income but also assume unlimited liability for the business (Box 13-4). The challenge of this type of arrangement is that two or more persons have to run the business together. Before you decide to enter a partnership,

Partnership Pros and Cons

+ Easy to organize, but the partners need to agree.
+ The partners receive all of the income.
+ More start-up money may be available.
+ Partners may have complementary skills.

− Partners have unlimited liability.
− Partners may disagree.
− The life of the business may be limited because of death or partner withdrawal.

Some of the tax forms you will need:

- Form 1040: Individual income tax
- Form 1040ES: Estimated tax for individuals
- Form 1065: Partnership return of income
- Form 1065K-1: Partner's share of income, credit, deductions
- Form 4562: Depreciation/amortization
- Schedule E: Supplemental income and loss
- Schedule SE: Self-employment tax

you and your partner(s) need to ensure that all current and future aspects of the business are acceptable to everyone:

- How will you make business decisions?
- How will you settle disputes?
- How will you go about buying out one of the partners?
- How will future partners join the business?
- How will you dissolve the business?

There are three general structures of partnership, including general partnership, limited partnership, and joint venture. A general partnership is an equal partnership in ownership and liability, unless otherwise stated. Limited partnerships limit the liability of the partners, the extent of their investment, or their decision-making input. Massage businesses and other service businesses typically do not enter limited partnerships. Joint ventures are generally short-term businesses or investment arrangements for single projects.

A **corporation** is a business arrangement with one or more owners who remain separate from the business (Box 13-5). Corporations are chartered by the state in which they are headquartered, they have a board of directors to make business decisions, and they do not dissolve when ownership changes. In essence, the owners are shareholders who own stock in the corporation and have limited liability for business transactions because the assets and liabilities belong to the business. The business pays taxes, can be sued, and can enter into contracts. Taxes are paid in accordance with how the owners take money out of the business. Again, if you are considering any of these arrangements, consult a tax advisor and/or an attorney.

There are different corporation structures. The most straightforward organization is a regular corporation, better known as a "C" corporation. Subchapter "S" corporations are taxed similarly to partnerships, which can be beneficial, but there are certain requirements for being designated an "S" corporation. Limited liability corporations are relatively new business structures that offer the tax efficiency and operational flexibility of a partnership with the limited liability of a corporation.

Working as an Employee

The details of starting a business can be overwhelming and more than many new massage therapists want to accept when starting a practice. Another option is to be employed by someone else, such as a spa, chiropractor, health club, or hospital. As an employee, you receive a paycheck from the employer, your taxes are withheld by the employer, and you may receive benefits such as insurance and paid time off for vacation, personal business, or sickness. The employer usually covers the overhead costs as well as manages the massage room, table,

sheets, lubricant, laundry, and scheduling, making it easier for you to focus on massage. On the other hand, you surrender control to your employer, possibly having less flexibility in scheduling, policies, and procedures. Employers generally tell their therapists when, where, and what hours to work. To cover the employer's overhead expenses, therapists receive only a portion of what the client pays for the massage session.

Even as an employee, you are in a professional practice, regardless of whether you are in charge of the daily operations, and thus you must maintain professionalism at all times. Be sure to clarify boundaries and expectations before starting work. The maximum number of massages performed on any given day, security, accessibility, fees, and safety issues should be clarified.

Writing a Resumé

A resumé (REHZ-oo-may) is generally a one-page written description of your personal contact information,

---

BOX 13-5
Corporations Pros and Cons

+ Shareholders (owners) have limited liability.
+ The corporation can raise funds by selling stock.
+ The life of the business is unlimited.
+ You can deduct the cost of benefits.

− The incorporation process takes time and money.
− You may pay higher taxes overall.

Some of the tax forms you will need for a "C" corporation:
- Form 1120 or 1120A: Corporation income tax return
- Form 1120W: Estimated tax for corporation
- Form 4625: Depreciation/amortization
- Form 8109-B: Deposit coupon
- Other forms as needed for capital gains, sale of assets, alternative minimum tax, etc.

Some of the tax forms you will need for an "S" corporation:
- Form 1040: Individual income tax
- Form 1040ES: Estimated tax for individuals
- Form 1120S: S Corporation income tax return
- Form 1120SK-1: Shareholder's share of income, credit, deductions
- Form 4625: Depreciation/amortization
- Schedule E: Supplemental income and loss
- Schedule SE: Self-employment tax
- Other forms as needed for capital gains, sale of assets, alternative minimum tax, etc.

educational background, professional experience and accomplishments, and volunteer work that you submit to potential employers when you are looking for a job or are promoting yourself. It may be the first impression someone has of you and your professionalism. A curriculum vitae (kuhr-IHK-yoo-luhm VAHY-tee), better known as a CV, is a detailed and structured list of your educational background, publications, projects, awards, and employment history. CVs tend to be longer than resumés, up to 10 pages, and are typically more appropriate for educators and scientists than for massage therapists.

A resumé usually includes:

- Your name

- Your address

- Your home, work, and cell phone numbers

- Your email address and web site, if applicable

- Your career objective or employment goal

- Your educational background information, listing schools, their locations, the degree or coursework completed and the dates of attendance, completion, or graduation

- Professional work experience, typically listed in reverse chronological order, starting with your current occupation

- Professional associations, memberships, awards, and accomplishments

- Volunteer contributions

Keep the format simple and easy to follow. Most computers are preloaded with programs that lead you through a step-by-step process for writing a resumé, and numerous books about writing resumés are available at libraries and bookstores.

People may read your resumé before they meet you, and they may use it to decide whether or not to interview you. Ask several people to look over your resumé and offer constructive criticism, looking for errors in grammar and spelling, suggesting content additions or deletions, and making sure your wording is clear and understandable. Your resumé is a paper representation of you and your qualifications, so you owe it to yourself to put a solid effort into writing and refining it before you submit it to anyone.

Business Start-up

The process of starting your own business can be complicated. Learn about the massage industry and the market, which is the local interest and demand for your services. Before opening the doors to your business, whether in an office or any other location, write a business plan, consider a place of business, choose and hire advisors, understand your

financial responsibilities, and have a plan for marketing and promoting your business. Box 13-6 has a sample business start-up checklist.

You will need to determine financing, legal structure, and local regulations that apply to massage therapy for your business; register your business name depending on your structure; explore and obtain insurance and benefits; open a business bank account; develop procedures for record keeping; and establish a set of policies and procedures. Following regulations, managing benefits, keeping your finances organized, and paying taxes are ongoing responsibilities that require constant time and attention. Learning about these business aspects before problems occur can help you avoid a painful and possibly expensive life lesson. Some of the many resources that can provide necessary information are the library; the internet; legal, tax, and accounting professionals; seminars; and networking groups.

Part of the preparation for starting a business is estimating the expenses necessary to get the business going. Set-up costs for a business vary, depending on the type of massage practice. Possible expenses may include:

- Down payment for rent

- Security deposit for space

- Establishing phone service and other utilities

- Membership in a professional organization

- Licenses, permits, insurance

- Professional service fees: accounting, legal, insurance, web designer/digital media consultant

- Equipment: massage table, massage chair, bolsters, lubricants, linens

- Office supplies and equipment: computer, printer, paper, envelopes, paper towels, toilet paper, pens, clipboard

- Furniture, mirrors, heater, fan, electric blanket, lamps

- Background music CDs and CD player

- Marketing: business cards, brochures, web site design and hosting

Knowing the costs of setting up a business ahead of time prepares you to meet those expenses. Running out of money could lead to phone service being disconnected, an inability to purchase lubricant, not having enough sets of sheets, or any number of problems.

Business Plan

Strongly consider writing a business plan before you begin your massage therapy practice. A good business plan provides a road map to help you realize and achieve your goals, leading you from your initial idea of starting a business through the development of a thriving massage therapy practice.

BOX 13-6
Business Start-up Checklist

REGULATIONS

☐ Obtain massage license from state, city, and/or county, if necessary.

☐ Obtain DBA (doing business as) permit from the appropriate agency.

☐ Obtain business license from city and/or county, if necessary.

☐ File necessary paperwork with appropriate state agencies for partnerships or corporations.

☐ Obtain federal identification numbers if operating as partnership or corporation.

☐ Check into local fire and safety codes, neighborhood rules, and property insurance.

☐ Obtain seller's permit and sales tax identification number if selling retail products.

INSURANCE

☐ Obtain professional and general liability insurance.

☐ Check into property insurance.

☐ Check into disability insurance.

☐ Check into medical insurance, if not currently covered under another policy.

☐ Check into workers' compensation insurance, if necessary.

BENEFITS

☐ Research and learn about providing your own benefits such as time off for being sick, vacation, bonus pay, and retirement funding.

☐ Consider setting up a "time-off" fund.

☐ Consider the "pay yourself first" principle of savings.

☐ Consult with an investment advisor regarding retirement planning.

RECORD KEEPING

☐ Create and copy client history forms.

☐ Create and copy SOAP forms.

☐ Buy a day planner, PDA, or calendar software.

☐ Create or obtain policies and procedures for the business where you will practice.

FINANCES

☐ Consult with a professional accountant regarding:

  ☐ Creating a system for recording income and expenses

  ☐ Creating a system for paying invoices

  ☐ Creating a good filing system for records retention: bank statements, invoices, tax returns, ledger sheets

  ☐ Setting up income and expenses categories

  ☐ Paying taxes

☐ Open checking and savings accounts for business use only.

☐ Obtain a credit card for business use only.

☐ Determine your fees.

SET-UP COSTS

☐ Down payment for rent

☐ Security deposit for space

☐ Equipment—massage table, massage chair, bolsters, lubricants, linens

☐ Business cards

☐ Membership in a professional organization

☐ Establishing phone service and other utilities

☐ Licenses, permits, insurance

☐ Furniture, mirrors, heater, fan, electric blanket, lamps

☐ Background music—CDs and CD player

☐ Professional service fees—accounting, legal, insurance, investment advisor

Additionally, it can prepare you for obstacles you may encounter along the way and can guide you toward alternate routes that can lead to success. Remember the saying, "Success is a journey, not a destination." The journey will bring conflicts, new information, and situations that require decisions. If you are prepared for the constant changes in business and in life, you can remain flexible and better able to make the appropriate adjustments to continue on your journey toward success.

A business plan is a set of written documents that defines your business, outlines your goals, and gives people an opportunity to thoroughly understand your business from a piece of paper. According to the SBA, business plans generally include the components listed in Box 13-7. The list may seem intimidating, but your local SBA office can be an excellent source of help and guidance through the process of writing a business plan. Use the resources that are available to you and continue working toward your goals.

There are personal, financial, and professional implications of starting a business. Initially, your massage practice

BOX 13-7
Components of a Business Plan

1. Cover sheet
2. Statement of purpose for your business
3. Details of the business
   a. Description
   b. Marketing
   c. Competition
   d. Operating procedures
   e. Business insurance
4. Financial information
   a. Loan applications
   b. Equipment and supply list
   c. Balance sheet
   d. Breakeven analysis
   e. Profit and loss projections
   f. Three-year plan, including monthly goals for the first year and quarterly goals thereafter
   g. Cash flow statement
5. Supporting documentation
   a. Individual income tax forms for the principal owner(s) for the previous 3 years
   b. Personal financial statement (available at banks)
   c. Copy of your proposed lease
   d. Copies of your licenses and other government documents
   e. Resumé for the principal owner(s)

will require a significant amount of personal energy, time, money, and attention, whether you perform one or several massages a week. One of the primary reasons for business failure is lack of preparation and poor management. A written business plan will help you distribute your energy expenditures evenly, learn about the massage therapy industry and market, and gain control of your business; it will also give you a competitive edge. If you look to an outside source such as a bank for funding, a prepared business plan will strongly increase your chances for procuring the funds. The written plan can also help you establish credit with suppliers, organize and manage business operations and finances, and identify your target market to focus your marketing and promotion. Start by asking yourself the following questions:

- What services will I provide?
- What needs are there for my service?
- Who are my potential customers?
- Why would they use me instead of someone else?
- How can I reach my potential customers to let them know my service is available?
- Where will I obtain the financing to start a business?

Regulations

Before opening your business, you must determine local zoning and governmental regulations that pertain to a massage practice. Even in a home-based business, you should abide by neighborhood rules and covenants and homeowner's association policies in addition to the governmental regulations. Contact your local SBA office, city hall, or other appropriate government office to find out if you need a professional license or certification to practice massage in your community. License regulations vary from state to state, and in the states that do not require licensure, a massage practice may be regulated by the city and/or county. A DBA permit is also required if you plan to work under a name other than your own first and last name. Appropriate paperwork must be filed with the state and federal agencies if the business will operate as a partnership or corporation, and a federal identification number is needed from the IRS.

As a professional therapist, you must follow the rules and scope of practice as outlined by all applicable state laws and county and city ordinances. Fire codes, safety codes, and property insurance are some of the issues that are regulated. The massage therapy scope of practice typically allows the use of specific massage techniques and does not allow diagnosis or prescriptions as part of treatment.

Massage businesses that sell retail products in addition to massage services must obtain a seller's permit or retail merchant permit as well as a sales tax identification number. Many responsibilities accompany retail sales, such as collecting and paying sales tax and property taxes and inventory accountability. Consult with a CPA or another financial advisor for guidance because these professionals stay current with the ever-changing tax laws and regulations. In addition to the business aspect of retail sales, you must know about the products you sell, including recommended usage, indications, and contraindications. For example, ginseng can have a negative effect on the body when certain pathological conditions exist or when it is combined with certain medications.

Insurance

Another major component of running a business is obtaining insurance. Although massage therapists are generally not subject to lawsuits, it is still wise to obtain professional and general liability insurance for your personal protection and security. Remember, in a sole proprietorship, therapists are personally held liable, but in a corporation, the business assumes liability. In either business structure, you need professional and general liability insurance to protect yourself and the practice to ensure that you can support a lawsuit if clients are injured on the premises.

Professional liability insurance offers therapists financial protection from clients who claim they were injured during a massage session. It is available through some of the professional massage organizations such as AMTA and ABMP, and you can purchase it through a private insurance company. General liability insurance protects the practice from clients who file a lawsuit claiming they were injured on the property by something other than the massage. For example, a client could slip in the parking lot, trip on the stairs, or get burned by hot water while washing hands in the bathroom.

Other types of insurance you might need or want include property insurance, disability insurance, medical insurance, and workers' compensation. Property insurance covers damage to your property and losses you incur due to theft, fire, or other hazards outside your control. Disability insurance provides you with some income if you are temporarily or permanently disabled. Although most massage therapists do not carry disability insurance, it is wise to seriously consider it. Without it, you earn no income when you cannot work. Medical insurance, which defrays the cost of medical treatment when you are hurt or ill, is worth considering. Consult with an insurance agent to find out possibilities for coverage.

The workers' compensation law requires most employers to provide medical, rehabilitation, and wage replacement benefits to their employees who are injured while performing within the normal scope of their job. Employers must pay for this form of insurance, called workers' compensation. States have slightly different rules and requirements, but workers' compensation generally covers employees while they are at work.

Benefits

Some employers offer benefits, including paid time off, bonus pay, and retirement funds, to employees. Frequently, benefits are only offered if you work a certain number of hours or perform a certain number of massages each week. Therapists who are self-employed must purchase and provide their own benefits and should take the time to learn about these, especially if their previous employment situation provided benefits. Missing work due to illness or taking a vacation usually means income lost. Therefore, you might want to set some money aside each week for a "time-off" or vacation fund.

Some therapists have the opportunity to earn bonus pay for completing a certain number of massages or selling a particular number of products to clients. If you employ other therapists, you have to decide whether you want to offer these kinds of incentives to your employees.

Retirement benefits are typically funds that a company or individual contributes into an employee's retirement fund. Most massage therapists are sole proprietors or employees of their own corporation and have to contribute to their own retirement fund. Follow the example set by many successful business people to "pay yourself first." Some experts suggest putting away 10% of your income for savings and/or retirement. When beginning a business, you may find this amount too steep, but it is a good habit to start, so save some portion, even if it is only 1% of your income. Certified financial planners and accounting professionals can inform you of different ways to invest for retirement.

Record Keeping

Every massage therapist should use some basic organizational tools in practice: written forms for client information and treatment documentation; a daily planner, calendar, smartphone, iPad®, netbook, or online charting service; and written forms listing business policies and procedures. Record keeping helps the business run smoothly, provides a paper trail, and allows you to see the overall picture of the practice. Have these forms in place before you start your practice.

Your clients' personal information, health history, and treatment records should be kept on paper, stored in a computer, or both. These specific forms are discussed in Chapter 6, Communication and Documentation, but are mentioned here as part of the business record keeping. Some of the client's personal information and health history is documented on client history forms. Informed consent for care is occasionally included at the end of the client history form because of its relevance to the client's health and any existing medical condition. Generally, informed consent for care explains the benefits and limits of massage therapy and the scope of practice and emphasizes that massage is not a substitute for medical treatment. The client is then given the opportunity to accept massage treatment with a signature and date. Keeping track of the client's treatments, progress, goals, and referrals to other healthcare professionals is managed with SOAP forms. At the time of this publication, there are also online services for keeping notes. Clients should understand that any conversation, personal information, treatment, and professional referrals will remain confidential unless they give their written permission to share the information. Under court order, you may be required to release confidential client files, but under no other circumstance should the information be shared with another person.

Any practice needs proof of appointments both in and outside the office. They can be recorded on a daily paper planner, calendar, smartphone, or online scheduling system. The paper versions provide written evidence that helps establish a paper trail for keeping track of business transactions, but some people find the electronic smartphone or online scheduling system more convenient and efficient. Online scheduling systems can send reminders to your client for their appointment times. Some also take payments for scheduled appointments. Both of these features increase the likelihood of clients keeping their appointments. Online scheduling also allows current and potential clients to schedule or reschedule at their convenience, which may be outside of your official office hours, potentially helping you save time in returning calls, emails, or text messages. This leaves time for other business activities or performing more massage sessions.

Policies and Procedures

Massage therapists need a set of business policies that lists client expectations, therapist expectations, and general information regarding business operation (Fig. 13-18 shows a sample Policies and Procedures form). Some therapists include the client's informed consent for care at the end of the policies form. Before treating new clients, review your policies and procedures with them. Encourage clients to ask questions to clarify any policy or procedure and to acknowledge agreement with a signature and date.

Therapeutic Massage Works Policies and Procedures

Office:
1. Office hours are by appointment only.
2. Fees are as follows:
   a. 1 hour session = $60
   b. Corporate Chair massage = $65 per hour
   c. Outcall fee = $40
3. Acceptable methods of payment: cash or check
4. Therapist requires a minimum of 3 hours notice for cancellation or client will be billed ½ the rate of the session.
5. Therapist will not treat clients with a fever or contagious condition and client is required to reschedule appointment.

Client:
1. Client reserves the right to discontinue treatment at any time during the session, however will be charged in full.
2. Clients may disrobe to their own level of comfort.
3. Client is strictly prohibited from any sexual advances or inappropriate behavior of any kind, however, will be charged in full for the session.

Therapist:
1. Therapist reserves the right to refuse treatment.
2. Therapist agrees that all information within the session will be kept confidential unless client releases therapist to disclose information or via court subpoena.
3. Therapist will refer client to another healthcare professional if she deems treatment is necessary that is out of her scope of practice.

Informed Consent:

I, _____, have read, fully understand and have discussed the above listed policies and procedures with Mary Therapist of Therapeutic Massage Works. I understand massage is not a substitute for medical treatment and that Mary Therapist does not diagnose nor prescribe medical treatment.

Signature: _____ Date: _____

Printed Name: _____

Figure 13-18. Sample Policies and Procedures form.

As a therapist, you may have some expectations of your clients' behavior. Your policies help clients understand your expectations and the way you run your practice. Some of the policies to consider include:

- Payment policies
  - Acceptable forms of payment
  - Fee schedules
  - Prompt payment
- Punctuality for scheduled appointments
  - Cancellation policy
- Choices for session duration
- Intolerance of any kind of sexual activity
- Referrals to other healthcare professionals
- Clients have permission to end the massage at any time for any reason
- Clients have permission to bring another person into the treatment room for peace of mind

Written policies regarding prompt payment and acceptable forms of payment convey a professional atmosphere. Because clients may cancel or not show up for a scheduled appointment, you may want to include a written cancellation policy that requires full or partial payment if an appointment slot cannot be filled.

Your policies can also describe your sanitation, safety, and hygiene practices. For instance, many clients are comforted to know that all equipment is disinfected between massage sessions and that you refuse any client who has a fever or contagious disease. You may even want to include, in writing, a list of contraindications for massage.

Choosing a Place of Business

Once you have decided to establish a business and collect income for your massage, you have to decide where you want to practice. Location is important in determining the success of any business, thus the saying "Location, location, location." The ease or difficulty with which clients can get to your place of business in terms of distance, traffic, and parking will influence your success, as will the appearance and atmosphere of the neighborhood and surroundings. Basically, the location of your practice sets the stage for the massage environment. Consider the following locations and think about how they influence the massage environment differently:

- Practicing in your own home
- Practicing in an office outside your home
- Traveling to your clients for outcalls

- Taking a massage chair to various public venues or corporate settings
- Working outdoors at sporting events
- Traveling with competitive sports teams

If you decide to occupy an office space, you will be spending many hours in your office, so it is important make sure you are comfortable in the surroundings. Finances might limit your choices, but wherever you locate your practice, make sure you project a professional image and atmosphere to your clients. Consider the following when contemplating your location:

- Are you comfortable in the location?
- Is it easily accessible for your clients?
- Is it in a safe neighborhood?
- Is there adequate parking?
- Is there adequate storage?
- Are there available restroom facilities?
- Does the space provide privacy and security?
- Is the noise level suitable for massage?
- Do you have direct access to temperature controls?
- Are the air conditioning and heating units in good working order?
- Does it need major improvements or remodeling for you to practice?
- Is the building in good condition and kept in good repair?
- Is the building properly zoned for a massage practice?
- Is the landlord easy to work with? (Ask other tenants, if possible.)
- What are the terms of the lease?
- Who is responsible for repairs and maintenance?
- Who is responsible for the upkeep of the premises: heating and cooling, water heater, snow removal, housekeeping?
- Who pays the utilities, taxes, and insurance?
- What are the renewal provisions?
- Can you sublease?

Consult your local SBA office or other government office to find out about zoning laws, consult your financial advisor for appropriate tax laws and regulations, and ask an attorney to review your lease agreement.

Setting up a practice in your own home creates an environment that is very personal and trusting. By inviting clients into your home for massage, you reveal where and how you live—your neighborhood, organization, and cleanliness. Therapists who practice massage in their own homes convey a sense of trust and openness because they allow clients into their personal space.

A massage business in someone's home feels very different from a massage practice in a hospital or at a sporting event. The atmosphere is different, and the environment affects the massage. For instance, getting a massage in a public venue will feel different from a massage you receive in your own home.

There are a number of opportunities to practice massage without an established treatment room. You can take your table to your clients at their homes, hotels, or offices for massage appointments known as outcalls. You can also take your massage table or chair to public venues, corporate offices, or outdoor sporting events. There are also growing opportunities to travel with competitive sports and auto racing teams and to perform veterinary massage.

Treatment Room Atmosphere

Most massage therapists work in a treatment room at home or in an office building, spa, clinical setting, or fitness center. Anything clients see, hear, smell, taste, and touch influences the atmosphere of the treatment room. All of those factors, in addition to your consideration of the client's level of comfort and safety, contribute to the massage environment. Have everything ready for clients before they arrive. Adjust the table properly, have the face cradle in place or readily available, put sheets or other draping on the table, have extra towels and blankets on top of the sheets or nearby, have bolsters nearby, have your music selected and playing or make sure it is ready to be played, and gather any necessary paperwork. Being prepared for clients demonstrates your commitment to professionalism and to your clients.

Privacy

One of the most important concerns for a treatment room should be privacy. To offer clients your focused attention, without distraction, privacy is important. Professional and ethical therapists want their clients to feel comfortable in the massage environment because comfort and relaxation can help people benefit from massage. Most importantly, clients must have privacy when they undress.

If at all possible, you should step out of the treatment room when clients undress, regardless of their modesty level. Some clients start undressing while you are still in the room, but you can simply say, "I'm going to step out and wash my hands while you undress and get on the table. I'll knock before I come back in just to make sure you are situated under the covers." Usually that stops them and gives you the opportunity to leave the room, close the door behind you, and wash your hands.

If you are using a space that does not have a door, offer clients a private area where they can undress and get onto the table without being seen by others. Set up a series of fabric screens or hang some long curtains to give clients privacy. Windows in the room should have blinds or drapes that can be closed while clients are undressed and on the table. Although there are exceptions, most people do not want to be watched while they are undressing or getting a massage.

Some therapists offer clients a separate room in which to undress. This creates an awkward scenario in which clients undress in one room and need to walk, undressed, to the treatment room. You need to pay more attention to sanitation, safety, and modesty issues in this situation, but it is possible to incorporate a separate dressing room into a professional massage practice (Box 13-8). After the massage is finished, you can use diaper draping to cover clients modestly enough or give them a robe so they can sit up, put their socks on, and walk to the dressing room without exposing themselves.

Even though privacy is important, treatment room doors should not be locked. Not only is the locked door a fire hazard, it may threaten your client's emotional safe space. Clients should always feel empowered to leave the treatment room of their own accord, and a locked door can take away their sense of control over the session. To keep people from walking into the treatment room during a massage, you can hang a sign that says, "Please do not disturb, massage in session" (or something like it) from the doorknob.

Visual Input

Clients may make judgments based on anything they see, so all of the visual aspects of your practice, from the parking area to the treatment room, must be considered. The neatness, lighting, and decor of the facility all play into clients' perceptions of your practice. Your practice reflects your personality, and if clients see messy piles of papers and overflowing trash cans, they may think you are messy and question the overall cleanliness of the practice. Pay attention to the type of shoes you wear and the cleanliness of the ceiling and corners of the treatment room. When the client lies on the table for their massage they see your shoes when prone and the ceiling when supine. These may seem like small things; however, they go a long way to ensure the client feels safe in the massage environment.

Ideally, the light fixtures are not directly over the massage table and the lights in your treatment room can be dimmed. During the client intake interview and during assessments, lights should be bright enough to read and fill out forms easily. During the massage, however, you want to dim the lights to help clients relax. If you cannot dim the overhead lights, use one or two lamps to provide a small amount of light. Relaxation massage and darkness cause the pupils of the eyes to dilate and let in more light. At the end of the massage, when clients are relaxed, gradually increase the amount of light in the room so as not to overwhelm the eyes with light.

Décor and furnishings create the scenery for your massage and let you express your personality. You can and should prominently display your diplomas, certifications, license (if applicable or required by law), and CE certificates.

BOX 13-8 **PROCEDURE** Instructions for Using a Separate Dressing Room

1   Show clients the treatment room, the table, and the separate dressing room.

2. Explain the draping on the table and show them how to use the draping to cover themselves after they get on the table. (See Chapter 9 for specific draping directions.)

3. Offer clients a clean robe and explain that they can go to the dressing room and:
    a. Undress, leaving their socks on and removing as many undergarments as they comfortably can; usually clients remove all clothing, but there are exceptions
    b. Put on the robe
    c. Walk to the treatment room
    d. Get on the table, with the robe on, under the appropriate drape

4. After clients are back in the treatment room, knock on the door to ask if they are situated and enter the room.

5. Create a tent with the top drape by holding it up with two hands.

6. Ask clients to take the robe off while you hold the tented drape.

7. Take the robe, lower the drape, and place the robe on a nearby chair or hook.

This helps assure the client that you are an appropriately credentialed, professional, legitimate massage therapist. Muscle and skeletal charts can be hung on the walls as sources for reference and client education. Because color can influence the atmosphere, pay attention to the colors in your treatment room: the floor, walls, your curtains or blinds, and your linens. Decorate the walls with things that you like to look at and that help you relax and focus because you will be looking at the walls more than anyone else. Depending on the quality, some white and lighter colored linens may be transparent, so patterns and darker solid colors may be more appropriate for draping purposes. Generally, linens are suitable as long as they are not transparent and the client's modesty is protected.

The size of your treatment room will determine how much furniture you need. Minimally, you need a massage table and something for clients to put their clothes on, such as a chair or a hook on the wall or door. Better yet, you can include:

- A table or desk
- A rolling stool for yourself
- A step stool to help clients on and off the table
- A clock
- A radio or sound system
- A trash can
- A box of Kleenex
- A bookshelf with some good references and self-help resource books

Because cleanliness is part of the atmosphere, make sure your décor and furniture are in good repair and are kept clean.

Auditory Input

Think about the sounds of dogs barking, babies crying, traffic, nearby conversation, a nearby television, a washing machine, clothes tumbling in the dryer, trains rushing by, kids playing, and birds singing. Depending on the person, any one of these sounds could promote relaxation or create stress, so try to minimize background noises. If some noise is unavoidable, use a small fan or white noise machine to reduce the noise. Most therapists use music in their massage sessions, which promotes relaxation and guides your timing for the session.

The physical properties of sound can be applied to human anatomy and physiology, resulting in some fascinating healing properties of music. The electrical activity of the brain can be measured objectively with an electroencephalogram and displayed on a chart as a wave pattern. Different forms of brain activity are associated with different frequencies of electrical activity, or brain waves:

- Beta (BAY-tuh) waves, 14 to 20 Hertz, are the highest frequency brain waves, which occur while people are awake and thinking and when they are experiencing strong negative emotions.

- Alpha (AL-fuh) waves, 8 to 13 Hertz, occur while people are in states of calm and heightened awareness.

- Theta (THAY-tuh) waves, 4 to 7 Hertz, occur while people are very creative, are meditating, and are sleeping.

- Delta (DEHL-tuh) waves, 0.5 to 3 Hertz, are the slowest frequency brain waves and occur during deep sleep, deep meditation, and unconsciousness.

Music with a pulse, or tempo, of about 60 beats per minute can cause brain waves to shift from beta waves to alpha waves. In other words, you can use music with a tempo of 60 beats per minute to help people relax or to ease them from a distracted mindset to a calm and clear-thinking mindset. Entrainment is the process by which specific kinds of music can encourage a change in the brain wave frequencies. For example[5]:

- Shamanic drumming can encourage theta waves.

- Mozart or baroque music can shift an unfocused mood to one more aware and calmer.

- Romantic, jazz, or New Age music can help an analytical mindset be more adaptable, flexible, or emotional.

- Fast, loud music can encourage beta waves and cause someone to lose concentration and make mistakes.

- Music with a slow tempo or long, slow tones can slow down brain waves and help someone calm down.

Music and sounds can affect our brain wave activity, heartbeat, breathing rate, and blood pressure. Paying attention to your clients' verbal and nonverbal messages can help you recognize if the music is encouraging relaxation or inducing stress. You can ask clients to choose the music or bring their own, but most clients want some kind of gentle, quiet music. If possible, collect a lot of music of different kinds, including instrumental, piano, vocals, chants, synthesized, and nature sounds. The sounds of a babbling brook are usually soothing sounds of nature, but some people respond to the sound of running water with an urge to go to the bathroom; be aware, whether the sounds of running water are in your massage music or from a nearby decorative fountain.

Olfactory Input

Olfactory input, or smells, can strongly affect a person's response to the environment. Smells are powerful memory triggers, and emotions can accompany those memories. Be aware of smells in or around your massage room that could offend clients: cooking smells, household chemicals, garbage odors, pet odors, cigarette smoke, cigar smoke, body odor, or breath odor. Scented products that you find pleasant may be offensive to others. Some clients may even be sensitive or allergic to your scented fabric softeners and detergents. To avoid a negative reaction to scents or odors, include a question on your intake form about sensitivities or allergies.

Practicing daily personal hygiene for your hair, teeth, and body will help you manage your body and breath odor. Before you use scented products to hide any breath or body odor, try using products that absorb or neutralize odors. Again, too many smells can overwhelm the client's nervous system and desensitize it, which could reduce the effects of any aromatherapy products you use.

True aromatherapy uses essential oils from flowers and plants to induce different physiological responses. Essential oils are frequently added to lubricants to make them more pleasant and therapeutic. Lavender and chamomile essences are especially popular and generally safe to use but not for everyone. **Ask clients about sensitivities and allergies before using any product.**

Tactile Sensations

Tactile sensations are things you physically feel with the sensory receptors in your skin. Anything that clients physically touch and feel is a factor of the massage environment. Pay attention to all surfaces clients touch, including the feel of the sheets, your skin and fingernails, temperature and humidity of the room, and even the amount of fresh air or breeze.

The primary consideration for tactile input is the fabric of your linens because most of the client's skin touches the draping. Material components and thread count, which are usually listed on the outside of the packaging, pertain to the quality of the sheets. All-cotton sheets tend to be softer than polyester and cotton blends. Flannel and jersey sheets feel especially soft and comfortable, but they may stick together during the massage and complicate the draping process. Thread counts refer to the density of the threads in the fabric: 200 or more is usually considered a high thread count, and 180 count is considered low. High-thread-count sheets feel silkier, they help clients feel substantially covered, and they hold up to repeated laundering better than lower thread-count sheets. The lower thread-count sheets sometimes have a gauzelike quality that can make them transparent and can feel thin and insubstantial to clients. Because draping is used to keep clients covered and comfortable and protect their modesty, you do not want see-through sheets.

Clients also feel the condition and temperature of your skin and hands. Make sure your skin and hands are soft, smooth, and clean, and that your nails are in good condition and kept short and smooth. Looking at your palm, your fingernails should be trimmed and filed so that you cannot see them extending beyond your fingertips, and there are no sharp or "pokey" edges.

Thoroughly wash and dry your hands while clients are getting undressed and on the table. After you dry your hands, the residual moisture on your hands quickly evaporates and cools your hands off. Initial touch with cold hands can be uncomfortable and startling, activating the sympathetic nervous system's fight or flight response. Before you initiate touch with cold hands, let your clients know that your hands are cold and reassure them that your hands will warm up very quickly during the massage. Conscious preparation for your cold hands can reduce the shock and the sympathetic nervous response and help a client relax sooner. Although the initial touch has a stimulating effect, your sustained touch soon stops that response and allows clients to relax. Initial touch with warm hands allows much faster relaxation. You can warm your hands with friction by briskly rubbing them together just before you initiate touch.

The room should be kept between 72° and 74°F, with moderate humidity. Although the temperature may feel too warm to you, it is comfortable for most clients during a massage. During the massage, clients are typically undressed and covered by a single sheet, and as they relax, the parasympathetic nervous response reduces their heart rate, breathing rate, and blood pressure. Consequently, they can easily feel cold and uncomfortable, which hinders relaxation. Heating pads can be placed on the massage table, underneath the draping, to provide a source of warmth to keep clients comfortable. When the humidity, or the amount of water vapor in the air, is low, it can dry out mucous membranes and skin. A humidifier or decorative water fountain can add moisture to the air, but make sure to keep it clean and sanitary to avoid transmission of pathogens. Pathogen transmission is covered in detail later in this chapter. High humidity can make the air feel oppressive and difficult to breathe; a dehumidifier or air conditioner can lower the humidity. Generally, fresh air is better than stagnant, recirculated air unless there are high levels of pollution and allergens outside. Stagnant air can make a room feel stuffy and oppressive. An open window or fan can move the air around, but a breeze that feels good to you may cause clients to feel cold. If you still want to feel a breeze, make sure you have extra blankets or covers to offer clients. For the most part, you want the air in your treatment room to feel comfortable and warm.

Advisors and Mentors

Before choosing your advisors, make sure they have experience and expertise in their given specialty and check their referrals. Talk with them about your needs. Try to determine if you can trust them, if they can best serve you, and if the two of you are compatible. If you have any doubts, continue interviewing other advisors.

An accountant will help you with the financial aspect of your business, including income, expenses, and taxes. A CPA must pass a rigorous examination and is required to stay current on the ever-changing tax laws. Better yet, you can talk to a CPA who specializes in small business because they may be more familiar with the challenges and obstacles you will face.

Before you sign any type of contract or lease, you should ask an attorney to review the contract. Legal terminology, like medical terminology, can be complicated for those who are unfamiliar with it. An attorney can help you understand exactly what is written into the contract, such as expectations, payments, responsibilities, penalties, and consequences.

If you decide to start investing for retirement, a financial advisor can help you understand the different types of investment avenues for small business owners. They can offer sound advice to help you reach your financial goals, and they can help you set up savings and investment accounts.

Part of doing business requires you to market your massage therapy practice and services. One of the main vehicles to do this is through a well-designed web site and digital marketing, which is essentially using the internet to market your business. It may help you to seek out an advisor to help you with your internet marketing. Done well, your internet presence will help people find you and your massage therapy services.

It may be helpful to find a veteran massage therapist who is willing to be your mentor or advisor. He or she may be able to give you some keen insight into how to run a massage practice and can offer encouragement and advice when you face inevitable challenges and obstacles. These mentors may be experienced therapists, former massage instructors, graduates of the massage school or program you attended, or fellow members of a professional association.

Finances

You will need to realistically assess your present and future financial situation to establish a solid foundation for your business. Consult with qualified financial advisors, learn the basics of accounting, set up your fee schedule, and determine how you will organize financial records. Additionally, set up a separate bank account for your business so you can clearly delineate business income and expenses.

Accounting

It is wise to consult a professional accountant or CPA when starting a business. Setting up the accounting and taxes for a business involves many steps that are unfamiliar to anyone without significant accounting knowledge. You may not realize that to run a business, you have to keep financial records organized and file taxes and tax forms on a timely basis. The key to a good record-keeping system is the ability to find information when necessary. One way to do this is to keep all records in one place and organize them by month. Keeping track of income and expenses may seem straightforward, but it is probably better to let a professional set up the accounting. Professional accountants can help ensure that all of the appropriate forms for your business are obtained and filed.

When your business has a lot of different expenses, your accountant will likely suggest and organize expense account categories. These categories simplify the accounting process, which in turn can simplify the tax calculations. A product called 13-column green bar paper, which can be found at office supply stores, can be used alone or in conjunction with a spreadsheet computer program to track income and expenses on a monthly basis. You may also use a computer program such as Intuit QuickBooks© or search for online resources specifically designed for massage therapists. At the time of this publication, one suggestion is www.massamio.com. The process itself is not so difficult, but it can be a challenge to take time to record income and expenses as they occur. **Do not wait until the end of the year to try to compile the accounting information you need.** Hold onto receipts for business purchases and keep copies of invoices that you pay in full. Because many expenses occur via electronic transaction, you may prefer storing your information on your computer. This allows you to conveniently track expenses electronically and print out a hard copy later, if necessary.

Taxes

All of the money you earn is not yours to keep. You are required to pay the government a percentage of your income in taxes. Every calendar year, as a business owner, you are required to file income tax forms with the IRS, and in most states, with the state's department of revenue. To fill out the forms correctly, you need to know the accounting details for your business.

Many expenses, but not all, associated with the business are deductible, meaning that the expenses can be subtracted from the income to determine the amount of tax you owe the government. All start-up costs may be deductible as well as other expenses incurred by the business throughout the year. Travel expenses, meals and entertainment, supplies, laundry, postage costs, utilities, and professional service fees related to the business are usually tax deductible, although some deductions are limited. Persons often question whether a particular expense is deductible. It is best to let a professional accountant determine your appropriate tax deductions and allowances.

Bookkeeping

It is a good idea to keep your business bank accounts and credit cards separate from your personal accounts because it simplifies the process of categorizing and keeping track of business transactions for bookkeeping and tax filing purposes. It is also much easier to keep track of business

income, enabling you to set aside the appropriate amount of money for quarterly estimated taxes. It is critical for a business to start out on the right foot. Otherwise, too much time will be spent managing the business and solving problems instead of acquiring and treating clients. Undoing mistakes can cost a lot of time and money. (Box 13-9 lists a sample of income and expense categories for a massage business.)

Financial Records

Therapists must keep track of their practice's income and expenses. When you receive any form of payment, provide clients with a formal receipt that includes the date, the amount received, and the form of payment, and keep a copy of the receipt for your own records. Use these receipts to keep track of income for tax purposes. You can purchase simple receipt booklets at most office supply stores or use a computer program to design your own. When you deposit

---

BOX 13-9
Sample Income and Expense Categories

INCOME CATEGORIES
- Fees

EXPENSE ACCOUNT CATEGORIES
- Office supplies
- Membership dues
- Subscriptions
- Mileage
- Health insurance
- Liability insurance
- Travel
- Meals and entertainment
- Rent
- Small equipment
  - Massage table
  - Computer
  - Printer
  - CD player
  - Storage cabinets
  - Desks
- Professional fees
  - Tax preparation fee
  - Accountant
- Laundry fees
- Massage supplies

funds into your business bank account, keep the deposit slips and file them for bookkeeping and tax purposes.

All business expenses and payments should be recorded as well. Expenses for practice-related supplies, laundry services, equipment, travel, gifts, education, meals and entertainment, repair costs, and any other services you pay for may be deductible with proof in the form of receipts. When you are given an invoice, which is a bill for goods or services provided, make sure that it identifies the items purchased and/or services rendered and the date. If any of this information is not clearly indicated, write it on the invoice. When you make a payment for an invoice, write down the amount, the form of payment, and the date of payment directly on the invoice (Fig. 13-19). Keep a copy of the invoice, with all

Therapeutic Massage Supplies and More, Inc.

123 West 45th Street Indianapolis, IN 46268 USA

Phone: 317-555-2165

Fax: 317-555-2185

Email: massagesuppliesandmore@internet.com

Invoice

Invoice #: 692
Invoice Date: October 24, 2012
Customer ID: 22721

Bill To:

Therapeutic Massage Works
7000 Cherry Lane
Zionsville, IN 48077

Ship To:

Keely S.
Therapeutic Massage Works
7000 Cherry Lane
Zionsville, IN 48077

Date	Your Order #	Our Order #	Sales Rep.	FOB	Ship Via	Terms	Tax ID
10/24/2012	TMW31	692-2012	Karen S.	Indianapolis	US Post	Net 30	35S-4237877

Quantity	Item	Units	Description	Discount %	Taxable	Unit Price	Total
2	DML	8 oz.	Deluxe massage lotion	none	yes	$10.00	$20.00

Paid $25.25 with check #3547
cjs 10/30/12

Subtotal	$ 20.00
Tax	$ 1.00
Shipping	$ 4.25
Miscellaneous	
Balance Due	$ 25.25

Figure 13-19. Sample invoice.

of your notations, in your files, and send a copy back with your payment. An organized system for paid invoices and receipts significantly reduces the time and energy required to prepare tax forms.

Setting Fees

The price you charge for your services will vary depending on the massage you provide, your education and experience, and the location of your practice. Your fees should be reasonable and should promote fairness and credibility. Typically, massage therapists charge fees similar to those of other local therapists. Consider the services you provide, your business overhead expenses, such as rent, utilities, cell phone usage, supplies, licenses, insurance, and laundry when you establish your fee schedule.

When starting a massage practice, you may want to offer special discounts to attract clients. Examples of discounts are:

- 25% to 50% discount for new clients
- $5 to $25 off the first massage
- Buy one massage, get one free or get the next massage for half off
- Packages such as three massage sessions for a lower fee
- Refer a friend, get your next massage for half price

Most importantly, keep your fee schedule simple. Offering too many options can confuse clients and complicate your bookkeeping and accounting. You might limit your services to 15-minute corporate massages; 30-, 60-, and 90-minute table massages; and outcalls. Again, research the local massage market and set your fees appropriately.

Marketing and Promotion

Your success in building and sustaining your massage practice depends on having a marketing plan. Marketing is the process of introducing your business and services to prospective clients. People must know what your business has to offer to take advantage of your services, so you must educate them. Generally, people do business with people they like and trust, making it necessary to build relationships as part of your marketing strategy. **Education and building relationships are the keys to any marketing tool.**

Branding

In massage therapy, whether you are a sole proprietor, have a corporation, or are an employee, you are your brand.

Branding consists of a number of factors including communication style, appearance, and print and online presence. The way you present yourself, in person or online, makes a difference in how people perceive you and your business. This all occurs before the client even shows up to get a massage.

Target Market

Your target market is the group of persons you are trying to attract as clients. Generally, when you first start a massage therapy practice, your target market will be anyone seeking health and well-being through massage, but the location of your practice may narrow the focus of your market. For example, if you work in a spa, you may attract more clients seeking massage for stress relief and relaxation. On the other hand, if you work in a medical setting such as a chiropractic office or hospital, you may attract clients seeking relief from pain or a particular medical condition such as low back tightness due to an overuse injury. Because you may work in several locations, you may have several markets to consider. As you continue your education and advance your skills, your target market may become even more focused as you specialize in certain techniques or special populations.

Types of Marketing

Self-promotion, printed materials, advertisements, digitally via the internet, networking, and chair massage are six ways to market your services. Because there are advantages and disadvantages to each, you should be familiar with all six marketing approaches and use whichever is best suited to you, your budget, your services, and your market.

Self-Promotion

Self-promotion is at the core of branding yourself and, ultimately, your success as a massage therapist, whether you are a business owner or employee. Branding is the emotional response and perception people have to you, your product or service, and your image. In order to successfully promote yourself, you need two things—to be passionate about the work you do and to be passionate about yourself. Passion breeds confidence in yourself, which emanates outward to potential and current clients. In order for others to know who you are and what you do, you need to tell them.

There are a number of methods for you to promote yourself. All methods include two essential things: education, and building and sustaining relationships. Education, not selling, helps people understand the benefits of massage and how it can help them. Building and sustaining relationships helps continually create opportunities for your business by raising your visibility and others' awareness of how you add value to people's lives through massage. All self-promotion will be void if you do not take action. Even a small step toward action will move you forward. Following are some simple ways to get the word out about who you are and what you do as a massage therapist.

Business Cards

At the very least, when starting your massage practice, business cards are a must. Business cards are compact, easy to carry, and you can customize them to reflect some of your personality and, ultimately, your brand. Your name, phone number(s), office address, email address, and web site address should be clearly listed so clients can easily contact you to make an appointment for a massage. You may also include a professional photo of yourself to begin to get people to associate you with your brand. Many therapists include titles and credentials next to their names to indicate professional affiliations or educational experience. These are the foundation to cultivating your image and position as an expert in massage therapy. You want to continually build the idea that you are the person who can help clients achieve the results they desire from massage therapy. The use of some titles, such as Certified Massage Therapist and Licensed Massage Practitioner, may be dictated by state or local regulations. Some credentials that are commonly included on massage therapists' business cards include:

- NCTMB—designation of national certification through the NCBTMB
- AMTA member
- ABMP member
- State license number
- Undergraduate and graduate degrees (BA, BS, RN, DC, PT)
- Certification or specialization in specific clientele and techniques

Attending a convention or taking an introductory weekend class in a massage or bodywork modality does not qualify a therapist as a specialist. Indicating special qualifications that are not completely valid falsely advertises a therapist's services. Effective use of techniques requires that therapist complete several classes and practice many hours to be considered proficient. Avoid false advertising and list only specialties for which you are qualified.

Brochures

Brochures are good marketing tools to educate prospective clients. They can educate the public about the various benefits of massage as well as what to expect during the first massage session. You can create brochures on a personal computer or use a professional marketing firm to design a unique brochure. Preprinted brochures are available from several different companies and professional massage organizations. Some promote specific techniques, some list services available, some include frequently asked questions and answers, and some allow therapists to customize the brochure with their own business card, personal information, or business policies.

Newsletters

Printed or email newsletters are an excellent way to educate clients about your qualifications, your practice, and the benefits of massage. Again, you can write your own newsletter or buy a professionally designed one with articles already written. Newsletters are good for keeping in touch with your clientele; educating them on the benefits of massage; and notifying them of special promotions, gift certificate availability, and any other business updates or changes.

Advertising

Advertising in the strictest sense is the use of various forms of media to attract people to your business, service, product, or event. Print ads in newspapers, magazines, journals, and phone books; large signs and banners; classified ads; and radio commercials are just some of the many advertising options. Generally, advertising can be expensive and is not very cost effective for you when beginning your massage therapy practice. If you have your heart set on advertising, the best approach is to run high-quality advertisements on a regular basis. As a general rule, people notice an ad only after they have seen it at least three times, and they take action to buy a product or use a service only after they have seen the advertisement at least seven times. Publications typically provide an advertiser's kit upon request that includes rates for print and classified ads, demographic statistics, and a sample of the publication. Examine these materials to determine whether your target market falls within the demographics of the publication.

The best form of advertising for massage therapists is word-of-mouth advertising. People who know you or have experienced the benefits of your massage are possibly some of your greatest promotional tools. When they tell people about you and your services, they tend to convey true excitement, trust, and belief in you. You can show your appreciation for client referrals by sending a thank you card or postcard or by offering a discount to people who refer new clients to your practice.

Web Site

In the globally connected world we live in, having a web site is a must if you are a business owner. Even if you are working as an employee, establishing a personal web site may be helpful in cultivating your brand within another business. Before doing this, you should check with your employer to ensure that this is acceptable within the structure of the business and your employment agreement.

There are three core components for establishing a web site—quality content, simplicity in design, and functionality. The first component is developing quality content. Developing quality content comes before and guides the design of your web site. A few guidelines for developing quality content include:

- The most important information should go on the top of the page.
- Less is more—if engaged, people spend an average of 7 minutes on a business web site, so be simple, direct, and to the point.
- Use bulleted lists—this helps readers scan more easily.
- Be polished—make sure text is well written and free from spelling and grammatical errors.
- Be client focused—connect readers with the value they will gain from your services.
- Include the following content:
  - Quality professional photo of yourself (head shot)
  - Logo
  - Contact information—physical address, phone number, and email address
  - Markers of expertise—education, credentials, and testimonials
  - Markers of trustworthiness—awards, volunteer involvement, testimonials, and CE (can be added as you build your practice)

You get a tenth of a second to make an impression on your web site so a simple design is critical in getting someone to delve further in. A busy-looking, cluttered site may turn people away from finding the value in what you have to offer via massage therapy. Functionality or the ease with which readers can find the information they want is equally important because a reader will decide to stay engaged on your site or leave it within 10 seconds. If your web site lacks these qualities, it is unlikely that readers will want to find out who you are and what you can offer them.

Social Media

In our global, 24/7 connected world, social media has become the norm in building and sustaining personal and professional relationships. In terms of building your massage therapy practice, it is a vehicle for online and relationship marketing. Social media provides potential clients a convenient way to connect with you or to learn about who you are and what you do. Further, it helps you create and

sustain relationships and gives you the opportunity, over time, to position yourself as an expert in massage therapy. Social media amplifies the content of your web site and, ultimately, your brand. To be successful in social media, you must participate consistently by posting quality content on a regular basis. Post content weekly, if not more often. A simple place to begin creating content is to share your passion about massage therapy, share the benefits of massage, describe the kinds of people you like to treat, or explain why you became a massage therapist. At the time of this publication there are four main social media outlets—Facebook®, LinkedIn®, Twitter®, and Pinterest. Facebook is informal and can be used for personal and business purposes. LinkedIn is a more formal, professional format that essentially hosts your online resumé and enables you to make professional connections. Twitter is a way for you to promote your business via tweets, which are short posts of up to 140 characters. Pinterest is a visual site that allows you to post pins or pictures of products, places, and services you like. You can choose one or all to start your business. In order to be successful on social media, you should:

- Include a professional head shot
- Fill out your profile completely
- Post regularly and consistently—fresh, quality content is key
- Convey who you are as well as your passions for your life and profession
- Collect and give recommendations
- Link to your web site

There are a myriad of resources that can help you establish your presence and brand on social media. You can start simply and expand your usage as you build your massage therapy business. The key is to take advantage of these outlets to build your authority and your brand by taking some action. If you do not know where to start, you may consider hiring a social media coach or expert to give you some advice.

Networking—The Importance of Building Relationships

Another way to promote your business is to network. **Networking** is the practice of establishing mutually beneficial professional relationships with other persons in a business or networking group. People tend to do business with people they know. Any time you personally promote your business, make sure to portray a friendly, trustworthy, professional image. **Business is essentially about building and sustaining relationships.** Building relationships helps create rapport and builds trust in you and your brand. As you begin your business, the easiest way to get the word out is to make a list of all your friends, family members, and businesses you frequent and ask for help. You can do this in several ways. You can mail everyone on the list an introductory letter that briefly summarizes your education, the benefits of massage, the services you offer, and some general business information, such as location, hours, and fees. You can enclose your business card and an introductory coupon for $10 off their first massage. You can connect with people on any of the social media outlets and link them back to your web site or Facebook page. You can "like" the Facebook page of the businesses you frequent.

Business Cards

More often than not, when people first meet each other, they ask each other what they do for a living. **You will frequently have the opportunity to educate a potential client about the benefits of massage, so it is wise to carry business cards with you at all times.** Whenever you hand someone your business card, briefly describe what you do and how massage is beneficial. People are often interested in receiving massage but are not ready enough to take the time to pursue it, so do not be discouraged if a person does not call right away. People come to massage when they are ready. When that time comes, you will have the opportunity to let them experience your massage to appreciate how it can improve the quality of their life.

Networking Groups

Another way to build relationships is to join business networking groups. You can search the internet for business networking groups in your area. People in all types of businesses build and become part of a business network, meeting consistently and periodically. The point of the group is to allow members to introduce themselves and educate each other about their particular businesses. Networking groups give you a chance to get used to public speaking, educating people about the benefits of massage. With regular meetings, the members of the group get to know each other and are more likely to take advantage of each other's services. It also increases the likelihood that the group's members will refer their friend and family to each other's businesses. Remember, people tend to do business with people they know, and word-of-mouth advertisement is often the best kind, especially for massage therapy.

Chair Massage

You can take relationship building to another level by actually giving people a sample of your massage therapy. Chair massage is an excellent marketing tool for introducing people to massage. It is relatively inexpensive, does not require a lot of space, can be set up quickly, provides prospective clients with a short hands-on experience, and familiarizes people with your touch. Because clients remain fully clothed for chair massage, some of the mystery and hesitance associated with full-body massage is eliminated. During the chair massage, you can educate clients about the benefits of receiving regular massage; afterward, offer your business card and an informational brochure. Businesses, health fairs, trade shows, professional business groups, and social gatherings are just a few of the many opportunities you have to use chair massage as a marketing tool.

You can search community calendars and tourism bureaus to find local events at which chair massage might be allowed. Talk to the event organizers about setting up a chair massage station. Some events will require you to pay a fee to reserve space, some events allow you to do chair massage without paying a fee, and other events will pay you to do chair massage. Make sure you take plenty of business cards and brochures in addition to your equipment and supplies.

LinkedIn

LinkedIn is the world's largest professional networking site. Along with providing an opportunity to network with other professionals, it gives you an opportunity to promote your business. LinkedIn is your online professional resumé and includes fields for professional experience, education, publications, and recommendations. To create a successful presence on LinkedIn, it is important to:

- Completely fill out your profile
- Upload a professional quality head shot
- Make connections
- Get recommendations
- Give recommendations

To get the most out of this professional networking site, spend a few minutes each week making connections and giving recommendations.

Long-term Business Development

Setting goals for your practice and defining a time frame for achieving those goals is another aspect to starting a business that can help you succeed in the long run. Identify some milestones that will allow you to recognize progress toward your goals and remain flexible as internal and external influences or challenges present themselves along the way.

Goals and Milestones

Goals are important whether you practice massage as an employee or you are self-employed because ultimately you are responsible for your own success. Before you set goals, envision your practice:

- Business structure
- Location and atmosphere of the business
- Preferred clientele
- Preferred massage techniques
- Size of your business, or the estimated number of weekly massages
- Your budget
- Marketing methods
- CE

The atmospheres in a hospital, physician's office, massage clinic, spa, and health club are very different, and the clientele may vary with the location. Consider these and other options when planning to start your own business. Clients will come from all walks of life. You must know yourself, the different populations you are trained to work with, and your comfort level with different people and health conditions. Some therapists find themselves drawn to a particular special population. Although many therapists enjoy the work and results of relaxation massage techniques, some prefer rehabilitative and therapeutic massage techniques. If your training or comfort level keeps you from treating someone, you must refer the client to another therapist who is better suited for that client. For example, therapists who are uncomfortable treating men, pregnant women, or elderly persons should encourage these people to seek massage from another local therapist.

The size of your business will grow as you increase your client base. The number of clients you have and the number of massages you perform will set your financial budget. Marketing methods you use may be limited by your budget or the amount of time you can allocate to self-promotion.

Incorporate CE into your practice. National certification has CE requirements, as do some professional associations and local and state regulations. There are classes, courses, and seminars offered nationwide in almost every aspect of massage and bodywork. In addition to considering what kind of education you want to pursue, you must factor the course fees into your budget, and you must take into account the lost income from being in class instead of working.

With an idea of how you want to run your business, spend some time organizing your thoughts to develop 1-month, 6-month, 1-year, and 3-year goals. Give some thought to how you want to achieve your goals. Just like short- and long-term treatment goals for clients that are recognizable and achievable, realistic business goals and the milestones leading up to the goals provide motivation while your business is growing. One goal to consider is the number of clients you would like to see each week in your massage practice.

Start by writing down the current condition of your business and the desired outcomes for your business. For example, you might be a new graduate of massage school who has no clients and wants to build up to 15 to 18 clients per week. You could set a 1-month goal to see 1 to 5 clients a week, a 6-month goal to see 5 to 10 clients a week, a 1-year goal to see 10 to 15 clients a week, and a 3-year goal to see 15 to 18 clients consistently each week. With these goals in mind, you have to devise a plan for achieving them with marketing strategies that will attract clients to your practice. The milestones at 1 month, 6 months, and 1 year give you an opportunity to evaluate your progress and adjust your marketing techniques or adjust your goals.

Flexibility

If one thing in life is certain, it is that change will occur. How you respond to change, challenges, and obstacles in your business will influence your success. Suppose you create a great advertisement for a publication, run it for 6 months, and gain no new clients. At the 6-month milestone, you need to evaluate the effectiveness of all of the marketing methods you are using. Rather than running your beautiful ad for an additional 6 months, set the ad aside and turn to the marketing tools that are attracting new clients or that you have not yet tried. Be flexible. If another 6 months goes by and your clientele has not increased, you should probably adjust your goals as well as your marketing tools. Each time you make adjustments to your goals, you will have learned something about your business and the market. Over time and with experience, that cumulative knowledge will help you remain flexible and respond to future changes more appropriately.

Competitive Edge

By developing and following a thorough business plan, your business will run more smoothly, allowing you to spend more time and energy on your massage. Consistently evaluating your business goals and making necessary adjustments will give you a better understanding of your business. This clear direction will keep you on a path that leads to success, and you will have a competitive edge over other therapists who are not as business savvy.

Organizational skills contribute significantly to the success of a business. Time management, client file management, and accounting are business practices that must be organized to be useful. Time management can be challenging for anyone, but especially for massage therapists who tend to be "givers" and have trouble limiting their time commitments. It is difficult to balance the time and energy you spend on your business, self-care, household, family, and friends. By being aware that you need to balance your commitments and by remaining flexible, you will have a competitive edge that helps you develop a successful business.

Self-Care

A business is influenced by the owner's physical, psychological, social, and spiritual health. Just as good health will support your practice as it grows, poor health can destroy it. As the general population becomes more interested in health and wellness, there is more public discussion and education regarding these topics. Wellness is a state when body, mind, and spirit are integrated and energy is used efficiently. You may recall that the Oriental approach to healthcare, based on dynamic and interactive processes, considers a person's health to be a process of responding and adapting to life's rewards and challenges. When body, mind, and spirit are integrated and energy is used efficiently, a person can achieve a higher level of wellness. **It is important to remember that wellness is not a constant state of existence.** The degree of wellness you attain is directly related to the degree to which you take care all parts of yourself. Education and awareness are tools that will assist you and your clients as you each continually strive for balance and high-level wellness.

"You can't give away what you don't have," Dr. Phil McGraw says in his book *Life Strategies*. This sums up the success or failure of a massage therapist. If you do not take care of yourself, you will not be able to take care of your personal life, clients, or business effectively. You can only give what you have. A massage therapist who works in the client's best interest is giving his or her valuable energy to the client during the entire session. Of course, the therapist may also receive energy from the client in the form of reward. Helping someone decrease pain or tension and gain an improved quality of life, even if just for an hour or so, is a great reward. To reap the rewards of massage, however, therapists must take care of themselves in order to have enough energy for clients. Most people who are attracted to massage are "givers" by nature, often giving more than they receive and finding little time for anything more than necessary self-care. Generally, burnout will occur if your level of giving exceeds your level of rest. Specifically, burnout in the massage therapy profession is more likely if a therapist does not begin and continue to practice self-care. Trying different forms of self-care and determining which work best can take time, but you should learn to take care of yourself so that you can take care of your clients.

Before engaging in any new activity, it is wise to assess your current balance of different life factors. Just as you assess a client's tissues prior to massage treatment, you must evaluate the balanced or imbalanced state of your own life before incorporating new or different forms of self-care. People are often unaware of an imbalance until a crisis occurs that highlights a problem. Life assessments are commonly made at the beginning of the calendar year. For example, New Year's resolutions often involve taking better care of one's health through diet, nutrition, and exercise. After 6 weeks or so, however, old habits often creep back, and no other assessment is made until the following January. To prevent this, massage therapists must develop an assessment process that endures the test of time.

Balance

Balance is a condition in which different parts of a whole are in harmony or equilibrium in proportion to each other. When a stack of blocks is balanced, minimal energy is required to maintain its stability. Likewise, when the components of life are balanced, minimal energy is required to maintain and benefit from good health. Evaluating one's physical, psychological, social, and spiritual components and determining whether each of them is receiving enough attention is a type of life assessment. Physical factors include body mechanics, exercise and activity, nutrition and hydration, and rest and sleep. Factors that influence psychological health include education, organization, work, and play. Human beings are social creatures affected by relationships and communication. The spiritual component of life is more difficult to pinpoint but is just as important as other factors. Taking an honest look at your physical, psychological, social, and spiritual components will help you identify areas that require more or less attention to achieve life balance (Fig. 13-20).

Make changes and additions of self-care activities gradually. If you change everything at once, the attempt may backfire and lead to disappointment. Worse yet, disappointment can easily cause you to abandon the quest for life balance. Making life changes and finding balance is a delicate process that should be approached carefully.

The relationships people have with themselves serve as the foundation for all energy exchange. The process of developing a relationship with yourself starts by recognizing your own behaviors and tendencies, understanding why they exist, and being able to change them to develop a healthier and more balanced life. Many factors may contribute to a massage therapist's tendency to give more than

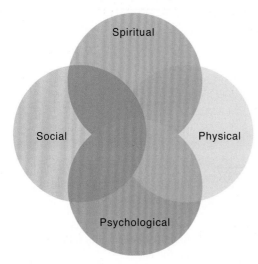

Figure 13-20. Life balance diagram.

receive. Because it can take years of self-examination, and sometimes counseling, to pinpoint those factors, it may be more effective to learn how to sustain a balance between giving and receiving. Massage therapists must take care of their own needs. One of the ways you can do this is by differentiating your needs from your wants and making sure you attend to your needs first. The relationship you have with yourself, or the level to which you know yourself, will help you devote the necessary time and energy to meet your needs, leaving you feeling enlightened and liberated (see Box 13-10).

Often, people are caught up in the "doingness" of life, becoming human "doings" instead of human beings. **The first step in forming a good relationship with yourself is to stop doing and start being.** Experiencing silence and solitude, trying meditation or yoga, and experimenting with activities that allow you to simply exist are good starting points for focusing on who you are rather than what you do. Using self-reflection and self-examination to learn about your physical, mental, social, and spiritual needs may be the most important thing you do in life. It is certainly one of the most important things massage therapists can do to understand how to save or expend energy. After making this evaluation, you can attempt to achieve the balance of these components that is vital for a successful massage practice.

Physical Self-Care

A good place to start making adjustments to your life balance is the physical factors. It is easier to know what changes to make, easier to understand how to accomplish the changes, and usually obvious when the changes have been achieved. More than anything, you must increase your massage work gradually. It is easy to overwork yourself as you try to build a clientele, but the physical work can quickly wear out your body and eventually lead to burnout. Any of the following symptoms may be a sign of burnout:

- Increased irritability and impatience
- Lack of energy
- Diminished satisfaction or passion with work
- Change in sleep or eating habits
- Increase in physical symptoms such as headaches or backaches

If you suspect you have burnout, take time to examine what you need to recharge your body, mind, and spirit. Burnout can lead to exhaustion and possibly injury. If your symptoms continue, seek help from your healthcare practitioner. The physical components of body mechanics, exercise and physical activity, nutrition and hydration, and rest and sleep are influential factors that might need attention in your physical self-care.

BOX 13-10
Life Balance Checklist

CORE SELF-CARE PRINCIPLES
- ☐ "You can't give away what you don't have"
- ☐ Determine which self-care activities work best for you
- ☐ Balance
- ☐ Make gradual changes and additions to your self-care routine

PHYSICAL SELF-CARE
- ☐ Good body mechanics
- ☐ Exercise and physical activity
- ☐ Nutrition and hydration
- ☐ Rest and sleep

PSYCHOLOGICAL SELF-CARE
- ☐ Grounding
- ☐ Centering
- ☐ Education
- ☐ Work and play

SOCIAL SELF-CARE
- ☐ Relationship with self
- ☐ Relationships with others

SPIRITUAL SELF-CARE
- ☐ Accept life's challenges and rewards

Table 13-2 Body Mechanics Problem Areas

Area of Discomfort	Possible Problematic Body Mechanics	Recommended Changes
Upper trapezius, levator scapulae (between head and shoulders)	Shrugged shoulders holding tension in the neck	Relax the neck and shoulders, making sure shoulders are dropped
Finger flexors (on the anterior forearm)	Excessive pétrissage or excessive individual finger work	Use the hand as if it were in a mitten, in which all four fingers work together
Wrist extensors, finger extensors (on the posterior forearm)	Holding fingers up while using the palm or heel of the hand to put pressure on the client	Relax the hands, wrists, and fingers, allowing the fingers to rest on the client
Quadratus lumborum, iliocostalis, longissimus, spinalis (low back)	Bending at the waist, requiring these muscles to continually lift and hold up the therapist	Keep the head, shoulders, hips, knee of the back leg and ankle of the back leg in a straight line

Body Mechanics

Massage therapists must take care of their bodies to sustain a successful practice. The physical nature of massage work can take its toll on your muscles, tendons, and fascia. Massage students often suffer from sore muscles a day or two after giving their first few massages. Most commonly, the upper trapezius, finger flexors, wrist extensors, and erector spinae feel the worst; usually, these muscles are sore as a result of poor body mechanics. Identifying body mechanics that need improvement may help you avoid muscle pain (Table 13-2).

Good body mechanics are critical to a therapist's physical condition. **In fact, good body mechanics is one of the most important factors in the longevity of a massage therapist's career.** When you use good body mechanics, you minimize your energy requirements, muscular misuse, and muscular overuse; you protect your joints from damage; and your work feels better to clients. Following are some key points to remember about good body mechanics (see Chapter 4 for more information about body mechanics):

- Make sure the equipment is adjusted properly.
- Use an asymmetric stance when possible.
- Keep your ears, shoulders, hips, and the heel of your back foot in as straight a line as possible.
- Keep your hips directed toward your work.
- Keep your wrist angle, or the angle between the back of your hand and your forearm, above 110°.
- Keep the axillary angle, or the angle between your humerus and the side of your body, below 90°.

- Keep your body as relaxed as possible, especially at the shoulders.
- Stand behind the point of contact and lean into the client instead of pushing.

Generally, body positions with "stacked" joints require the least energy and should be used when possible. For example, when applying an effleurage stroke with the heel of your hand, try to keep your fingers, wrist, elbow, and shoulder in as straight a line as possible to minimize muscular tension and joint stress. When these joints are stacked, like a straight stack of blocks, they form a stable structure that can deliver a substantial amount of force.

Most persons are unaware of their body positioning when learning a new activity. Seeing your own body in a mirror, positioned with poor body mechanics, is sometimes the best way to recognize problem areas. Truth can be harsh, especially in the form of a mirror reflection, but truth can also be helpful. It may be uncomfortable to see yourself in the mirror, bending over or shrugging your shoulders, but acknowledging and correcting these positions early in your education will minimize future problems. Full-length mirrors mounted on the wall or held by someone nearby are best because they allow you to see all aspects of your body mechanics, including the head-to-heel line.

Exercise and Physical Activity

Exercise is a key component for maintaining physical energy and endurance. Exercise increases one's circulation, bringing more oxygen to the cells and providing more energy. It is generally accepted that a person should get a physician's approval prior to beginning an exercise program. When beginning a new exercise program, start slowly and increase the activity gradually. Increase your activity over time to help build endurance for performing back-to-back massages. You can start by taking short walks; taking the stairs instead of elevators; taking walks during lunch or coffee breaks; doing light calisthenics during television commercials; and taking a series of full, deep breaths when there is a spare moment. Some people prefer the group interaction of an exercise class and the subtle obligation of showing up for a class. Classes and personal trainers can be excellent resources to make sure you are exercising safely, avoiding injury, and using correct techniques.

With everything you know about muscles developing shorter resting lengths when they are held in passive contraction and when they repeatedly perform active contractions and everything you know about the behavior of fascia and the results of fascial restrictions, you should know how important it is to lengthen and stretch your soft tissues. Stretch slowly and gradually, and wait for the tendon reflex to lengthen the muscle. Relaxation techniques, hydrotherapy, massage, and bodywork modalities are your specialties. Use them appropriately to keep yourself in good physical condition.

Nutrition and Hydration

Nutrition is a component of health widely discussed in the media, sometimes to the point of confusion. Contradicting statements are frequently made, making it difficult to know the truth about what is best for your body. It is common knowledge that surviving on coffee and sugary and fast food is not healthy. Likewise, almost everyone knows the general recommendations for what we should and should not consume. A balanced food program that consists of appropriate amounts of water, fruits, vegetables, lean meats and proteins, whole grains, and minimal fat and sugar will help sustain a person's core energy. The key is to gear your nutrition to your unique body and lifestyle.

Because the word "diet" usually carries the negative connotation of deprivation, nutritional changes may be easier to accept when they are thought of as an exploration of a healthy food program. A myriad of fad diets tend to be extreme, concentrating on a particular food group or supplemental pills. It can be unhealthy and potentially dangerous to follow this kind of unbalanced food program. Consulting a physician and/or a nutritionist or dietitian before embarking on a new food program or any other significant lifestyle change is always a good idea.

Massage therapists will do their bodies and health a favor by drinking plenty of water. By setting a good example for clients, you encourage them to follow your recommendations. Drinking adequate amounts of water helps

the body function at an optimal level with minimal energy requirements. Maintaining one's energy is critical for performing numerous high-quality massage sessions.

Recommendations for water consumption vary greatly, depending on the source. Nutritionists and doctors generally recommend about 8 cups, or 64 ounces, of water daily for the average adult, or 0.5 ounces per pound of your body weight. The intake should be increased with physical exercise, salty food, alcoholic beverages, exposure to sun or heat, and illness.

The question of whether liquid intake must be in the form of plain water is also controversial. The best choice is water, but many persons find it challenging to drink 64 ounces of water daily. Drinking liquids that have any kind of additives or chemicals in them can be problematic because processing those chemicals requires more energy from the body. Alcohol actually causes the body to shed water. For persons who dislike water, however, drinking the same amount of another liquid may be the best option. One easy way to get enough water is to carry water in a bottle with you everywhere you go. Water has become increasingly popular and is available almost everywhere. Staying hydrated is easier to do now than ever, and there are few excuses for not drinking several glasses of water each day.

Rest and Sleep

Rest and sleep are crucial to health. Feeling fatigued or overtired negatively affects how a person thinks and acts, and it can hamper bodily processes. Rest is a period of inactivity or refreshing quiet. You can incorporate rest into your daily routine by taking a midafternoon nap or short breaks between massages. Regardless of how much rest you get, your body needs a certain amount of sleep to function properly. Sleep is a bodily process during which consciousness is partially or completely suspended and the parasympathetic nervous system sets the body's rejuvenation mechanism into action. Many scientific studies have proven that without sufficient sleep, there are severe health consequences. Different persons require different amounts of sleep, and people generally know when they are not getting enough. There are a number of small adjustments you can make to lifestyle and daily habits that can improve the quality and quantity of sleep.

Psychological Self-Care

Massage therapists and their clients have a professional relationship that requires them to share personal space. Although many persons reject the idea that emotions and thoughts can be shared through touch and without words, just as many persons believe it to be fact. Either way, therapists have an obligation to provide a client-focused massage session, without giving or receiving any kind of psychological or physical discord or stress. Grounding and centering techniques can help you share space with your clients in a healthy way. As a reminder, grounding techniques provide a sort of psychological barrier between you and your clients, and centering techniques help you stay focused on your clients. Psychologically stimulating activities such as education, work, and play can go a long way toward helping you create and maintain mental wellness.

Grounding

By using grounding before or during a massage, you can remind yourself that you are only a facilitator for the client's healing process. When you take on sole responsibility for healing your clients, curing their ills, and repairing the soft tissues of their bodies, you use your own core energy, which can leave you mentally and physically drained. It is more productive to create a partnership with your client, in which you are a facilitator, redirecting the client's own energies toward better health and more efficient healing. With this philosophy in mind, you can remain humble while empowering your clients to participate in their health and well-being. This is a subtle difference in your intent and approach that can affect your massage practice in the long term.

Centering

Mental centering is a good technique that clears the mind of distraction and helps therapists focus on the client and the massage. Visualization and breathing techniques are most common. Some persons envision a specific place that brings them feelings of peace and relaxation, free of noise and distraction. Other persons take slow and rhythmic breaths, focusing on the body and its response to the breath. After reaching a state of mental quiet, you can turn your attention to the present and approach the massage session with a clear focus.

Education

Education also stimulates the mind, whether in the form of reading, writing, or learning a new activity. Many magazines, journals, and books cover topics on massage and bodywork. Being familiar with the changes and new developments in the field can boost your confidence and increase client trust. Learning about business practices and how to streamline a business can help your business run more smoothly and efficiently. Education and training should not stop at graduation. Your initial training just scratches the surface of knowledge about massage and the structures and functions of soft tissues. CE broadens your knowledge base and often rekindles enthusiasm for practicing massage.

Work and Play

A person's perceptions of work and play are influenced more by his or her attitude than by the activity itself, as demonstrated by kids who love to play house and sweep floors. Once the child considers sweeping to be work, it can seem torturous and dreadful. The activity of sweeping did not change; only the perception changed. Work and play are components of life that significantly affect one's mental health. Massage therapists may need to examine the amount of work they do and compare it with the amount of fun or playful activities in an effort to balance the two.

Social Self-Care

Although social self-care is often overlooked, it can also influence the success of a massage practice. Social and personal relationships and communication are important for social self-care, and massage therapists should evaluate how they affect their life.

Relationships with partners, friends, and family members become important as one discovers more about energy distribution. Relationships ebb and flow, sometimes giving energy and sometimes costing energy. Friends and family members may find it difficult to accept less energy from you as you venture into a massage practice, and you may find it difficult to devote less energy to your relationships as you build a practice. Adjusting your energy distribution is easier said than done. Changing dynamics within relationships involves special challenges, but true friends and family members who support you will eventually understand the need for change. Be aware that this may occur, and monitor your energy as you move through this sometimes delicate process.

On the positive side, socializing with people can be a tremendous source of energy. Include social gatherings, dining experiences, and any other social activities that are fun for you in your social self-care plan. Humans are social by nature and need human interaction, and social activities can give you a tremendous energy boost.

Good communication skills are very helpful as you reorganize your time and energy commitments. Listening carefully to others and reiterating their statements to ensure that you understand them are important elements of good communication. If your friends feel left out or rejected, explain the need for changes in the relationship's dynamics.

Spiritual Self-Care

Life has a spiritual component even for persons who do not attend church or practice a religion. Spirituality is a very personal matter about which many persons are sensitive, and it plays an important role in our wellness. Some believe spirituality to be an issue of whether a person believes in a higher power, whether one follows a set of religious rules, or whether one believes in heaven or reincarnation. In a way, spirituality is an acceptance of life's challenges and rewards, and it can help you move toward wellness.

CHAPTER SUMMARY

Massage therapy is a business. In addition to understanding anatomy, physiology, and massage techniques, you must understand how to start and sustain a successful business. Many massage therapists begin their practices with zeal and excitement, only to soon find out that they are not prepared for what it takes to be a professional massage therapist as well as the business demands of such an endeavor. As a result, many therapists eventually drop out of the profession.

Massage therapists can burn out physically, financially, emotionally, or from lack of perseverance. Improper body mechanics and poor physical self-care are common factors in physical burnout, but almost as common is attempting to give too many massages too soon. Financially, therapists may run out of money before their practice is thriving. Emotionally, therapists may find that they have given beyond their means and have not conserved their energy, leaving nothing for themselves. We must remember that we are facilitators for healing, not healers. Finally, therapists may lose interest or fail to persevere while establishing a massage practice. To avoid burnout, thoroughly examine how you want to set up your practice, learn and practice good approaches to self-care, set up a plan for success, and persevere until you meet your business goals. Begin the practice carefully, gradually increasing the number of massages given in a day and in a week.

Physical, psychological, social, and spiritual aspects of self-care and wellness are dynamic, interactive processes. Their effects on each other influence a person's health and well-being. Ultimately, your health will affect your massage practice. Keeping up your education and awareness of wellness, learning and comprehending business basics and government regulations, and practicing self-care help you establish a stronger foundation upon which you can build a successful massage practice.

CHAPTER EXERCISES

1. Write at least a paragraph describing why it is important to have a business plan when beginning your massage therapy practice.

2. Compare and contrast self-employment with working as an employee, including the different tax responsibilities, set-up requirements, levels of liability, and levels of control over your work.

3. Write your resumé.

4. Write a list of policies and procedures for your own massage therapy practice.

5. Describe in detail at least three different ways you plan on marketing yourself.

6. Design your business card.

7. Explain the importance of self-care for the massage therapist.

8. Write a description of the locations of at least five different massage practices you have seen or visited. Compare and contrast the locations and your perception of the massage environment.

9. Write a description of your ideal massage treatment room, including the location, all of the equipment, and environmental factors.

10. Massage equipment manufacturers typically offer equipment packages that include an adjustable massage table and some accessories such as a bolster and/or carrying case. Research the massage equipment packages offered by at least four different companies and write down the similarities and differences between them.

11. Describe each of the three different levels of infection control.

12. How much household bleach should you add to a wash cycle of laundry that has been contaminated with bodily fluids?

13. Describe the five steps of proper handwashing.

14. Identify the four concepts of standard precautions you need to follow.

15. Describe the four steps for primary assessment in an emergency situation.

CRITICAL THINKING EXERCISES

Below is a sample of a critical thinking format that helped Jane design her plan for success as a massage therapist. On a separate sheet of paper, use the same format to design your own plan for success.

Sample Personal Plan for Success and Self-Care

Name: Jane Therapist   **Date: May 1, 2006**

Objective	Critical Thinking Questions and Activities	Outcomes	Plan
Develop a plan for success	Research the benefits of joining a professional organization	Search the web: www.aboutmassage.com/associations-main.htm. Research all associations for the one the fits best for me. Main benefit: liability insurance Other benefits: trade magazine, marketing materials, etc.	Join AMTA as a professional member.
	List at least three techniques you are interested in learning more about	Identify techniques and web resources. Find resources (magazine articles, books, web site information). Search the web for more information on each technique.	Sign up for Craniosacral class from the Upledger Institute. (www.Upledger.com) Find and read references on myofascial and Shiatsu techniques.
	Copy Business Start-up Checklist (Box 13-6)	If applicable, complete each step on the business start-up checklist.	First steps: Obtain appropriate licenses and permits. Set up appointment with professional accountant. Design and have business cards printed.
	Find at least one mentor	Search the local area for business networking groups. Ask your instructor/school owner for a list of names of people who might be willing to be a mentor.	Set up an initial meeting with at least one potential mentor.
Develop a plan for self-care	Research the concept of life balance	Search the local library or bookstore for references on life balance. Search the web for more information on life balance.	Buy a notebook/journal. Sign up for www.maximumbalance.com. Buy a book on avoiding burnout. Talk to my massage mentor for tips on how to avoid burnout. Preplan time off and vacation.
	Develop a plan for physical self-care	Determine what exercises and/or physical activity you enjoy. Determine your nutritional and hydration needs. Determine how much rest and sleep you require.	Write down my plan for each activity in my self-care notebook/journal. Revise as needed.

Objective	Critical Thinking Questions and Activities	Outcomes	Plan
Develop a plan for psychological self-care		Determine how you will ground and center yourself before each massage session.	Write down my plan for each activity in my self-care notebook/journal.
		Determine how you would like to continue your education (books, magazines, classes).	Revise as needed.
		Determine activities that enrich you outside of the massage practice or workplace.	
Develop a plan for social self-care		Examine how you will prioritize yourself and time alone.	Schedule at least 1 day a month for time off to spend doing whatever I enjoy.
		Determine your sources of social and personal support (significant other, family, friends, and/or coworkers, etc.).	Schedule social time with my sources of support.
			Write down my thoughts and feelings in my self-care notebook/ journal at least once a week. Revise as needed.

REFERENCES

1. http://www.osha-slc.gov/SLTC/healthguidelines/oilmist/, accessed 3.5.06.
2. http://www.preventcancer.com/consumers/cosmetics/cosmetics_personal_care.htm, accessed 3.5.06.
3. http://www.nlm.nih.gov/medlineplus/ency/article/002771.htm, accessed 3.5.06.
4. http://www.nlm.nih.gov/medlineplus/ency/article/002719.htm, accessed 3.5.06.
5. Campbell D. *The Mozart Effect*. New York: Avon Books, 1997.

SUGGESTED READINGS

American Massage Therapy Association. *The Business of Massage: The Complete Guide to Establishing Your Massage Career*. Evanston, IL: American Massage Therapy Association, 2002.

American Massage Therapy Association. *Career Guide*. Evanston, IL: American Massage Therapy Association, 1999.

Ashton J, Cassel D. *Review for Therapeutic Massage and Bodywork Certification*. Baltimore: Lippincott Williams & Wilkins, 2002.

Be well: Therapist self-care. *Massage Magazine*. 2003:101.

Boyce-Tillman J. *Constructing Musical Healing*. Philadelphia: Jessica Kingsley, 2000.

Brown J. *Don't Touch That Doorknob!: How Germs Can Zap You and How You Can Zap Back*. New York: Warner Books, 2001.

Campbell D. *The Mozart Effect*. New York: Avon Books, 1997.

Carter P, Lewsen S. *Lippincott's Textbook for Nursing Assistants, A Humanistic Approach to Caregiving*. Philadelphia: Lippincott Williams & Wilkins, 2005.

Covey S. *The Seven Habits of Highly Effective People*. New York: Simon & Schuster, 1989.

Deckers E, Lacy K. *Branding Yourself: How to Use Social Media to Invent or Reinvent Yourself*. Upper Saddle River, NJ: Pearson Education, Inc., 2011.

Evans DH. *The Ultimate Handbook: Self-Care for Bodyworkers and Massage Therapists*. San Francisco: Self-published, 1992.

Greene L. *Save Your Hands: Injury Prevention for Massage Therapists*. Seattle: Infinity Press, 1995.

Jackson R. *Holistic Massage, The Holistic Way to Physical and Mental Health*. New York: Sterling Publishing, 1987.

MacDonald G. *Massage for the Hospital Patient and Medically Frail Client*. Baltimore: Lippincott Williams & Wilkins, 2005.

McGraw P. *Life Strategies*. New York: Hyperion Press, 1999.

Molle E, Kronenberger J, Durham LS, et al. *Comprehensive Medical Assisting*. 2nd ed. Baltimore: Lippincott Williams & Wilkins, 2005.

Osborne-Sheets C. *Deep Tissue Sculpting*. 2nd ed. Poway, CA: Body Therapy Associates, 1990.

Pagliarulo, MA. *Introduction to Physical Therapy*. 2nd ed. St. Louis: Mosby, 2001.

Ruud E. *Music Therapy: Improvisation, Communication and Culture*. Gilsum, NH: Barcelona Publishers, 1998.

Sohnen-Moe CM. *Business Mastery: A Guide for Creating a Fulfilling, Thriving Business and Keeping It Successful*. 3rd ed. Tucson, AZ: Sohnen-Moe & Associates, 1997.

Tracy B. *The 100 Absolutely Unbreakable Laws of Business Success*. San Francisco: Berrett-Koehler Publishers, 2002.

Travis JW, Ryan RS. *The Wellness Workbook*. 2nd ed. Berkeley, CA: Ten Speed Press, 1988.

Werner R. *A Massage Therapist's Guide to Pathology*. Baltimore: Lippincott Williams & Wilkins, 1998.

http://aolsvc.homeworkhelp.search.aol.com/homeworkhelp/search?source=webster&query=sepsis, accessed 10.30.05.

http://digestive.niddk.nih.gov/ddiseases/pubs/viralhepatitis/, accessed 9.11.05.

http://editiondigital.net/publication/?i;EQ64159, accessed 10.20.12.

http://encarta.msn.com/encnet/refpages/search.aspx?q=human+disease&Submit2=Go, accessed 3.5.06.

http://kylelacy.com, accessed 10.21.12.

http://seattlepi.nwsource.com/national/cra30.shtml, accessed 3.5.06.

http://writingabluestreak.com, accessed 10.20.12.

http://www.abmp.com/home/index.html, accessed 3.5.06.

http://www.amtamassage.org, accessed 3.5.06.

http://www.apic.org, accessed 3.5.06.

http://www.biotone.com, accessed 3.5.06.

http://www.britannica.com, accessed 3.5.06.

http://www.bt.cdc.gov/disasters/extremeheat/faq.asp, accessed 9.17.06.

http://www.cdc.gov/HAI/pdfs/ppe/PPEslides6-29-04.pdf, accessed 10.20.12.

http://www.cdc.gov/mmwr/preview/mmwrhtml/rr5116a1.htm, accessed 3.5.06.

http://www.cdc.gov/ncidod/dhqp/bp_laundry.html, accessed 3.5.06.

http://www.cdc.gov/ncidod/dhqp/bp_sterilization_medDevices.html, accessed 3.5.06.

http://www.cdc.gov/ncidod/dhqp/bp_universal_precautions.html, accessed 3.5.06.

http://www.cdc.gov/ncidod/op/handwashing.htm, accessed 3.5.06.

http://www.cdc.gov/niosh/hcwold5.html, accessed 3.5.06.

http://www.cdc.gov/od/oc/media/pressrel/fs021025.htm, accessed 3.5.06.

http://www.chrisbrogan.com, accessed 10.21.12.

http://www.cinetwork.com/otero/cdc.html, accessed 3.5.06.

http://www.clorox.com/solutions_reg_bleach.php, accessed 3.5.06.

http://www.customcraftworks.com, accessed 3.5.06.

http://www.earthlite.com, accessed 3.5.06.

http://www.eatwell.gov.uk/healthydiet/nutritionessentials/drinks/drinkingenough/, accessed 3.5.06.

http://www.epa.gov/oppad001/chemregindex.htm, accessed 10.20.12.

http://www.epa.gov/oppad001/list_b_tuberculocide.pdf, accessed 3.5.06.

http://www.geologyshop.co.uk/chalk.htm, accessed 3.5.06.

http://www.info4people.com, accessed 3.5.06.

http://www.in.gov/sos/business/2428.htm, accessed 9.3.12.

http://www.ivillage.com/food/experts/hltheat/qas/0,11749,242248_17843,00.html, accessed 3.5.06.

http://www.mansfield.ohio-state.edu/sabedon/biol2050.htm, accessed 3.5.06.

http://www.massagetherapy.com/careers/stateboards.php, accessed 10.20.12.

http://www.mayoclinic.com/health/burnout/wl00062, accessed 10.22.12.

http://www.mayoclinic.com/invoke.cfm?id=FA00061, accessed 9.13.06.

http://www.niaid.nih.gov/factsheets/hivinf.htm, accessed 9.11.06.

http://www.nlm.nih.gov/medlineplus/ency/article/002719.htm, accessed 3.5.06.

http://www.nlm.nih.gov/medlineplus/ency/article/002771.htm, accessed 3.5.06.

http://www.nlm.nih.gov/medlineplus/heatillness.html, accessed 9.17.06.

http://www.nohsc.gov.au/OHSInformation/Databases/Exposure Standards/az/Oil_mist_refined_mineral.htm, accessed 3.5.06.

http://www.nursingworld.org/AJN/2000/aug/Health.htm, accessed 3.5.06.

http://www.osha.gov/pls/oshaweb/owadisp.show_document?p_table=standards&p_id=10051, accessed 10.20.12.

http://www.osha.gov/SLTC/etools/hospital/hazards/univprec/univ.html, accessed 10.20.12.

http://www.osha.gov/SLTC/healthguidelines/oilmist/recognition.html, accessed 3.5.06.

http://www.ou.edu/oupd/choke.htm, accessed 9.13.06.

http://www.preventcancer.com/consumers/cosmetics/talc.htm, accessed 3.5.06.

http://www.redcross.org/services/hss/tips/universal.html, accessed 3.5.06.

http://www.redcrossstore.org/shopper/product.aspx?uniqueitemid=584&viewsource=xxx, accessed 10.20.12.

http://www.saveyourhands.com, accessed 3.5.06.

http://www.sba.gov, accessed 9.3.12.

http://www.score.org, accessed 9.3.12.

http://www.sohnen-moe.com/, accessed 3.5.06.

http://www.stayingintouch.net, accessed 3.5.06.

http://www.useit.com, accessed 10.21.12.

http://www.watercolorscards.com, accessed 3.5.06.

http://www.wdghu.org/topics/cd/cd_handwashing.html, accessed 3.5.06.

https://massage.bloomfire.com, accessed 10.20.12.

https://sohnen-moe.com/t-tools/student-success-guide.pdf, accessed 10.20.12.

https://www.fsmtb.org, accessed 9.3.12.

www.imassageinc.com, accessed 10.20.12.

www.spinweb.net, accessed 10.20.12.

Glossary

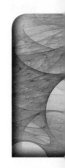

Accountability The quality of accepting the consequences of your actions and claiming responsibility for your decisions.

Active range of motion (AROM) Joint movement that requires clients to actively use their own energy to demonstrate how much of the full range can be completed comfortably and without restriction.

Activity and analysis information The massage activity and an analysis of the treatment session documented on the SOAP note.

Acupoints Specifically located points on the body that influence, and are influenced by, body energies.

Acupressure (AK-yoo-preh-sher) A bodywork modality in which firm fingertip pressure is applied to acupoints along the energy meridians to regulate the flow of Qi.

Acute Refers to a condition that has developed very quickly and severely, or has a short duration.

Anatomical position Describes a person standing up, feet shoulder-width apart, arms at the sides, and palms facing forward.

Anatomy The study of the structures of plants and animals.

Anointing Ritualistic or religious activity of rubbing oil into the skin.

Antagonist A muscle that moves in opposition to the prime mover.

Artery A tube that carries blood away from the heart.

Artificial respiration (also called **artificial resuscitation**, **mouth-to-mouth respiration**, and **rescue breathing**) A mechanical or manual technique of forcing air into a person's lungs if he/she is not breathing but has a pulse.

Asian Bodywork Therapy (ABT) The term used to encompass all bodywork modalities that have their theoretical roots in Chinese medicine.

Assessment The process of evaluating a client's condition.

Asymmetric stance (also **one-foot-forward stance**) Standing position in which both feet are on the ground, shoulder-width apart, one foot is in front of the other, and the back foot is laterally rotated.

Athlete A person who participates in sports on an amateur or professional level.

Bioenergy The electrical, electromagnetic, and/or bioelectromagnetic qualities of living tissue.

Biomechanics The study of how movement of living creatures is affected by both internal and external factors.

Body mechanics The efficient and effective use of your body when performing massage.

Body of knowledge The essential knowledge, concepts, skills, and attitudes of a profession, as defined by the relevant professional association, which must be mastered to achieve success.

Bodywork Treatment that involves manipulation of the client's body as a way to maintain or improve health.

Bony landmark Site for muscle attachment or safe passageway for nerves and blood vessels; bony landmarks can usually be externally palpated.

Cardiopulmonary resuscitation (CPR) A combination of artificial respiration and chest compressions that restores circulation for a person who is not breathing and has no pulse.

Centering A technique that helps you focus your attention on your clients.

Certification The act of issuing someone a certificate of completion or validation of authenticity.

Chair massage A massage for persons who are fully clothed that is delivered while the client is seated in a specially designed chair, also called seated massage, onsite massage, corporate massage, and event massage.

Chronic Refers to a condition that has persisted for a long time, develops slowly, or recurs.

Chronic illness Illness that lasts a year or longer, usually limits a patient's physical activity, and may require ongoing medical care and treatment.

Client-centered When attitudes, decisions, and activities of a practice are in the best interest of the client's health and well-being.

Code of ethics Commonly accepted guidelines or principles of conduct that govern professional conduct.

Compensation pattern A postural offset that is the body's attempt to correct an imbalance or protect a primary dysfunction or injury.

Compression A stroke that applies pressure to soft tissues to squeeze them together without any slip.

Concentric contraction A muscle contraction in which the muscle shortens and the attachment sites of the muscle move closer together.

Confidentiality The principle that client information revealed to a health professional during an appointment is to be kept private and has limits on how and when it can be disclosed to a third party.

Contraindication A situation or condition in which massage could worsen the condition.

Contrast therapy Heat application followed by cold application, also called alternating therapy.

Corporation A business arrangement that has one or more owners who are legally separate from the business.

Deep Refers to something farther from the surface of the skin, or deeper inside the body.

Deep-fiber friction A stroke that is applied with deep, localized pressure without any slip on the skin to break up fascial adhesions and separate the muscle fibers.

Deficiency The term used to describe a depleted condition in Chinese medicine.

Direct manipulation (DM) A proprioceptive neuromuscular facilitation (PNF) technique in which you use the muscle spindles and Golgi tendon organs to relax a hypertonic muscle.

Direction of ease The direction in which tissues move with least resistance.

Direction of restriction The direction in which tissues resist movement the most.

Distal Refers to something that is farther away from the torso, toward the fingers or toes.

Eccentric contraction A muscle contraction in which the distance between the muscle attachments increases and the muscle effectively gets longer.

Effleurage (EF-lur-ahzh) A slow, gliding stroke along the client's skin.

End feel A unique feel when a joint reaches the end of its passive range of motion (PROM) determined by specific structures that stop the movement.

Ergonomics The science that designs and coordinates people's activities with the equipment they use and the working conditions of their environment.

Ethics Conduct rules based on integrity and differentiating right from wrong.

Etiology The study of the source or cause of disease.

Event massage Administered on the day of the event to help the athlete prepare for and recover from the activity, it includes pre-event, inter-event, and post-event massage.

Excess The term used to describe an overly strong condition in Chinese medicine.

Fascia (FASH-uh) A fibrous band or sheetlike tissue membrane that provides support and protection for the body organs.

Fascial adhesion (fascial restriction) An area where the fascia has adhered to nearby tissues or has been crumpled or kinked.

Five Vital Substances Defined by Chinese medicine as the five basic substances that supplement the tissues in a human body: Qi, Blood, Essence, body fluids, and Shen (consciousness).

Flow A routine-like sequence of steps that leads the massage from one body part to the next in a systematic, fluid pattern that often specifies stroke sequences.

Gait A walking pattern.

Grounding A technique you can use to establish an emotional and energetic boundary between you and your clients.

Gymnastics Activity at ancient gymnasiums that included exercise, massage, and baths.

HIPAA Health Insurance Portability and Accountability Act, enacted in 1996 to help employees and their families obtain and transfer health insurance coverage when their employment changes or is terminated.

Homeostasis (HOH-mee-oh-STAY-sis) The process by which the body continually adjusts to changes in order to maintain chemical, physiological, and structural balance.

Hospice A healthcare approach that caters to the quality of remaining life rather than the quantity of life when a person's life expectancy is limited by a life-threatening illness with no known cure.

Hydrotherapy The external or internal use of water for therapeutic use.

Hypertonic (HAHY-per-TAHN-ik) Excessively tense or tight.

Indication A condition for which massage could be beneficial and is recommended.

Inferior (also caudad) Refers to something more toward the feet, or below.

Informed consent A client's agreement to participate in an activity after the purpose, methods, benefits, risks, and rights to withdraw at any time have been explained.

Insertion of a muscle The point of attachment that moves most during contraction, often at the distal end.

Inter-event massage Performed in between events that occur on the same day and within a given time period, focusing on areas of increased muscular tension that have occurred as a direct result of participation in the activity.

Joint The mechanical structure where neighboring bones are attached, often with connective tissue and cartilage.

Kinesiology The study of human movement.

Lateral Refers to something farther away from the midline of the body

Lengthening The neurological process that lengthens myofibrils and results in a longer muscle.

Licensure Legal authority or permission to practice massage when the state laws or regulations require it.

Local contraindication A situation in which massage would be considered therapeutic except in a localized area, whereby using massage could cause further harm.

Lymph The fluid that started out as blood plasma, leaked out through the capillaries to become interstitial fluid, and is picked up by the very delicate ends of the lymphatic vessels from tissues all over the body.

Lymphatic fluid (lymph) The interstitial fluid that is taken from the all over the body into the lymphatic system.

Maintenance massage Performed in between sporting events to maintain flexibility and ensure that muscles are relaxed and lengthened to prevent injuries from occurring during training.

Massage Manual therapy involving pressure applied with the hands (term started by the French explorers in the 1700s).

Massage treatment record The document containing input from clients, your objective assessments of the clients' condition, the massage techniques you use, results of the treatment session, and plans for future massage treatment.

Mechanical effects Therapist applies pressure or manipulation to physically change the shape or condition of the client's tissues.

Medial Refers to something closer to the midline of the body.

Meridians Precise and orderly channels or pathways through which Qi flows.

Meridian therapy The art of working to open and move the joints, release blockages in tissue, balance the Qi moving in the meridians, and stimulate the actions of acupoints as needed.

Metabolic effects Combined result of mechanical and reflex effects on the whole body.

Metabolism The overall cellular activity that breaks down nutrients to generate energy to build essential molecules.

Modality A collection of manual therapies that tends to use similar applications of movement or massage strokes to reach a similar goal.

Motor neuron (efferent neuron) Neuron that carries messages away from the central nervous system to the muscle or organs that must react.

Motor unit One motor neuron and all of the muscle cells it stimulates.

Movement Cure American version of Ling's movement system.

Muscle A specially organized and packaged group of muscle cells, connective tissue wrappings, and blood vessels.

Muscle energy techniques (METs) Bodywork applications that use the nervous system to change a muscle's resting length, also called proprioceptive neuromuscular facilitation.

Muscle guarding Hypertonic muscles stabilizing or splinting an injured area.

Nerve A specially organized and packaged bundle of neurons, connective tissue wrappings, and blood vessels.

Nerve plexus Large network of intertwined nerves.

Networking The practice of establishing mutually beneficial professional relationships with other persons in a business or networking group.

Neuron (nerve cell) The basic unit of the nervous system.

Objective information Your visual, palpation, range-of-motion, and gait assessments of the client's body and soft tissues documented on the SOAP note.

Origin of a muscle The attachment on the bone or connective tissue structure that is more stationary during muscle contraction.

Palpation The skillful art of client evaluation that uses touch to locate and assess the quality of different structures.

Parasympathetic response Autonomic nervous system response that stimulates organs to work in a relaxing "rest and digest" mode.

Partnership A company in which two or more persons share ownership and personal liability for all business transactions.

Passive range of motion (PROM) Joint movement that requires the therapist to move the relaxed client through a range of motion to determine how much of the full range can be completed comfortably and without restriction.

Pathology The study of disease processes or of any deviation from a normal, healthy condition.

Petrissage (PET-rih-sahzh) A stroke that kneads soft tissues with a grasping and lifting action.

Pharmacology The study of the preparation, mechanisms, applications, and effects of medications.

Physiology The study of the functions of a living organism or any of its parts.

Plan information The section of the SOAP note including plans for future treatment and self-care recommendations.

Polarity (poh-LAIR-ih-tee) therapy A modality in which very light massage strokes and energy movements are applied on and off the client's body to balance electromagnetic fields, energy nutrition, and develop a higher consciousness.

Positional release (PR) A PNF technique that relieves hypertonicity by holding the body in a painless position and waiting for the nervous system to trigger relaxation, also called strain/counterstrain.

Post-event massage Performed within 2 hours of the athletic performance, it focuses on circulatory enhancement to aid in recovery from the activity as well as decrease muscle and connective tissue tension.

Post-isometric relaxation (PIR) A PNF technique that uses active contraction and relaxation of the target muscle to lengthen the muscle.

Pre-event massage Performed just before the client participates in an athletic event, it focuses on circulatory enhancement and warming up the tissues.

Prime mover (also agonist) The muscle that performs most of the intended movement.

Privacy Rule (Standards for Privacy of Individually Identifiable Health Information) A modification of the original HIPAA that legally protects health-related information from being shared without clients' written permission by requiring all healthcare practitioners to keep their clients' health information private and protected.

Professionalism Ethical conduct, goals, and qualities characterized by a profession.

Prone Lying face down.

Proprioceptive neuromuscular facilitation (PROH-pree-oh-SEP-tive NOO-roh-MUSS-kyoo-lar fah-SIHL-ih-TAY-shun) (PNF) Bodywork applications that use the nervous system to change a muscle's resting length, also called muscle energy techniques.

Proprioceptor (PROH-pree-oh-SEP-tor) Sensory neuron responsible for detecting body position, muscle tone, and equilibrium.

Proximal Describes something toward the attachment point of the limb to the body.

Qi (C'hi, Ki) (pronounced CHEE) Life force or vital energy; the bioenergy of living things.

Qi (CHEE) A dynamic, changing energy force that runs through the whole body, supplying and being supplied by body processes and activities.

Range of motion (ROM) The end-to-end distance of a specific joint movement that is structurally possible.

Reciprocal inhibition (RI) A PNF technique in which the client contracts a target muscle's antagonists to reflexively relax the target muscle.

Refer Recommend that someone see a specific healthcare practitioner.

Reflex effects Therapist stimulates the client's sensory neurons, which triggers the client's nervous system to change the shape or condition of the tissues in areas that were addressed as well as other, related areas.

Reflexology (REE-fleks-AH-loh-jee) A modality in which fingertip compression is applied to reflex points on the hand, foot, or ear that affect other parts of the body.

Registration The act of enrolling in a system or database that keeps track of recorded information.

Resting length The length to which a relaxed, inactive muscle can be safely extended.

Resting stroke A stroke that requires you to stop moving and lightly rest your relaxed hands, fingers, or arms on your client for several seconds.

Restorative massage Performed 6 to 72 hours after the athletic performance, it is intended to increase circulation and restore the normal resting length of muscles; also called curative massage and post-recovery massage.

Right lymphatic duct A major drain that collects all of the lymph from the upper right quadrant of the body, including everything on the right side of the body above the diaphragm, and empties it into the right subclavian vein.

Scope of practice A practitioner's service limits and boundaries as determined by legal, educational, competency, and accountability factors.

Self-care (self-help) Activities that clients can use between massage sessions to participate in their healing process and help them achieve their treatment goals.

Sensory neuron (afferent neuron) Neuron that receives sensory input and transmits that information to the central nervous system.

Side-lying (laterally recumbent) Lying on one's side.

Slip The sliding of your skin over the surface of the client's skin.

SOAP An acronym for Subjective, Objective, Activity and analysis, and Plan that refers to a format for documentation.

Sole proprietorship A business arrangement in which one person owns the business and is personally liable for all business transactions.

Special populations Segments of the population whose massage requires special considerations.

Standard precautions Specific procedures that maintain a hygienic and sanitary practice and reduce the risk for germ transmission.

Standards of practice Specific rules and procedures for professional conduct and quality of care that are to be followed by all members of a profession.

Strain/counterstrain (SCS) A PNF technique that relieves hypertonicity by holding the body in a painless position and waiting for the nervous system to trigger relaxation, also called positional release.

Stretch reflex A protective muscle contraction that occurs when the tissues are stretched too far and/or too fast.

Stretching An elastic deformation of the fascia that extends its length.

Subacute The period from about 3 days to 3 weeks after a condition started.

Subjective information Verbal and written information clients share with you regarding their health documented in the SOAP note.

Superficial Refers to something closer to the surface of the skin.

Superficial friction A brisk variation of light effleurage that increases circulation in the superficial tissues and dissipates body heat.

Superior (also cephalad) Refers to something closer to a person's head, or above.

Supine Lying face up, on back or spine.

Swedish Gymnastics A therapeutic movement system developed by Per Henrik Ling.

Swedish Movements Europe's version of Ling's movement system.

Symmetric stance (also parallel stance) Standing position in which both feet face forward about shoulder-width apart, hips face forward, and knees are bent.

Sympathetic response Autonomic nervous system response that prepares the body for a stressful situation, sometimes called the "fight or flight" response.

Synergist Assists the prime mover by contracting at the same time to facilitate more effective movement, also called an accessory muscle.

Systemic contraindication A condition or situation in which massage should be avoided altogether.

Tapotement (tuh-POHT-ment) A fast rhythmic stroke that uses both hands, like rapid drumming.

Target muscle The muscle being treated in a therapeutic technique.

Tender point A small, painful area of hypertonicity, also called a tender spot.

Tendon reflex A reflex that relaxes a muscle when a muscle and its tendon are subjected to slow and gentle tension.

Thoracic duct A major drain that collects the lymph from everywhere in the body, except the right side of the head and thorax, and empties it into the left subclavian vein.

Tissue An organized group or layer of cells with similar structure and function.

Treatment goal A specific goal that is determined after therapeutic massage treatment to clarify progress toward overcoming functional limitations.

Treatment massage Intended to facilitate the healing process when an injury has occurred or when chronic strain has diminished the athlete's performance.

Treatment plan Your recommendations for future treatment, self-care activities, and referrals to other healthcare professionals.

Trigger point (TrP) A localized area of hypertonicity at the motor end unit, or neuromuscular junction, that refers symptoms to other areas of the body.

Unwinding (myofascial unwinding) The process in which soft tissues move in different directions, circles, or wavy lines as the collagen fibers change shape and the fascia softens.

Vein A tube that transports blood from the capillaries of the body back to the heart.

Vibration A stroke that involves high-frequency shaky hand movements and is capable of deep effects.

Yang (YAHNG) Energy that flows down from the sun and is associated with the active, bright, warm, consumptive, and outward activities of the body.

Yin (YIHN) Energy that flows upward from the earth and is associated with the passive, dark, cool, supportive, and inward activities of the body.

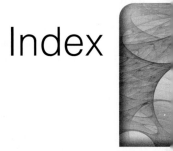

Index

NOTE: Page numbers in *italic* indicate figures; page numbers followed by *t* indicate tables; *b* indicates boxes.

A

Abdominal aponeurosis, *98*
Abdominal region, 149–152, *150–151*
Abnormal spinal curvature, 306–307
Accountability, definition, 30, 41
Accounting, 572–573
Acetaminophen, 181
Acetylcholine, 102
Achilles tendon, *99*
Acne vulgaris, 185
Acromion process, 304
Action potential. *see* Nerve impulses
Active range of motion (AROM), 156, 309–311, *310*
    definition, 295
Active transport mechanisms, 60, *62*
Activity and analysis information, 276–277, *278b*
    definition, 253
Acupoints, 485–486
    definition, 466
Acupressure, 494–496
    definition, 466, 482
    points for self-care, 494–495*t*
Acute, definition, 179
Adams, Francis, *7b*
Adductors, *98*
Adenosine diphosphate, *157, 158*
Adenosine triphosphate, 157, *157*
Adipose tissue, *66, 67*
Adrenal glands, 136
Adrenocorticotropic hormone (ACTH), 135
Advertising, 576
Advisors and mentors, 572
Aerobic respiration, *157, 158*
Agonist, definition, 147
Agonist (muscles), 161
Air, 497
Ajna chakra, 499*t*, 500
Al-Razi, 9
Alexander technique, 16*t*, *18*
Algotherapy, 473*t*
Alimentary canal, 131
Alkylamines, 183
Alprazolam (Xanax), 182
Alveoli, 129, *129*
Alzheimer's disease, 531
American Association of Masseurs and Masseuses (AAMM), 49
American Cancer Society, 183
American Massage Therapy Association (AMTA), 21–22, 32, 49
    Code of Ethics, 34*b*
    Standards of Practice document, 36*b*

American Organization for Bodywork Therapies of Asia (AOBTA), 481–482
Aminoglycosides, 182
Amitriptyline (Elavil), 182
Amma, 2*t*
    definition, 482
Amobarbital (Amytal), 182
Amphiarthrotic joints, 155
Amphotericin B, 183
Amputation, 532
Anaerobic mechanism, *157, 158*
Anahata chakra, 499*t*, 500
Analgesics, 181
Anaphase, 59, *59*
Anatomical position, 147, *147. see also* Client position; Positioning the body
    definition, 146
Anatomical terminology, 147–152
    incorporating into a session, 152
Anatomy, 57
    definition, 55
    levels of organization, *57*
Anatripsis, 2*t*
Ancient civilizations, *3,* 3–6
Angiotensin-converting enzyme inhibitors (Accupril, Monopril, Vasotec, Lotensin), 182
Anisindione (Miradon), 183
Anma, 2*t*
Anmo, 2*t*
Anointing, definition, 1, 3
Antagonist, definition, 146
Antagonists (muscles), 161
Antebrachial region, 149–152, *150–151*
Anterior superior iliac spine (ASIS), 304
Anti-anxiety medications, 182
Anti-inflammatory drugs, 181
Antianginal drugs, 182
Antibacterial drugs, 182
Anticoagulant therapy, 183
Antidepressants, 182
Antidiuretic hormone (ADH), 135
Antiherpesvirus drugs, 182–183
Antihistamines, 183
Antihypertensive drugs, 182
Antiinfectives, 182–183
Antilipemics, 182
Antimycotic drugs, 183
Antiviral drugs, 182–183
Anxiety, 368*t*
Aponeuroses, 70
Appendicular skeleton, 91–94
Arab world, middle ages, 9

Arachnoid mater, 113
Areolar connective tissue, *67, 70*
Arizona Center for Integrative Medicine, 23
Aroma bath, 473*t*
The Art of Massage (Kellogg), 14, 26
Arterial enhancement, 427, 427*b*
Arteries, 121–122, *122*
    definition, 55
Arthritis, 531
Arthrology, 152–156
Articular cartilage, knee joint, *95*
Artificial respiration, 556
    definition, 535
Asclepiades of Bithynia, 8
Asian Bodywork Therapy (ABT), 481–496, 482*b*
    basic routine (shaitsu), 490–493*b*
    definition, 466
    massage therapy differences, 481–482
    principles of treatment, 489–493
    professional association and national certification, 482
    self-care, 494–496
Asking, 487
Aspirin, 181
Assessment
    definition, 295
    documentation, 301–303, *303*
    emergency situation, 555–556
    wellness *versus* therapeutic massage, 296–297
Assistance, on and off table, 360–364, *361–364b*
Associated Bodywork & Massage Professionals (ABMP), 32, 34, 49
    Code of Ethics, 35*b*
Asthma, 200, 531
Astrocytes, 106, *106*
Asymmetric stance, 171–173, *172, 173*
    definition, 146
Atharva Veda, 4
Athletes, 516–526
    common injuries, 525
    definition, 515
    self-care for, 525
Atom, 57
Atrophy, muscle, 161
Auditory cues of conduct, 43–44
Auditory input, treatment room, 570–571
Aulus Cornelius Celsus, 8
Authorization to Use and Disclose Health Care Information, 254, *266*
Autonomic nervous system, 116–117
    responses, 118*t*
Axial skeleton, 84–85, 85–86*t*
Axillary region, 149–152, *150–151*

Axons, 73, *80*, 102
Ayurvedic healthcare, 496–500
    definition of health, 496*b*
    doshas, 497
    energy and chakras, *498*, 498–501
    five elements, 497

B

Ball-and-socket joints, 155–156
Balneotherapy, 473*t*
Barbiturates, 182
Baths, 472
    local, 476
Benzodiazepines, 182
Beta-adrenergic anti-anginals, 182
Beta-blockers (Inderal, Toprol XI, Betaloc,
        Lopressor, Tenormin, Corgard), 182
Biceps brachii, *98*, *100*, 161, *161*
    direct manipulation, 444*b*
Biceps femoris, *99*, *100*
Bile-sequencing drugs (Colestid, Prevalite), 182
Bioenergy, definition, 466, 481
Biomechanics, 168–177
    definition, 146
Blisters, 368*t*
Blood circuits, 122–123
Blood thinner therapy. *see* Anticoagulant therapy
Blood vessels, *66*, *67*, 121–122
Body awareness, 175, 335
Body mechanics, 147
    components of, *169*, 169–170, *170*
    definition, 146
    improper, 176
    injury, 176
    injury prevention, 176–177
    massage therapists, 582, 582*t*
Body movements, 169–175
    pairs, *168*, *168*
Body of knowledge, 32
    definition, 30, 31
Body regions, 149–152, *150–151*
Body systems, 55–145
Body wraps, in hydrotherapy, 476
Bodywork
    definition, 1, 2
    modalities, 14–19, 16*t*
    timeline, *15*
Bolstering, in client positioning, 354
Bolsters, *544*
Bone, *66*, *67*, 69
    shapes, 83, *84*
    structure, 82–84, *83–84*
    visible structure, 83–84, *84*
Bone formation, 95–96
Bone growth, 96
Bone remodeling, 96
Bony landmark, 83, *84*
    definition, 55
Bony thorax, 89, *90*
Bookkeeping, *574*, 574–575
Brachial plexus, *107*, 157
Brachial region, 149–152, *150–151*
Brachialis, *100*
Brachioradialis, *98*
Brain, 111, *111*
Brainstem, 111, *111*
Branding, 575
Breast cancer, 202–203
Breast recess table, *538*

Breathing rhythm, 315
Brine baths, 473*t*
Brochures, 576
Brompheniramine maleate (Dimetapp), 183
Bronchi, 129
Brossage, 473*t*
Brow (third eye) chakra, 499*t*, 500
Bruises, 368*t*
Bruising, 197
Brush and tone, 473*t*
Bulk transport mechanisms, 60, *62*
Bunions, 368*t*
Burns, subacute and postacute, 368*t*
Bursae, 155
Business cards, 576, 578
Business development, long-term, 578–580
Business options, 560–563
Business practices, 44
Business start-up, 563–568, 564*b*
    benefits, 566
    business plan components, 565*b*
    choosing a place of business, 568–572
    insurance, 565–566
    policies and procedures, 567–568
    record keeping, 566
    regulations, 565
Buspirone (BuSpar), 182

C

Calcaneus, *94*
Calcium channel blockers (Norval, Candene,
        Calan, Procardia, Cardizem), 182
Cancer, 183–184, 531
Cancer symptoms, 368*t*
Canon of Medicine (Ibn Sina), 9
Capillaries, 122, *123*
Carcinogens, 183
Cardiac muscle, *71*, 72, 96–97, *97*
Cardiac pulse rhythm, 315
Cardiopulmonary resuscitation (CPR),
        definition, 535, 556
Cardiovascular disease, 196–198
    management, 182
Cardiovascular system, 119–125
    effects of massage, 125
    functions, 123–125
Carpal bones, *92*
Carpal region, 149–152, *150–151*
Carpal tunnel syndrome, 368*t*
Cartilage, *66*, *67*, 67–69, 94–95, *95*
    types, *68*
Cartilaginous (amphiarthrotic) joints, 155
Case studies, 283–289, 316–317, 342–343
Caudad, *148*, 149
    definition, 146
Cell membrane, 59–60, *63*
    structure, 60, *60*
Cells, *57*, 58–63
    components of, 59–63, *63*
    homeostasis, 58
    stages of division, 58–59, *59*
Cells and tissues, abnormal conditions, 183–184
Centering, 386*t*
    definition, 349, 370–371
    massage therapists, 584
Central nervous system (CNS), 73, 111–113
Cephalad, *148*, 149
    definition, 147
Cephalosporins, 182

Cerebellum, 111, *111*
Cerebrospinal fluid (CSF), 74
Cerebrum, 111, *111*
Certification
    definition, 30, 37
    versus licensure, 38*t*
Cervical plexus, *107*, 157
Cervical region, 149–152, *150–151*
Cervical vertebrae, 89, *89*
Cetrizine (Zyrtec), 183
Chair massage, 405–416, 543, *543–544*
    business relationships and, 578
    client positioning, *406*
    corporate chair accounts, 413
    definition, 349
    face cradle coverings, *413*
    highlights, 406*b*
    indications and contraindications, 413, 414*b*
    safety and sanitation for, 406
    sample flow, 407–412*b*
Chakras, 499*t*
Chartered Society of Massage and Remedial
        Gymnastics, 14
Chi Nei Tsang, definition, 482
China, ancient, 3–4, *4*
Chinese medicine, 482–489
    assessment, 487
    disease origin and prevention, 486–487
    eight principles, 487–488
    five phase theory, 488, 488*t*
    four examinations, 487
Chlorpheniramine maleate (Chlor-Trimeton),
        183
Choking, 556
Cholesterol synthesis inhibitors (Lipitor, Zocor,
        Mevacor, Pravachol), 182
Chondrocytes, 69, *69*
Chromatin, *63*
Chronic, definition, 179
Chronic fatigue, 368*t*
Chronic illness, 531
    definition, 515
Cibot, P. M., 11
Circular friction, *454*
Circulation of light, *498*
Circulatory enhancement, 17, 426–438
Circulatory system, effects of massage, 366*t*
Citalopram (Celexa), 182
Clear boundaries, 558–559
Clemastine fumarate (Tavist, Dayhist), 183
Client-centered, definition, 30
Client history, 270, 272, 285–292
Client interview, 272
    procedure, 275*b*
Client positioning, 350–354. *see also* Anatomical
        position; Positioning the body
    communication for, 359–360
    determination of, 354
Client relationships, 52–53
Client's condition, discussion of, 337
Coccyx, 89, *89*
Code of ethics, 33–34
    definition, 30, 31
Cold applications, indications for, 470*b*
Cold plunge, 473*t*
Cold-related conditions, 557–558
Collagen, *66*, *67*
Combination medications, 181
Comminuted fracture, *187*

Common cold, 199
Communication, 261–270
    client positioning and draping, 359–360
    describe a massage session to a new client, 360b
    follow-up, 336–337
    referral and insurance reimbursement, 337
Compensation patterns, 297–301, 301, 302b
    definition, 295
    procedure, 318b
Competency, 38–39
Competitive edge, 579
Complementary and alternative medicine (CAM), 20
Compresses, hot, 477
Compression, 372, 372–373, 386t, 469–470
    definition, 349
Concentric contractions, 160, 160
    definitions, 146
Conceptual boundaries, 50
Conduct, as a professional, 43, 43–44
Conductivity, nerve cells, 109–110
Condyloid joints, 155
Confidence, 558
Confidentiality, 45–46, 264
    definition, 30, 253
Cong Fou, 3, 11
Connective tissue, 64, 66, 67, 421–422
    areolar, 67, 70
    examples, 66
    fibrous, 69–70
    hard, 67, 69
    liquid, 70
    soft, 70
Connective tissue membranes, 75–76
    coverings, 75
Connective tissue techniques
    45° stroke, 445, 449
    C-stroke, S-stroke, 450
    skin rolling, 449–450, 451b, 452
Contagious skin conditions, 368t
Continuing education, 559
Contraindication, definition, 179
Contrast foot bath, routine, 476b
Contrast therapy, 470
    definition, 466
Corporations, 561–562, 562b
    definition, 535
Corticosteroids, 181
Cortisol, 119
Countertransference, 53
Cramping, 525
Cranial nerves, 114, 114
Cranial region, 149–152, 150–151
Craniosacral rhythm, 315
Craniosacral system, 116–117
Craniosacral therapy (CST), 17, 453
Creams, 535
Crenotherapy, 473t
Cross-fiber friction, 454
Crounotherapy, 473t
Crown chakra, 499t, 500
Cuboid, 94
Cuneiforms, 94
Current Procedural Terminology codebook, 269
Cutaneous glands, 81
Cutaneous membranes, 74, 74–75
Cuts and open wounds, 368t
Cyriax, James, 17

Cysts, 368t
Cytokinesis, 59, 59
Cytoplasm, 62, 63
Cytoplasmic organelles, 62–63
Cytosol, 63

D

Da Vinci, Leonardo, 9, 9
Dantrium, 181
De Humani Corporis Fabrica (Vesalius), 10
De Medicina, 8
Dead Sea mud treatment, 473t
Deep, 148, 149
    definition, 146
Deep breathing, lymphatic flow and, 431
Deep fascia, 76, 77
Deep-fiber friction, 380, 381
    definition, 349
Deep tissue modalities, 16t 16–17
Deficiency, definition, 466
Dehydration, 480–481
Deltoid, 98, 99, 100
Deltoid region, 149–152, 150–151
Dendrites, 73, 80
Depression, 368t
Dermatomes, 116
Dermis, 79, 79
Descartes, Rene, 10
Desloratadine (Clarinex), 183
Diabetes, 368t, 531
Diabetes mellitus, 202
Diaphragm muscle, 168, 168
Diaphragmatic breathing, 371
Diarthrotic joints, 155
Diazepam, 181–182
Diencephalon, 111, 111
Diffusion, 60, 60
    passive transport mechanism, 60, 60
Digestive system, 130–133
    accessory organs, 132
    conditions, 201
    effects of massage, 133, 366t
    functions, 132
    structures, 131, 131–132
Dimenhydrinate (Dramamine), 183
Diphenhydramine hydrochloride (Benadryl, Hydramine), 183
Direct manipulation (DM)
    biceps brachii, 444b
    definition, 419
Direct phosphorylation, 157, 157
Direction of ease, 312–313, 425
    definition, 295, 443
Direction of restriction, definition, 419, 450
Directional terms, 148, 148–149, 149t
Disabled clients, 531–533
Disease, 548–550
Distal, 148, 149
    definition, 146
Diuretics, 182
Documentation, 268–270
Dopamine, 119
Doshas, 497
    comparing to Ancient Greek humours, 497b
Douche massage, 473t
Draping, 354–360
    assisting client off table, 362–364b
    communication for, 359–360
    uncovering different areas, 356–358b

Dual relationships, 52
Ducts, 139–140
Duke Integrative Medicine program, 23
Dulse scrub, 473t
Dura mater, 113
Dynamic contractions, 160, 160

E

Earth, 497
Eccentric contraction, 160, 161
    definition, 146
Edema, 198–199
Education. see Massage education
    massage therapists, 584
Efferent neuron. see Motor neuron
Effleurage, 11, 12t, 373–376, 375, 386t
    definition, 349
Effleurer, 11, 12t
Egypt, ancient, 5–6, 6
Eighteenth Century, 11
Elastic cartilage, 68, 94–95, 95
Elastin, 66, 67
Electric lift table, 539
Elevation, 469–470
Emergency situation, primary assessment of, 555–556
Emotions, 50
Employment, 560–563
    working as an employee, 562
End feel, 311–312, 312t
    definition, 295
Endangerment sites, 193, 194, 383–385, 384
Endocrine system, 135, 135–137
    conditions, 201–202
    effects of massage, 137, 367t
    structures, 135–136
Endocytosis, 60, 62
Endomysium, 103
Endoneurium, 106, 107
Endoplasmic reticulum, 119, 120
Endorphins, 119
Energy, 51
Energy modalities, 17–18
Enkephalins, 119
Ependymal cells, 106, 106
Epidermis, 78–79, 79
Epilepsy, 531
Epineurium, 103, 107
Epiphyseal plates, 96
Epithelia, examples of, 65
Epithelial membranes, 74, 74–75
Epithelial tissue, 64
Equipment, 173–175, 174, 536–545
    event sports massage, 521
    specifications, 536–537
Ergonomics, 173–174, 335–336
    definition, 326
Erythrocytes. see Red Blood cells
Escitalopram (Lexapro), 182
Esophagus, 132
Ethanolamines, 183
Ether, 497
Ethical responsibilities, 44–45
Ethics, 40–42. see also Code of ethics
    definition, 30
    professional, 41
    reporting unethical activity, 41–42
    resolving dilemmas, 42, 42b
Ethmoid bone, 87

Etiology, definition, 179
Europe
    middle ages (dark ages), 8–9
    19th Century, 11–12
Event massage
    definition, 515, 517
    sports, 517–521
        contraindications for, 521
        equipment for, 521
Excess, definition, 466
Excursion, definition, 369
Exercise and physical activity, massage
    therapists, 582–583
Exhalation (expiration), 130
Exocytosis, 60, *62*
Extensor carpi, *98*
Extensor digitorum longus, *100*
External auditory meatus, *87*
External genitalia, 141
External oblique, *100*
External obliques, *98*
Exteroceptors, 107–108, *108*
Extremities. *see* Lower extremities; Upper
    extremities

F

Face cradles, 542, *543*
    coverings, *413*
Facial region, 149–152, *150–151*
Facilitated diffusion, 60, *60*
    passive transport mechanism, *60*, 61
Fallopian tubes, 137
Fango, *473t*
Fascia, 75–76, 297, *301*, 425
    definition, 55
Fascial adhesion (fascial restriction), definition,
    295, 297
Fascicle, 103, *107*
Fast-twitch fibers, 158, *159*
Federation of State Massage Therapy Boards
    (FSMTB), 32, 39–40
Fees, setting of, 575
Feet, 308
Feldenkrais, Moshe, *16t*, 18
Femoral region, 149–152, *150–151*
Femur, *94*
Fever, 199
Fexofenadine hydrochloride (Allegra,
    Allegra-D), 183
Fibric acid derivatives (Tricor, Lopid), 182
Fibrils, *100*
Fibrocartilage, *68*, 94–95, *95*
Fibromyalgia, *191*, 191–192, *368t*
Fibrous (synarthrotic) joints, 154–155
Fibula, *94*
Field, Tiffany, 20, *20*
Filtration, 60, *60*
    passive transport mechanism, *60*, 61
Finances, 572–575
Financial records, *573*
Finish sauna, *473t*
Fire, 497
Fire safety, *555*
Five phase theory, 488, *488t*
    creation cycle, *488*
Five Vital Substances, 484–485
    definition, 466

Flat-back posture, 306, *307*
Flexeril, 181
Flexibility, in business, 579
Flexor carpi, *98*
Flexor reflexes, 112
Florida State Massage Therapy Association, 49
Flow, 386–387t, 395–396
    definition, 349
    sample sequences for specific areas, 397–404
Fluconazole, 183
Fluoroquinolones, 182
Fluoxetine (Prozac, Sarafem), 182
Foramen magnum, *88*
Fractures, 187, *187*, *368t*
Free nerve endings, *108*
Friction, *386t*
    in hydrotherapy, 475
    myofascial techniques, 453, *454b*
    principles of, *386t*, *454b*
Frontal bone, *87*
Frontal plane, 148, *148*
Full-body massage, flows, 390
Functional assessments, 315–316
Functional limitations, prioritizing, 276
Functional stress assessment, 272, 274
Fungal infections, 186, *368t*
Future treatment, 329–331
    duration of sessions, 330
    frequency, 330
    length, 330–331

G

Gait
    assessment, 308–309, *309*
    definition, 295
Ganglia, 106
Gas exchange, 129, *129*
Gastrocnemius, *98*, *99*, *100*
    reciprocal inhibition, *447b*
Gels, 535
General adaptation syndrome (GAS), 196
General assessments, 296–302
    forms, *303*, *319*, *322*
    procedure, 298–300b
Geriatric massage, 530, *530b*
Glaucoma, 531
Gliding joints, 155
Gluteal region, 149–152, *150–151*
Gluteus maximus, *99*, *100*
Gluteus medius, *100*
Golgi apparatus, *63*
Golgi tendon organs, 107, *108*, *159*
Goniometer, 309
Gouty joints, *368t*
Greece, ancient, 6–7
Greenstick fracture, *187*
Grounding, *386t*
    definition, 349, 369–370
    massage therapists, 584
Growth hormone (GH), 135
Gymnastics, 6
    definition, 1

H

Hair, 80, *81*
Hamstring group, *99*
Hand hygiene, 551, *552b*

Handbook of Massage (Kleen), 12
Haysack wrap, *473t*
Headaches, 194–195
Healing
    phase I, 421–422
    phase II, 422
    phase III, 422
Healing time, 329–330
Health Insurance Portability and Accountability
    Act. *see* HIPAA
Health report, *273*
Hearing, 142
Hearing impairment, 531–532
Heart, 120–121, *121*
Heart chakra, *499t*, 500
Heart disease, 531
Heat applications
    indications and contraindications, *471b*
    moist, 477, *478b*
Heat production, muscular system, 104–105
Heat-related conditions, 557
Hellerwork, *16t*, 18
Hematopoiesis, skeletal and, 95
Hemostasis, 421
Hepatitis, 531, 549–550
Herbal wrap, *473t*
High blood pressure. *see* Hypertension
Hinge joints, 155
HIPAA, 253, 269–270
    compliance, 269–270
    documentation forms, 270
    HSS website, 269
Hippocrates of Cos, 6–7
Hippocratic Oath, 7, *7b*
HIV, 531, 549–550
Homeostasis, 56, 58, 127
    definition, 55
Hospice, definition, 515, 531
Human immunodeficiency virus. *see* HIV
Humerus, *85*, *86*, 92
Humours, Ancient Greece, *497b*
Hyaline cartilage, *68*, *69*, 94–95, *95*
Hydromassage (hydrotub), *473t*
Hydrotherapy, 332, 467–481
    applications, 471–481
    chronic low back pain, *471b*
    cold, 468–469
    contrast therapy, 470
    definition, 326, 466
    external, 333
    heat, 470
    internal, 332–333, 480–481
    local applications, 476–480
    medication and, 481
    muscle spasms, *472b*
    neutral, 470–471
    physiological effects of cold and heat, *469b*
    upper extremity muscles, *472b*
    water temperature, *468t*
    whole-body applications, 471–472
Hygiene, 547–555
    aseptic techniques, 551–552
    barrier techniques, 551, *553*
    disease and, 548–550
    hand, 551, *552b*
    preventing transmission of
        pathogens, 550–553

Hypertension (high blood pressure), 198, 368*t*
    massage and, 125*b*
Hypertonic, definition, 419, 423
Hypertonic muscles, 189
Hypertonic solution, 61, *61*
Hypertrophy, muscle, 161
Hypotonic solution, 61, *61*

I

Ibn Sina, 9
Ice, 469–470
    applications, 477
    massage routine, 479–480*b*
Iliac crest, 304
Iliac region, 149–152, *150–151*
Iliotibial band, *99*, *100*
Imipramine (Apo-Imipramine), 182
Independent contractor, 561
India, ancient, 4
Indication, definition, 179
Infants, massage in, *528*, 528–529
Infectious diseases, 549–550
Inferior, *148*, 149
    definition, 146
Inflammation, 421
Influenza drugs, 182–183
Informed consent, 44–45, *46*
    definition, 30
Inguinal region, 149–152, *150–151*
Inhalation (inspiration), 130
Initial session of treatment plan, 327–328, *328*
    report, *340*
Injury, tissue repair and, 420–422
Insertion of a muscle, definition, 146
Insurance, 565–566
Insurance reimbursement, 337
Integrative medicine centers, 22–23
Integrative Medicine Service at Memorial
        Sloan-Kettering Cancer Center, 23
Integumentary system (skin), 76–82
    conditions, 184–186
    effects of massage, 81–82, 366*t*
    functions, 76, 78
    sensory receptors, *108*
    structures, 78–81
Intellect, 50
Inter-event massage, 518–519
    definition, 515
Intercostals, *98*
Internal oblique, *98*
International Classification of Diseases, 269
International Spa Association (ISPA), 24, *25*
Interphase, 59, *59*
Interviewing skills, 263–268
Irritable bowel syndrome (IBS), 201
    peptic ulcers and, 201
Irritability, nerve cells, 109–110
Isocarboxazid (Marplan), 182
Isotonic solution, 61, *61*

J

Japanese enzyme bath, 474*t*
Joint
    definition, 55, 146
    movement, 381–382, *382*
    types, 152, 153–154*t*
Joint capsule, 155

Joint cavity, 155
Jostling, 382, *382*

K

Kampo, 2*t*
Kellogg, John Harvey, 13, 26
    physiological effects of massage, 13, 13*t*
Ketoconazole, 183
Kidneys, *133*, 133–134
Kinesiology, 147, 152–168
    definition, 146
Kleen, Emil, 12
Knee joint, articular cartilage, *95*
Kneipp, Father Sebastian, 467, *468*
Kneipp therapy, 474*t*
Kyphosis, 187
Kyphosis-lordosis, 306, *308*

L

Lacrimal bone, *87*
Large intestine, 132
Larynx, 128, 130
Lateral, *148*, 148–149
    definition, 146
Latex gloves, 551, *553*
Latissimus dorsi, *99*, *100*
    trigger point map, *455*
Leading questions, 267
Leaning, 169–170
Legal requirements, 44–45
Lengthening, definition, 419, 426
Leukocytes, *119*, 120, *120*
Licensure
    versus certification, 38*t*
    definition, 30, 37
Life balance, 580–581, *581*, 581*b*
Lifting, 170, *170*
Ligaments, *66*, 155
Limits of practice, 40
Linens and laundry, 554–555
Ling, Per Henrik, 11
LinkedIn, 578
Listening, 487
Local contraindication, definition, 179
Local inflammation, 368*t*
Long-term goals, 277, 328
Longitudinal friction, *454*
Loofah body scrub, 474*t*
Looking, 487
Loop diuretics (Lasix, Bumex), 182
Loratadine (Alavert, Claritin), 183
Lorazepam (Ativan), 182
Lordosis, 187
Lotions, 535
Low back pain
    chronic, 457
    hydrotherapy, 471*b*
    moist hot pack application, 478*b*
Lower extremities, 92–94, *94*
    nerves, 117
Lower respiratory tract, 128–129
Lower trapezius, positional release of, 448*b*
Lubricants, *545*, 545–547
    application of, 547
    storage, 535
Lumbar plexus, *107*, 157
Lumbar region, 149–152, *150–151*

Lumbar vertebrae, 89, *89*
Lupus, 531
Luteinizing hormone (LH), 135
Lymph, 125, *126*
    definition, 419
Lymph drainage, 428–438, *429–430*
    benefits and contraindications, 431*b*
    enhancement, 433–438*b*
    techniques, *432*
Lymph Drainage Therapy (LDT), 431
Lymph nodes, 125, *126*
Lymph organs and tissues, 126–127
Lymph vessels, 125, *126*
Lymphatic and immune system conditions,
        198–199
Lymphatic fluid (lymph), definition, 55
Lymphatic system, 125–127
    effects of massage, 127
    functions, 127
Lysosome, *63*

M

Macrolides, 182
Maintenance massage, 523–524
    definition, 515, 517
Makeh, 2*t*
Mammary glands, 137
Mandible, *87*
Manipura chakra, 499*t*, 500
Manubrium, 91
Marine hydrotherapy, 474*t*
Marketing and promotion, 575–577
Mass, 2*t*
Massa, 2*t*
Massage. *see also* specific type
    abbreviations and symbols, 280–282*t*
    ABT differences, 481–482
    acne vulgaris, 185
    ancient Greece, 6
    anticoagulant therapy and, 183
    antihistamines and, 183
    asthma and, 200
    athletes, 516–525
    breast cancer and, 202–203
    cancer and, 23, 183
    cardiovascular system and, 125, 143*t*, 196–198
    common cold and, 199
    contemporary, 14
    contraindications for, 368*t*
    definition, 1–2
    diabetes mellitus and, 202
    digestive system and, 133, 144*t*
    disabled clients, 531–533
    edema and, 198–199
    endangerment sites and, 193, *194*
    endocrine system and, 137, 144*t*
    fever and, 199
    fibromyalgia and, *191*, 191–192
    fractures and, 187
    as French term, 11, 12*t*
    fungal infections and, 186
    general effects, 365–368
    geriatric, 530, 530*b*
    headaches and, 194–195
    high blood pressure and, 125*b*
    hospice, 531
    IBS and, 201

Massage (*continued*)
incorporating terminology into session, 152
incorporation of reflexology, 501
indications for, 368t
infants, 528, 528–529
integumentary system and, 81–82, 143t
legitimization of, 12–13
lubricants, 545, 545–547
lymphatic system and, 127, 143t
modalities, 14–19
muscle spasms and cramps, 189–190
muscle strains and, 192, 192–193
muscles and, 189–193
muscular system and, 104, 143t
myofascial pain syndrome, 190–191
NCCAM-funded research, 56
nervous system and, 118–119, 143t
open wounds or sores, 184–185
osteoarthritis and, 188–189
pain and, 367b
parasympathetic nervous system and, 82b
part of the American healthcare system, 22–23
plantar fasciitis and, 183
pregnancy and, 203–204
pregnant women, 525–528
prostate cancer and, 203
reproductive system and, 141–142, 144it
respiratory system and, 130, 144t
roots and terms, 2t
scar tissue and, 185
sciatica and, 193–194
sinusitis and, 200
skeletal muscle tissue and, 70–72
skeletal system and, 96, 143t
special senses and, 142, 144t
sprains and, 188
stress and, 196, 367b
tendinopathy and, 193
terms with French roots, 11, 12t
20th Century, 14
19th Century America, 13–14
19th Century Europe, 11–12
thoracic outlet syndrome, 195–196
timeline, 15
touch research, 19, 19
urinary system and, 135, 143t
weather-related conditions, 557–558
Massage Act (Florida), 49
Massage Certificate, 14
Massage chairs. *see* Chair massage
Massage education, 24
current perspective of, 32
historical perspective of, 31–32
legalities, 38
trends in, 26
Massage mats, 544
bolsters, 544
Massage practice, 535–588
Massage Registration Act (AAMM), 49
Massage stroke, 370
basic, 371–382
components, 369
lymphatic drainage, 432–438
stationary, 369
Massage table, 537–543
accessories, 541
asymmetric stance next to, 172b
electric lift, 539
extensions, 542–543, 543

face cradles, 542, 543
foam padding, 538
portable, 540–541, 540–542
proper height, 539, 540
sanitizing of, 554
specialty, 538
stationary, 539–540, 540
support, 539
symmetric stance, 171
tabletop, 537–538, 538
Massage Therapy and Medications (Persad), 181
Massage Therapy Body of Knowledge
Stewardship group, 32
Massage Therapy Foundation, 32
Massage Therapy Research Database, 22
Massage tools, 544, 544–545
Massage treatment record, 270, 286–287
definition, 253
Massein, 2t
Masser, 2t, 11, 12t
Masseter, 98
Masseur, 11, 12t
Masseuse, 11, 12t
Mass'h, 2t
Masso, 2t
Mastoid process of temporal bone, 87
Maxilla, 87, 88
Mayo Clinic's Complementary and Integrative
Medicine program, 23
Mechanical effects
definition, 1
Kellogg, 13
Medial, 148, 148–149
definition, 146
Medical Qigong therapy, 482
Medical records, requesting copies of, 337
Medical Spas, 24
Medical terminology, 254–261
Medications VI (Descartes), 10
Meissner's corpuscles, 109
Meninges, 75, 113, 113
Meridian Qi flow directions, 489
Meridian therapy, 489
definition, 466
Meridians, 484–485, 484
definition, 466
primary pathway descriptions, 486t
Merkel cells, 109
Mesopotamia, ancient, 4–5, 4–5
Metabolic effects
definition, 1
Kellogg, 13
Metabolism, definition, 55
Metacarpal bones, 92
Metaphase, 59, 59
Metatarsal bones, 94
Mezger, Johan Georg, 11
MICE (mobilization, ice, compression,
elevation), 470
Microglia, 106, 106
Microvilli, 63
Middle Ages, 8–9
Mineral water (baths), 474t
Mitochondrion, 63
Modality, definition, 1, 16
Molecule, 57
Monoamine oxidase inhibitors, 182
Moor baths, 474t
Mordan, 2t

Motor neuron (efferent neuron), 108, 109
definition, 55
Motor unit, 102
definition, 55
Movement
muscular system, 103–104, 104
skeletal and, 95
Movement cure
definition, 1
Taylor, 13
Movement modalities, 18
Mucous membranes, 74, 75
Muladhara chakra, 498, 499t
Multiple sclerosis, 531
Muscle attachment, 104
Muscle cells, 67
Muscle energy techniques (METs), definition,
419
Muscle fibers
attachments: origin and insertion, 160
types, 157–158, 159
Muscle guarding, definition, 419, 424
Muscle relaxants, 181
Muscle spasms
and cramps, 189–1907
hydrotherapy, 472b
Muscle spindles, 159
Muscle strain, 192, 192–193
Muscle tissue, 70–72
types, 71, 96–97
Muscles, 66, 70. *see also* specific type
definition, 55
effects of exercise, 162
effects of stretching, 162
energy requirement for contraction, 157, 157
functions of, 103–104
involved in some common sports, 516b
movement and coordination, 161–162
movement and stability, 439, 440–442t
myology, 156–162
nerve supply to, 157
origin of, definition, 146
restorative massage to increase circulation,
523b
texture and movement, 314
Muscular control mechanism, 101–102
Muscular system, 96–104
conditions, 189–193
effect of massage, 104
effects of massage, 366t
Myelin, 105, 106
Myofascial pain syndrome, 190–191
Myofascial techniques, 449–453
friction, 453
Myofibrils, 100
Myology, 156–162
Myosin, 100

N

Nails, 80, 81
Narcotics, 181
Nasal bone, 87
National Center for Complementary and
Alternative Medicine (NCCAM), 20, 56b
National Certification Board for Therapeutic
Massage and Bodywork
(NCBTMB), 32, 39
Examination of Therapeutic Massage and
Bodywork (NCETMB), 39

Examination of Therapeutic Massage (NCETM), 39
National Certification Commission for Acupuncture and Oriental Medicine (NCCAOM), 482
National Institutes of Health (NIH), Office of Alternative Medicine, 19
Navicular, *94*
Neck, chronic pain, 457
Nei Ching, 3
Nerve, definition, 55
Nerve cells. *see* Neurons
Nerve impulses, *109,* 109–110
Nerve plexus, 106, *107*
    definition, 55
Nerve tissue, organization, 106
Nervous system, 104–119. *see also* specific system
    conditions, 193–196
    effects of massage, 118–119, *366t*
    functions, 117–118
    organization, 111
    tissue, 105–109
Nervous tissue, 72–74
Networking
    building relationships, 577–578
    definition, 535
    groups, 578
Neurilemma, 105, *107*
Neuroglia, 74, 106, *106*
Neurological memory, 114
Neuromuscular junction, 102, *102,* 157
Neuromuscular modalities, 17
Neuromuscular techniques, 435–460
Neurons (nerve cell), *72,* 72–73, 105, *105.*
    see also specific type
    classification by function, 107–109
    definition, 55
    mixed nerves, 109
New York State Society of Medical Massage Therapists, 49
Newsletters, 576
Nineteenth Century, 11–12
Nitrates (Nitrodisc, Nitrostat, Cedocard, Monoket), 182
Nitrofurantoin, 182
Nociceptors, 108
Nodes of Ranvier
Noninfectious disease, 548–549, *548t*
Nonverbal communication, 267–268
Nortriptyline (Anti-Nortriptyline), 182
Nose and nasal cavity, 128
Nuad Bo 'Rarn, 482
Nuclear membrane, *63*
Nucleolus, *63*
Nucleus, *63*
Nutrition, 335
Nutrition and hydration, massage therapists, 583

O

Objective information, 274–276
    definition, 253
Oblique, *98*
    fracture, *187*
Occipital bone, 87, *88*
Occipital condyle, *88*
Occipital region, 149–152, *150–151*
Oils, 535
Olfactory cues of conduct, 44
Olfactory input, treatment room, 571

Oligodendrocytes, 106, *106*
Oncology massage, 23
One-foot-forward stance, definition, 146, 171
Onsen, *474t*
Open-ended questions, 264–265
Oral cavity, 132
Orbicularis oculi, *98*
Orbicularis oris, *98*
Organ, *57*
Organ system, *57*
Organism, *57*
Oriental/Eastern modalities, 18
Osmosis, 60, *60*
    effects on red blood cells, *61*
    passive transport mechanism, *60,* 60–61
Osteoarthritis, 188–189
Osteoblasts, 69, *69*
Osteoclasts, 69, *69*
Osteocytes, 69, *69*
Ova, 139
Ovaries, 137
Oxytocin, 119, 135
Ozonized baths, *474t*

P

Pacinian corpuscles, 109
Pain, 423–424
    massage and, *367b*
Pain-spasm cycle, *189,* 423
Palpation, 487
    assessment, 313–314
    definition, 295
Panadol. *see* Acetaminophen
Parafango, *474t*
Parallel stance, 171
    definition, 147
Paralysis, 532
Parasympathetic nervous system, 116–117
Parasympathetic response
    definition, 55
    massage and, *82b*
Parathyroid glands, 136
Parietal bone, 87
Parkinson's disease, 531
Paroxetine (Paxil), 182
Partnership, 561–562, *561b*
    definition, 535
Passive range of motion (PROM), 156, 309, *310,* 311
    definition, 295
Passive transport, 60–61
Patella, *94*
Patellar region, 149–152, *150–151*
Pathogens, preventing transmission, 550–553
Pathological headaches, 195
Pathology, 180
    definition, 179
Patient's Release of Health Care Information, 264, *265*
Peat bath, *474t*
Pectoralis major, *98*
Peloid therapy, *474t*
Pelvic girdle, 92, *93*
Pelvic region, 149–152, *150–151*
Penicillins, 182
Pennsylvania's State Board of Massage Therapy Scope of Practice, *33b*
Peptic ulcers, 201
Pericardium, *74, 75*

Perineurium, 106, *107*
Peripheral nervous system, 113–117
Peristalsis, 132–133
Peritoneum, *74, 75*
Peroneus longus, *98, 99,* 100
Perseverance, 559–560
Pétrir, 11, *12t*
Pétrissage, 11, *12t, 376,* 376–378, *378, 386t*
    definition, 349
pH maintenance, 130, 134–135
Phagocytosis, 421–422
Phalangeal region, 149–152, *150–151*
Phalanges, *92, 94*
Pharmacology, 180–181
    definition, 179
Pharmacology for Massage Therapy (Wible), 181
Pharynx, 128, 132
Phenelzine (Nardil), 182
Phenobarbital (Luminal), 182
Physical boundaries, 50
Physical disabilities, 532
Physicians' Desk Reference (PDR), 181
Physiology, 57
    definition, 55
Pia mater, 113
Pineal gland, 136–137
Piperidines, 183
Pitting edema, *368t*
Pituitary gland, 135, *136*
Pivot joints, 155
Plan information, 277
    definition, 253
Planes, 148, *148*
Planning process, 327–329
Plantar fasciitis, 184
Plantar region, 149–152, *150–151*
Plasma membrane, *60, 63*
Platelets, *119,* 120
Platysma, *100*
Pleura, *74, 75*
Polarity therapy, 17, 511–513
    definition, 467
Popliteal region, 149–152, *150–151*
Portable tables, 540–541, *540–541*
    set-up and takedown, 541–542, *542b*
Position change
    sheet draping for, 355
    towel draping for, 359
Positional release (PR)
    definition, 419, 443
    lower trapezius, *419,* 448b
Positioning the body. *see also* Anatomical position; Client position
    for PIR, 445
    pregnant women, 526–527
Post-event massage, 520–521, *520b*
    definition, 515
    long-distance runner, 522–523b
Post-isometric relaxation (PIR)
    definition, 419, 445
    gastrocnemius, 447b
Posterior superior iliac spine (PSIS), 304
Postpartum massage, 528
Posttreatment assessment, 316
Posture
    anterior assessment, 305
    assessment, 302–308, *303*
    deviations, 186–187, *187,* 306–308
    ideal, 304, *304*

Posture (*continued*)
    lateral, 305–306
    posterior assessment, 305
Potassium-sparing diuretics (Spiractin, Inspra),
    182
Powders, 535
Pre-event massage, 517–518, 518*b*
    definition, 515
    long-distance runner, 519–520*b*
Prefixes, 255, 257–259, 258–259*t*
Pregnant women, 203–204, 525–528
    considerations for massage, 527–528
    first trimester, 526
    postpartum massage, 528
    second trimester, 526–527
    third trimester, 527
Prenatal bolstering, *352*
Prescription and referral form, *339*
*The Prevention and Cure of Many Chronic Diseases
    by Movements* (Roth), 11
Prime mover, definition, 147
Prime movers (muscles), 161
Privacy, treatment room, 569
Privacy Rule, definition, 253, 269
Professional associations
    America, 49
    Britain, 49
Professional massage therapist, 558–585
Professional relationships, 53
    advisors and mentors, 572
    networking, 577–578
Professionalism
    characteristics, 31–37
    clear boundaries, 558–560
    competitive edge, 579
    conduct, goals, and qualities, 43–49
    continued learning, 559
    definition, 30
    employment and business options, 560–563
    flexibility, 579
    goals and milestones, 579
    perseverance, 559–560
    self-awareness and confidence, 558
    support from others, 559
    web sites, 33*b*
Prolactin, 135
Prone position, 352–353, *353*
    assisting client onto table, 361*b*
    definition, 349
    flow, 387, 391*b*
    leg and foot, 404, 405*b*
Pronunciation and spelling, 261, 263*t*
Prophase, 59, *59*
Proprioception, 142
Proprioceptive neuromuscular facilitation (PNF)
    definition, 419
    techniques, 439, 443–449
Proprioceptors, 107–108, *108*
    definition, 55, 147, 158
Prostate cancer, 203
Proximal, *148*, 149
    definition, 147
Psychological issues, 533
Pulmonary circuit, 122–123

Q

Qi (C'hi, Ki), 18, 484–485
    definition, 1, 467

Qigong exercise, 496*b*
Quadriceps femoris, reciprocal inhibition, 448*b*

R

Radius, *92*
Range of motion (ROM)
    assessment, 309–313
    definition, 147, 156, 295
Rapport, in effective communication, 263
Reciprocal inhibition (RI)
    definition, 420, 446–449
    quadriceps femoris, 448*b*
Rectus abdominis, *98*, *100*
Rectus femoris, *98*, *100*
Red blood cells, *119*, *120*
    formation, 135
    osmosis and, *61*
Refer, definition, 326
Referral
    communication for, 337
    form, *339*
    other healthcare professionals, 336–341
    recommendations, 342
Reflective listening, 264–265
Reflex arcs, 111–112, *112*
Reflex effects
    definition, 1
    Kellogg, 13
Reflexology, 500–504
    basic flow, 504–511*b*
    basic techniques, *503*
    definition, 467
    footcharts, *502*
    indications and contraindications, 501
    in a massage session, 501
Registration, definition, 30, 37
Reiki, 17, 37
Relationships, 50–51
Release forms, *47–48*
Renaissance, 9–10
Repaichage massage/facial, 474*t*
Reproductive system, 137–142
    conditions, 203–204
    effects of massage, 141–142
    female, 137–139
        functions, 139
        structures, 137–138, *138–139*
    male, 139–142
        functions, 1410142
        structures, 139–140, *140–141*
Resisted ROM (manual resistance), 156
Respiration, 130
Respiratory system, 127–130
    conditions, 199–200
    effects of massage, 130, 366*t*
    functions, 129–130
    structures, 127–128, *128*
Rest, 334–335
Rest and sleep, massage therapists, 583
Resting, 386*t*
Resting length, definition, 420, 423
Resting stroke, definition, 349, 371
Restorative massage, 521–523
    definition, 515, 517
    increase circulation, 523*b*
Resumé writing, 562–563
Reticular fibers, 66
Rhythms, 314–315

Ribonucleic acid, *63*
Ribosomes, *63*
RICE (rest, ice, compression, elevation), 470
Right lymphatic duct, definition, 420, 428
Rik Veda, 4
Rocking, 381
Rolfing, 16*t*, 18, 439
Roman bath, 474*t*
Rome, 7–8
    fall of, 8
    Greek physicians in, 8
Root chakra, 498, 499*t*
Roots, 255, 256–257*t*
Rotation, 307–308
Roth, Mathias, 11
Ruffini end organs, 109
Russian bath, 474*t*

S

Sacral (pelvic) chakra, 499*t*, 500
Sacral plexus, *107*, 157
Sacral region, 149–152, *150–151*
Sacrum, 89, *89*
Saddle joints, 155
Safe space, 52
Safety, 555–558
Sagittal plane, 148, *148*
Sahasrara chakra, 499*t*, 500
Salicylates, 181
Salt glow, 474*t*
Saltwater bath, 474*t*
Sama Veda, 4
Samvahana, 2*t*
Sanitation, 547–555
    cleaning and sanitizing techniques, 553–554
    linens and laundry, 554–555
    massage table, *554*
Sarcolemma, 100
Sarcomeres, 100
Satorius, *98*
Sauna, 473*t*, 474*t*, 475
Scapular region, 149–152, *150–151*
Scar release, 450–452, 452*b*
Scar tissue, 70, 185
Schwann cells, 105, 106, *106*
Sciatic nerve, 109
Sciatica, 193–194
Scoliosis, *187*, 306, *307*
Scope of practice, 32–33, 37–40
    definition, 30, 31
    therapeutic massage, 40
    wellness massage, 40
Scotch hose, 474*t*
Seated position, flow, 387, 396*b*
Seaweed wrap, 474*t*
Selective serotonin reuptake inhibitors
    (SSRIs), 182
Self-care, 494–496
    athletes, 525
    considerations for, 332
    definition, 326
    in professional massage therapists, 580–585
        physical, 581–584
        psychological, 583–584
        social, 584
        spiritual, 584–585
    recommendations, 331–336
Self-employment, 560

Self-promotion, 575–576
Semimembranosus, *99*
Semitendinosus, *99*
Sensory neurons, 105, *108*
    definition, 56
Sensory receptors
    integument, *108*
    skin, *80*
Serotonin, 119
Serous membranes, *74*, 74–75
Serratus anterior, *98*, *100*
Sertraline (Zoloft), 182
Session-to-session treatment plan, 328*b*
Sexuality, massage and, 51
Sheet draping, 355
    changing from prone to supine, 359*b*
    for position change, 355
Shiatsu, 482, 490–493*b*
Short-term goals, 277, 328
Shoulder girdle, 91, *91*
Showers, 472
Side-lying (laterally recumbent), *353*, 353–354
    definition, 349
    position flow, 387, 392–395*b*
Sinusitis, 200
Skelaxin, 181
Skeletal muscle, 70, *71*, *97*, 97–98
    contraction, 157–158
    microscopic structures of cell, 100–103
    pump for venous blood flow, *124*
    structures, *97*, *99*–100
    whole, structures of cell, 103, *103*
Skeletal muscles, activity, 159–160
    extreme conditions of, 161, *161*
Skeletal support, muscles and, 104
Skeletal system, 82–96
    conditions, 186–189
    effects of massage, 96, 366*t*
Skin, 78, *79*
    assessment of temperature, 314
    sensory receptors, *80*
Skin glow rub, 474*t*
Skull, 84–85, *87*
Sleep, 334–335
Selenium wrap, 475*t*
Sliding filament theory, 100–101, *101*
Slip, definition, 349
Slow-twitch fibers, 157–158, *159*
Small intestine, 132
Smell, 142
Smooth muscle, *71*, 72, *97*, *97*
SOAP, 270–283
    definition, 253
    guidelines for putting together,
        278–283, *279*
    plan information, 277
SOAP NOTE, *271*
    variations, 283, *285*
Social media, 577
Society of Trained Masseuses, 12
Soft tissues, texture and movement, 314
Solar plexus chakra, 499*t*, 500
Sole proprietorship, 560–561, 561*b*
    definition, 535
Soleus, *98*, *100*
Soma, 181
Somatic nervous system, 114
Spa glossary, 473–475*t*

Spa industry
    history of, 24
    massage education, 24
    massage in, 23–26
    medical spas, 24
Special populations, 18, 515–534
Special senses, 142
    conditions of, 204
    effects of massage, 142
Speech production, 130
Spelling and pronunciation, 261, 263*t*
Sperm, 141
Sphenoid bone, 87, 88
Spinal cord, *72*, 72–73, 111
    curves of adult and fetus, 89, *89*
    sections, 89, *90*
Spinal nerves, *115*
Spiral fracture, *187*
Spleen, 126–127
Splenius capitis, *100*
Sports, major muscles involved in, 516*b*
Sprains/strains, 187–188, 368*t*
St. John Method of Neuromuscular Therapy
        (NMT), 17
Standard precautions, definition, 535, 547
Standards for Privacy of Individually
        Identifiable Health Information. *see*
        Privacy Rule
Standards of practice, 34–36
    definition, 30, 31
Static contractions, 160, *160*
Steam room, 475*t*
Sternocleidomastoid, *98*, *99*, *100*
Sternum, 91
Stomach, 132
Stools, *545*
Storage, skeletal and, 95
Strain-counterstrain (SCS), definition, 420, 443
Stress, 195–196
    cumulative effects, 274
    massage and, 367*b*
Stretch reflex, 112
    definition, 56
Stretches, 333–334
Stretching, definition, 420, 426
Structural alignment, inefficient, 169, *170*
Structural and postural integration
        modalities, 18
Strumming, 456
Styloid process of temporal bone, *87*
Subacute, definition, 179
Subcutaneous layer, 80
Subjective, Objective, Activity and
        Analysis. *see* SOAP
Subjective information, 270–274
    definition, 254
Subsequent sessions of treatment plan, 328–329
Substance P, 119
Suffixes, 259–260, 260*t*
Superficial, *148*, 149
    definition, 147
Superficial friction, 380
    definition, 350
Superior, *148*, 149
    definition, 147
Supine position, 351
    abdomen, 400–403, *401*, 401–402*b*
    arm, 400, 400*b*

    chest, neck and head, 397–399*b*
    definition, 350
    flow, 387, 388–390*b*
    leg and foot, 403, 403*b*
    with neck and knee bolsters, *351*
    prenatal bolstering, *352*
Svadisthana chakra, 499*t*, 500
Sway-back posture, 306
Swedish Gymnastics, definition, 1, 11
Swedish massage, 11
Swedish modalities, 16, 16*t*
Swedish Movements, definition, 1, 11
Swiss shower, 475*t*
Symmetric stance, *170–171*, 171
    definition, 147
Sympathetic nervous system, 116
Sympathetic response, 116
    definition, 56
Sympatholytic drugs (Cardura, Tenex,
        Dopamet, Hytrin), 182
Synapses, *80*, 110, *110*
Synaptic transmission. *see* Conductivity
Synarthrotic joints, 154–155
Synergists (accessory muscles), 161
    definition, 147
Synovial (diarthrotic) joints, 155
Synovial membrane, 155
Systemic circuit, 123
Systemic contraindication, definition, 179

T

Tactile sensations, treatment
        room, 571–572
Tai Ji symbol, *484*
Talus, *94*
Tapotement, 11, 12*t*, 378–380, *379*, 386*t*
    definition, 350
Tapoter, 11, 12*t*
Target market, 575
Target muscle
    definition, 420, 424
    relaxing, 445–446
Tarsal region, 149–152, *150–151*
Taste, 142
Taxes, 573, 573*b*
Taylor, George H., 13
Telophase, 59, *59*
Temporal bone, *87*, 88
Temporalis, *98*
Temporomandibular joint (TMJ), 94, 156*b*
Tempra. *see* Acetaminophen
Tender point
    definition, 420
    monitoring of, 443–444
    releasing of, 445
Tendinopathy, 193
Tendon reflex, 112
    definition, 56
Tendons, 66, *67*
Tension headaches, 195
Tensor fascia latae, *100*
Teres major, *99*, *100*
Teres minor, *99*
Testes, 139
Testosterone, 141
Tetany, muscle, 161
Tetracyclines, 182
Thalassotherapy, 475*t*

Therapeutic massage. *see also* Massage
    design, 415–416*t*
    policies and procedures, 567–568
Therapeutic techniques, 424–426, 424*b*
Thermal wrap, 475*t*
Thermoregulatory conditions, 525
Thiazide (Lozol, Lozide, Naturetin,
    Renese), 182
Thoracic duct, definition, 420, 428
Thoracic outlet syndrome, 195–196
Thoracic region, 149–152, *150–151*
Thoracic vertebrae, 89, *89*
Thoracolumbar fascia, *99, 100*
Throat chakra, 499*t, 500*
Thrombocytes. *see* Platelets
Thymus gland, 137
Thyroid gland, 135–136, *136*
Thyroid-stimulating hormone (TSH),
    135
Tibia, *94*
Tibialis anterior, *98, 100*
Tissue, *57, 63–76. see also* Connective tissue;
    Soft tissue; specific type
    appearance of, 313
    definition, 56
    repair, 420–422
    types, 64*t*
Tissue membranes, 74–76
Tonalastil wrap, 475*t*
Torque. *see* Rotation
Touch, 19–22
    interpretation, 22
    physiology, 19
Touch Research Institute (TRI), 20, *20*, 21*b*
Towel draping, 355–356
    position change, 359, *359*
Trachea
    lower, 129
    upper, 128
Trager, 16*t, 18*
Transference, 53
Translating terms, 261, 262*t*
Transverse fracture, *187*
Transverse plane, 148, *148*
Tranylcypromine (Parnate), 182
Trapezius, *98, 99, 100*
Treatment goal, 276–277
    definition, 254
Treatment massage, 524
    definition, 515
Treatment plan
    definition, 326
    future treatment, 329–331
    initial report, *340*

initial session, 327–328, *328*
presentation of, 342
progress report, *341*
reevaluation, 331
session-to-session, 328*b*
subsequent sessions, 328–329
techniques and areas to include or
    avoid, 331
Treatment recommendations, 342
Treatment room
    atmosphere, 569–572
    separate dressing room, 570*b*
Triazolam (Halcion), 182
Triceps brachii, *99, 100*
Tricyclic antidepressants, 182
Trigger point (TrP), *458–459*
    chronic low back pain, 457
    chronic neck pain, 457
    combined techniques, 456
    definition, 420
    map for latissimus dorsi, *455*
    pressure release, 455–456
    specific conditions, 457
    strumming, 456
    techniques, 455
    techniques for palpation, *456*
Tui-na, 482
Twentieth Century, 14
Tylenol. *see* Acetaminophen

U

Ulna, *92*
Unethical activity, reporting of,
    41–42
Unwinding (myofascial unwinding),
    definition, 420, 449
Upper extremities, 9–92*1, 92*
    nerves, 117
    pain and fatigue in muscles, hydrotherapy
        for, 472*b*
Upper respiratory tract, 128
Ureter, 134
Urethra, 134
Urinary bladder, 134
Urinary system, 133–135
    effects of massage, 135, 367*t*
    functions, 134–135
    structures, *133*, 133–134
Uterus, 137

V

Vagina, 137
Valium, 181. *see also* Diazepam
Vancomycin, 182

Varicose veins, 197–198
    moderate to severe, 368*t*
Vascular headaches, 195
Vasodilating drugs (Hyperstat, Nu-Hydral,
    Nitropress), 182
Vastus lateralis, *98, 100*
Vastus medialis, *98*
Vein, 122, *123*
    definition, 56
Venous blood flow, *124*
Venous enhancement, 427–428, 428*b*
Ventilation, 129–130
Ventricles, brain, 112
Vertebral column, *88*, 88–89
Very cold applications, indications for, 470*b*
Vesalius, Andreas, 10, *10*
Vibration, 381–382, *382*, 386*t*
    definition, 350
Vichy shower, 475*t*
Vishuddha chakra, 499*t*, 500
Vision, 142
Visual cues of conduct, 43
Visual impairment, 531–532
Visual input, treatment room, 569
Vitamin D, 78
Vomer, *87, 88*

W

Walking with stroke, *173*
Warfarin (Coumadin), 183
Water, 497
Web site, 576–577
Whirlpool, 475*t*
White House Commission on Complementary
    and Alternative Medicine Policy
    (WHCCAMP), 20
Word elements, 255–261
    combining vowels, 260
Work and play, massage therapists, 584
Workplace design, 174–175, *175*
Wounds, open, 368*t*
Wounds or sores, massage and, 184–185

X

Xiphoid process, 91

Y

Yajur Veda, 4
Yang (YAHNG), definition, 467, 483*t*, 484
Yin/Yang theory, 483–484, 483*t*, *484*
Yin (YIHN), definition, 467, 483, 483*t*

Z

Zygomatic bone, *87, 88*